Differential Diagnoses in Surgical Pathology
Gynecologic Tract

SECOND EDITION

Differential Diagnoses in Surgical Pathology
Gynecologic Tract

SECOND EDITION

Russell Vang, MD

Professor of Pathology and Gynecology and Obstetrics
Director, Gynecologic Pathology In-house Service
Co-director, Gynecologic Pathology Consultation Service
Co-director, Gynecologic Pathology Fellowship Training Program
Division of Gynecologic Pathology
Department of Pathology
The Johns Hopkins Medical Institutions
Baltimore, Maryland

Anna Yemelyanova, MD

Professor of Pathology
Chief of Gynecologic Pathology
Director, Gynecologic Pathology Fellowship Training Program
Department of Pathology and Laboratory Medicine
Weill Cornell Medical College/New York Presbyterian Hospital
New York, New York

Jeffrey D. Seidman, MD

Medical Officer/Pathologist
Division of Molecular Genetics and Pathology
Office of In Vitro Diagnostics
Office of Product Evaluation and Quality
Center for Devices and Radiological Health
Food and Drug Administration
Silver Spring, Maryland

SERIES EDITOR

Jonathan I. Epstein, MD

Professor of Pathology, Urology and Oncology
The Reinhard Professor of Urological Pathology
Director of Surgical Pathology
The Johns Hopkins Medical Institutions
Baltimore, Maryland

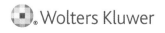. Wolters Kluwer

Philadelphia • Baltimore • New York • London
Buenos Aires • Hong Kong • Sydney • Tokyo

Acquisitions Editor: Nicole Dernoski
Development Editor: Ariel S. Winter
Editorial Coordinator: Varshaanaa SM
Editorial Assistant: Kristen Kardoley
Marketing Manager: Kirsten Watrud
Production Project Manager: Justin Wright
Manager, Graphic Arts & Design: Stephen Druding
Manufacturing Coordinator: Beth Welsh
Prepress Vendor: Straive

Second Edition

Cataloging-in-Publication Data available on request from the Publisher

ISBN: 978-1-9751-9901-2

shop.lww.com

PREFACE

A multitude of lesions in the different anatomic sites within the gynecologic tract can display a wide range of histologic appearances, including neoplasms that have several recognized variants. Given that these may mimic one another and that application of existing diagnostic criteria for several categories of lesions in the gynecologic tract can be challenging, differential diagnosis often can be problematic.

This book provides a focused approach to differential diagnosis in gynecologic pathology. Each chapter is devoted to either one anatomic site or one related group of lesions within the gynecologic tract. Furthermore, each of the several sections within every chapter addresses a specific differential diagnosis, in which two lesions are directly compared and contrasted with respect to clinicopathologic features and ancillary tests. This format highlights not only why certain lesions can closely simulate one another but also how they may be distinguished.

It is not the intention of this book to deal with every single lesion/diagnosis that has been described in the gynecologic tract. Rather, it is meant to be practical in that the most frequently encountered differential diagnoses in gynecologic pathology are presented. However, less common lesions that may create extremely difficult diagnostic problems are also discussed.

This volume in the *Differential Diagnoses in Surgical Pathology* series is intended not only for pathology trainees but also for pathologists who frequently handle gynecologic specimens in routine practice. In this second edition of the book, new entities have been added. In addition, significant updates have been made to reflect new information in the literature, including molecular alterations. Lastly, nomenclature has been modified to be consistent with the current 2020 WHO Classification for Female Genital Tumors, particularly for ovarian tumors.

Russell Vang, MD
Anna Yemelyanova, MD
Jeffrey D. Seidman, MD

ACKNOWLEDGMENTS

Dr. Vang's Acknowledgments

I would like to thank: Roberta Knox (Administrative Coordinator, Division of Gynecologic Pathology, The Johns Hopkins Hospital) for her invaluable administrative support; Drs. Brigitte M. Ronnett, Deyin Xing, and Trish Murdock (Division of Gynecologic Pathology, The Johns Hopkins Hospital) for their collegiality and collaborations over the years; the Gynecologic Pathology fellows at The Johns Hopkins Hospital (2003-2022) for their assistance with administrative, service work, educational, and academic matters; and all the pathologists at outside hospitals who submitted cases for consultation to the Gynecologic Pathology Consultation Service at The Johns Hopkins Hospital.

Dr. Yemelyanova's Acknowledgments

For their collegiality and support in bringing this work to fruition, I would like to thank my colleagues Drs. Seidman and Vang as well as all my colleagues at Weill Cornell and all the trainees, whose astute questions helped formulate the differential diagnoses. Finally, I thank my son, Venya Gushchin, who has been a source of inspiration for all my endeavors.

Dr. Seidman's Acknowledgments

I would like to thank my colleagues Drs. Yemelyanova and Vang for their tremendous efforts in shouldering the lion's share of this endeavor. I also thank my family, Aimee, Melanie, and Mike, for their unwavering support.

CONTENTS

1

Vulva and Vagina

	Vestibular Papillomatosis (Hymenal Tag)	Condyloma Acuminatum
Age	Young women of reproductive age, upon onset of sexual activity	Adults and sexually active adolescents; peak age 20-39 y
Location	Vaginal vestibulum, inner aspects of the labia minora	Vulva, mucosal and skin surfaces, vagina, less commonly cervix
Symptoms	Generally asymptomatic, symptoms can be related to irritation, secondary infection, and local trauma, occasionally dyspareunia	Generally asymptomatic, symptoms can be related to irritation and local trauma
Signs	Incidental finding during speculum examination: delicate, skin or mucosa colored, nearly translucent, finger-like projections in small clusters, some in linear arrangement, often symmetrical	Papillary, verrucous, or warty lesions and cauliflower-like projections fused at the base; often multiple or multifocal; no symmetry in distribution
Etiology	Unknown; considered a normal anatomical variant of the vulva	Low-risk human papillomavirus infection, most commonly implicated viral types 6 and 11
Histology	1. Branching "villiform" papillae *(Fig. 1.1.1)* 2. Normal-appearing, nonkeratinizing squamous epithelium *(Fig. 1.1.2)* 3. Papillae can appear fused in tangential sections *(Fig. 1.1.3)* 4. No atypia/viral cytopathic effect, small hyperchromatic nuclei *(Fig. 1.1.4)*	1. Verrucous/warty architecture; at nonkeratinized site, papillae can appear delicate *(Fig. 1.1.5)* 2. Broad papillary fronds with pointed or rounded ends; hyperkeratosis and parakeratosis 3. Papillae are often fused at the base 4. Viral cytopathic changes/koilocytosis; enlarged hyperchromatic nuclei with irregular contours surrounded by cytoplasmic halo *(Figs. 1.1.6 and 1.1.7)*
Special studies	• None required • Absence of low-risk HPV by *in situ* hybridization • Ki-67 proliferative activity limited to the parabasal epithelial layers	• None required • HPV *in situ* hybridization for low-risk HPV can be done for confirmation • Ki-67 proliferative activity can be increased with scattered cells labeled in the upper epithelial layers *(Fig. 1.1.8)*
Treatment	None required; lesions causing symptoms can be removed	Can regress spontaneously; conservative excision, immunomodulating topical agents can be used for large persisting lesions
Prognosis	Unremarkable	Benign; however, recurrences are common even after spontaneous regression

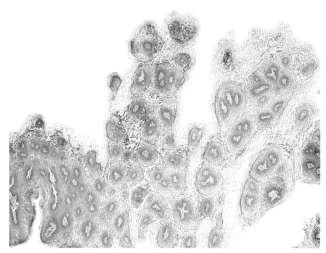

Figure 1.1.1   Vestibular papillomatosis. Multiple branching delicate villiform papillae.

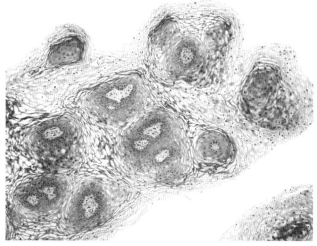

Figure 1.1.2   Vestibular papillomatosis. Same case as *Figure 1.1.1*, higher magnification. Delicate papillae are lined by normal nonkeratinizing squamous epithelium. No hyperkeratosis is seen.

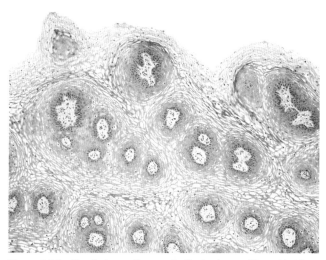

Figure 1.1.3   Vestibular papillomatosis. Coalescing papillae with thin fibrovascular cores.

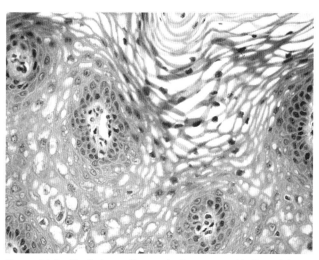

Figure 1.1.4   Vestibular papillomatosis. Squamous epithelium without viral cytopathic change (koilocytosis).

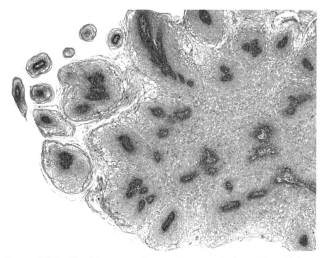

Figure 1.1.5   Condyloma acuminatum. Verrucous lesion with multiple papillary projections lined by nonkeratinizing squamous epithelium.

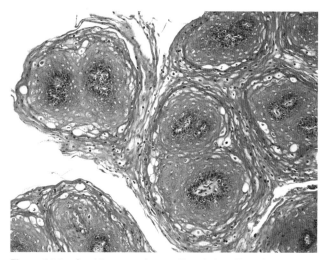

Figure 1.1.6   Condyloma acuminatum. Rounded papillae with some degree of hyperkeratosis and parakeratosis. Occasional atypical, binucleate cells are present.

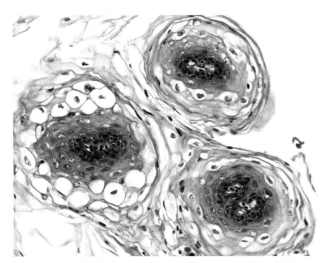

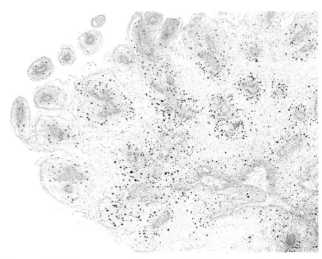

Figure 1.1.7   Condyloma acuminatum. Same case as *Figure 1.1.5*, higher magnification. Koilocytes: large cells with abundant cytoplasm, typical perinuclear halo, and enlarged hyperchromatic nuclei with irregular contours.

Figure 1.1.8   Same case as *Figure 1.1.5*. Condyloma acuminatum. Increased Ki-67 labeling in midzone and superficial epithelial layers.

	Condyloma Acuminatum	Squamous Papilloma
Age	Adults and sexually active adolescents; peak age 20-39 y	Reproductive age and postmenopausal women
Location	Vulva, mucosal and skin surfaces, vagina, less commonly cervix	Vagina, vulva, less commonly cervix
Symptoms	Generally asymptomatic; symptoms can be related to irritation and local trauma	Usually asymptomatic; symptoms can be related to irritation and local trauma
Signs	Papillary, verrucous, or warty lesions and cauliflower-like projections fused at the base; often multiple/multifocal	Polypoid growth, single or multiple
Etiology	Low-risk human papillomavirus infection, most commonly implicated viral types 6 and 11	Considered normal anatomic variant
Histology	1. Verrucous/warty architecture; multiple papillae are often fused at the base *(Fig. 1.2.1)* 2. Broad papillary fronds with pointed or rounded ends *(Fig. 1.2.2)* 3. Mature squamous epithelium 4. Hyperkeratosis, hypergranulosis *(Fig. 1.2.3)* 5. Koilocytosis is seen at least focally, often in the creases between the papillae *(Fig. 1.2.4)* Also see Sections 1.1 and 1.3	1. Polypoid lesion with central fibrovascular core *(Figs. 1.2.5-1.2.7)* 2. No significant arborization; rounded contour *(Fig. 1.2.6)* 3. Mature squamous epithelial lining 4. Depending on the location, hyperkeratosis can be variably present; hypergranulosis is not typical 5. No cytologic atypia, koilocytosis *(Fig. 1.2.8)*
Special studies	• None • HPV *in situ* hybridization for low-risk HPV can be done for confirmation • Ki-67 proliferative activity is increased with scattered positive cells in the upper epithelial layers (see *Fig. 1.1.8)*	• None • No evidence of HPV by *in situ* hybridization • No increase in Ki-67 labeling above the parabasal areas
Treatment	Can regress spontaneously; conservative excision, laser fulguration, or immunomodulating topical agents for persisting lesions	None required; diagnostic biopsy is usually curative
Prognosis	Benign; however, recurrences are common even after spontaneous regression	Unremarkable

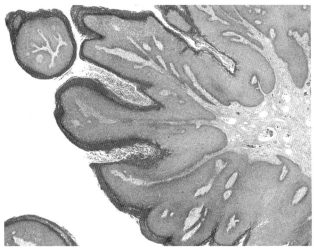

Figure 1.2.1   Condyloma acuminatum. Verrucous lesion with multiple papillary projections with pointed or rounded ends.

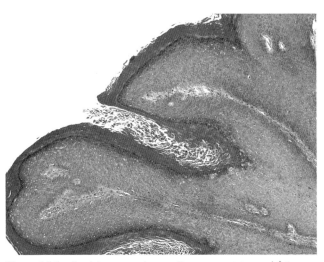

Figure 1.2.2   Condyloma acuminatum. Same case as *Figure 1.2.1*, higher magnification.

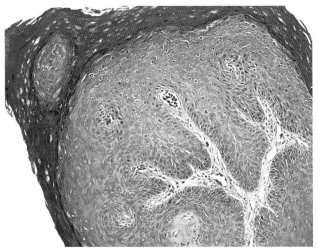

Figure 1.2.3   Condyloma acuminatum. Same case as *Figure 1.2.1*, higher magnification. Marked hyperkeratosis.

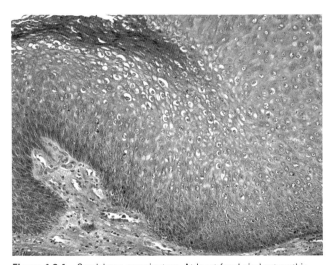

Figure 1.2.4   Condyloma acuminatum. At least focal viral cytopathic change (koilocytes) is seen in the creases between the papillae.

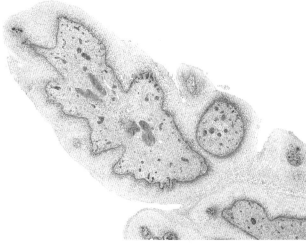

Figure 1.2.5   Squamous papilloma. Polypoid lesion with central fibrovascular core.

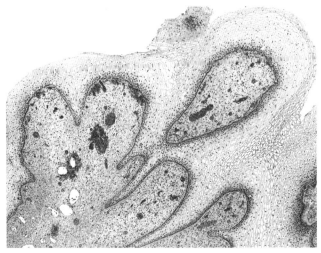

Figure 1.2.6   Squamous papilloma. Same case as in *Figure 1.2.5*. Minimal arborization is present.

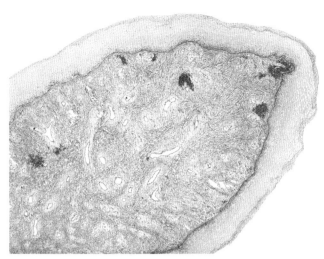

Figure 1.2.7   Squamous papilloma. Single polypoid lesion with fibrovascular core and rounded end.

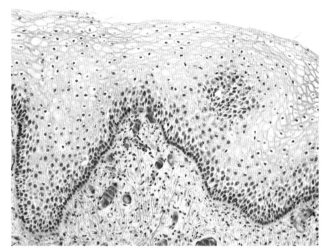

Figure 1.2.8   Squamous papilloma. Same case as in *Figure 1.2.5*, higher magnification. Mature squamous epithelium lacking cytologic atypia.

	Condyloma Acuminatum	Seborrheic Keratosis
Age	Adults and sexually active adolescents; peak age 20-39 y	Middle-aged and postmenopausal women
Location	Vulva, vagina, skin, and mucosal surface	Vulvar skin (keratinized portions)
Symptoms	Often asymptomatic, some present with pruritus, irritation	Often asymptomatic, some present with pruritus, irritation
Signs	Cauliflower-like lesion(s), skin colored or white	Papular lesion(s), waxy skin colored, or pigmented with stuck-on appearance, often multiple
Etiology	Low-risk HPV, HPV types 6 and 11 are most common; some vulvar lesions with seborrheic keratosis (SK)–like features can harbor low-risk HPV and are considered variants of condyloma acuminatum	Generally is not associated with HPV
Histology	1. Complex verrucous architecture *(Fig. 1.3.1)*; a subset can have areas with SK-like features *(Fig. 1.3.2)* 2. Acanthosis, elongation, and thickening of rete ridges 3. Compact hyperkeratosis, hypergranulosis 4. Epithelial maturation is preserved; koilocytosis is seen at least focally *(Fig. 1.3.3)* Also see *Figures 1.2.1, 1.2.2, 1.2.3, 1.2.4, 1.6.7, and 1.6.8*	1. Polypoid or papillary architecture is not uncommon *(Fig. 1.3.4)* 2. Epithelial hyperplasia, acanthosis; invaginations of the epithelial surface with flattened base *(Fig. 1.3.5)*; pseudohorn cysts *(Fig. 1.3.6)*; squamous eddies and mitosis in irritated seborrheic keratosis 3. Laminated hyperkeratosis; hypergranulosis is minimal or absent 4. Expansion of small monomorphic basophilic keratinocytes without viral cytopathic change (koilocytosis) *(Fig. 1.3.7)*
Special studies	• *In situ* hybridization for HPV 6/11, positive diffuse nuclear signal • Increased Ki-67 labeling in upper epithelial layers	• Usually, no detectable HPV by *in situ* hybridization • Increased Ki-67 labeling
Treatment	Can regress spontaneously; conservative excision, laser fulguration, or topical immunomodulating agents can be used for persistent lesions	None required; shave biopsy is often curative, and large lesions causing discomfort can be removed via local excision or laser fulguration
Prognosis	Benign; however, recurrences are common even after spontaneous regression	Unremarkable

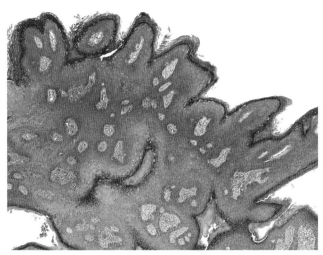

Figure 1.3.1   Condyloma acuminatum. Verrucous architecture with multiple papillary projections.

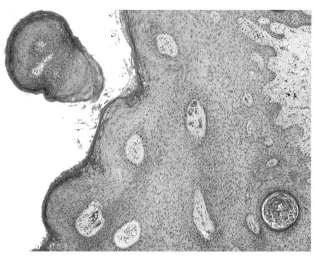

Figure 1.3.2   Condyloma acuminatum with SK-like features. Note both koilocytotic change and horn cysts. HPV 6/11 was detected by *in situ* hybridization (not shown).

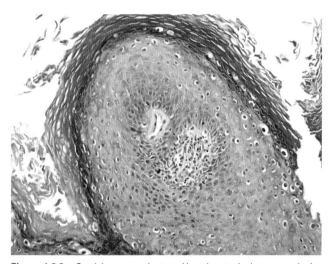

Figure 1.3.3   Condyloma acuminatum. Hyperkeratosis, hypergranulosis, and preserved squamous maturation. Koilocytes are seen in the superficial epithelial layers.

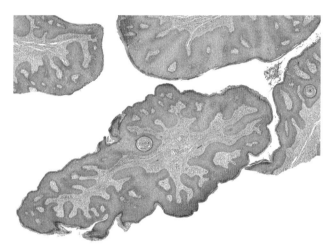

Figure 1.3.4   Seborrheic keratosis with polypoid architecture.

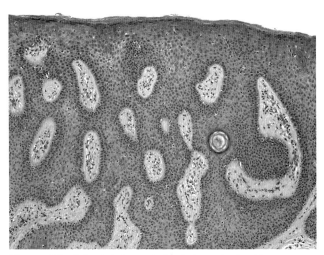

Figure 1.3.5   Seborrheic keratosis. Marked acanthosis with anastomosing rete ridges.

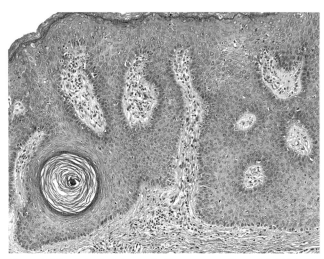

Figure 1.3.6   Seborrheic keratosis. Same case as *Figure 1.3.3,* higher magnification. Pseudohorn cyst.

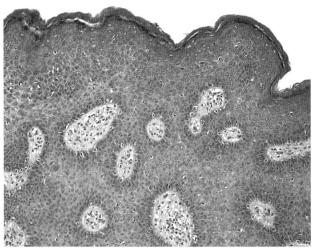

Figure 1.3.7   Seborrheic keratosis. Proliferation of monotonous small basophilic keratinocytes. Lack of atypia/koilocytosis.

	Condyloma Acuminatum	Verruca Vulgaris (Common Wart)
Age	Adults and sexually active adolescents; peak age 20-39 y	Children, including infants, and adolescents; can be seen in adults. Girls are more commonly affected than boys
Location	Vulva, mucosal and skin surfaces, as well as vagina and cervix	Vulva, perineum; also on the hands/fingers, toes, knees
Symptoms	Generally asymptomatic, symptoms can be related to irritation and local trauma	Generally asymptomatic, symptoms can be related to irritation and local trauma
Signs	Papillary, verrucous, or sessile lesions; can turn white after application of acetic acid; often multiple; in children raises concern for sexual abuse	Rough keratotic papules
Etiology	Low-risk HPV infection; viral types 6 and 11 cause 90% of lesions	HPV infection; viral types 2 and 4 cause majority of the lesions
Histology	1. Complex branching architecture, usually asymmetrical (*Fig. 1.4.1*) 2. Rounded and pointed papillary projections; acanthosis, elongation and thickening of rete ridges, irregular or flattened lesion base 3. Hyperkeratosis 4. Hypergranulosis is present, but not as prominent as in verruca 5. Koilocytosis at least focally seen, often in the creases between the papillae (*Fig. 1.4.2*) Also see *Figures 1.2.1, 1.2.2, 1.2.3, 1.2.4*	1. Warty architecture with some degree of symmetry; peripheral rete ridges pointing toward the center of the lesion (*Fig. 1.4.3*) 2. Pointed ends of filiform papillae 3. Hyper- and parakeratosis (*Fig. 1.4.4*) 4. Hypergranulosis; variation is size and shape of keratohyalin granules (*Fig. 1.4.5*) 5. Koilocytotic atypia absent or very focal (*Fig. 1.4.6*)
Special studies	• *In situ* hybridization for HPV 6/11, diffuse nuclear signals • Ki-67 proliferative activity can be increased in upper epithelial layers	• Generally not needed • HPV typing can be considered in medicolegal cases
Treatment	Can regress spontaneously; conservative excision, laser fulguration, or topical immunomodulating agents can be used for persistent lesions	Biopsy is often curative; for extensive or persistent lesions, topical agents, cryotherapy, laser, and surgical excision can be used
Prognosis	Benign; however, recurrences are common even after spontaneous regression	Benign, usually resolve spontaneously with time. Do not raise suspicion for sexual abuse when present on the vulva of female infants and young girls

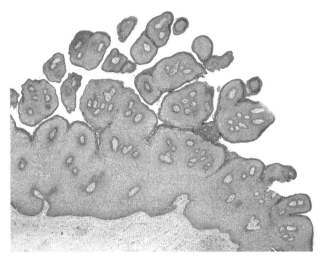

Figure 1.4.1 Condyloma acuminatum. Verrucous lesion with multiple papillary projections with pointed or rounded ends. Broad-based lesion with no apparent symmetry.

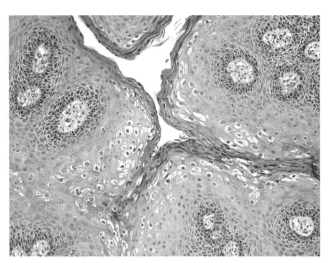

Figure 1.4.2 Condyloma acuminatum. Same case as *Figure 1.4.1*, higher magnification. Prominent koilocytosis.

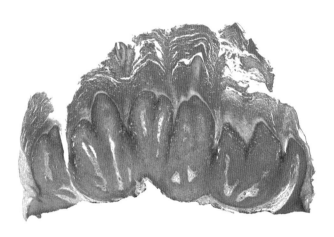

Figure 1.4.3 Verruca vulgaris. Symmetrical lesion with peripheral rete ridges pointing toward the center of the lesion. Mature squamous epithelium with marked hyperkeratosis.

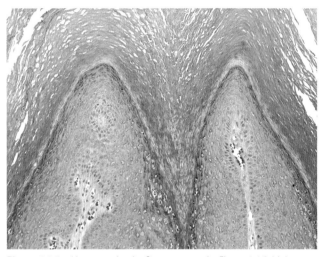

Figure 1.4.4 Verruca vulgaris. Same case as in *Figure 1.4.3*, higher magnification. Filiform papillae with marked hyper- and parakeratosis.

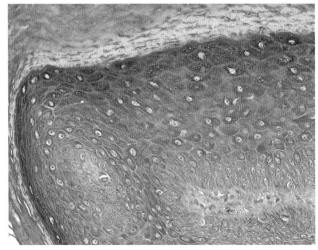

Figure 1.4.5 Verruca vulgaris. Same case as in *Figure 1.4.3*, higher magnification. Prominent hypergranulosis and thick compact hyperkeratosis.

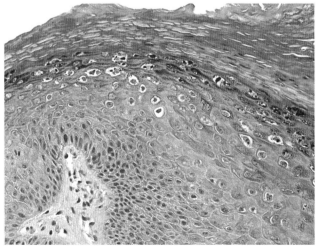

Figure 1.4.6 Verruca vulgaris. Same case as in *Figure 1.4.3*, higher magnification. Very focal koilocytotic change can be seen.

	Verrucous Carcinoma	Condyloma Acuminatum
Age	Postmenopausal women	Adults and sexually active adolescents; peak age 20-39 y
Location	Vulva, uncommonly cervix	Vulva, vagina, less commonly cervix
Symptoms	Vulvar mass, symptoms related to secondary infection and local trauma	Related to local irritation and trauma
Signs	Broad-based exophytic vulvar mass	Exophytic papillomatous lesion
Etiology	Unknown; some cases reportedly are associated with HPV 6; vulvar acanthosis with altered differentiation (VAAD) *(Figs. 1.5.1 and 1.5.2)* and differentiated exophytic vulvar intraepithelial lesion (DEVIL) have been suggested as putative precursor	Low-risk HPV, most commonly types 6 and 11
Histology	1. Downward invasive growth pattern with some exophytic component *(Figs. 1.5.3-1.5.6)* 2. Prominent acanthosis, expansion of rete ridges, and compression of dermal papillae; lack of true fibrovascular cores *(Fig. 1.5.5)* 3. Broad epithelial nests, pushing-border invasion *(Fig. 1.5.6)* 4. Hyperkeratosis can be seen; hypergranulosis is not typical 5. Bland cytologic features, lack of overt viral epithelial changes *(Fig. 1.5.7)* 6. Inflammatory infiltrate with eosinophils in the stroma *(Fig. 1.5.8)*	1. Exophytic growth; complex branching architecture *(Fig. 1.5.9)* 2. Acanthosis, elongation, and thickening of rete ridges; papillary projections 3. Base of the lesion can be flat or irregular due to tangential orientation; no invasion 4. Hyperkeratosis and hypergranulosis 5. Koilocytosis at least focally seen, often in the creases between the papillae *(Fig. 1.5.10)* 6. Stromal inflammation is not typical Also see *Figures 1.1.6, 1.1.7, 1.1.8 and 1.2.1, 1.2.2, 1.2.3, 1.2.4*
Special studies	• None helpful in this differential • Presence of low-risk HPV does not preclude the diagnosis	• None helpful in this differential • *In situ* hybridization for low-risk HPV can be considered
Treatment	Wide/radical local excision; radiation therapy can be considered for advanced and recurrent tumors	Conservative excision may be necessary in large lesions
Prognosis	Locally invasive tumor; regional lymph node involvement and distant metastases are rare	Benign; morbidity is related to local irritation, trauma, and secondary infection

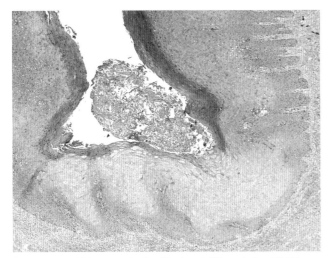

Figure 1.5.1   Vulvar acanthosis with altered differentiation (VAAD) displays acanthosis, hypogranulosis, and plaque-like hyperkeratosis.

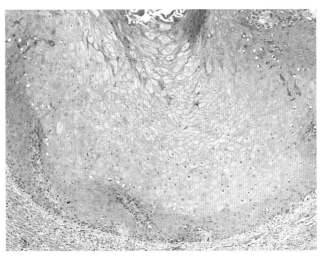

Figure 1.5.2   Vulvar acanthosis with altered differentiation (VAAD). Markedly thickened epithelium with cytoplasmic pallor; no evidence of atypia, same case as in *Figure 1.5.1*.

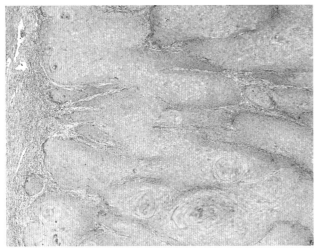

Figure 1.5.3   Verrucous carcinoma. Pale lesion with verrucous architecture and "pushing-border" stromal invasion.

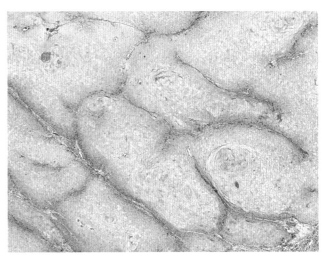

Figure 1.5.4   Verrucous carcinoma. Same case as in *Figure 1.5.3*.

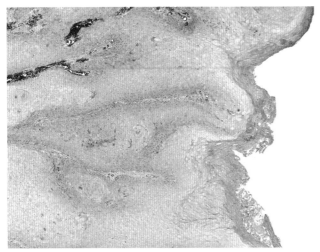

Figure 1.5.5   Verrucous carcinoma. Same case as in *Figure 1.5.3*, surface. Mature bland squamous epithelium with surface hyperkeratosis.

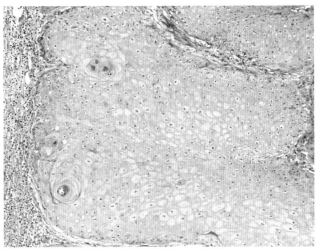

Figure 1.5.6   Verrucous carcinoma. Same case as in *Figure 1.5.3*, higher magnification. Broad epithelial nests extend into the stroma.

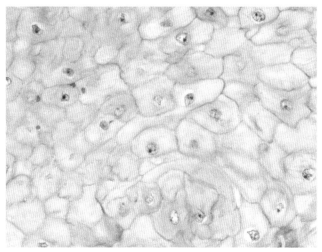

Figure 1.5.7   Verrucous carcinoma. Same case as in *Figure 1.5.3*, higher magnification. Mature keratinocytes lacking cytologic atypia.

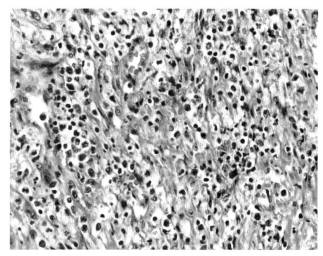

Figure 1.5.8   Verrucous carcinoma. Stromal inflammatory infiltrate with eosinophils is seen at the deep edge.

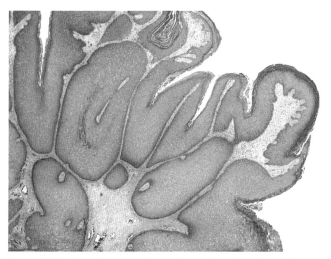

Figure 1.5.9   Condyloma acuminatum. Exophytic lesion with warty architecture; prominent acanthosis.

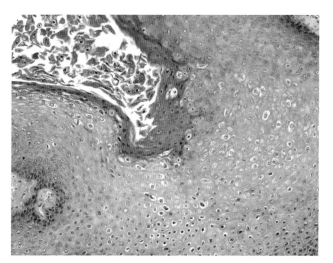

Figure 1.5.10   Condyloma acuminatum. Koilocytosis is seen on the surface of the lesion.

	High-Grade Squamous Intraepithelial Lesion (HSIL, VIN 2-3) With Condylomatous Features	Condyloma Acuminatum
Age	Adults; peak age 45-50 y	Adults and sexually active adolescents; peak age 20-39 y
Location	Vulva	Vulva, vagina
Symptoms	Related to irritation, local trauma, or underlying immunosuppressive condition	Related to irritation or local trauma
Signs	Warty/papillomatous lesion	Warty/papillomatous lesion
Etiology	High-risk HPV infection, types 16 and 18 are most common; frequently in immunocompromised patients	Low-risk HPV infection, types 6 and 11 are most common
Histology	1. Epithelial immaturity *(Figs. 1.6.1 and 1.6.2)* 2. Minimal or absent koilocytosis; significant cytologic squamous atypia throughout epithelial thickness *(Figs. 1.6.3 and 1.6.4)* 3. Mitotic figures in the upper epithelial layers *(Fig. 1.6.5)*	1. Retained epithelial maturation *(Fig. 1.6.7)* 2. Cytologic atypia is limited to superficial epithelial layers/koilocytes *(Fig. 1.6.8)* 3. Mitotic figures are infrequent; if present, observed exclusively in parabasal layers
Special studies	• p16, strong and diffuse *(Fig. 1.6.6,* **left***)* • Ki-67 labeling increased in upper epithelial layers *(Fig. 1.6.6,* **right***)* • *In situ* hybridization positive for high-risk HPV	• p16 patchy or negative • Ki-67 labels individual cells in upper epithelial layers • *In situ* hybridization positive for low-risk HPV; high-risk HPV not detected
Treatment	Local excision	Conservative excision may be necessary in large lesions
Prognosis	Considered a precursor of HPV-related squamous cell carcinoma; can progress to invasive carcinoma if not removed	Benign; morbidity is related to local irritation, trauma, and secondary infection

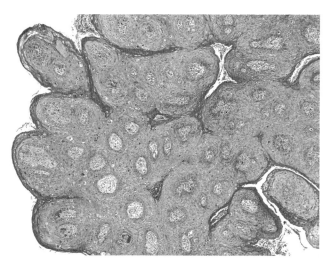

Figure 1.6.1 High-grade squamous intraepithelial lesion (HSIL/VIN 2-3) with prominent condylomatous architecture. Lesion with wart-like architecture appears "blue," immature at low power.

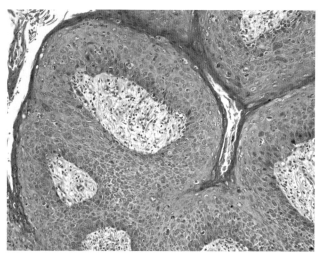

Figure 1.6.2 High-grade squamous intraepithelial lesion (HSIL/VIN 2-3) with prominent condylomatous architecture. Same case as in *Figure 1.6.1*, higher magnification. Full-thickness epithelial immaturity.

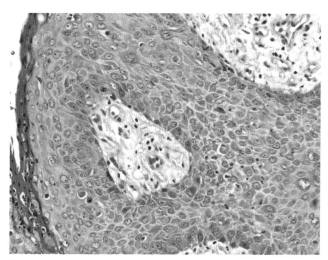

Figure 1.6.3 High-grade squamous intraepithelial lesion (HSIL/VIN 2-3) with prominent condylomatous architecture. Same case as in *Figure 1.6.1*, higher magnification. Epithelial immaturity and notable cytologic atypia.

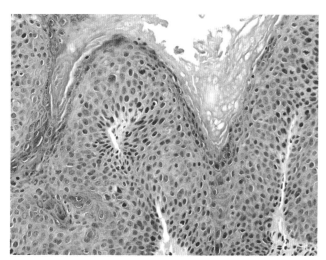

Figure 1.6.4 High-grade squamous intraepithelial lesion (HSIL/VIN 2-3) with prominent condylomatous architecture. Hyperchromasia and atypia throughout epithelial thickness.

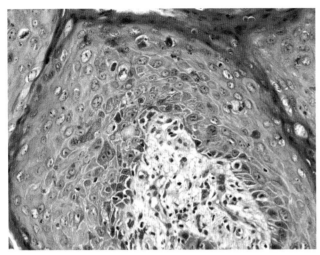

Figure 1.6.5 High-grade squamous intraepithelial lesion (HSIL/VIN 2-3) with prominent condylomatous architecture. Mitotic figures in the midzone and upper epithelial layers.

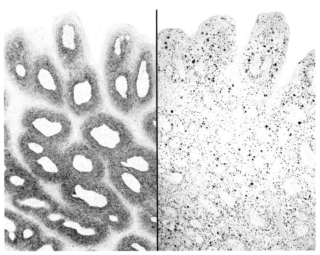

Figure 1.6.6 High-grade squamous intraepithelial lesion (HSIL/VIN 2-3) with prominent condylomatous architecture. Same case as in *Figure 1.6.1*. Diffuse p16 expression in at least lower one-third of the epithelial thickness **(left)**; markedly increased Ki-67 labeling throughout epithelial thickness **(right)**.

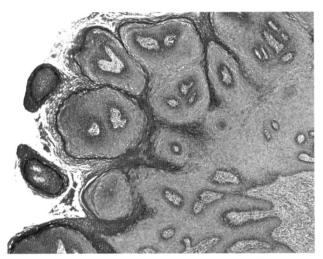

Figure 1.6.7 Condyloma acuminatum. Verrucous lesion with multiple papillary projections with pointed or rounded ends.

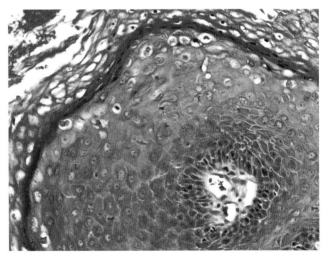

Figure 1.6.8 Condyloma acuminatum. Same case as *Figure 1.6.7*, higher magnification. Preserved epithelial maturation. Focal koilocytosis on the surface.

	High-Grade Squamous Intraepithelial Lesion (HSIL, VIN 2-3)	Benign Squamous Epithelium (Vulvar Skin)
Age	Adults; peak age 45-50 y	N/A
Location	Vulva	Vulva
Symptoms	Often asymptomatic	N/A
Signs	Papule, plaque; can be raised pale, pigmented, or red	Usually none; pigmentation or keratotic plaque can be seen; frequently in vulvar excisions with adjacent HSIL or invasive squamous cell carcinoma
Etiology	High-risk HPV infection, most commonly HPV type 16	N/A
Histology	1. Epithelial thickening; acanthosis is often seen 2. Hyperchromatic/basophilic-appearing epithelium at low power *(Figs. 1.7.1-1.7.3)* 3. Immature cell expansion and disorganization in parabasal zone 4. Surface maturation is often preserved; hyperkeratosis is often present *(Figs. 1.7.4 and 1.7.5)* 5. Enlarged, hyperchromatic nuclei with nuclear contour irregularities pointing in different directions; nucleoli are typically not seen *(Fig. 1.7.6)* 6. Mitoses are common and extend above the parabasal zone	1. Epithelial thickening; acanthosis may be seen 2. Blue/basophilic-appearing epithelium *(Figs. 1.7.8 and 1.7.9)* 3. Quiescent parabasal zone; can appear expanded if tangentially sectioned *(Fig. 1.7.10)* 4. Preserved epithelial maturation; hyperkeratosis is usually not prominent 5. Uniform normal size nuclei with small nucleoli and smooth nuclear membranes *(Fig. 1.7.11)*; occasional atypical multinucleated cells can be seen in the epithelium 6. Mitoses are rare; in parabasal zone, if present
Special studies	• Strong and diffuse expression of p16 (block-like), at least 1/3 of the epithelial thickness *(Fig. 1.7.7, **left**)* • Increased Ki-67 labeling in the upper epithelial layers *(Fig. 1.7.7, **right**)*	• Negative or weak, focal p16 staining *(Fig 1.7.12, **left**)* • Ki-67 labeling is limited to basal parabasal layers *(Fig. 1.7.12, **right**)*
Treatment	Local excision, laser evaporation	None required
Prognosis	Considered a precursor of HPV-related squamous cell carcinoma; can progress to invasive carcinoma if not removed	Unremarkable

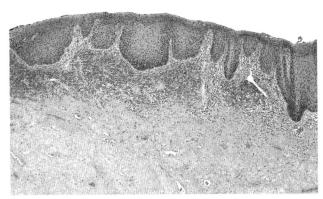

Figure 1.7.1 High-grade squamous intraepithelial lesion (high-grade VIN). Acanthosis, broadening of the rete ridges.

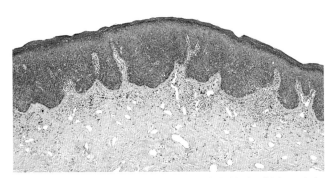

Figure 1.7.2 High-grade squamous intraepithelial lesion (high-grade VIN). Hyperchromatic/basophilic epithelium with acanthosis and broadening of the rete ridges.

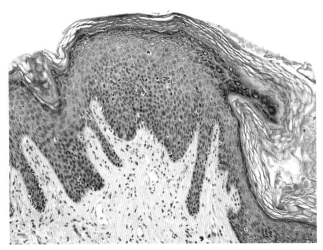

Figure 1.7.3 Focal high-grade squamous intraepithelial lesion (high-grade VIN). Expanded parabasal zone **(center)**.

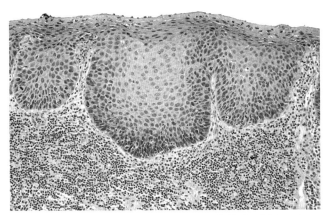

Figure 1.7.4 High-grade squamous intraepithelial lesion (high-grade VIN). Same case as in *Figure 1.7.1*, higher magnification. Expansion of parabasal zone. Maturation is preserved in upper epithelial layers.

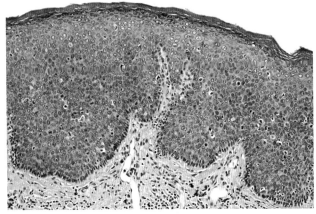

Figure 1.7.5 High-grade squamous intraepithelial lesion (high-grade VIN). Same case as in *Figure 1.7.2*, higher magnification. Loss of epithelial maturation; however, granular and corneal layers are still present.

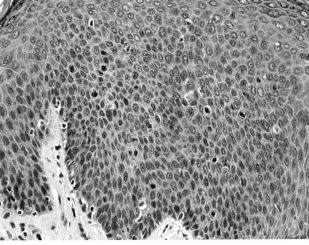

Figure 1.7.6 High-grade squamous intraepithelial lesion (high-grade VIN). Same case as in *Figure 1.7.3*, higher magnification. Expansion of the parabasal zone, atypical keratinocytes with increased nucleocytoplasmic ratio, and frequent mitotic figures above the parabasal zone.

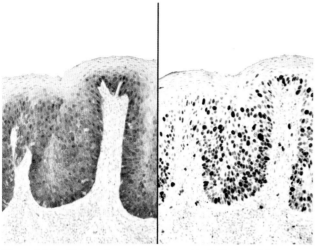

Figure 1.7.7 High-grade squamous intraepithelial lesion (high-grade VIN). Same case as in *Figure 1.7.1*. Diffuse "block-like" expression of p16 in at least two-thirds of epithelial thickness **(left)** and increased Ki-67 labeling above the parabasal layers **(right)**.

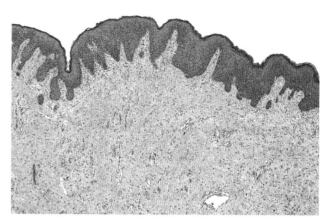

Figure 1.7.8 Normal (nonlesional) skin adjacent to HSIL in a vulvar excision specimen. Acanthosis, broadening of the rete ridges, and hyperkeratosis.

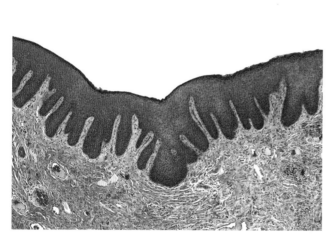

Figure 1.7.9 Normal (nonlesional) skin adjacent to HSIL in a vulvar excision specimen. Acanthosis, broadening of the rete ridges, and basophilic-appearing epithelium.

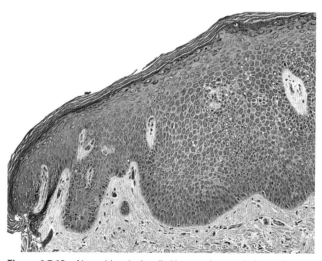

Figure 1.7.10 Normal (nonlesional) skin near the margin in a vulvar excision for squamous cell carcinoma. Parabasal zone appears expanded due to tangential sectioning; no cytologic atypia is seen.

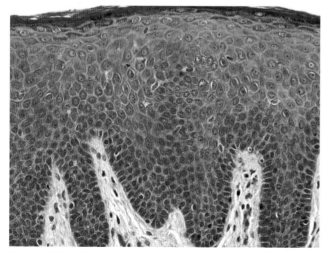

Figure 1.7.11 Normal (nonlesional) skin. Same case as in *Figure 1.7.9*, higher magnification. Normal epithelial maturation; keratinocytes lack cytologic atypia.

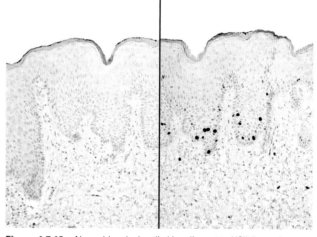

Figure 1.7.12 Normal (nonlesional) skin adjacent to HSIL in a vulvar excision specimen. Same case as in *Figure 1.7.8*. No expression of p16 **(left)** and low Ki-67 proliferative activity limited to parabasal zone **(right)**.

	Differentiated-Type Vulvar Intraepithelial Neoplasia	Reactive/Reparative Atypia
Age	Adults, postmenopausal, usually 6th to 8th decade	Adults, no specific age predilection
Location	Vulva	Vulva
Symptoms	Vulvar irritation and itching	Vulvar irritation and itching
Signs	Lichen sclerosus–like appearance, inflammatory/dermatitis-like changes, no distinct lesional borders	Erythematous skin, appearance of dermatitis; adjacent erosion/ulceration can be seen
Etiology	Unknown, *TP53* mutations are frequently detected; mutations in *PIK3CA*, *NOTCH1*, and *HRAS* are also seen	Related to the underlying condition
Histology	1. Elongation and anastomosis or thickening of rete ridges *(Figs. 1.8.1 and 1.8.2)*; dermal or interface inflammation can be present 2. Variable hyperkeratosis; prominent intercellular bridges *(Fig. 1.8.3)* 3. Abnormal keratinization, abundant eosinophilic cytoplasm in the basal and parabasal epithelial layers *(Figs. 1.8.4 and 1.8.5)* 4. Marked nuclear atypia in basal/parabasal layers, dyskeratotic keratinocytes *(Fig. 1.8.6)* 5. Ulceration can be occasionally seen, particularly in cases with adjacent invasive carcinoma 6. Background of lichen sclerosus–type changes can be seen	1. Acanthosis is common; hyperkeratosis can be seen; dermal/interface inflammation *(Fig. 1.8.8)* 2. Variable hyperkeratosis; intercellular bridges can be seen in cases with intraepithelial inflammation, but generally not prominent *(Fig. 1.8.9)* 3. No abnormal keratinization/cytoplasmic eosinophilia 4. Enlarged relatively uniform vesicular nuclei with inconspicuous nucleoli *(Fig. 1.8.10)* 5. Epithelial attenuation at the edge of an ulcer with surface exudate *(Fig. 1.8.11)* 6. Association with lichen sclerosus is not consistent
Special studies	• Strong p53 expression in basal keratinocytes nuclei extending to the middle epithelial layers can be seen in some cases *(Fig. 1.8.7, **left**)* • Variable Ki-67 proliferative activity *(Fig. 1.8.7, **right**)*	• p53 labeling usually limited to the basal layer, "wild-type pattern"*(Fig. 1.8.12, **left**)* • Some increase in Ki-67 proliferative activity can be observed *(Fig. 1.8.12, **right**)*
Treatment	Local excision with clear margins	Treatment of the underlying cause (fungal, bacterial infection, etc.)
Prognosis	Considered a precursor of non–HPV-related vulvar squamous cell carcinoma; quick progression to invasive carcinoma	Benign; prognosis related to the underlying condition

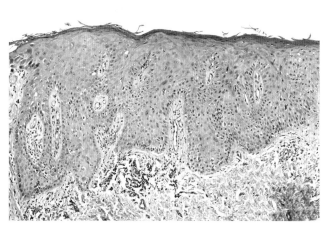

Figure 1.8.1   Differentiated vulvar intraepithelial neoplasia (simplex VIN). Prominent acanthosis and hyperkeratosis.

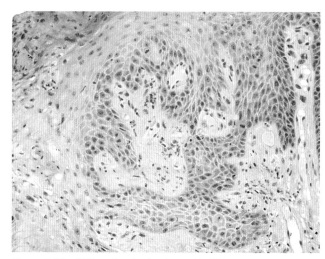

Figure 1.8.2   Differentiated vulvar intraepithelial neoplasia. Elongated anastomosing rete ridges.

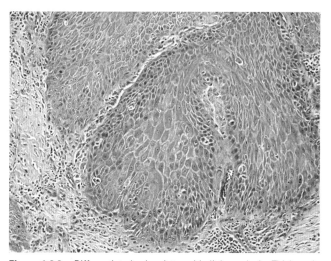

Figure 1.8.3   Differentiated vulvar intraepithelial neoplasia. Thickened rete ridges; prominent intercellular bridges. Parabasal zone appears disorganized.

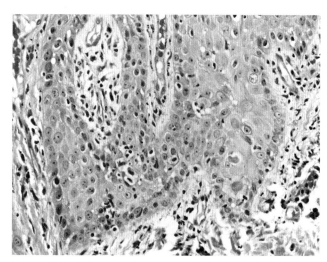

Figure 1.8.4   Differentiated vulvar intraepithelial neoplasia. Same case as in *Figure 1.8.1*, higher magnification. Atypical parabasal keratinocytes with prominent nucleoli. Cytoplasmic hypereosinophilia **(right)**.

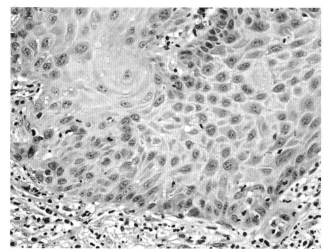

Figure 1.8.5   Differentiated vulvar intraepithelial neoplasia. Atypical parabasal keratinocytes with cytoplasmic keratinization (hypereosinophilia).

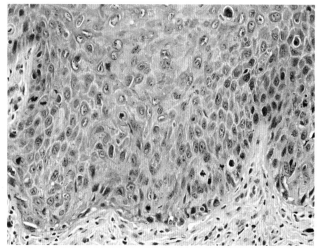

Figure 1.8.6   Differentiated vulvar intraepithelial neoplasia. Basal and parabasal atypia and brisk mitotic activity.

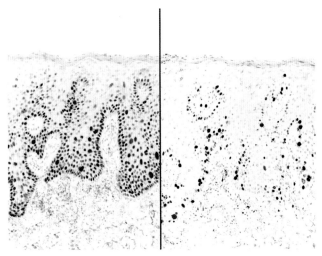

Figure 1.8.7 Differentiated vulvar intraepithelial neoplasia. Same case as in *Figure 1.8.1*. Increased p53 labeling **(left)** and only mildly increased Ki-67 proliferative activity **(right)**.

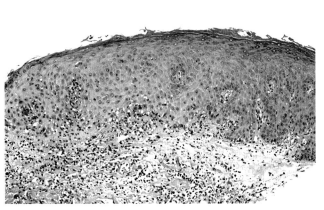

Figure 1.8.8 Vulvar skin with reactive changes at the edge of erosion. Interface and dermal mixed inflammatory infiltrate.

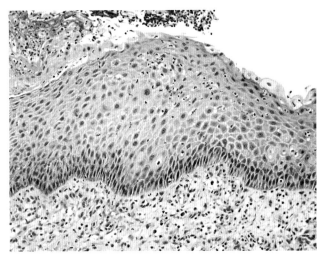

Figure 1.8.9 Vulvar skin with reactive changes. Neutrophils in the epidermis. Notable intercellular bridges. Nuclear enlargement and some degree of pleomorphism in the middle epithelial layers.

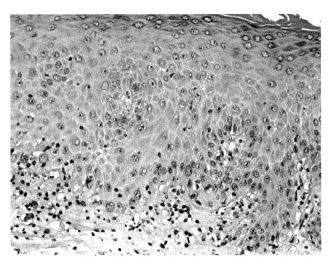

Figure 1.8.10 Vulvar skin with reactive changes at the edge of erosion. Same case as in *Figure 1.8.8*, higher magnification. Keratinocytes with uniform enlarged nuclei and nucleoli.

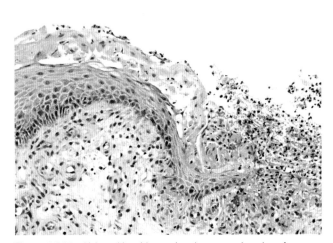

Figure 1.8.11 Vulvar skin with reactive changes at the edge of an ulcer. Basal and parabasal hyperchromasia, but no significant atypia.

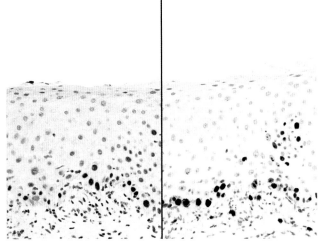

Figure 1.8.12 Vulvar skin with reactive changes at the edge of erosion. Same case as in *Figure 1.8.8*. Rare cells in basal/parabasal layers staining for p53 **(left)** and mild increase in Ki-67 labeling **(right)**.

	High-Grade Squamous Intraepithelial Lesion (HSIL, VIN 2-3)	Differentiated-Type Vulvar Intraepithelial Neoplasia
Age	Adults; peak age 45-50 y	Adults, postmenopausal, usually 6th to 8th decade
Location	Vulva	Vulva
Symptoms	Often asymptomatic	Vulvar irritation and itching
Signs	Papule, plaque; can be raised pale, pigmented, or red	Lichen sclerosus–like appearance, inflammatory/dermatitis-like changes, no distinct lesional borders
Etiology	High-risk HPV infection, most commonly HPV type 16	Unknown; *TP53* mutations are frequently detected; mutations in *PIK3CA, NOTCH1,* and *HRAS* are also seen
Histology	1. Epithelial thickening; acanthosis is often seen. Surface maturation is often preserved; hyperkeratosis is often present *(Figs. 1.9.1-1.9.3)* 2. Hyperchromatic/basophilic-appearing epithelium at low power *(Figs. 1.9.1-1.9.3)* 3. Immature cell expansion throughout epithelial thickness and disorganization in parabasal zone *(Fig. 1.9.2)* 4. Enlarged, hyperchromatic nuclei with nuclear contour irregularities pointing in different directions; nucleoli are typically not prominent *(Fig. 1.9.4)* 5. Mitoses are common and extend above the parabasal zone *(Fig. 1.9.4)* 6. Variable nonspecific inflammation in the background can be seen; lichen sclerosus–type changes are not typical	1. Elongation and anastomosis or thickening of rete ridges. Variable hyperkeratosis; dermal or interface inflammation can be present *(Figs. 1.9.6 and 1.9.7)* 2. Eosinophilic-appearing epithelium; no basophilia/immaturity at low power *(Figs. 1.9.6 and 1.9.7)* 3. Epithelial maturation is retained; abnormal keratinization, abundant eosinophilic cytoplasm in the basal and parabasal epithelial layers *(Figs. 1.9.8 and 1.9.9)* 4. Marked nuclear atypia in basal/parabasal layers with prominent nucleoli and notable intercellular bridges *(Figs. 1.9.8 and 1.9.9)* 5. Increased mitotic activity can be seen in basal/parabasal epithelial layers *(Fig. 1.9.9)* 6. Background of lichen sclerosus–type changes can be seen
Special studies	• P53 "overexpression" can be seen in midepithelial layers; basal layer is negative/"wild-type" pattern *(Fig. 1.9.5)* • Strong and diffuse expression of p16 (block-like), at least 1/3 of the epithelial thickness • Increased Ki-67 labeling throughout the epithelial thickness, including upper epithelial layers • Positive high-risk HPV by *in situ* hybridization	• Strong p53 expression in basal keratinocytes nuclei extending to the middle epithelial layers can be seen in some cases • Usually patchy or negative p16 • Variable Ki-67 proliferative activity • No detectable high-risk HPV by *in situ* hybridization
Treatment	Local excision, laser evaporation	Local excision with clear margins
Prognosis	Considered a precursor of HPV-related squamous cell carcinoma; can progress to invasive carcinoma if not removed	Considered a precursor of non–HPV-related vulvar squamous cell carcinoma; quick progression to invasive carcinoma

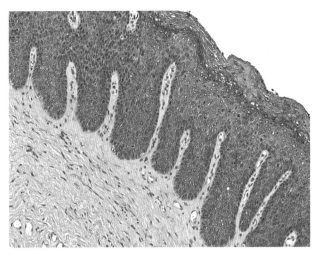

Figure 1.9.1   High-grade squamous intraepithelial lesion (VIN 2-3). Prominent acanthosis, lack of maturation, and diffuse epithelial basophilia. Prominent hyperkeratosis.

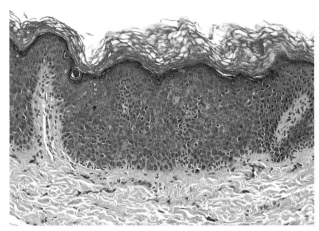

Figure 1.9.2   High-grade squamous intraepithelial lesion (VIN 2-3). Atypical squamous epithelium with immaturity and nuclear hyperchromasia.

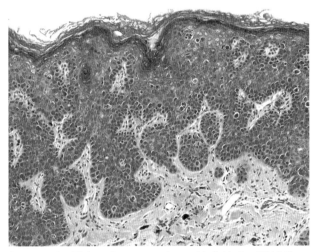

Figure 1.9.3   High-grade squamous intraepithelial lesion (VIN 2-3). Atypical immature squamous epithelium with acanthosis, tangentially oriented.

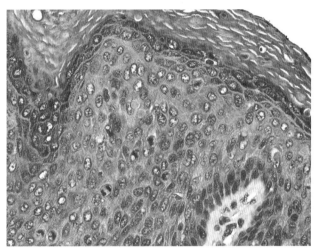

Figure 1.9.4   High-grade squamous intraepithelial lesion (VIN 2-3). Same case as in *Figure 1.9.1*. Higher magnification. Atypical immature keratinocytes with increased nucleocytoplasmic ratio and hyperchromatic nuclei with coarse chromatin. Mitotic figures in the midepithelial layers.

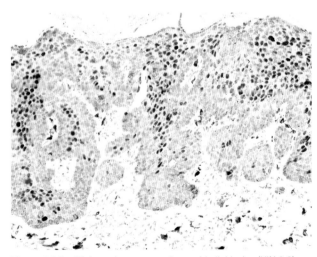

Figure 1.9.5   High-grade squamous intraepithelial lesion (VIN 2-3). Same case as in *Figure 1.9.3*. Immunohistochemical staining for p53 with mid epithelial/basal sparing pattern that can be confused with patterns seen in non–HPV-related intraepithelial neoplasia/differentiated-type vulvar intraepithelial neoplasia.

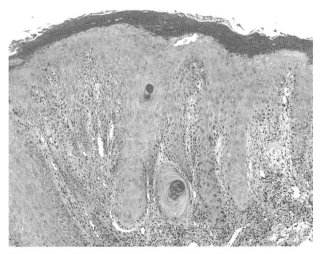

Figure 1.9.6   Differentiated-type vulvar intraepithelial neoplasia. Marked acanthosis and hyperkeratosis. Epithelial eosinophilia and abnormal keratinization in the lower epithelial layers.

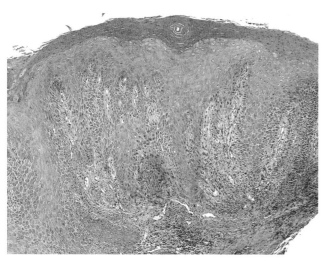

Figure 1.9.7 Differentiated-type vulvar intraepithelial neoplasia. Elongation and anastomosis or thickening of rete ridges. Marked hyper- and parakeratosis.

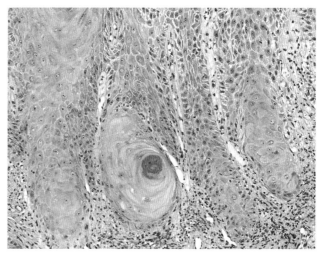

Figure 1.9.8 Differentiated-type vulvar intraepithelial neoplasia. Same case as in *Figure 1.9.6*, higher magnification. Abnormal intracellular keratinization and keratin pearl formation. Atypical basal/parabasal nuclei with prominent nucleoli.

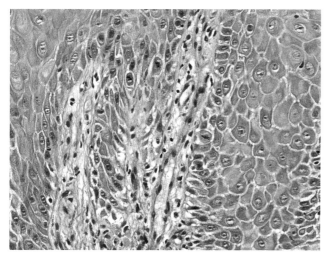

Figure 1.9.9 Differentiated-type vulvar intraepithelial neoplasia. Same case as in *Figure 1.9.7*, higher magnification. Atypical nuclei with prominent nucleoli and intercellular bridges. Mitotic figures in the basal/parabasal layers.

	Basal Cell Carcinoma	Basaloid Squamous Cell Carcinoma
Age	Adults over 40 y of age	Adults, peak incidence 6th decade
Location	Vulva	Vulva
Symptoms	Vulvar irritation, pruritus, ulcer	Vulvar irritation and/or mass
Signs	Raised nodule or ulcerated lesion, slow growing; can be pigmented	Vulvar mass or raised plaque, occasionally ulcerated
Etiology	Cutaneous lesions are associated with significant UV exposure; etiology of vulvar BCC is unclear; environmental exposures such as ionizing radiation and arsenic may be implicated; increased incidence in organ transplant recipients. Germline and somatic mutations in *PTCH1* gene may be implicated	High-risk HPV infection; HPV 16 is the most commonly implicated viral type. Risk factors include immunosuppression and smoking
Histology	1. Overlying epidermis is typically unremarkable; basaloid nests are contiguous with the basal layer *(Figs. 1.10.1-1.10.3)* 2. Stromal clefting and loose/myxoid stroma; necrosis is not common 3. Squamoid-appearing areas can be seen, but overt keratinization is usually absent 4. Consistent peripheral palisading *(Fig. 1.10.4)* 5. Monotonous elongated hyperchromatic nuclei and clear cytoplasm *(Fig. 1.10.5)* 6. Mitotic activity can be brisk accompanied by variable number of apoptotic bodies	1. Associated high-grade squamous intraepithelial lesion (HSIL, vulvar intraepithelial neoplasia 3 [VIN 3]) in the majority of cases 2. Stromal desmoplasia; stromal clefting can be seen but less frequent; necrosis can be seen *(Figs. 1.10.7 and 1.10.8)* 3. Overt squamous differentiation and keratinization in the middle of the invasive nests *(Fig. 1.10.9)* 4. Peripheral palisading can be seen but not a consistent feature 5. Enlarged hyperchromatic atypical nuclei with at least some degree of pleomorphism; dense eosinophilic cytoplasm 6. Frequent mitosis; apoptotic bodies can be seen
Special studies	• BerEP4 positive *(Fig. 1.10.6, **left**)* • p16 patchy/negative *(Fig. 1.10.6, **right**)* • No detection of high-risk HPV by *in situ* hybridization	• Negative or focal BerEP4 *(Fig. 1.10.10, **right**)* • p16 strong and diffuse *(Fig. 1.10.10, **left**)* • High-risk HPV detected by *in situ* hybridization
Treatment	Conservative excision with clear margins	Wide/radical local excision; regional lymph node dissection in cases with the depth of invasion >1 mm
Prognosis	Local recurrences are uncommon; lymph node metastases are exceedingly rare	Recurrences (local or in regional lymph nodes) in up to 24% of cases; lymph node metastases in up to 15% of cases with the depth of invasion >1 mm

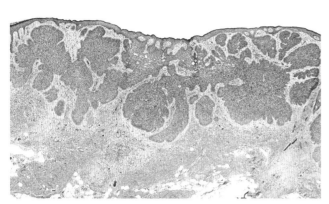

Figure 1.10.1   Basal cell carcinoma. Nodular growth pattern with epidermal connection. Loose stroma surrounding the nests.

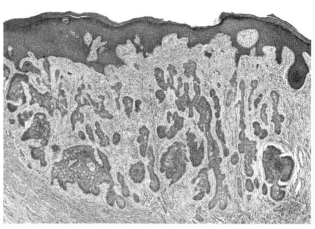

Figure 1.10.2   Basal cell carcinoma. Irregular epithelial nests in the stroma with focal epithelial connection and peripheral clefting. Overlying epidermis is uninvolved.

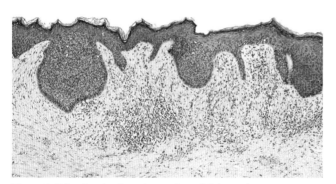

Figure 1.10.3   Basal cell carcinoma. Superficial growth pattern. Overlying epidermis is uninvolved.

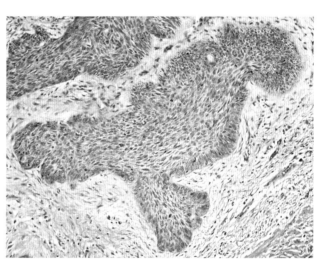

Figure 1.10.4   Basal cell carcinoma. Same case as in *Figure 1.10.2*, higher magnification. Tumor nests with prominent peripheral palisading and loose stroma.

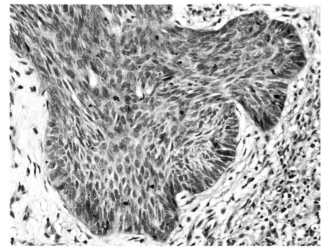

Figure 1.10.5   Basal cell carcinoma. Same case as in *Figure 1.10.2*, higher magnification. Brisk mitotic activity and frequent apoptotic bodies.

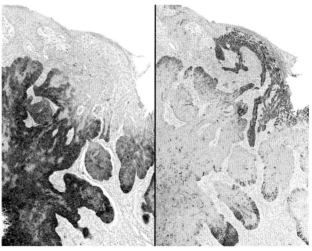

Figure 1.10.6   Basal cell carcinoma. Extensive expression of BerEP4 **(left)** and patchy staining for p16 **(right)**.

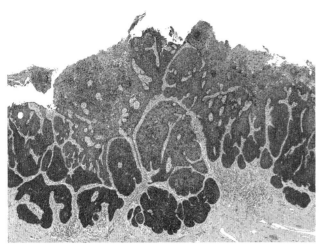

Figure 1.10.7 Basaloid squamous cell carcinoma. Some keratinization is evident in the superficial areas of the tumor.

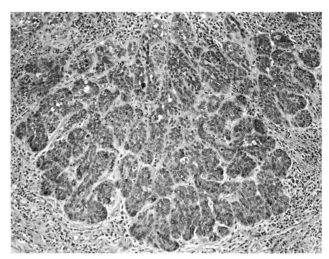

Figure 1.10.8 Squamous cell carcinoma. Tumor cells contain scant amount of eosinophilic cytoplasm and hyperchromatic nuclei with some degree of pleomorphism.

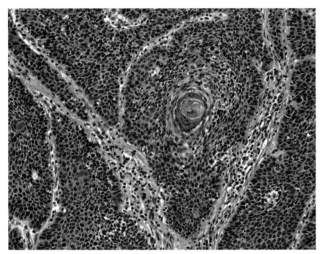

Figure 1.10.9 Basaloid squamous cell carcinoma. Same case as in *Figure 1.10.7*, higher magnification. Deeply basophilic cells with focus of keratinization in the center of the nest. Basal palisading is not prominent.

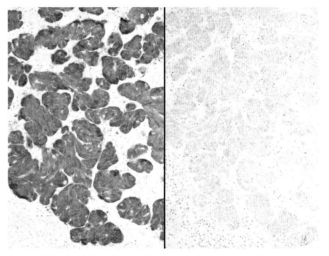

Figure 1.10.10 Squamous cell carcinoma. Same case as in *Figure 1.10.8*. Strong and diffuse expression of p16 **(left)** and essentially negative staining for BerEP4 **(right)**.

	Invasive Squamous Cell Carcinoma	High-Grade Squamous Intraepithelial Lesion (HSIL, VIN 2-3) With Extension Into Skin Adnexal Structures
Age	Mean age 50 y	Most common in 5th to 6th decade
Location	Vulva	Vulva
Symptoms	Vulvar mass, raised lesion, pain, bleeding	Often asymptomatic or vulvar papule, change in skin color, irritation
Signs	Mass lesion, raised, polypoid, or ulcerated	Papule, plaque; can be raised pale, pigmented, or red
Etiology	High-risk HPV infection, most commonly HPV 16	High-risk HPV infection, most commonly HPV 16
Histology	1. Invasive epithelial nests in a reasonably well-oriented section *(Fig. 1.11.1)* 2. Epithelial nests in the stroma independent of the adjacent adnexal structure 3. Small irregular tumor nests and single tumor cells in the stroma *(Fig. 1.11.2)* 4. Paradoxical maturation *(Fig. 1.11.3)* 5. Desmoplastic stromal reaction	1. Evidence of tangential sectioning; cross-sectionally cut dermal papillae 2. Presence of adnexal structure in the tissue section with partial involvement by intraepithelial lesion *(Fig. 1.11.4)* 3. Lesional nests follow the outlines of the skin adnexal structures *(Figs. 1.11.5-1.11.8)*; lack of small irregular nests, individual tumor cells in the stroma 4. Lack of paradoxical maturation 5. True desmoplastic stromal reaction is not typical; however, stroma surrounding adnexal structures can appear loose; inflammation can be present
Special studies	• Not helpful in this differential • Additional H&E levels are often helpful	• Not helpful in this differential • Additional H&E levels are often helpful
Treatment	Wide/radical local excision; regional lymph node dissection in cases with the depth of invasion >1 mm	Local excision with clear margins
Prognosis	Dependent on the stage. Cases with superficially invasive carcinoma can be cured by surgery alone. Recurrences (local or in regional lymph nodes) in up to 24% of cases; lymph node metastases in up to 15% of cases with the depth of invasion >1 mm	Can progress to invasive squamous cell carcinoma if untreated; excision with clear margins can be curative; however, recurrences are common Large clinically apparent lesions often harbor foci of invasive carcinoma and need to be exhaustively sampled

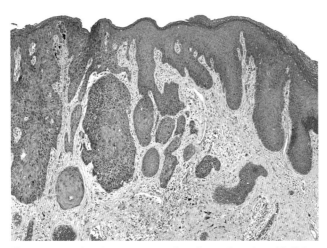

Figure 1.11.1 Invasive squamous cell carcinoma. Irregular epithelial nests with paradoxical maturation invading stroma.

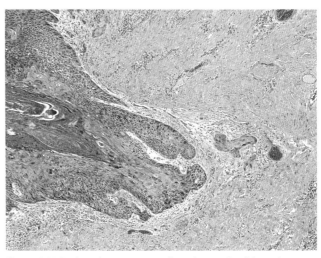

Figure 1.11.2 Invasive squamous cell carcinoma. Small irregular carcinoma nests associated with desmoplastic stromal response.

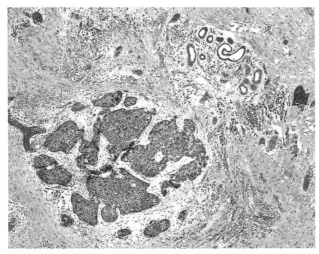

Figure 1.11.3 Invasive squamous cell carcinoma. The focus of invasive carcinoma resembles the outline of the adjacent skin adnexal structure. However, irregular outlines of the epithelial nests, paradoxical maturation, and associated stromal reaction are diagnostic of invasion.

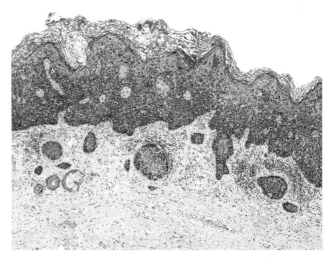

Figure 1.11.4 High-grade squamous intraepithelial lesion (high-grade VIN) extending into skin adnexal structures. Partial adnexal structure involvement is seen. Cytoplasmic eosinophilia in the center of some of the squamous nests in the stroma represents residual maturation of the intraepithelial lesion.

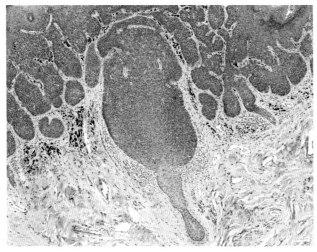

Figure 1.11.5 High-grade squamous intraepithelial lesion (high-grade VIN). Tangentially sectioned lesion extending into follicular structure.

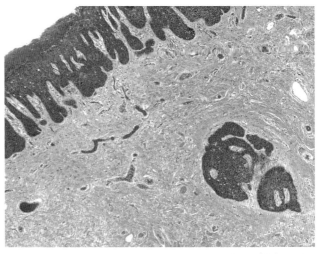

Figure 1.11.6 High-grade squamous intraepithelial lesion (high-grade VIN) extending into skin adnexal structures. Somewhat irregularly shaped epithelial nest in the stroma some distance away from the surface intraepithelial lesion.

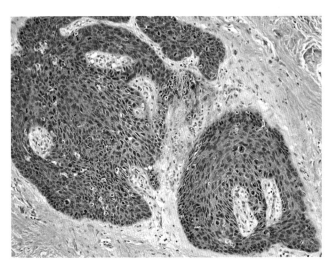

Figure 1.11.7 High-grade squamous intraepithelial lesion (high-grade VIN). Same focus as in *Figure 1.10.6*, higher magnification.

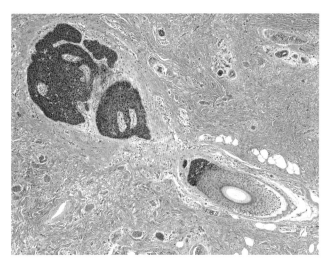

Figure 1.11.8 High-grade squamous intraepithelial lesion (high-grade VIN). Same focus as in *Figure 1.11.6*; deeper level reveals tangentially oriented hair follicle partially involved by HSIL aligned with detached stromal focus.

1.12

INVASIVE SQUAMOUS CELL CARCINOMA VS HIGH-GRADE SQUAMOUS INTRAEPITHELIAL LESION (HSIL, VIN 2-3) WITH CONVOLUTED ARCHITECTURE AND/OR TANGENTIAL ORIENTATION

	Invasive Squamous Cell Carcinoma	High-Grade Squamous Intraepithelial Lesion (HSIL, VIN 2-3) With Convoluted Architecture and/or Tangential Orientation
Age	Mean age 50 y	Peak age 45-50 y
Location	Vulva	Vulva
Symptoms	Vulvar mass, raised lesion, pain, bleeding	Often asymptomatic or vulvar papule, change in skin color, irritation
Signs	Mass lesion, raised, polypoid, or ulcerated	Papule, plaque; can be raised pale, pigmented, or red
Etiology	High-risk HPV infection, most commonly HPV 16	High-risk HPV infection, most commonly HPV 16
Histology	1. Irregular invasive squamous nests of different size and shape haphazardly situated in the stroma *(Fig. 1.12.1)* 2. Paradoxical maturation *(Fig. 1.12.2)* 3. Stromal desmoplastic reaction *(Fig. 1.12.3)* 4. Small epithelial nests with irregular contours and single cells in the stroma *(Fig. 1.12.4)*	1. Exophytic growth; evidence of tangential sectioning: cross-sectionally cut dermal papillae *(Fig. 1.12.5)*; regular outline of the epithelial nests in the stroma with retention of linear arrangement *(Fig. 1.12.6)*; merging and interconnected epithelial nests with rounded outline of the lesion *(Fig. 1.12.7)* 2. Rounded nests; maturation in the middle of tangentially cut epithelial pegs and squamous eddies can be present *(Fig. 1.12.8)*; no paradoxical maturation 3. Stromal inflammation may be present, but generally no true desmoplasia is seen 4. No single tumor cells infiltrating stroma
Special studies	• Not helpful in this differential • Additional H&E levels are often helpful	• Not helpful in this differential • Additional H&E levels are often helpful
Treatment	Wide/radical local excision; regional lymph node dissection in cases with the depth of invasion >1 mm	Local excision with clear margins
Prognosis	Dependent on the stage. Cases with superficially invasive carcinoma can be cured by surgery alone. Recurrences (local or in regional lymph nodes) in up to 24% of cases; lymph node metastases in up to 15% of cases with the depth of invasion >1 mm	Can progress to invasive squamous cell carcinoma if untreated; excision with clear margins can be curative; however, recurrences are common Large clinically apparent lesions often harbor foci of invasive carcinoma and need to be exhaustively sampled

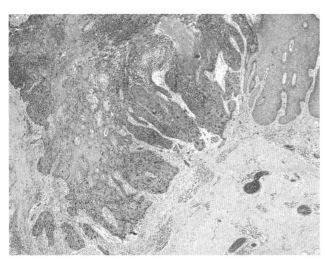

Figure 1.12.1   Invasive squamous cell carcinoma. Irregular epithelial nests haphazardly distributed in the stroma.

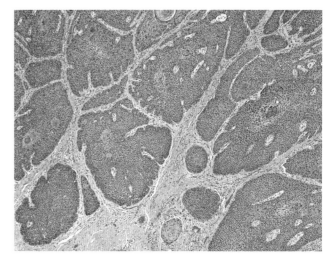

Figure 1.12.2   Invasive squamous cell carcinoma. Broad basaloid epithelial nests with foci of keratinization and a small eosinophilic nest at the leading edge representing paradoxical maturation.

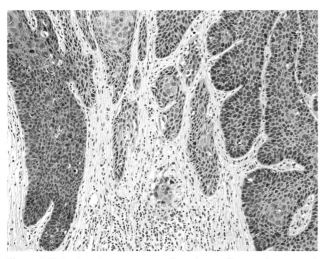

Figure 1.12.3   Invasive squamous cell carcinoma. Elongated tongues of invasive carcinoma in desmoplastic stroma.

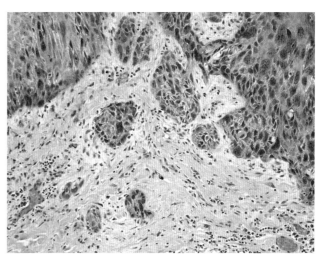

Figure 1.12.4   Invasive squamous cell carcinoma. Small irregular nests comprised atypical cells with eosinophilic cytoplasm, associated focal desmoplastic reaction.

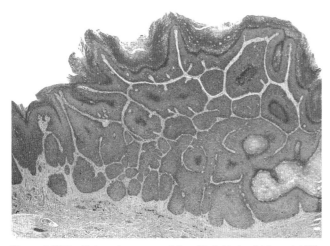

Figure 1.12.5   High-grade squamous intraepithelial lesion (high-grade VIN). Tangentially sectioned warty exophytic lesion. Epithelial nests with relatively smooth contours and "cut in" islands of the stratum corneum in the **center**.

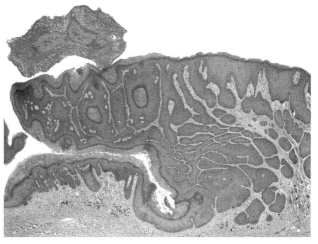

Figure 1.12.6   High-grade squamous intraepithelial lesion (high-grade VIN). Polypoid exophytic lesion. Epithelial nests in the stroma follow "linear" arrangement.

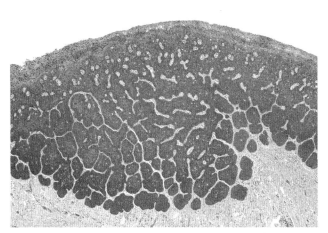

Figure 1.12.7 High-grade squamous intraepithelial lesion (high-grade VIN). Flat lesion overlying a stromal bulge is tangentially oriented. Interconnected epithelial nests; overall rounded outline of the focus. Additional levels help recover better oriented intraepithelial lesion.

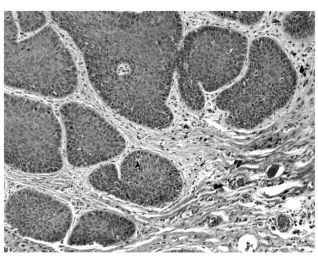

Figure 1.12.8 High-grade squamous intraepithelial lesion (high-grade VIN). Same case as in *Figure 1.12.6*, higher magnification. Rounded epithelial nests with preserved basal palisading; lack of surrounding stromal reaction.

	Primary Extramammary Paget Disease	Pagetoid High-Grade Squamous Intraepithelial Lesion (Pagetoid HSIL, VIN 2-3)
Age	Postmenopausal women, median age 65 y, occasionally in reproductive age women	Women in 5th and 6th decades, becoming more frequent in younger women
Location	Vulva (cutaneous and mucosal surfaces), vagina	Vulva, vagina
Symptoms	Pruritus, pain	Often asymptomatic; occasionally may present with pruritus
Signs	Eczematous-appearing plaque; moist, raised, white, or red areas, can be ulcerated; mimics dermatitis	Raised plaque-like lesion, pale, skin colored, or pigmented
Etiology	Cell of origin: pluripotent epidermal or adnexal stem cells, Toker cells. Amplification in ch Xcent-q21 and 19 and loss of 10q24-qter; *ERBB2* (HER2) amplification in some cases. Mutations in PI3K/AKT pathway genes in correlation with CDH1 hypermethylation	High-risk HPV infection; most commonly HPV 16
Histology	1. Epithelial thickness is variably increased 2. Intraepithelial nest or single cells in basal and parabasal epithelial layers *(Figs. 1.13.1 and 1.13.2)* 3. Extension into superficial epithelial layers and adnexal structures 4. Large cells with abundant pale basophilic cytoplasm *(Fig. 1.13.3)* 5. Large vesicular nuclei occasionally with prominent nucleoli 6. Mitotic figures can be seen, but not frequent *(Fig. 1.13.4)*	1. Epithelial hyperplasia, acanthosis 2. Basophilic intraepithelial nests distributed throughout epithelial thickness *(Figs. 1.13.5-1.13.7)* 3. Involvement of superficial epithelial layers and extension into skin adnexal structures can be seen 4. Scant eosinophilic cytoplasm 5. Increased nucleocytoplasmic ratio; enlarged hyperchromatic nuclei *(Figs. 1.13.8 and 1.13.9)* 6. Mitosis is common and can be seen in superficial epitholial layers
Special studies	• p16 patchy or negative • No detection of high-risk HPV by *in situ* hybridization • Cytokeratin 7, diffusely positive *(see Fig. 1.14.12)* • Can be GCDFP-15, GATA-3 positive	• p16 strong and diffuse *(Fig. 1.13.10)* • High-risk HPV detected by *in situ* hybridization *(Fig. 1.13.10,* **inset***)* • Cytokeratin 7 can be positive, but often focal • Negative for GCDFP-15, GATA-3
Treatment	Local excision; clear margins are often difficult to achieve	Conservative excision with clear margins; laser vaporization
Prognosis	Considered a form of adenocarcinoma *in situ* with slow protracted course; multifocality and recurrences are common. Invasion can be seen in up to 12% of cases; in such cases, depth of invasion would determine prognosis	Premalignant lesion; can progress to invasive carcinoma if untreated

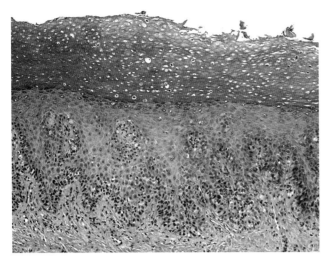

Figure 1.13.1 Primary extramammary Paget disease with extensive epidermal involvement.

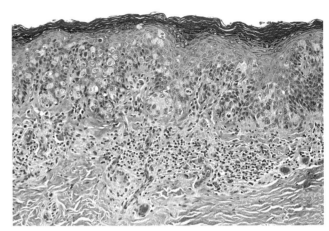

Figure 1.13.2 Primary extramammary Paget disease with extensive epidermal involvement. Intraepithelial cell nest and single cells with upward migration.

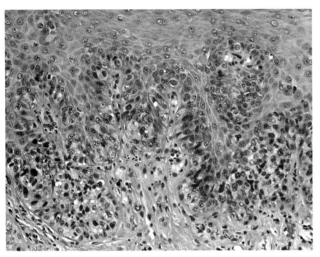

Figure 1.13.3 Primary extramammary Paget disease. Same case as in *Figure 1.13.1*, higher magnification. Clusters of cells with basophilic cytoplasm along the dermal epidermal junction.

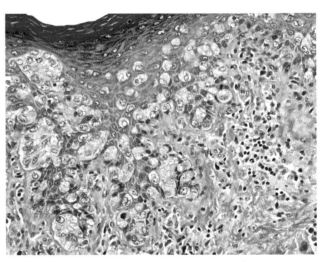

Figure 1.13.4 Primary extramammary Paget disease. Same case as in *Figure 1.13.2*, higher magnification. Pale cell nests in the epidermis. Occasional mitotic figure is seen

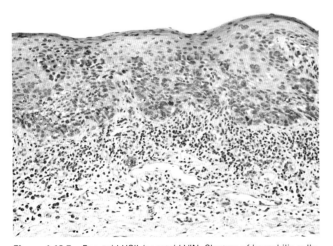

Figure 1.13.5 Pagetoid HSIL/pagetoid VIN. Clusters of basophilic cells in the epidermis.

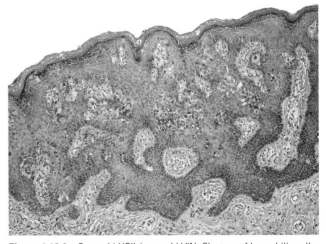

Figure 1.13.6 Pagetoid HSIL/pagetoid VIN. Clusters of basophilic cells in the epidermis.

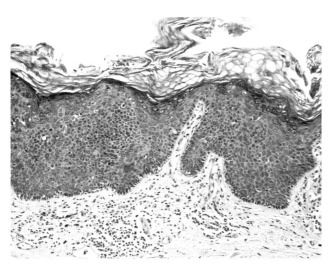

Figure 1.13.7   Pagetoid HSIL/pagetoid VIN. Islands and nests of cells with hyperchromatic nuclei and scant cytoplasm paler than that of surrounding normal keratinocytes.

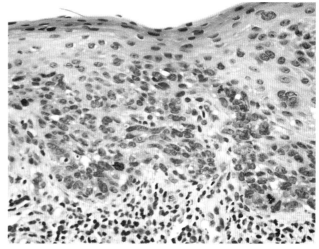

Figure 1.13.8   Pagetoid HSIL/pagetoid VIN. Same case as in *Figure 1.13.5,* higher magnification.

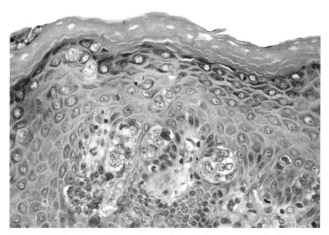

Figure 1.13.9   Pagetoid HSIL/pagetoid VIN. Same case as in *Figure 1.13.6,* higher magnification. Clusters of cells with scant cytoplasm and atypical hyperchromatic nuclei.

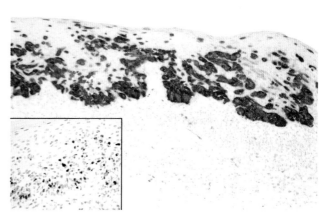

Figure 1.13.10   Pagetoid HSIL/pagetoid VIN. Same case as in *Figure 1.13.5.* Diffuse expression of p16 and punctate nuclear signals on high-risk HPV *in situ* hybridization preparation **(inset)**.

	Melanoma *In situ*	Primary Extramammary Paget Disease
Age	Women in 4th through 8th decades; median age in 6th decade	Postmenopausal women, median age 65 y, occasionally in reproductive age women
Location	Vulva, vagina	Vulva (cutaneous and mucosal surfaces), vagina
Symptoms	Asymptomatic; may present with pruritus or bleeding	Pruritus, pain
Signs	Pigmented flat or raised lesion, usually asymmetrical; up to 35% amelanotic	Eczematous-appearing plaque; moist, raised, white, or red areas; can be ulcerated; mimics dermatitis
Etiology	Low TMB, lack of UV signature. Numerous chromosomal structural variants and copy-number changes. Somatic mutations in *SF3B1, KIT, ATRX, TP53, ARID2, SETD2,* and *BRAF* less prevalent than in cutaneous melanomas	Cell of origin: pluripotent epidermal or adnexal stem cells, Toker cells. Amplification in ch Xcent-q21 and 19 and loss of 10q24-qter; *ERBB2* (HER2) amplification in some cases. Mutation in PI3K/AKT pathway genes in correlation with CDH1 hypermethylation
Histology	1. Confluent intraepithelial proliferation of atypical single and nested melanocytes *(Figs. 1.14.1 and 1.14.2)* 2. Extension into superficial epithelial layers/pagetoid spread *(Figs. 1.14.3 and 1.14.4)* 3. Melanoma cells are present along the dermal epidermal junction within basal layer 4. Extension into skin adnexal structures *(Fig. 1.14.5)* 5. Eosinophilic or amphophilic cytoplasm 6. Dusty cytoplasmic brown pigment can be seen, but not constant feature; no mucin in the cytoplasm *(Fig. 1.14.6)* 7. Hyperchromatic or vesicular nuclei with prominent nucleoli	1. Nests or single cells in the epithelium *(Figs. 1.14.7 and 1.14.8)* 2. Extension into superficial epithelial layers *(Fig. 1.14.9)* 3. Preserved layer of compressed basal keratinocytes seen in some areas *(Fig. 1.14.10)* 4. Extension into skin adnexal structures 5. Large cells with pale basophilic cytoplasm *(Fig. 1.14.11)* 6. Intracytoplasmic mucin/vacuoles; pigmented forms infrequent, but occur 7. Large vesicular nuclei with prominent nucleoli
Special studies	• HMB-45, Melan-A, MART1, MITF, SOX10 positive *(Fig. 1.14.1,* **right***)* • Negative cytokeratins, GCDFP-15, GATA-3	• Cytokeratins, cytokeratin 7, positive *(Fig. 1.14.12)* • Can be GCDFP-15, GATA-3 positive
Treatment	Wide local excision with negative margins (at least 0.5 cm)	Local excision; clear margins are often difficult to achieve
Prognosis	Recurrences are common in cases not completely excised. Can be associated with invasive malignant melanoma	Considered a form of adenocarcinoma *in situ* with slow protracted course; multifocality and recurrences are common. Invasion can be seen in up to 12% of cases; in such cases, depth of invasion/tumor stage determines prognosis

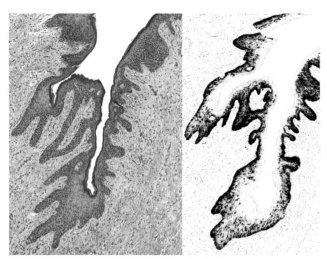

Figure 1.14.1 Melanoma *in situ.* Atypical intraepithelial melanocytic proliferation highlighted by melanoma cocktail immunohistochemical stain (HMB-45 and tyrosinase).

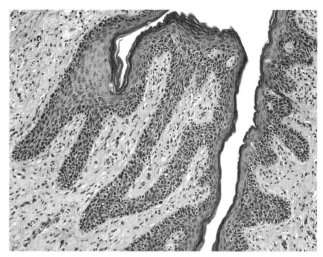

Figure 1.14.2 Melanoma *in situ.* Same case as in *Figure 1.14.1,* higher magnification. Atypical intraepithelial melanocytic proliferation with junctional confluence.

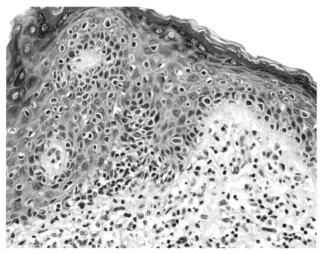

Figure 1.14.3 Melanoma *in situ.* Atypical intraepithelial melanocytic proliferation with junctional confluence and upward migration of melanocytes.

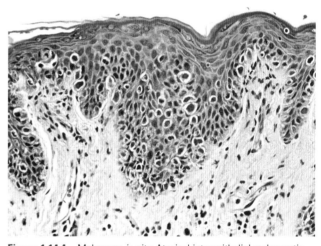

Figure 1.14.4 Melanoma *in situ.* Atypical intraepithelial melanocytic proliferation with junctional confluence and marked nuclear pleomorphism.

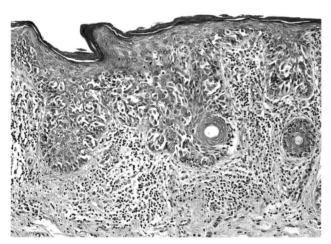

Figure 1.14.5 Melanoma *in situ.* Intraepithelial nests of atypical melanocytes and extension into adnexal structure.

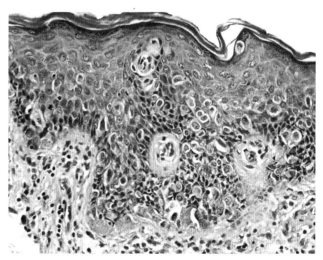

Figure 1.14.6 Melanoma *in situ.* Atypical melanocytes with prominent nucleoli and dusty intracytoplasmic brown pigment.

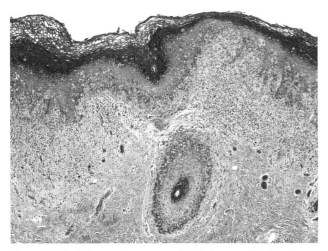

Figure 1.14.7 Primary extramammary Paget disease with extensive epidermal involvement and extension into skin adnexal structures.

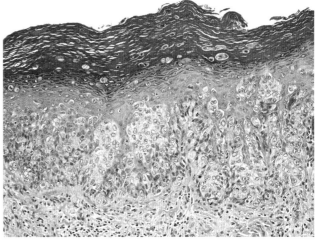

Figure 1.14.8 Primary extramammary Paget disease. Same case as in *Figure 1.14.7*, higher magnification. Paget nests in the epidermis.

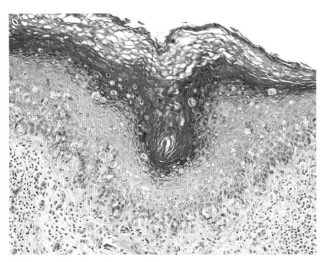

Figure 1.14.9 Primary extramammary Paget disease. Same case as in *Figure 1.14.7*, higher magnification. Individual cells extend into the stratum corneum.

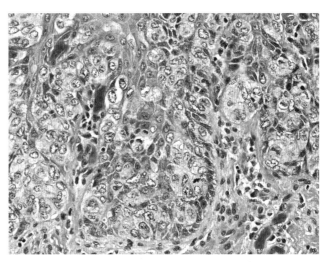

Figure 1.14.10 Primary extramammary Paget disease. Large cells with abundant basophilic cytoplasm and vesicular nuclei. A layer of compressed basal keratinocytes is underlying Paget cell nests.

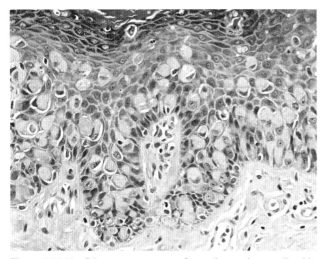

Figure 1.14.11 Primary extramammary Paget disease. Large cells with abundant pale cytoplasm and signet ring–like appearance.

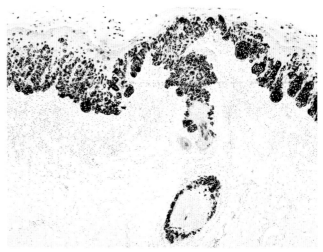

Figure 1.14.12 Primary extramammary Paget disease. Same case as in *Figure 1.14.7*. Immunohistochemical stain for cytokeratin 7 highlights numerous Paget cells.

	Ectopic Prostatic Tissue	Primary Vaginal Adenocarcinoma
Age	Wide age range; most cases in premenopausal women	4th to 7th decade
Location	Cervix, vagina	Anterior upper third of vagina (for clear cell carcinoma); posterior vaginal wall
Symptoms	Asymptomatic	Pelvic pain, vaginal discharge or bleeding, occasionally abnormal Pap smear
Signs	Usually incidental finding; occasionally mass lesion	Vaginal mass, polypoid exophytic, ulcerated, or deep
Etiology	Misplaced Skene glands or metaplastic process involving endocervical glands have been suggested	Vaginal primaries are rare; arise in vagina from endometriosis, vaginal adenosis, some associated with *in utero* DES exposure. More commonly metastasis from other sites
Histology	1. Proliferation of large mucinous glands/acini within the stroma; no stromal desmoplasia *(Fig. 1.15.1)* 2. Often prominent squamous differentiation 3. Duct-like structures can be present; large glands with wide patent lumina and intraglandular papillary infoldings *(Fig. 1.15.2)* 4. Two cell layers: basal layer composed of flattened cells with scant cytoplasm is apparent in some glands *(Fig. 1.15.3)* 5. Abundant pale cytoplasm 6. Luminal cells with abundant foamy cytoplasm and basally placed small uniform round nuclei	1. Large glandular spaces can be present, usually with complex true papillary structures *(Fig. 1.15.5)*; stromal desmoplasia can be present 2. Squamous differentiation can be seen in endometrioid carcinoma arising in endometriosis 3. No distinct duct-like structures; glandular dilatation can be seen 4. Single cell layer forming glands 5. Mucinous differentiation can be seen in cases of either endocervical or gastrointestinal types *(Fig. 1.15.6)* 6. Clear cell carcinoma can have pale cytoplasm, mimicking mucinous differentiation; some degree of cytologic atypia is usually present (also see Section 1.16)
Special studies	• PSA and/or PSAP positive *(Fig. 1.15.4,* **left***)*; double negative cases have been described; CD10, androgen receptor, NKX3.1, AMACR positive; basal layer positive for 34βE12 *(Fig. 1.15.4,* **right***)* • PAX8, ER, and PR negative	• Negative for PSA, NKX3.1, AMACR • PAX8, ER, and PR variably positive
Treatment	None required	Surgery with lymphadenectomy vs radiation therapy +/− chemotherapy
Prognosis	Benign/nonneoplastic condition	Prognosis is stage dependent; DES exposure–related tumors have better prognosis (84% 5-y survival, compared to 69% 5-y survival in non–DES-exposed cases). Recurrences are seen in 25% of cases

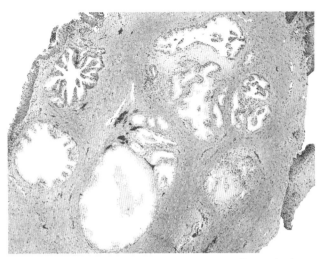

Figure 1.15.1 Ectopic prostatic tissue. Proliferation of large glands, some architecturally complex in cervical stroma.

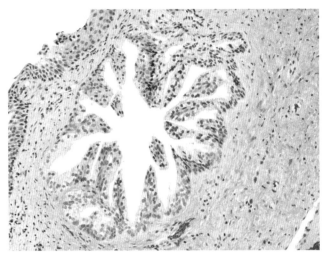

Figure 1.15.2 Ectopic prostatic tissue. Same case as in *Figure 1.15.1*, higher magnification. Large glands with prominent intraglandular infoldings.

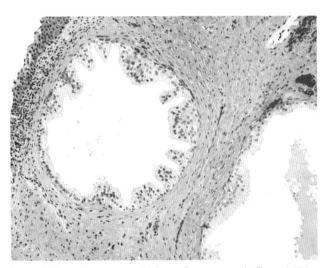

Figure 1.15.3 Ectopic prostatic tissue. Same case as in *Figure 1.15.1*, higher magnification. Basal layer is present around the glands.

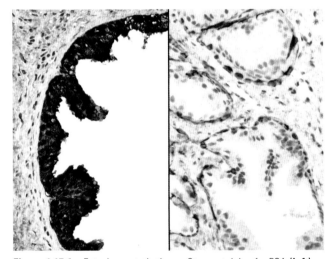

Figure 1.15.4 Ectopic prostatic tissue. Strong staining for PSA **(left)**; 34βE12 stain highlights basal cells **(right)**.

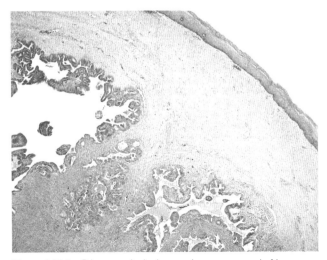

Figure 1.15.5 Primary vaginal adenocarcinoma composed of large glands with complex papillary infoldings.

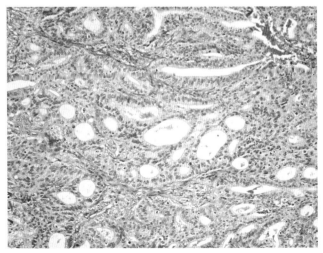

Figure 1.15.6 Primary vaginal adenocarcinoma with mucinous features. Complex cribriforming architecture.

	Metastatic Adenocarcinoma	Primary Vaginal Adenocarcinoma
Age	Older women, most commonly postmenopausal	4th to 7th decade
Location	Vagina, vaginal cuff	Anterior upper third of vagina (for clear cell carcinoma); posterior vaginal wall
Symptoms	Vaginal bleeding, discharge, dyspareunia, urinary symptoms	Vaginal bleeding, discharge, dyspareunia, urinary symptoms; small tumor can be asymptomatic
Signs	More common than primary; knowledge of the history of prior malignancy is crucial to the diagnosis	Metastatic carcinoma from other sites should be excluded first
Etiology	Direct extension or hematogenous spread from cervical, endometrial, colorectal, ovarian/tubal, pancreatic primary, etc.	History of *in utero* DES exposure, associations with adenosis, endometriosis, endocervicosis, mesonephric remnants, enteric-type adenoma, and high-risk HPV infection
Histology	1. Comparison with pathology materials from prior malignancy 2. Endometrial carcinoma with all respective histologic types (*Figs. 1.16.1 and 1.16.2*) 3. Colorectal adenocarcinoma, mucinous differentiation; occasionally surface disruption with mucosal involvement (*Figs. 1.16.3 and 1.16.4*) 4. Ovarian/fallopian tube carcinoma; usually in a setting of recurrence; morphologic features can be altered by prior chemotherapy (*Figs. 1.16.5 and 1.16.6*)	1. Histologic features identical to those seen in tumors of respective histologic types at other locations 2. Clear cell carcinoma; tubulocystic, papillary, solid patterns (*Fig. 1.16.7*) 3. Endometrioid carcinoma (*Fig. 1.16.8*), background of endometriosis can be seen (*Fig. 1.16.9*) 4. Mucinous carcinoma; resembles endocervical-type epithelium or enteric type with goblet cells 5. Mesonephric carcinoma, tubular pattern with eosinophilic secretions
Special studies	• Metastasis from GYN tract adenocarcinoma—no studies are helpful (except serous carcinoma of ovary/fallopian tube are WT-1 positive) • Colorectal adenocarcinoma are CK20, CDX2 positive; CK7, ER, PR, PAX8 negative	• Endometrioid carcinoma, positive for PAX8, ER, and PR • Clear cell carcinoma, negative for ER and PR • Mesonephric carcinoma, positive for CD10, GATA-3, PAX8; negative for ER, PR
Treatment	Surgery vs radiation therapy +/− chemotherapy	Surgery with lymphadenectomy vs radiation therapy +/− chemotherapy
Prognosis	Poor; however, in case of isolated vaginal metastasis/recurrence, radical surgery (pelvic exenteration can be curative)	Prognosis is stage dependent; DES exposure–related tumors have better prognosis (84% 5-y survival, compared to 69% 5-y survival in non–DES-exposed cases). Recurrences are seen in 25% of cases

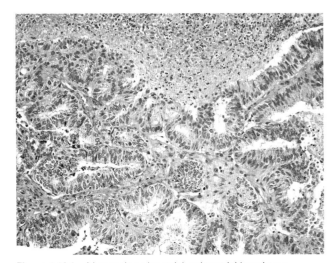

Figure 1.16.1 Metastatic endometrial endometrioid carcinoma. Necrosis is present; this would be not typical of the primary well-differentiated tumor.

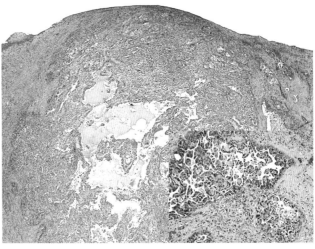

Figure 1.16.2 Metastatic uterine carcinosarcoma (epithelial component). Nodule in vaginal wall with mucosal erosion. High-grade carcinoma, higher magnification **(inset)**.

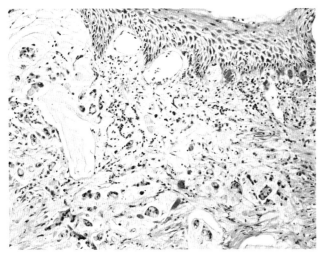

Figure 1.16.3 Metastatic mucinous appendiceal adenocarcinoma. Dissecting mucin with fragments of mucinous epithelium beneath squamous epithelium.

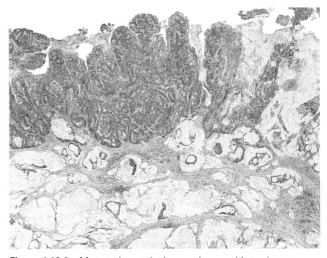

Figure 1.16.4 Metastatic rectal adenocarcinoma with mucinous features. Tumor colonizes mucosal surface and can mimic primary vaginal adenocarcinoma arising from vaginal villous adenoma.

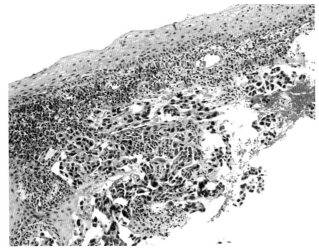

Figure 1.16.5 Metastatic ovarian high-grade serous carcinoma. Cytologic features are altered by prior chemotherapy.

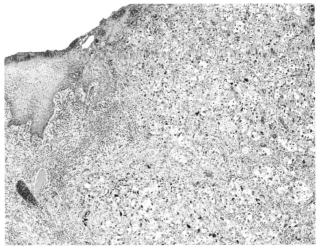

Figure 1.16.6 Metastatic ovarian clear cell carcinoma. Primary vaginal clear cell carcinoma can have similar appearance.

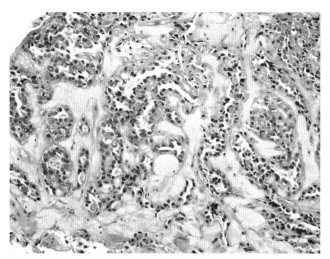

Figure 1.16.7   Primary vaginal clear cell carcinoma in a patient with history of DES exposure.

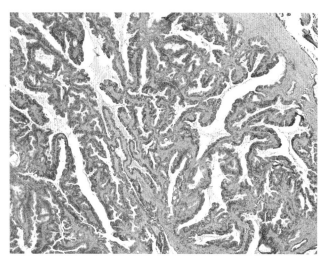

Figure 1.16.8   Primary vaginal adenocarcinoma arising in endometriosis with glandular and papillary architecture.

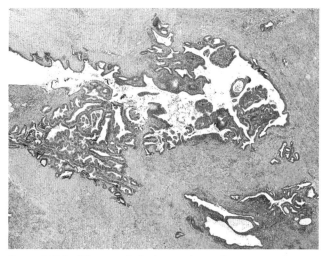

Figure 1.16.9   Primary vaginal adenocarcinoma. Same case as in *Figure 1.16.8*. Focus of endometriosis is seen deep in the vaginal wall **(lower right)**.

	Prolapsed Fallopian Tube	**Vaginal Adenocarcinoma**
Age	Adults, months to years posthysterectomy; median 6 mo	4th to 7th decade
Location	Vaginal apex	Anterior upper third of the vagina (for clear cell carcinoma); posterior vaginal wall
Symptoms	Status post hysterectomy, abdominal pain, vaginal discharge or bleeding, dyspareunia; abnormal Pap smear	Pelvic pain, vaginal discharge or bleeding, occasionally abnormal Pap smear
Signs	Red granular nodule or mass up to 2 cm in size; appearance of granulation tissue or malignancy; often painful with manipulation	Vaginal mass, polypoid exophytic, ulcerated, or deep
Etiology	Complication of vaginal (more commonly) or abdominal hysterectomy; particularly after postoperative complications, infections, delayed peritoneal closure, cul-de-sac drains	Vaginal primaries are rare; arise in vagina from endometriosis, vaginal adenosis, some associated with *in utero* DES exposure. More commonly metastasis from other sites
Histology	1. Tubular–glandular or papillary architecture with blunted, clubbed plicae *(Fig. 1.17.1)*; in some cases, retained recognizable intact fallopian tube plicae *(Fig. 1.17.2)* 2. Thick-walled vessels and bundles of smooth muscle tissue at the base of the lesion *(Fig. 1.17.3)* 3. Hyperplastic epithelium with cribriforming and intraglandular infoldings *(Fig. 1.17.4)* 4. At least focally retained tubal-serous differentiation with ciliated and secretory cells 5. Cytologic atypia very mild, if present 6. Granulation tissue–like stroma with mixed inflammatory infiltrate with plasma cells and eosinophils *(Fig. 1.17.5)*	1. Haphazardly arranged infiltrating glands *(Fig. 1.17.6)*; architectural patterns resembling fallopian tube are not present 2. Thick-walled vessels are not typical; can be seen deep in the vaginal wall 3. Glandular crowding *(Fig. 1.17.7)* and cribriform patterns 4. Tubal differentiation can be seen in cases arising from endometriosis *(Fig. 1.17.8)* 5. Cytologic atypia is usually present, but can be mild 6. Stromal desmoplasia and inflammation can be seen, but not a constant feature Also see Section 1.16
Special studies	• Generally not needed • WT-1 immunostain can be used to confirm tubal-/serous-type epithelium	• WT-1 negative; unless serous carcinoma, metastatic from ovary/fallopian tube
Treatment	Initial conservative measures often fail to control the symptoms; most cases require total salpingectomy with vaginal repair (closure of the vaginal vault)	Surgery +/– lymphadenectomy vs radiation therapy +/– chemotherapy
Prognosis	Benign	Prognosis is stage dependent; DES exposure–related tumors have better prognosis, 84% 5-y survival, compared to 69% 5-y survival in non–DES-exposed cases. Recurrences are seen in 25% of cases

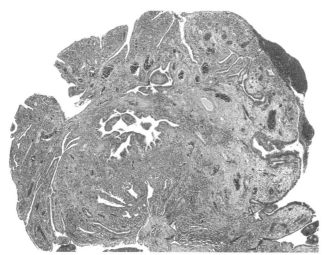

Figure 1.17.1 Prolapsed fallopian tube. Nodule with glandular proliferation and blunted papillary structures on the surface.

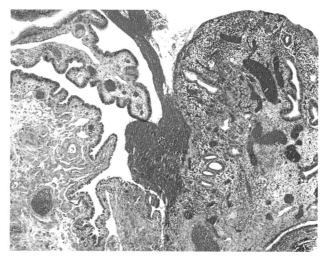

Figure 1.17.2 Prolapsed fallopian tube. Recognizable fallopian tube plicae **(left)** and small glandular structures in inflamed congested stroma **(right)**.

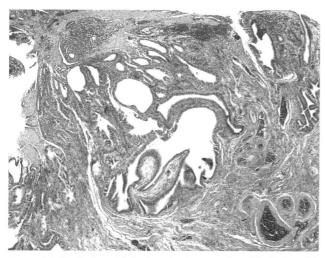

Figure 1.17.3 Prolapsed fallopian tube. Deep portion of the lesion with larger caliber vessels and smooth muscle bundles **(lower right)**.

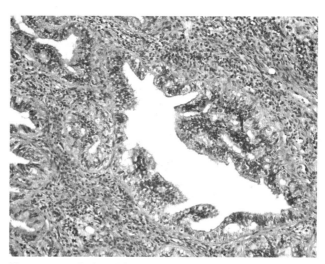

Figure 1.17.4 Prolapsed fallopian tube. Same case as in *Figure 1.17.1*, higher magnification. Intraglandular infoldings simulate cribriforming.

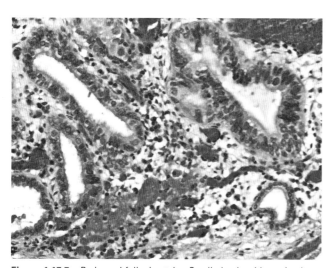

Figure 1.17.5 Prolapsed fallopian tube. Small glands with retained tubal-type epithelium in the stroma with plasma cells and eosinophils.

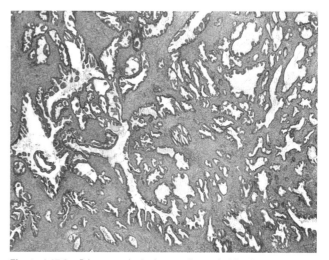

Figure 1.17.6 Primary vaginal adenocarcinoma (arising in endometriosis, not shown). Haphazard infiltrating growth.

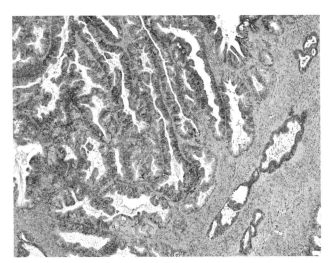

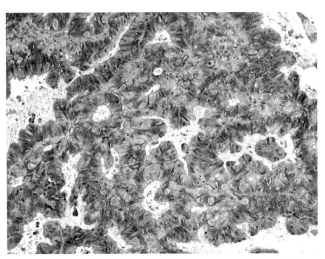

Figure 1.17.7   *Primary vaginal adenocarcinoma. Same case as in* Figure *1.17.6,* higher magnification. Crowded complex glands.

Figure 1.17.8   *Primary vaginal adenocarcinoma. Same case as in* Figure *1.17.6,* higher magnification. Back-to-back glands with prominent tubal differentiation.

	Bartholin Gland Hyperplasia/Adenoma	Primary Mucinous Carcinoma (Bartholin Gland Carcinoma)
Age	Wide age range, more common in young adults	Most between 40 and 70 y, mean age 50 y
Location	Lower vagina, vestibule, lateral	Lower vagina, vestibule, lateral
Symptoms	Asymptomatic or mass lesion	Mass at the site of Bartholin gland; may simulate Bartholin gland cyst, pain, and bleeding
Signs	Mass-forming lesion in some cases	Vaginal vestibular mass, surface ulceration
Etiology	Originates in the Bartholin gland	Often originates in the Bartholin gland; may be associated with vulvar Paget disease; some cases are associated with high-risk HPV
Histology	1. Increased number of mucinous glands in lobular arrangement; maintained gland architecture with preserved duct-acinar relationship *(Fig. 1.18.1)* in hyperplasia; densely packed proliferation of small glands and tubules and absent ducts in adenoma 2. Uniform glands with little variation in size and shape forming lobules; stromal reaction is absent *(Fig. 1.18.2)*; in adenoma two cell layers with preserved myoepithelial cells 3. Stromal desmoplasia is generally absent 4. Glandular epithelium with abundant mucinous cytoplasm and small bland uniform basally placed nuclei *(Fig. 1.18.3)* in hyperplasia; cuboidal cells with depleted mucin, round nuclei with small nucleoli in adenoma	1. Irregular borders, infiltrative growth pattern, and papillary architecture can be present *(Figs. 1.18.4 and 1.18.5)* 2. Mucinous differentiation is common; adenosquamous features and adenoid cystic morphology can be seen 3. Stromal desmoplastic response 4. Cytologic atypia is present but can be mild; increased mitotic activity *(Fig. 1.18.6)*
Special studies	• None for hyperplasia • Myoepithelial markers: p63, smooth muscle myosin heavy chain can be used to highlight myoepithelial cells in adenoma	• None for carcinoma vs hyperplasia • Negative myoepithelial markers: p63, smooth muscle myosin heavy chain
Treatment	Local excision is curative	Partial to total vulvectomy with lymphadenectomy; +/− radiation therapy
Prognosis	Bartholin hyperplasia is benign; some cases of adenoma were seen in association with adenoid cystic carcinoma; thus, careful evaluation and thorough sampling are warranted	Dependent on stage; 20% are metastatic to inguinal–femoral lymph nodes; recurrences are seen in more than 50% of patients. 5-y survival is 66%-67%

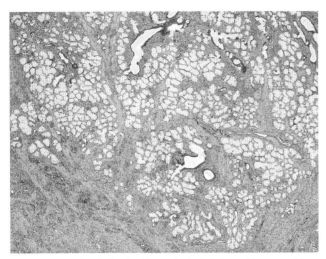

Figure 1.18.1 Bartholin gland hyperplasia. Lobular architecture with central ducts.

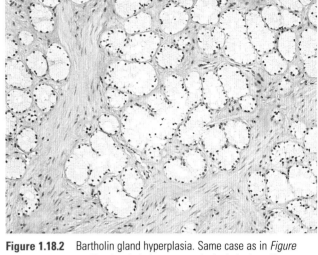

Figure 1.18.2 Bartholin gland hyperplasia. Same case as in *Figure 1.18.1*, higher magnification. Lobule composed of relatively uniform mucinous glands. No stromal reaction is present.

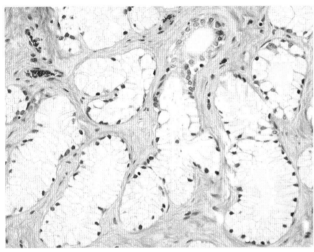

Figure 1.18.3 Bartholin gland hyperplasia. Same case as in *Figure 1.18.1*, higher magnification. Abundant mucinous cytoplasm and small basally placed uniform nuclei.

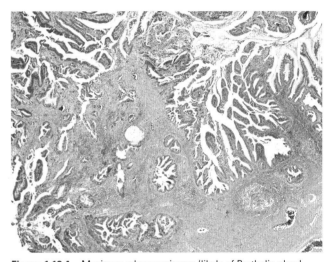

Figure 1.18.4 Mucinous adenocarcinoma (likely of Bartholin gland origin). Irregularly shaped glands infiltrate stroma. Large areas of papillary formations.

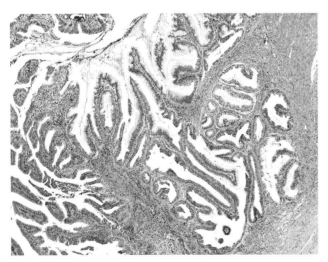

Figure 1.18.5 Mucinous adenocarcinoma (likely of Bartholin gland origin). Same case as in *Figure 1.18.4*, higher magnification.

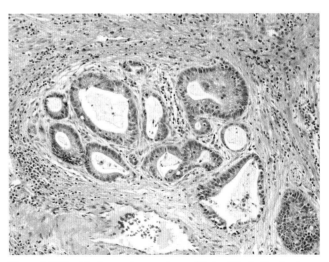

Figure 1.18.6 Mucinous adenocarcinoma (likely of Bartholin gland origin). Same case as in *Figure 1.18.4*, higher magnification. Small irregular glands with some nuclear stratification and cytologic atypia. Surrounding stroma with desmoplastic changes.

	Hidradenoma Papilliferum (Papillary Hidradenoma)	Vulvar Adenocarcinoma Arising From Mammary-like Glands
Age	Adults	Most patients are older than 60 y; age ranges from 4th to 8th decades
Location	Vulva, lateral aspects of the labia or interlabial sulcus	Vulva, labium majus
Symptoms	Often asymptomatic, small nodule, bleeding related to surface ulceration is uncommon	Mass lesion, pain
Signs	Circumscribed nodule, usually <2 cm; overlying intact epidermis, ulceration is uncommon	Vulvar mass, subcutaneous nodule, associated skin changes, ulceration, or dermatitis-like changes when associated with Paget disease
Etiology	Arises from anogenital mammary-like sweat glands; alterations in PI3K/AKT pathway have been reported	Arises from anogenital mammary-like sweat glands; alterations in PI3K/AKT pathway genes have been reported
Histology	1. Well-circumscribed, unencapsulated *(Fig. 1.19.1)*; complex papillary architecture with delicate fibrovascular cores *(Fig. 1.19.2)* 2. Overlying epidermis is usually intact 3. Uniform columnar secretory cells; apocrine-like differentiation *(Fig. 1.19.3)*; absent or mild atypia 4. Presence of two cell layers, epithelial and myoepithelial cells *(Fig. 1.19.4)* 5. Mitoses are generally infrequent but can be present and focally prominent	1. Circumscribed or irregular/infiltrative borders; low-grade papillary carcinoma: complex papillary architecture and lack of myoepithelial cells *(Fig. 1.19.5)* or infiltrative growth pattern *(Figs. 1.19.6 and 1.19.7)* 2. Subepithelial extension and surface ulceration can be seen *(Fig. 1.19.8)* 3. Features resembling different variants of mammary carcinoma can be seen *(Figs. 1.19.9-1.19.11)* 4. Lack of myoepithelial cells 5. Variable mitotic activity
Special studies	• Myoepithelial markers: p63, smooth muscle myosin heavy chain can be used to highlight myoepithelial cells • Positive GATA-3	• Myoepithelial markers: p63, smooth muscle myosin heavy chain are negative *(Fig. 1.19.12,* **right***)* • Positive GATA-3 *(Fig. 1.19.12,* **left***)*
Treatment	Local complete excision	Total or partial vulvectomy, lymphadenectomy; chemotherapy and radiation therapy depending on the stage
Prognosis	Benign; may recur locally if incompletely excised. Malignant transformation is rare but can occur with development of DCIS-like lesions or low-grade phyllodes tumor	Deep invasion and regional lymph node metastases are seen in more than 50% of cases

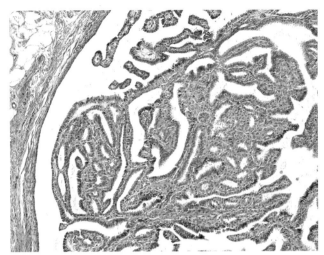

Figure 1.19.1 Hidradenoma papilliferum. Circumscribed, intracystic lesion with complex papillary architecture.

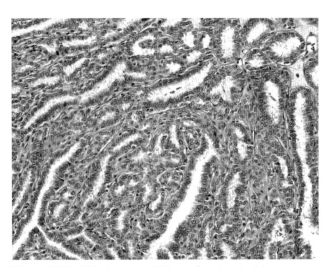

Figure 1.19.2 Hidradenoma papilliferum. Complex glandular pattern.

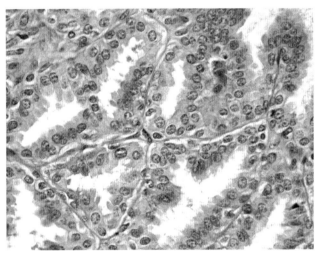

Figure 1.19.3 Hidradenoma papilliferum. Same case as in *Figure 1.19.1*, higher magnification. Cuboidal cells with apocrine features.

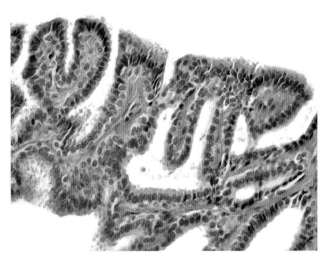

Figure 1.19.4 Hidradenoma papilliferum. Same case as in *Figure 1.19.1*, higher magnification. Fused papillary structures. Two cells layers are evident: luminal columnar cells and basal myoepithelial cells with pale cytoplasm.

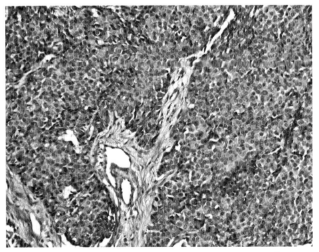

Figure 1.19.5 Vulvar adenocarcinoma arising from mammary-like glands. Papillary (intraductal) carcinoma. Also see *Figure 1.19.12* for corresponding immunostains.

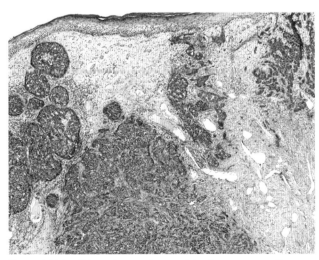

Figure 1.19.6 Vulvar adenocarcinoma arising from mammary-like glands. Infiltrative growth pattern.

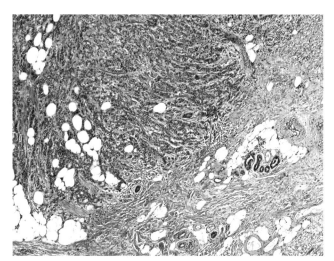

Figure 1.19.7   Vulvar adenocarcinoma arising from mammary-like glands. Infiltrative growth pattern. Mammary-like glands are seen at the periphery of the tumor.

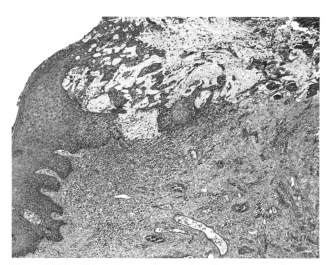

Figure 1.19.8   Vulvar adenocarcinoma arising from mammary-like glands (resembling colloid carcinoma) eroding through the skin.

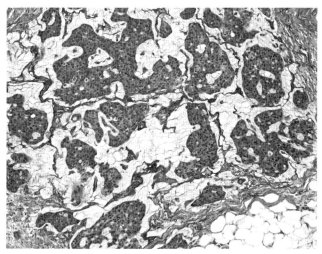

Figure 1.19.9   Vulvar adenocarcinoma arising from mammary-like glands. Same case as in *Figure 1.19.8*, higher magnification. Tumor resembles colloid carcinoma of the breast.

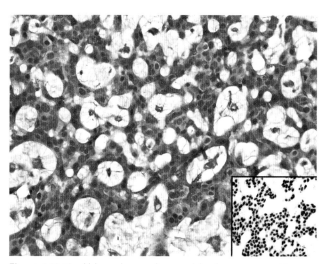

Figure 1.19.10   Vulvar adenocarcinoma arising from mammary-like glands. Positive GATA-3 staining **(inset)**.

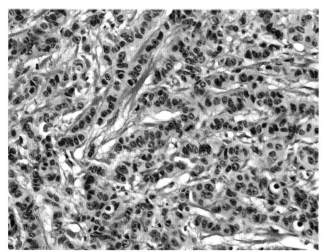

Figure 1.19.11   Vulvar adenocarcinoma arising from mammary-like glands. Same case as in *Figure 1.19.7*, higher magnification. Carcinoma cells infiltrate in single-file pattern.

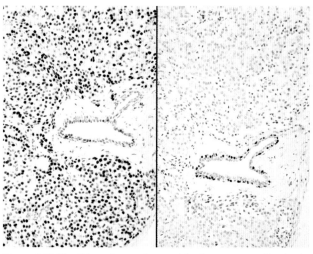

Figure 1.19.12   Vulvar adenocarcinoma arising from mammary-like glands. Same case as in *Figure 1.19.5*. Tumor cells are positive for GATA-3 **(left)**; p63 expression is absent **(right)** except for the normal ductal structure.

	Fibroepithelial (Mesodermal) Stromal Polyp	Aggressive Angiomyxoma
Age	All age groups (newborn to 77 y), most common in reproductive age women, mean age 40 y	Young adults, mean age 35 y
Location	Vagina, commonly lower third, lateral wall; less commonly vulva, cervix	Vulva, perineum, pelvic soft tissue
Symptoms	Usually asymptomatic	Unilateral vulvar mass
Signs	Incidental finding during pelvic examination, polypoid lesion, usually <5 cm in size; common during pregnancy	Vaguely circumscribed non–encapsulated deep-seated mass, usually >5 cm
Etiology	Unknown, likely represents reactive process; possibly hormonally induced	Unknown; translocations involving 12q15, 12q14.3 region/high mobility group (HMG) protein/HMGA2 has been reported in one third of tumors; rearrangement partners include ch 1, 5, 7, 8, 11, and 21
Histology	1. Superficially located exophytic polypoid lesion *(Fig. 1.20.1)* 2. Fibroblastic stroma with a central fibrovascular core; no extension into the underlying tissue *(Fig. 1.20.2)* 3. Myxoid stromal change can be present in subepithelial areas 4. Small to medium caliber vessels 5. Stellate and multinucleated stromal fibroblasts *(Fig. 1.20.3)*	1. Deep mass with extension to subepithelial area in some cases *(Fig. 1.20.4)* 2. Diffuse infiltrative growth pattern 3. Paucicellular; loose myxoid stroma 4. Haphazardly arranged and widely distributed varying caliber vessels with patent lumina *(Fig. 1.20.5)* 5. Monotonous spindle cells with round to oval nuclei *(Fig. 1.20.6)*
Special studies	• Positive for desmin, ER, and PR	• Weakly Alcian blue positive • HMGA2 positive • Variably positive for ER and PR
Treatment	Polypectomy for diagnosis is generally curative	Local excision, negative margins are difficult to achieve; gonadotropin-releasing hormone agonists are an alternative emerging therapy
Prognosis	Benign/nonneoplastic; pregnancy-associated polyps can regress spontaneously postpartum, local recurrences are rare, but have been described	Local recurrences are common, distant metastases are exceedingly rare

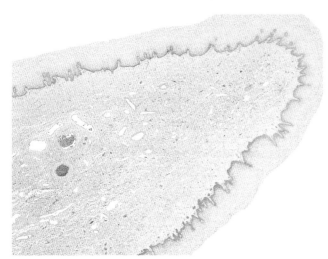

Figure 1.20.1   Fibroepithelial/mesodermal stromal polyp. Loose subepithelial stroma becoming denser toward the center of the lesion.

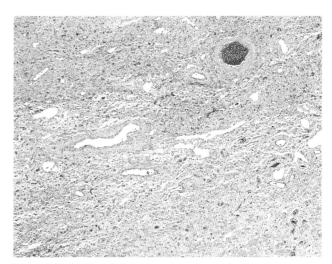

Figure 1.20.2   Fibroepithelial/mesodermal stromal polyp. Central fibrovascular core.

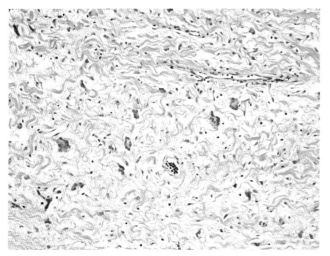

Figure 1.20.3   Fibroepithelial/mesodermal stromal polyp. Same case as in *Figure 1.20.1*, higher magnification. Atypical fibroblasts in finely collagenous matrix.

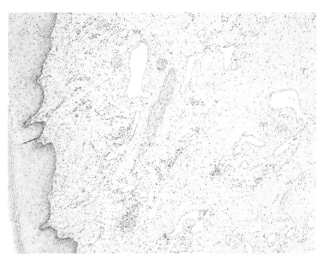

Figure 1.20.4   Aggressive angiomyxoma. Paucicellular tumor with variably distributed vessels extends to vaginal mucosa.

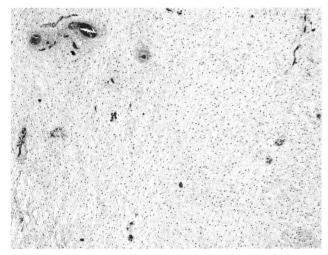

Figure 1.20.5   Aggressive angiomyxoma. Same case as in *Figure 1.20.4*. Variably distributed vessels with wide patent lumina, some in small clusters.

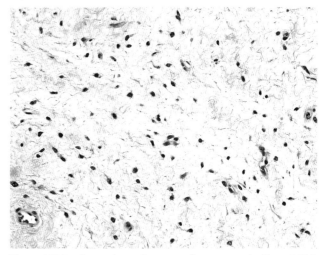

Figure 1.20.6   Aggressive angiomyxoma. Same case as in *Figure 1.20.4*, higher magnification. Concentric condensation of collagen bundles around the vessel. Bland tumor cells with uniform round to ovoid nuclei.

	Vulvar Lymphedema	Aggressive Angiomyxoma
Age	Adults, usually older women	Young adults, mean age 35 y
Location	Vulva, extension to inner thighs	Vulva, perineum, pelvic soft tissue
Symptoms	Bilateral vulvar swelling	Unilateral vulvar mass
Signs	Swelling of superficial vulvar tissue; no deep tissue involvement	Vaguely circumscribed non–encapsulated deep-seated mass, usually larger than 5 cm
Etiology	Presumed chronic lymphatic obstruction, associated with morbid obesity, decreased ambulation; pregnancy, preeclampsia, infection, and Crohn disease	Unknown; translocations involving 12q15, 12q14.3 region/high mobility group (HMG) protein/IIMGA2 has been reported in one-third of tumors; rearrangement partners include ch 1, 5, 7, 8, 11, and 21
Histology	1. Stromal edema without distinct borders *(Fig. 1.21.1)* 2. Dilated and tortuous vascular channels; perivascular lymphocytic infiltrates *(Fig. 1.21.2)* 3. Bland stromal fibroblasts with elongated nuclei *(Fig. 1.21.3)*; scattered multinucleated stromal cells can be seen	1. Infiltrative growth pattern, extension into surrounding fibroadipose tissues *(Fig. 1.21.4)*; however, lipomatous variants have been described 2. Haphazardly arranged and widely distributed varying caliber vessels with widely patent lumens; occasional vascular clusters with "myoid bundles" *(Fig. 1.21.5)* 3. Monotonous spindle cells with round to oval nuclei *(Fig. 1.21.6)* Also see *Figures 1.20.4, 1.20.5, 1.20.6*
Special studies	• Alcian blue negative • HMGA2 has not been studied	• Weakly Alcian blue positive • HMGA2 positive, sensitive but not very specific
Treatment	Treatment of the underlying causes; simple excision with vulvoplasty may be necessary and is usually curative	Local excision; negative margins are difficult to achieve; gonadotropin-releasing hormone agonists are an alternative emerging therapy
Prognosis	Prognosis is related to underlying comorbidities	Local recurrences are common; distant metastases are exceedingly rare

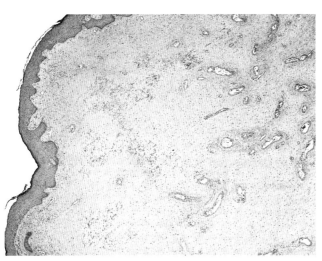

Figure 1.21.1 Vulvar lymphedema. Edema/expansion of subepithelial and deep stroma with prominent vascular proliferation.

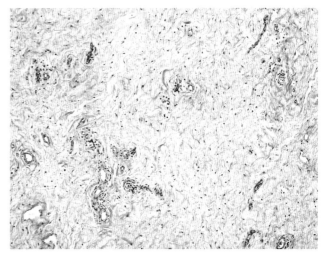

Figure 1.21.2 Vulvar lymphedema. Prominent vascular proliferation with perivascular chronic inflammatory infiltrate.

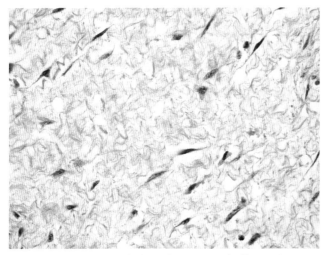

Figure 1.21.3 Vulvar lymphedema. Same case as in *Figure 1.21.1,* higher magnification. Bland spindle cells in edematous stroma.

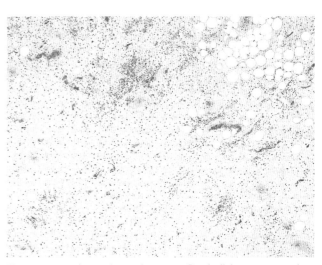

Figure 1.21.4 Aggressive angiomyxoma. Paucicellular tumor extends into deep adipose tissue.

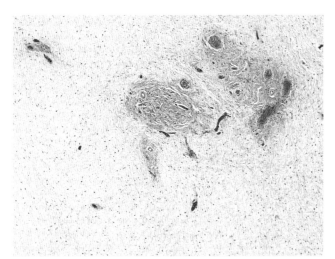

Figure 1.21.5 Aggressive angiomyxoma. Vascular clusters with collections of "myoid bundles."

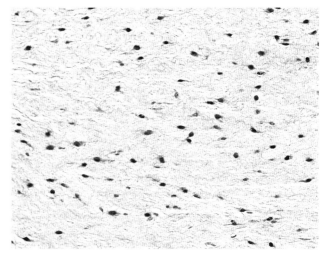

Figure 1.21.6 Aggressive angiomyxoma. Same case as in *Figure 1.21.4,* higher magnification. Bland cells with uniform round to ovoid nuclei.

	Aggressive Angiomyxoma	Angiomyofibroblastoma
Age	Young adults, mean age 35 y	Reproductive age women; can be seen in postmenopausal women
Location	Vulva, perineum, pelvic soft tissue	Vulva, vaginal vestibule
Symptoms	Unilateral vulvar mass	Painless vulvar mass
Signs	Vaguely circumscribed non–encapsulated deep-seated mass, usually larger than 5 cm	Circumscribed mass, usually <5 cm; can mimic Bartholin gland cyst
Etiology	Unknown; translocations involving 12q15, 12q14.3 region/high mobility group (HMG) protein/HMGA2 has been reported in one-third of tumors; rearrangement partners include ch 1, 5, 7, 8, 11, and 21	Unknown; arises from subepithelial stroma of gynecologic tract
Histology	1. Usually >5 cm in size; deep mass with extension to subepithelial area in some cases; diffuse infiltrative growth pattern 2. Uniformly paucicellular tumor with loose myxoid stroma 3. Haphazardly arranged and widely distributed varying caliber vessels *(Fig. 1.22.1)* 4. Uniformly widely distributed tumor cells 5. No perivascular sclerotic rim 6. Bland small round to ovoid nuclei Also see *Figures 1.20.4-1.20.6 and 1.21.4-1.21.6*	1. Usually <5 cm in size; well-demarcated non–encapsulated tumor; intralesional fat can be present (lipomatous variant) 2. Alternating zones of cellularity and edematous collagenous matrix *(Fig. 1.22.2)* 3. Thin-walled, capillary-like small to medium caliber vessels 4. Clusters of stromal cells, some in perivascular distribution *(Fig. 1.22.3)* 5. Sclerotic rim around vascular structures *(Fig. 1.22.4)* 6. Bland often epithelioid or plasmacytoid stromal cells *(Fig. 1.22.5)*
Special studies	• Weakly Alcian blue positive • Positive for HMGA2, sensitive but not very specific	• HMGA2 can be negative
Treatment	Local excision, negative margins are difficult to achieve; gonadotropin-releasing hormone agonists are an alternative emerging therapy	Local excision is generally curative
Prognosis	Local recurrences are common; distant metastases are rare	Benign; malignant transformation is reported, but exceedingly rare

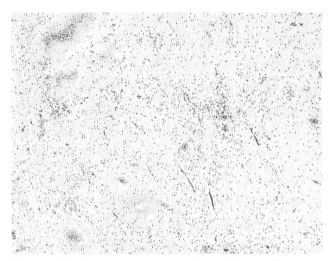

Figure 1.22.1 Aggressive angiomyxoma. Paucicellular myxoid neoplasm with variably distributed vessels.

Figure 1.22.2 Angiomyofibroblastoma. Variably cellular tumor with prominent thin-walled vessels.

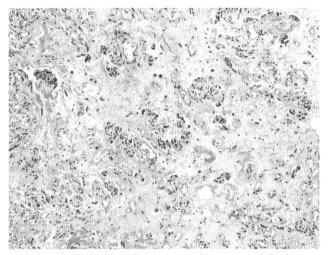

Figure 1.22.3 Angiomyofibroblastoma. Clusters of stromal cells within edematous and collagenous matrix.

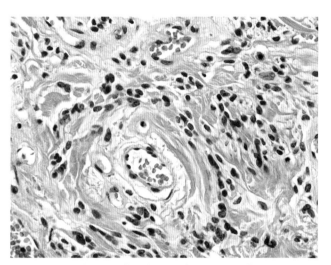

Figure 1.22.4 Angiomyofibroblastoma. Same case as *Figure 1.22.2*, higher magnification. Sclerotic rim around the vessel in the center of the image. Bland stromal cells in perivascular distribution.

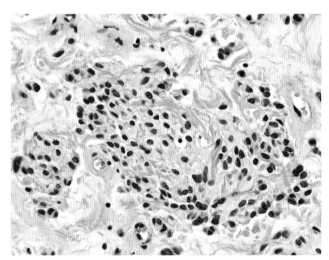

Figure 1.22.5 Angiomyofibroblastoma. Same case as *Figure 1.22.2*, higher magnification. Clusters of bland epithelioid stromal cells.

	Cellular Angiofibroma	Leiomyoma
Age	Mean age 54 y	Wide age range; most cases between 38 and 48 y
Location	Vulva, occasionally, vagina, subcutaneous tissue, or more superficial in the dermis	Vulva or vagina (most common in the uterus; also occurs in the cervix)
Symptoms	Usually painless mass, occasionally painful	Painless mass
Signs	Superficial vulvar mass, most reported cases are <3 cm	Superficial or deep; can simulate Bartholin cyst; most reported cases are <5 cm
Etiology	Unknown; complete or partial loss of ch 13 (including *RB1* locus) and/or ch 16	Unknown; rare cases are associated with Alport syndrome (germline deletion of *COL4A5* and *COL4A6*)
Histology	1. Usually well circumscribed; some contour irregularity can be seen 2. Uniformly increased cellularity *(Figs. 1.23.1 and 1.23.2)* 3. Spindle cells forming short intersecting fascicles *(Fig. 1.23.3)* 4. Small to medium caliber vessels distributed throughout the tumor; prominent hyalinization of the vessel wall *(Fig. 1.23.4)* 5. Pale eosinophilic cytoplasm and elongated/ovoid uniform nuclei *(Fig. 1.23.5)* 6. Mitotic activity is variable, but generally mitoses are infrequent 7. May contain mature adipose tissue, usually at the periphery of the lesion	1. Well circumscribed; infiltrative margin should raise concern for a more aggressive smooth muscle tumor 2. Most tumors are not highly cellular; cellular variants do occur 3. Long interlacing fascicles of spindle cells *(Fig. 1.23.6)* 4. Variably distributed thick-walled vessels occasionally in clusters *(Fig. 1.23.7)*; hyalinization (as degenerative change) is not uncommon, but hyalinization of vessel wall is infrequent 5. Eosinophilic fibrillary cytoplasm and cigar-shaped nuclei *(Fig. 1.23.8)* 6. Up to 5 mitotic figure/10 HPF
Special studies	• Most cases are negative for desmin • CD34 (50% of cases)	• Positive for desmin • Negative for CD34 (marker will highlight vascular structures)
Treatment	Local excision	Local excision
Prognosis	Benign; malignant transformation has been described, most commonly in lipomatous component	Benign; local recurrences are possible

Figure 1.23.1   Cellular angiofibroma. Uniformly cellular neoplasm with numerous variably distributed medium- to small-caliber vessels.

Figure 1.23.2   Cellular angiofibroma. Highly cellular spindle cell neoplasm with prominent vessels.

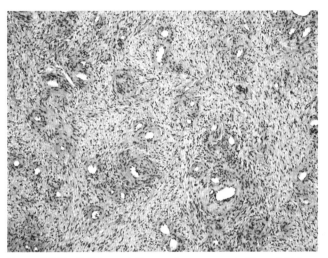

Figure 1.23.3   Cellular angiofibroma. Same case as in *Figure 1.23.2*, higher magnification. Short intersecting fascicles of spindle cells.

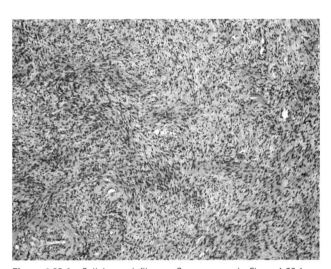

Figure 1.23.4   Cellular angiofibroma. Same case as in *Figure 1.23.1*, higher magnification. Numerous medium- and small-caliber vessels with hyalinization of the vessel wall.

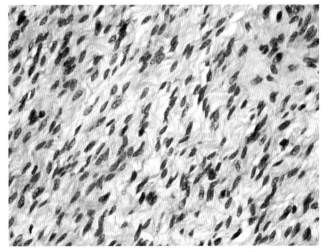

Figure 1.23.5   Cellular angiofibroma. Same case as in *Figure 1.23.1*, higher magnification. Spindle cells with pale eosinophilic cytoplasm and uniform ovoid/elongated nuclei.

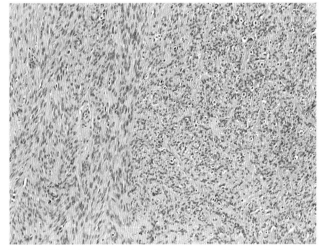

Figure 1.23.6   Leiomyoma. Long intersecting fascicles of spindle cells.

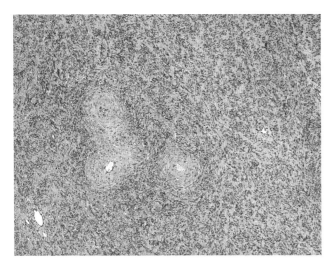

Figure 1.23.7 Leiomyoma. Cellular variant. A cluster of thick-walled vessels.

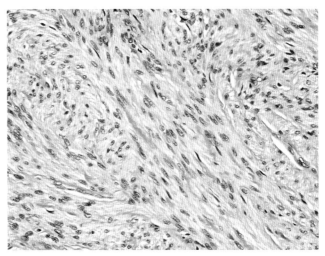

Figure 1.23.8 Leiomyoma. Intersecting bundles of spindle cells with eosinophilic fibrillary cytoplasm and cigar-shaped nuclei.

	Myofibroblastoma	Leiomyoma
Age	Reproductive age and postmenopausal women, mean age 57 y	Wide age range; most cases between 38 and 48 y
Location	Vagina; less commonly vulva and cervix; arises from superficial lamina propria	Vulva or vagina (most common in the uterus; also occurs in the cervix)
Symptoms	Usually asymptomatic; occasionally, symptoms can be related to compression of surrounding structures	Painless mass
Signs	Circumscribed mass, usually solitary	Can simulate Bartholin cyst, most reported cases are <5 cm
Etiology	Unknown; monoallelic deletion of 13q14, including *RB1*, has been reported in some cases; reported in tamoxifen-treated patients	Unknown; rare cases are associated with Alport syndrome (germline deletion of *COL4A5* and *COL4A6*)
Histology	1. Circumscribed unencapsulated nodular mass in the superficial stroma lifting overlying squamous epithelium *(Fig. 1.24.1)* 2. Variegated growth pattern *(Fig. 1.24.2)* 3. Lace-like or sieve-like architecture, cellular central areas, regions of myxoid changes *(Fig. 1.24.3)* 4. Spindled and stellate-shaped mesenchymal cells in finely collagenous matrix and thick collagenous bundles *(Fig. 1.24.4)* 5. Mitoses are uncommon	1. Well-circumscribed, lobulated growth can be seen; infiltrative margin should raise concern for a more aggressive smooth muscle tumor *(Fig. 1.24.5)* 2. Most tumors not highly cellular; cellular variants do occur 3. Long interlacing fascicles of uniform spindle cells *(Fig. 1.24.6)*; in cross-sectionally cut bundles, cells can have pseudoepithelioid appearance *(Fig. 1.24.7)*; hyalinization (as degenerative change) can be seen *(Figs. 1.24.8 and 1.24.9)* 4. Cells with eosinophilic fibrillary cytoplasm and cigar-shaped nuclei *(Fig. 1.24.10)* 5. Up to 5 mitotic figures/10 HPF
Special studies	• Positive for desmin, ER, PR; focal expression of smooth muscle actin and muscle-specific actin • Positive for CD34	• Positive desmin, smooth muscle actin, muscle-specific actin, ER, and PR • CD34 is negative in the tumor cells (vessels provide internal positive control)
Treatment	Local excision	Local excision
Prognosis	Benign; no recurrences reported after excision with negative margins	Benign; can recur locally

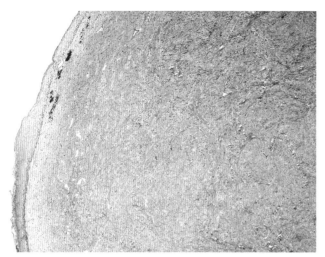

Figure 1.24.1   Myofibroblastoma. Circumscribed spindle cell neoplasm in the subepithelial stroma.

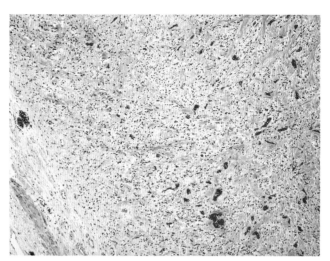

Figure 1.24.2   Myofibroblastoma. Variegated growth pattern.

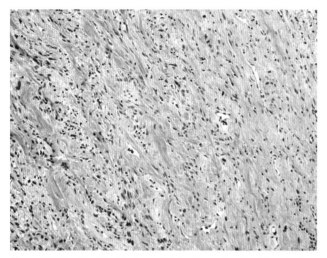

Figure 1.24.3   Myofibroblastoma. Thick collagen bundles intermixed with bundles and islands of bland spindle cells.

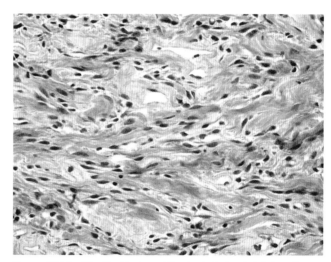

Figure 1.24.4   Myofibroblastoma. Bland spindled and stellate cells with oval or elongated nuclei.

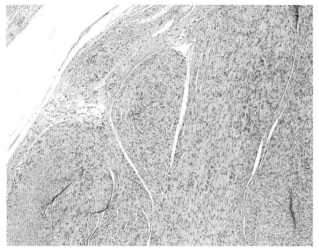

Figure 1.24.5   Leiomyoma. Circumscribed neoplasm with some lobulation at the periphery.

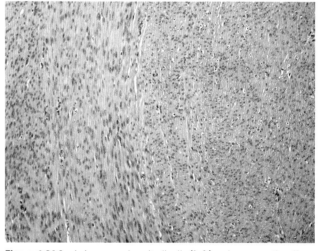

Figure 1.24.6   Leiomyoma. Longitudinally **(left)** and cross-sectionally **(right)** cut interlacing long bundles of spindle cells.

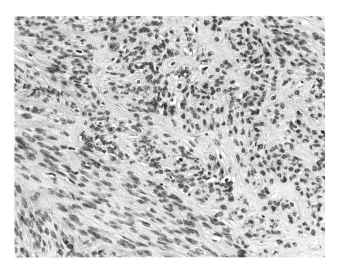

Figure 1.24.7   Leiomyoma. Interlacing long bundles of spindle cells. Cells in cross-sectionally cut bundles have pseudoepithelioid appearance.

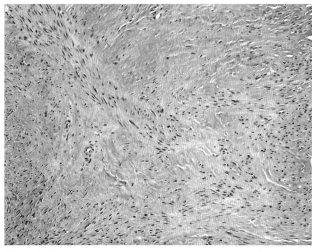

Figure 1.24.8   Leiomyoma. Large virtually acellular areas of hyalinization. Cells in remaining cellular areas retain fascicular growth pattern.

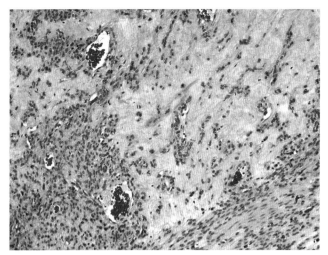

Figure 1.24.9   Leiomyoma. Large area of hyalinization with entrapped cells having pseudoepithelioid appearance.

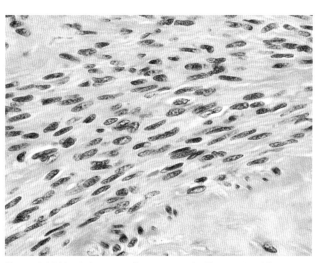

Figure 1.24.10   Leiomyoma. Same case as in *Figure 1.24.7*, higher magnification. Spindle cells with eosinophilic fibrillary cytoplasm and cigar-shaped nuclei.

	Neurofibroma	Myofibroblastoma
Age	Sporadic tumors are uncommon before the age of 20; syndrome-associated tumors are seen in children and young adults	Reproductive age and postmenopausal women, mean age 57 y
Location	Vulva; much less common in the vagina, cervix, and other gynecologic sites; clitoral tumors are often congenital	Vagina; less common in vulva and cervix; arises from superficial lamina propria
Symptoms	Painless, cosmetic defect; symptoms can be related to irritation/local trauma; urinary symptoms and vaginal obstruction during pregnancy	Usually asymptomatic; occasionally, symptoms can be related to compression of surrounding structures
Signs	Firm nodular growth. In the pediatric population, it may be confused with ambiguous genitalia. Other signs of neurofibromatosis (café au lait, etc.)	Circumscribed mass, usually solitary
Etiology	May be sporadic or associated with neurofibromatosis type I (autosomal dominant disorder with nearly 100% penetrance)	Unknown; monoallelic deletion of 13q14, including *RB1*, has been reported in some cases; reported in tamoxifen-treated patients
Histology	1. Lack of sharp circumscription, abuts overlying epidermis *(Fig. 1.25.1)*; can entrap skin adnexal structures, epithelial hyperplasia 2. Relatively uniformly cellular tumor with randomly distributed spindle cells arranged in bundles *(Fig. 1.25.2)*; vague storiform pattern can be seen 3. Longitudinally cut bundles have wave-like appearance *(Fig. 1.25.3)*; thin collagen bundles admixed with tumor cells *(Fig. 1.25.4)* 4. Small dark nuclei; some with tapered/pointed ends *(Fig. 1.25.5)* 5. Wagner-Meissner–like bodies	1. Circumscribed unencapsulated nodular mass in the superficial stroma lifting overlying squamous epithelium *(Fig. 1.25.7)* 2. Variegated growth pattern *(Fig. 1.25.8)* 3. Lace-like or sieve-like architecture, cellular central areas, areas of myxoid changes 4. Spindled and stellate-shaped mesenchymal cells in finely collagenous matrix and thick collagen bundles *(Figs. 1.25.9 and 1.25.10)* 5. Wagner-Meissner–like bodies are not seen
Special studies	• Negative muscle markers, CD34, ER, and PR • S100 positive *(Fig. 1.25.6)*	• Positive desmin, CD34, ER, and PR; focal expression of smooth muscle actin and muscle-specific actin • Negative S100
Treatment	Conservative resection in enlarging symptomatic tumors	Local excision
Prognosis	Benign; may undergo malignant transformation (should be suspected in rapidly growing tumors)	Benign; no recurrences reported after excision with negative margins

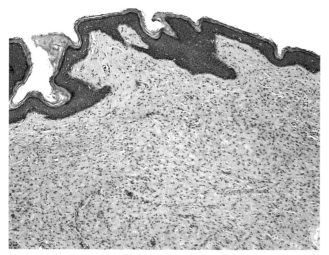

Figure 1.25.1 Neurofibroma. Moderately cellular neoplasm abuts overlying hyperplastic epidermis.

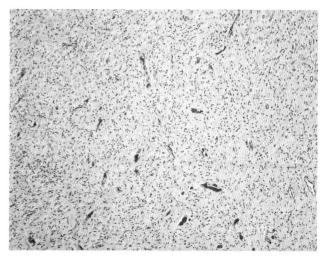

Figure 1.25.2 Neurofibroma. Uniformly cellular spindle cell neoplasm with small randomly distributed vessels.

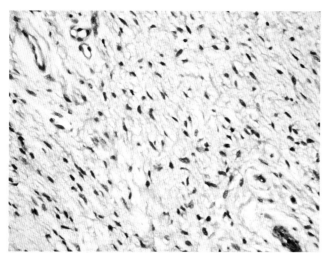

Figure 1.25.3 Neurofibroma. Bundles of spindle cells with wavy appearance.

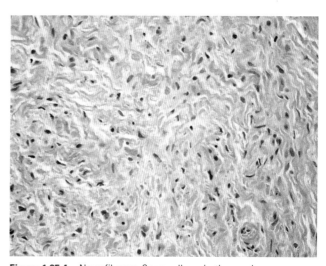

Figure 1.25.4 Neurofibroma. Some collagenization can be seen.

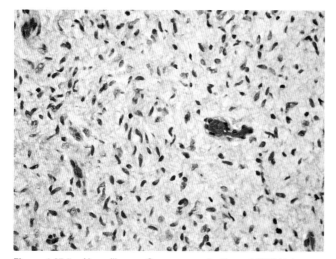

Figure 1.25.5 Neurofibroma. Same case as in *Figure 1.25.2*, higher magnification. Spindle cells, dark nuclei with tapered/pointed ends.

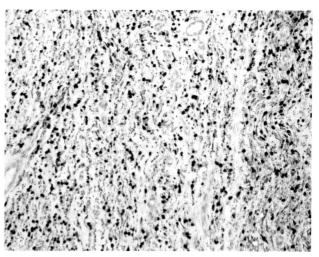

Figure 1.25.6 Neurofibroma. Diffuse expression of S100 in tumor cells.

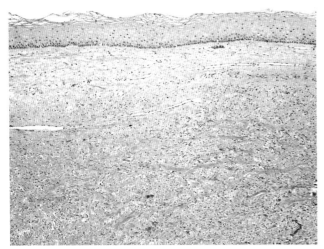

Figure 1.25.7 Myofibroblastoma. Circumscribed spindle cell neoplasm in the subepithelial stroma.

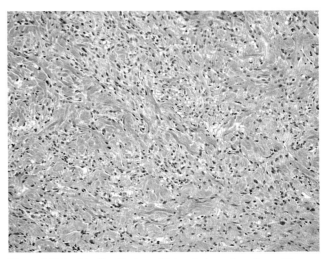

Figure 1.25.8 Myofibroblastoma. Variegated growth pattern with cellular and collagenous areas.

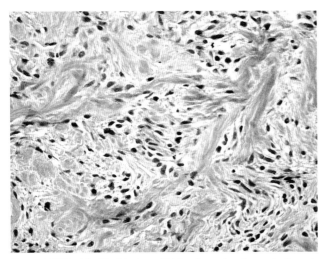

Figure 1.25.9 Myofibroblastoma. Thick collagen bundles and adjacent islands of bland spindle cells.

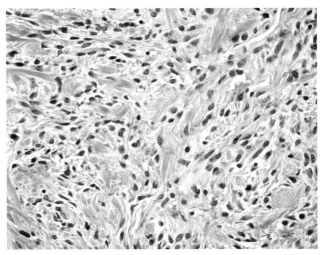

Figure 1.25.10 Myofibroblastoma. Same case as in *Figure 1.25.8*, higher magnification. Bland spindled and stellate cells with elongated nuclei.

	Spindle Cell Melanoma	Leiomyosarcoma
Age	Wide age range (4th to 9th decades); more commonly postmenopausal women	Wide age range (4th to 9th decades); most women are older than 40 y
Location	Vagina (more common in lower third, anterior, and lateral walls) vulva	Vagina (most common in posterior wall) vulva
Symptoms	Vaginal bleeding, discharge, mass lesion	Enlarging mass, vaginal or rectal bleeding, dyspareunia
Signs	Polypoid or flat lesion; can be ulcerated; commonly pigmented	Vaginal or vulvar mass; most are >5 cm in size
Etiology	Low TMB, lack of UV signature. Numerous chromosomal structural variants and copy-number changes. Somatic mutations in *SF3B1*, *KIT*, *ATRX*, *TP53*, *ARID2*, *SETD2*, and *BRAF* (less prevalent than in cutaneous melanomas)	Unknown; derived from smooth muscle tissue Frequent mutations in *TP53*, *ATRX*, and *MED12*; complex numerical and structural chromosomal aberrations
Histology	1. Cellular neoplasm with solid, nested, and trabecular patterns *(Figs. 1.26.1 and 1.26.2)* 2. Necrosis can be seen *(Fig. 1.26.3)* 3. Cells forming solid sheets, nests, and fascicles; epithelioid and spindle cell morphology can be seen *(Figs. 1.26.3-1.26.6)* 4. Pigment is variably present *(Fig. 1.26.4)* 5. Pale amphophilic to eosinophilic cytoplasm *(Figs. 1.26.4, 1.25.6, and 1.26.7)* 6. Pleomorphic hyperchromatic nuclei with prominent often multiple red nucleoli *(Fig. 1.26.7)* 7. Melanoma *in situ* can be seen at the periphery of the lesion	1. Intersecting fascicles of markedly atypical cells *(Fig. 1.26.9)* 2. Necrosis with abrupt transition from viable to necrotic tumor is common 3. Spindled cell morphology is apparent in longitudinally cut bundles; cross-sectionally cut bundles appear pseudoepithelioid *(Fig. 1.26.10)*; epithelioid morphology can be seen 4. Pigment is absent 5. Abundant fibrillary eosinophilic cytoplasm *(Fig. 1.26.11)* 6. Markedly pleomorphic nuclei with coarse chromatin; occasional cells with prominent nucleoli can be seen *(Fig. 1.26.11)* 7. No intraepithelial component or precursor
Special studies	• Positive S100 (most sensitive), variably positive for Melan-A, tyrosinase, HMB-45, SOX10, MITF *(Fig. 1.26.8)* • Negative for desmin and/or other smooth muscle markers • Negative for ER and PR	• Negative for melanocytic markers • Positive for desmin *(Fig. 1.26.12,* **left***)* and/or other smooth muscle markers • Variably positive for ER and PR *(Fig. 1.26.12,* **right***)*
Treatment	Radical resection; primary radiation therapy in unresectable cases	Radical surgery with/without adjuvant chemotherapy and radiation therapy
Prognosis	Prognosis is stage dependent, but generally poor; median survival is 20 mo; 5-y survival is up to 20%	The overall 5-y survival is <50%. Local recurrences and distant metastases (lung) are common

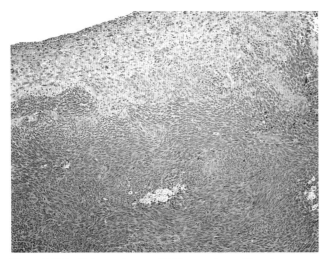

Figure 1.26.1   Vulvar melanoma. Cellular neoplasm with surface ulceration and spindled areas.

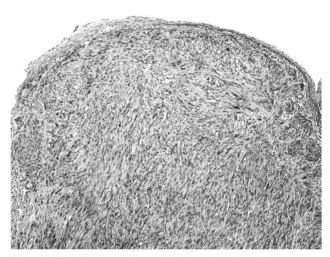

Figure 1.26.2   Vaginal melanoma. Spindle cell neoplasm forming a nodule beneath squamous mucosa.

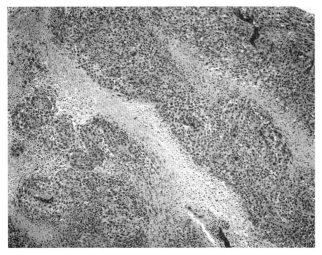

Figure 1.26.3   Vulvar melanoma. Cellular neoplasm with areas of geographic necrosis.

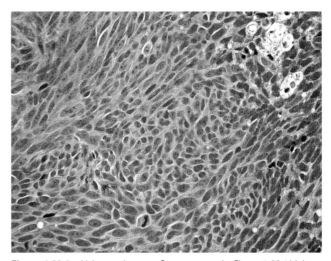

Figure 1.26.4   Vulvar melanoma. Same case as in *Figure 1.26.1* higher magnification. Atypical spindle cells with prominent nucleoli; frequent mitotic figures. Focal fine cytoplasmic brown pigment **(upper right)**.

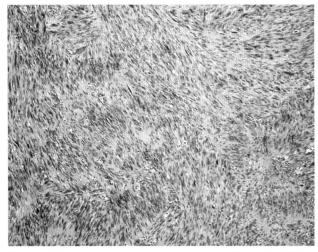

Figure 1.26.5   Vaginal melanoma. Same case as in *Figure 1.26.2* higher magnification. Fascicles of atypical spindle cells.

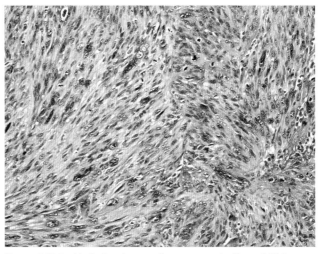

Figure 1.26.6   Vaginal melanoma. Same case as in *Figure 1.26.2* higher magnification. Marked nuclear pleomorphism and frequent mitotic figures.

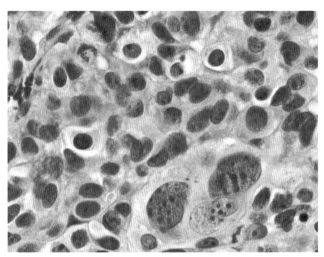

Figure 1.26.7 Vulvar melanoma. Same case as in *Figure 1.26.3*, higher magnification. Marked nuclear pleomorphism, hyperchromasia, and multiple prominent nucleoli.

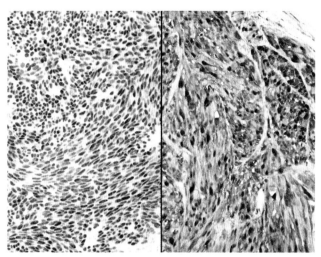

Figure 1.26.8 Melanoma. Diffuse expression of MITF **(left)** and S100 **(right)**.

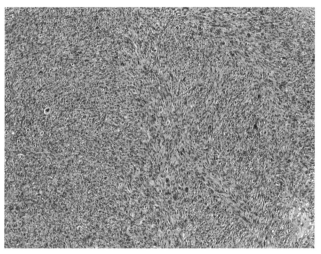

Figure 1.26.9 Vulvar leiomyosarcoma. Cellular neoplasm composed of sheets of spindle cells.

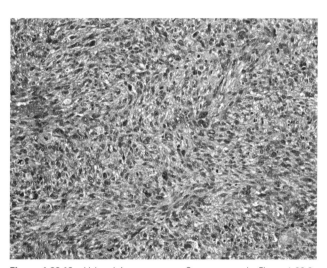

Figure 1.26.10 Vulvar leiomyosarcoma. Same case as in *Figure 1.26.9*, higher magnification. Cellular neoplasm composed of bundles of spindle cells.

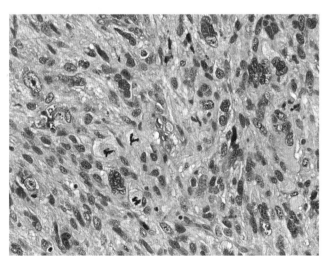

Figure 1.26.11 Vulvar leiomyosarcoma. Same case as in *Figure 1.26.9*, higher magnification. Marked nuclear atypia and pleomorphism; occasional cells with prominent nucleoli. Brisk mitotic activity.

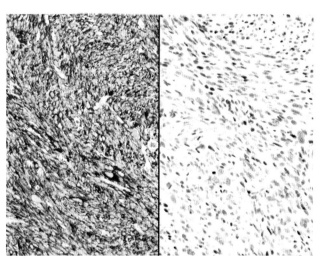

Figure 1.26.12 Vulvar leiomyosarcoma. Same case as in *Figure 1.26.11*. Diffuse expression of desmin **(left)** and some expression of ER **(right)**.

	Kaposi Sarcoma	Sarcomatoid (Spindled) Squamous Cell Carcinoma
Age	2nd to 4th decades	HPV related: mean age 50 y HPV independent: peak incidence 7th to 8th decades
Location	Vulva, also mucosal sites, viscera, and lymph nodes	Vulva, vagina, cervix
Symptoms	Vulvar mass, raised lesion, pruritis, or pain	Vulvar mass, raised lesion, pain, bleeding; occasionally in recurrent setting
Signs	Mass lesion, raised, nodular, or polypoid	Mass lesion, raised, polypoid, or ulcerated
Etiology	Human herpesvirus HHV8 infection Often HIV/AIDS associated; subset of cases in HIV-negative women	HPV related: commonly, HPV 16 HPV independent: *TP53* mutations in up to 80% of cases; mutations in *NOTCH1/2, HRAS, PIK3CA* are also detected
Histology	1. No intraepithelial precursor lesion; surface ulceration can be seen *(Figs. 1.27.1 and 1.27.2)* 2. Vaguely nodular spindle cell proliferation; ectatic and congested vessels *(Figs. 1.27.1 and 1.27.2)* 3. Relatively bland spindle to epithelioid cells arranged in fascicles; erythrocytes in slit-like spaces *(Fig. 1.27.3)* 4. Foci of lymphoplasmacytic infiltrate *(Fig. 1.27.4)* 5. Occasional mitotic figures *(Fig. 1.27.5)*	1. Overlying/adjacent skin with differentiated VIN/Lichen sclerosus or HSIL/high-grade VIN can be seen *(Figs. 1.27.7 and 1.27.8)* 2. Spindle cell proliferation with variable atypia in subepithelial stroma; stromal hemorrhage and congestion may be seen, but not a constant feature *(Figs. 1.27.9 and 1.27.10)* 3. Haphazardly arranged atypical spindle cells with prominent nucleoli *(Figs. 1.27.11 and 1.27.12)* 4. Mixed inflammation may be seen, particularly, in cases with ulceration 5. Usually brisk mitotic activity *(Fig. 1.27.11)*
Special studies	• HHV8 (LANA-1), positive *(Fig. 1.27.6)* • Endothelial markers: CD31, CD34, ERG, positive • Keratins may be focally positive • P63/p40, expected negative	• HHV8 (LANA-1) negative • Endothelial markers, negative • Keratins positive, often focal • P63/p40 positive, often focal
Treatment	Antiretroviral therapy in HIV/AIDS associated lesions; local excision or radiation therapy	Wide/radical local excision; regional lymph node dissection in cases with depth of invasion >1 mm
Prognosis	Depends on KS type and extent; metastases are rare	Dependent on stage. Recurrences (local or in regional lymph nodes) in up to 24% of cases; lymph node metastases in up to 15% of cases with depth of invasion >1 mm

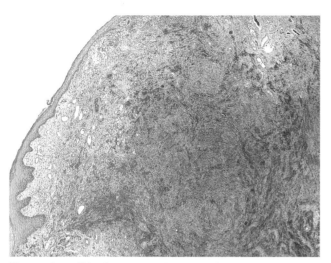

Figure 1.27.1   Kaposi sarcoma, nodular stage. Cellular spindle cell proliferation in subepithelial stroma. Overlying squamous epithelium appears normal.

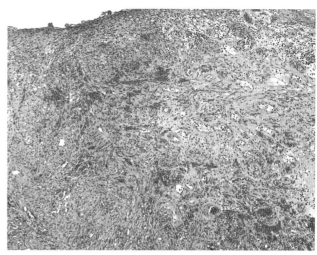

Figure 1.27.2   Kaposi sarcoma, nodular stage. Surface ulceration. Spindle cell proliferation with dispersed ectatic vessels.

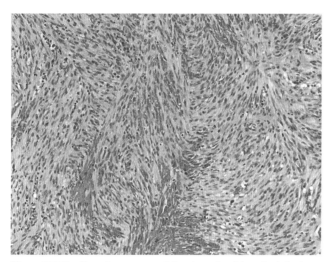

Figure 1.27.3   Kaposi sarcoma, nodular stage. Fascicles of relatively monotonous spindle cells with erythrocytes in slit-like spaces.

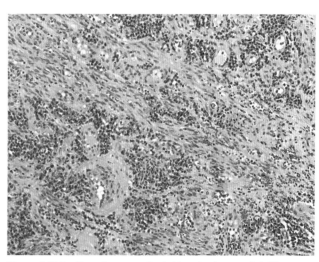

Figure 1.27.4   Kaposi sarcoma. Foci of lymphoplasmacytic infiltrate.

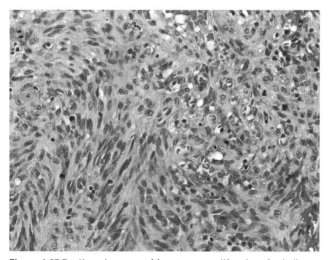

Figure 1.27.5   Kaposi sarcoma. Monotonous proliferation of spindle cells with occasional mitotic figures; extravasated erythrocytes.

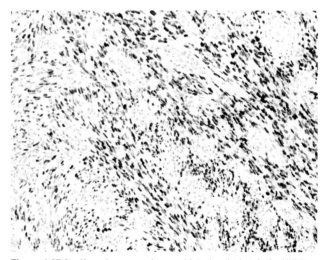

Figure 1.27.6   Kaposi sarcoma. Immunohistochemical stain for HHV8 (LANA) shows strong nuclear expression.

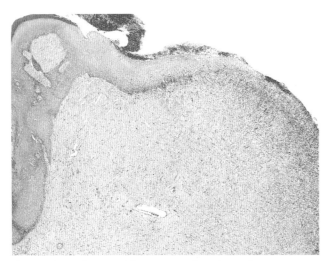

Figure 1.27.7   Sarcomatoid squamous cell carcinoma. Squamous mucosa with surface ulceration and inflammation in subepithelial stroma.

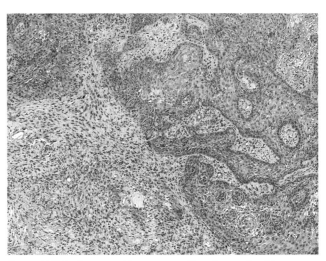

Figure 1.27.8   Sarcomatoid squamous cell carcinoma. Overlying atypical squamous proliferation, consistent with dVIN.

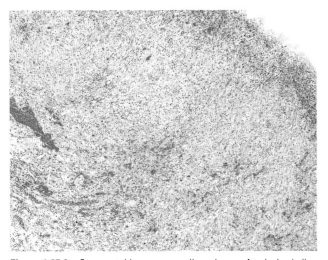

Figure 1.27.9   Sarcomatoid squamous cell carcinoma. Atypical spindle cell proliferation beneath ulcer bed.

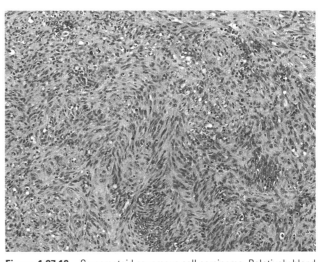

Figure 1.27.10   Sarcomatoid squamous cell carcinoma. Relatively bland spindle cell proliferation with foci of stromal hemorrhage.

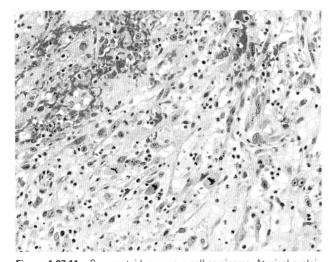

Figure 1.27.11   Sarcomatoid squamous cell carcinoma. Atypical nuclei with prominent nucleoli; readily identifiable mitotic figures.

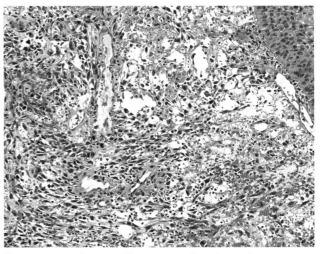

Figure 1.27.12   Sarcomatoid squamous cell carcinoma. Same case as in *Figure 1.27.8*, higher magnification. Atypical pleomorphic spindle cells stomal hemorrhage. Intraepithelial component, dVIN **(upper right)**.

SUGGESTED READINGS

1.1-1.6

Aguilera-Barrantes I, Magro C, Nuovo GJ. Verruca vulgaris of the vulva in children and adults: a nonvenereal type of vulvar wart. *Am J Surg Pathol.* 2007;31:529-535.

Bai H, Cviko A, Granter S, et al. Immunophenotypic and viral (human papillomavirus) correlates of vulvar seborrheic keratosis. *Hum Pathol.* 2003;34:559-564.

Brisigotti M, Moreno A, Murcia C, et al. Verrucous carcinoma of the vulva. A clinicopathologic and immunohistochemical study of five cases. *Int J Gynecol Pathol.* 1989;8:1-7.

Li J, Ackerman AB. "Seborrheic keratoses" that contain human papillomavirus are condylomata acuminata. *Am J Dermatopathol.* 1994;16:398-405; discussion 406-408.

Maniar KP, Ronnett BM, Vang R, et al. Coexisting high-grade vulvar intraepithelial neoplasia (VIN) and condyloma acuminatum: independent lesions due to different HPV types occurring in immunocompromised patients. *Am J Surg Pathol.* 2013;37:53-60.

Moyal-Barracco M, Leibowitch M, Orth G. Vestibular papillae of the vulva. Lack of evidence for human papillomavirus etiology. *Arch Dermatol.* 1990;126:1594-1598.

Nascimento AF, Granter SR, Cviko A, et al. Vulvar acanthosis with altered differentiation: a precursor to verrucous carcinoma? *Am J Surg Pathol.* 2004;28:638-643.

Potkul RK, Lancaster WD, Kurman RJ, et al. Vulvar condylomas and squamous vestibular micropapilloma. Differences in appearance and response to treatment. *J Reprod Med.* 1990;35:1019-1022.

Rush DS, Wilkinson EJ. Benign diseases of the vulva. In: Kurman RJ, Ellenson LH, Ronnett BM, eds. *Blaustein's Pathology of the Female Genital Tract.* 7th ed. Springer; 2019:3-59.

Talia KL, McCluggage WG. Seborrheic keratosis-like lesions of the cervix and vagina: report of a new entity possibly related to low-risk human papillomavirus infection. *Am J Surg Pathol.* 2017;41(4):517-524.

Tumors of the vulva. In: Kurman RJ, Ronnett BM, Sherman ME, et al., eds. *Atlas of Tumor Pathology*, 4th series, Fasc 13. Tumors of the Cervix, Vagina, and Vulva. Armed Forces Institute of Pathology; 2010:67-237.

Wilkinson EJ, Rush DS. Precursors and malignant tumors of the vulva. In: Kurman RJ, Ellenson LH, Ronnett BM, eds. *Blaustein's Pathology of the Female Genital Tract.* 7th ed. Springer; 2019:66-122.

1.7

Darragh TM, Colgan TJ, Thomas Cox J, et al. The lower anogenital squamous terminology standardization project for HPV-associated lesions: background and consensus recommendations from the College of American Pathologists and the American Society for Colposcopy and Cervical Pathology. *Int J Gynecol Pathol.* 2013;32:76-115.

Del Pino M, Rodriguez-Carunchio L, Ordi J. Pathways of vulvar intraepithelial neoplasia and squamous cell carcinoma. *Histopathology.* 2013;62:161-175.

Hoevenaars BM, van der Avoort IA, de Wilde PC, et al. A panel of p16(ink4a), mib1 and p53 proteins can distinguish between the 2 pathways leading to vulvar squamous cell carcinoma. *Int J Cancer.* 2008;123:2767-2773.

van de Nieuwenhof HP, van der Avoort IA, de Hullu JA. Review of squamous premalignant vulvar lesions. *Crit Rev Oncol Hematol.* 2008;68:131-156.

1.8 and 1.9

Akbari A, Pinto A, Amemiya Y, et al. Differentiated exophytic vulvar intraepithelial lesion: clinicopathologic and molecular analysis documenting its relationship with verrucous carcinoma of the vulva. *Mod Pathol.* 2020;33(10):2011-2018.

Chiesa-Vottero A, Dvoretsky PM, Hart WR. Histopathologic study of thin vulvar squamous cell carcinomas and associated cutaneous lesions: a correlative study of 48 tumors in 44 patients with analysis of adjacent vulvar intraepithelial neoplasia types and lichen sclerosus. *Am J Surg Pathol.* 2006;30:310-318.

Del Pino M, Rodriguez-Carunchio L, Ordi J. Pathways of vulvar intraepithelial neoplasia and squamous cell carcinoma. *Histopathology.* 2013;62:161-175.

Griesinger LM, Walline H, Wang GY, et al. Expanding the morphologic, immunohistochemical, and HPV genotypic features of high-grade squamous intraepithelial lesions of the vulva with morphology mimicking differentiated vulvar intraepithelial neoplasia and/or lichen sclerosus. *Int J Gynecol Pathol.* 2021;40(3):205-213.

Hoevenaars BM, van der Avoort IA, de Wilde PC, et al. A panel of p16(ink4a), mib1 and p53 proteins can distinguish between the 2 pathways leading to vulvar squamous cell carcinoma. *Int J Cancer.* 2008;123:2767-2773.

Liu YA, Ji JX, Almadani N, et al. Comparison of p53 immunohistochemical staining in differentiated vulvar intraepithelial neoplasia (dVIN) with that in inflammatory dermatoses and benign squamous lesions in the vulva. *Histopathology.* 2021;78(3):424-433.

Tessier-Cloutier B, Kortekaas KE, Thompson E, et al. Major p53 immunohistochemical patterns in in situ and invasive squamous cell carcinomas of the vulva and correlation with TP53 mutation status. *Mod Pathol.* 2020;33(8):1595-1605.

Tessier-Cloutier B, Pors J, Thompson E, et al. Molecular characterization of invasive and in situ squamous neoplasia of the vulva and implications for morphologic diagnosis and outcome. *Mod Pathol.* 2021;34(2):508-518.

Thompson EF, Chen J, Huvila J, et al. p53 Immunohistochemical patterns in HPV-related neoplasms of the female lower genital tract can be mistaken for TP53 null or missense mutational patterns. *Mod Pathol.* 2020;33(9):1649-1659.

van de Nieuwenhof HP, Bulten J, Hollema H, et al. Differentiated vulvar intraepithelial neoplasia is often found in lesions, previously diagnosed as lichen sclerosus, which have progressed to vulvar squamous cell carcinoma. *Mod Pathol.* 2011;24:297-305.

van de Nieuwenhof HP, van der Avoort IA, de Hullu JA. Review of squamous premalignant vulvar lesions. *Crit Rev Oncol Hematol.* 2008;68:131-156.

1   VULVA AND VAGINA

Watkins JC, Howitt BE, Horowitz NS, et al. Differentiated exophytic vulvar intraepithelial lesions are genetically distinct from keratinizing squamous cell carcinomas and contain mutations in PIK3CA. *Mod Pathol*. 2017;30(3):448-458.

Watkins JC, Yang E, Crum CP, et al. Classic vulvar intraepithelial neoplasia with superimposed lichen simplex chronicus: a unique variant mimicking differentiated vulvar intraepithelial neoplasia. *Int J Gynecol Pathol*. 2019;38(2):175-182.

Yang B, Hart WR. Vulvar intraepithelial neoplasia of the simplex (differentiated) type: a clinicopathologic study including analysis of HPV and p53 expression. *Am J Surg Pathol*. 2000;24:429-441.

1.10

Elwood H, Kim J, Yemelyanova A, et al. Basal cell carcinomas of the vulva: high-risk human papillomavirus DNA detection, p16 and Ber-EP4 expression. *Am J Surg Pathol*. 2014;38:542-547.

Flipo R, Bani MA, Rejaibi S, et al. Vulvar basal cell carcinoma: clinical and histopathologic features. *Int J Gynecol Pathol*. 2022;41(1):86-92.

Mulvany NJ, Rayoo M, Allen DG. Basal cell carcinoma of the vulva: a case series. *Pathology*. 2012;44:528-533.

Renati S, Henderson C, Aluko A, Burgin S. Basal cell carcinoma of the vulva: a case report and systematic review of the literature. *Int J Dermatol*. 2019;58:892-902.

1.11 and 1.12

Abdel-Mesih A, Daya D, Onuma K, et al. Interobserver agreement for assessing invasion in stage 1a vulvar squamous cell carcinoma. *Am J Surg Pathol*. 2013;37:1336-1341.

Tumors of the vulva. In: Kurman RJ, Ronnett BM, Sherman ME, et al., eds. *Atlas of Tumor Pathology*, 4th series, Fasc 13. Tumors of the Cervix, Vagina, and Vulva. Armed Forces Institute of Pathology; 2010:67-237.

Wilkinson EJ, Rush DS. Precursors and malignant tumors of the vulva. In: Kurman RJ, Ellenson LH, Ronnett BM, eds. *Blaustein's Pathology of the Female Genital Tract*. 7th ed. Springer; 2019:66-122.

1.13 and 1.14

Cai Y, Sheng W, Xiang L, et al. Primary extramammary Paget's disease of the vulva: the clinicopathological features and treatment outcomes in a series of 43 patients. *Gynecol Oncol*. 2013;129:412-416.

De la Garza Bravo MM, Curry JL, Torres-Cabala CA, et al. Pigmented extramammary Paget disease of the thigh mimicking a melanocytic tumor: report of a case and review of the literature. *J Cutan Pathol*. 2014;41:529-535.

Fabrizi G, Zannoni GF, Lopez LI, et al. Melanocytic dysplasia and multiple melanoma of the vulva. *Eur J Gynaecol Oncol*. 2002;23:323-324.

Garganese G, Inzani F, Mantovani G, et al. The vulvar immunohistochemical panel (VIP) project: molecular profiles of vulvar Paget's disease. *J Cancer Res Clin Oncol*. 2019;145(9):2211-2225.

Higgins HW II, Lee KC, Galan A, et al. Melanoma in situ: part II. Histopathology, treatment, and clinical management. *J Am Acad Dermatol*. 2015;73:193-203.

Raju RR, Goldblum JR, Hart WR. Pagetoid squamous cell carcinoma in situ (pagetoid Bowen's disease) of the external genitalia. *Int J Gynecol Pathol*. 2003;22:127-135.

Shaco-Levy R, Bean SM, Vollmer RT, et al. Paget disease of the vulva: a histologic study of 56 cases correlating pathologic features and disease course. *Int J Gynecol Pathol*. 2010;29:69-78.

Terlou A, Blok LJ, Helmerhorst TJ, et al. Premalignant epithelial disorders of the vulva: squamous vulvar intraepithelial neoplasia, vulvar Paget's disease and melanoma in situ. *Acta Obstet Gynecol Scand*. 2010;89:741-748.

Vincent J, Taube JM. Pigmented extramammary Paget disease of the abdomen: a potential mimicker of melanoma. *Dermatol Online J*. 2011;17:13.

1.15 and 1.16

Carleton C, Hoang L, Sah S, et al. A detailed immunohistochemical analysis of a large series of cervical and vaginal gastric-type adenocarcinomas. *Am J Surg Pathol*. 2016;40(5):636-644.

DeMars LR, Van Le L, Huang I, et al. Primary non-clear-cell adenocarcinomas of the vagina in older DES-exposed women. *Gynecol Oncol*. 1995;58:389-392.

Ebrahim S, Daponte A, Smith TH, et al. Primary mucinous adenocarcinoma of the vagina. *Gynecol Oncol*. 2001;80:89-92.

Frank SJ, Deavers MT, Jhingran A, et al. Primary adenocarcinoma of the vagina not associated with diethylstilbestrol (des) exposure. *Gynecol Oncol*. 2007;105:470-474.

Halat S, Eble JN, Grignon DJ, et al. Ectopic prostatic tissue: histogenesis and histopathological characteristics. *Histopathology*. 2011;58:750-758.

Kelly P, McBride HA, Kennedy K, et al. Misplaced Skene's glands: glandular elements in the lower female genital tract that are variably immunoreactive with prostate markers and that encompass vaginal tubulosquamous polyp and cervical ectopic prostatic tissue. *Int J Gynecol Pathol*. 2011;30(6):605-612.

Mazur MT, Hsueh S, Gersell DJ. Metastases to the female genital tract. Analysis of 325 cases. *Cancer*. 1984;53:1978-1984.

McCluggage WG, Ganesan R, Hirschowitz L, et al. Ectopic prostatic tissue in the uterine cervix and vagina: report of a series with a detailed immunohistochemical analysis. *Am J Surg Pathol*. 2006;30:209-215.

Mudhar HS, Smith JH, Tidy J. Primary vaginal adenocarcinoma of intestinal type arising from an adenoma: case report and review of the literature. *Int J Gynecol Pathol*. 2001;20:204-209.

Ng HJ, Aly EH. Vaginal metastases from colorectal cancer. *Int J Surg*. 2013;11:1048-1055.

Nucci MR, Ferry JA, Young RH. Ectopic prostatic tissue in the uterine cervix: a report of four cases and review of ectopic prostatic tissue. *Am J Surg Pathol*. 2000;24:1224-1230.

Staats PN, Clement PB, Young RH. Primary endometrioid adenocarcinoma of the vagina: a clinicopathologic study of 18 cases. *Am J Surg Pathol.* 2007;31:1490-1501.

Staats PN, McCluggage WG, Clement PB, et al. Primary intestinal-type glandular lesions of the vagina: clinical, pathologic, and immunohistochemical features of 14 cases ranging from benign polyp to adenoma to adenocarcinoma. *Am J Surg Pathol.* 2014;38:593-603.

Wong RW, Moore M, Talia KL, et al. Primary vaginal gastric-type adenocarcinoma and vaginal adenosis exhibiting gastric differentiation: report of a series with detailed immunohistochemical analysis. *Am J Surg Pathol.* 2018;42(7):958-970.

1.17

Ouldamer L, Caille A, Body G. Fallopian tube prolapse after hysterectomy: a systematic review. *PLoS One.* 2013;8:e76543.

Silverberg SG, Frable WJ. Prolapse of fallopian tube into vaginal vault after hysterectomy. Histopathology, cytopathology, and differential diagnosis. *Arch Pathol.* 1974;97:100-103.

Staats PN, Clement PB, Young RH. Primary endometrioid adenocarcinoma of the vagina: a clinicopathologic study of 18 cases. *Am J Surg Pathol.* 2007;31:1490-1501.

Wheelock JB, Schneider V, Goplerud DR. Prolapsed fallopian tube masquerading as adenocarcinoma of the vagina in a postmenopausal woman. *Gynecol Oncol.* 1985;21:369-375.

1.18 and 1.19

Abbott JJ, Ahmed I. Adenocarcinoma of mammary-like glands of the vulva: report of a case and review of the literature. *Am J Dermatopathol.* 2006;28(2):127-133.

Chamlian DL, Taylor HB. Primary carcinoma of Bartholin's gland. A report of 24 patients. *Obstet Gynecol.* 1972;39:489-494.

Kazakov DV, Spagnolo DV, Kacerovska D, et al. Lesions of anogenital mammary-like glands: an update. *Adv Anat Pathol.* 2011;18:1-28.

Koenig C, Tavassoli FA. Nodular hyperplasia, adenoma, and adenomyoma of Bartholin's gland. *Int J Gynecol Pathol.* 1998;17:289-294.

Meeker JH, Neubecker RD, Helwig EB. Hidradenoma papilliferum. *Am J Clin Pathol.* 1962;37:182-195.

Nazeran T, Cheng AS, Karnezis AN, et al. Bartholin gland carcinoma: clinicopathologic features, including p16 expression and clinical outcome. *Int J Gynecol Pathol.* 2019;38(2):189-195.

Pfarr N, Allgäuer M, Steiger K, et al. Several genotypes, one phenotype: PIK3CA/AKT1 mutation-negative hidradenoma papilliferum show genetic lesions in other components of the signalling network. *Pathology.* 2019;51(4):362-368.

Santos LD, Kennerson AR, Killingsworth MC. Nodular hyperplasia of Bartholin's gland. *Pathology.* 2006;38:223-228.

Tessier-Cloutier B, Asleh-Aburaya K, Shah V, et al. Molecular subtyping of mammary-like adenocarcinoma of the vulva shows molecular similarity to breast carcinomas. *Histopathology.* 2017;71(3):446-452.

Wilkinson EJ, Rush DS. Precursors and malignant tumors of the vulva. In: Kurman RJ, Ellenson LH, Ronnett BM, eds. *Blaustein's Pathology of the Female Genital Tract.* 7th ed. Springer; 2019:66-122.

1.20-1.22

Dahiya K, Jain S, Duhan N, et al. Aggressive angiomyxoma of vulva and vagina: a series of three cases and review of literature. *Arch Gynecol Obstet.* 2011;283:1145-1148.

Fadare O, Brannan SM, Arin-Silasi D, et al. Localized lymphedema of the vulva: a clinicopathologic study of 2 cases and a review of the literature. *Int J Gynecol Pathol.* 2011;30:306-313.

Fetsch JF, Laskin WB, Lefkowitz M, et al. Aggressive angiomyxoma: a clinicopathologic study of 29 female patients. *Cancer.* 1996;78:79-90.

Laskin WB, Fetsch JF, Tavassoli FA. Angiomyofibroblastoma of the female genital tract: analysis of 17 cases including a lipomatous variant. *Hum Pathol.* 1997;28:1046-1055.

McCluggage WG, Connolly L, McBride HA. Hmga2 is a sensitive but not specific immunohistochemical marker of vulvovaginal aggressive angiomyxoma. *Am J Surg Pathol.* 2010;34:1037-1042.

McCluggage WG, Nielsen GP, Young RH. Massive vulval edema secondary to obesity and immobilization: a potential mimic of aggressive angiomyxoma. *Int J Gynecol Pathol.* 2008;27:447-452.

Miettinen M, Wahlstrom T, Vesterinen E, et al. Vaginal polyps with pseudosarcomatous features. A clinicopathologic study of seven cases. *Cancer.* 1983;51:1148-1151.

Nielsen GP, Rosenberg AE, Young RH, et al. Angiomyofibroblastoma of the vulva and vagina. *Mod Pathol.* 1996;9:284-291.

Nucci MR, Young RH, Fletcher CD. Cellular pseudosarcomatous fibroepithelial stromal polyps of the lower female genital tract: an underrecognized lesion often misdiagnosed as sarcoma. *Am J Surg Pathol.* 2000;24:231-240.

Ockner DM, Sayadi H, Swanson PE, et al. Genital angiomyofibroblastoma. Comparison with aggressive angiomyxoma and other myxoid neoplasms of skin and soft tissue. *Am J Clin Pathol.* 1997;107:36-44.

Rabban JT, Dal Cin P, Oliva E. Hmga2 rearrangement in a case of vulvar aggressive angiomyxoma. *Int J Gynecol Pathol.* 2006;25:403-407.

Silverman JS, Albukerk J, Tamsen A. Comparison of angiomyofibroblastoma and aggressive angiomyxoma in both sexes: four cases composed of bimodal CD34 and factor xiiia positive dendritic cell subsets. *Pathol Res Pract.* 1997;193:673-682.

Sims SM, Stinson K, McLean FW, et al. Angiomyofibroblastoma of the vulva: a case report of a pedunculated variant and review of the literature. *J Low Genit Tract Dis.* 2012;16:149-154.

Steeper TA, Rosai J. Aggressive angiomyxoma of the female pelvis and perineum. Report of nine cases of a distinctive type of gynecologic soft-tissue neoplasm. *Am J Surg Pathol.* 1983;7:463-475.

Sutton BJ, Laudadio J. Aggressive angiomyxoma. *Arch Pathol Lab Med.* 2012;136:217-221.

Vang R, Connelly JH, Hammill HA, et al. Vulvar hypertrophy with lymphedema. A mimicker of aggressive angiomyxoma. *Arch Pathol Lab Med.* 2000;124:1697-1699.

1.23-1.25

Flucke U, van Krieken JH, Mentzel T. Cellular angiofibroma: analysis of 25 cases emphasizing its relationship to spindle cell lipoma and mammary-type myofibroblastoma. *Mod Pathol.* 2011;24(1):82-89.

Gutmann DH, Aylsworth A, Carey JC, et al. The diagnostic evaluation and multidisciplinary management of neurofibromatosis 1 and neurofibromatosis 2. *JAMA.* 1997;278:51-57.

Howitt BE, Fletcher CD. Mammary-type myofibroblastoma: clinicopathologic characterization in a series of 143 cases. *Am J Surg Pathol.* 2016;40(3):361-367.

Laskin WB, Fetsch JF, Tavassoli FA. Superficial cervicovaginal myofibroblastoma: fourteen cases of a distinctive mesenchymal tumor arising from the specialized subepithelial stroma of the lower female genital tract. *Hum Pathol.* 2001;32:715-725.

Magro G, Caltabiano R, Kacerovska D, et al. Vulvovaginal myofibroblastoma: expanding the morphological and immunohistochemical spectrum. A clinicopathologic study of 10 cases. *Hum Pathol.* 2012;43:243-253.

Magro G, Righi A, Caltabiano R, et al. Vulvovaginal angiomyofibroblastomas: morphologic, immunohistochemical, and fluorescence in situ hybridization analysis for deletion of 13q14 region. *Hum Pathol.* 2014;45(8):1647-1655.

Mandato VD, Santagni S, Cavazza A, et al. Cellular angiofibroma in women: a review of the literature. *Diagn Pathol.* 2015;10:114.

McCluggage WG, Ganesan R, Hirschowitz L, et al. Cellular angiofibroma and related fibromatous lesions of the vulva: report of a series of cases with a morphological spectrum wider than previously described. *Histopathology.* 2004;45:360-368.

Nielsen GP, Rosenberg AE, Koerner FC, et al. Smooth-muscle tumors of the vulva. A clinicopathological study of 25 cases and review of the literature. *Am J Surg Pathol.* 1996;20:779-793.

Nucci MR, Granter SR, Fletcher CD. Cellular angiofibroma: a benign neoplasm distinct from angiomyofibroblastoma and spindle cell lipoma. *Am J Surg Pathol.* 1997;21:636-644.

Schoolmeester JK, Fritchie KJ. Genital soft tissue tumors. *J Cutan Pathol.* 2015;42:441-451.

1.26

Aulmann S, Sinn HP, Penzel R, et al. Comparison of molecular abnormalities in vulvar and vaginal melanomas. *Mod Pathol* 2014;27:1386-1393.

Benda JA, Platz CE, Anderson B. Malignant melanoma of the vulva: a clinical-pathologic review of 16 cases. *Int J Gynecol Pathol* 1986;5:202-216.

Gonzalez-Bugatto F, Anon-Requena MJ, Lopez-Guerrero MA, et al. Vulvar leiomyosarcoma in Bartholin's gland area: a case report and literature review. *Arch Gynecol Obstet.* 2009;279:171-174.

Mills AM, Longacre TA. Smooth muscle tumors of the female genital tract. *Surg Pathol Clin.* 2009;2:625-677.

Nielsen GP, Rosenberg AE, Koerner FC, et al. Smooth-muscle tumors of the vulva. A clinicopathological study of 25 cases and review of the literature. *Am J Surg Pathol.* 1996;20:779-793.

Ordonez NG. Value of melanocytic-associated immunohistochemical markers in the diagnosis of malignant melanoma: a review and update. *Hum Pathol.* 2014;45:191-205.

Ragnarsson-Olding BK, Kanter-Lewensohn LR, Lagerlof B, et al. Malignant melanoma of the vulva in a nationwide, 25 year study of 219 Swedish females: clinical observations and histopathologic features. *Cancer.* 1999;86:1273-1284.

Rouzbahman M, Kamel-Reid S, Al Habeeb A, et al. Malignant melanoma of vulva and vagina: a histomorphological review and mutation analysis—a single-center study. *J Low Genit Tract Dis.* 2015;19:350-353.

Sayeed S, Xing D, Jenkins SM, et al. Criteria for risk stratification of vulvar and vaginal smooth muscle tumors: an evaluation of 71 cases comparing proposed classification systems. *Am J Surg Pathol.* 2018;42(1):84-94.

Seifried S, Haydu LE, Quinn MJ, et al. Melanoma of the vulva and vagina: principles of staging and their relevance to management based on a clinicopathologic analysis of 85 cases. *Ann Surg Oncol.* 2015;22:1959-1966.

Swanson AA, Howitt BE, Schoolmeester JK. Criteria for risk stratification of vulvar and vaginal smooth muscle tumors: a follow-up study with application to leiomyoma variants, smooth muscle tumors of uncertain malignant potential, and leiomyosarcomas. *Hum Pathol.* 2020;103:83-94.

1.27

Choi DS, Lee JW, Lee SJ, et al. Squamous cell carcinoma with sarcomatoid features of the vulva: a case report and review of literature. *Gynecol Oncol.* 2006;103(1):363-367.

Comerio C, Jaconi M, Zambetti B, et al. Recurrence of vulvar squamous cell carcinoma as an undifferentiated sarcomatoid carcinoma. *Int J Gynecol Cancer.* 2021;31(4):627-630.

Errichetti E, Stinco G, Pegolo E, et al. Primary classic Kaposi's sarcoma confined to the vulva in an HIV negative patient. *Ann Dermatol.* 2015;27(3):336-337.

Iavazzo C, Karavioti E, Kokkali K, et al. Sarcomatoid squamous cell carcinoma of the vulva: a case report. *Clin Ter.* 2021;172(5):392-394.

Laartz BW, Cooper C, Degryse A, et al. Wolf in sheep's clothing: advanced Kaposi sarcoma mimicking vulvar abscess. *South Med J.* 2005;98(4):475-477.

Troncoso A, Gulotta H, Benetucci J, et al. Genital manifestations in women with AIDS. *J Int Assoc Physicians AIDS Care (Chic).* 2005;4(1):16-19.

2

Cervix

	Low-Grade Squamous Intraepithelial Lesion (LSIL)	Nondiagnostic Squamous Atypia
Age	Wide age range, from teenage to postmenopausal years	Wide age range, from teenage to postmenopausal years
Location	Cervix, transformation zone, ectocervix	Cervix, transformation zone, ectocervix
Symptoms	None	None
Signs	Abnormal Pap, high-risk HPV variably detected, acetowhite changes or other abnormal findings at colposcopy	Abnormal Pap, abnormal findings at colposcopy
Etiology	HPV, low- and high-risk types	Broad category, including variety of conditions; reactive changes and HPV-driven processes that do not meet criteria for LSIL
Histology	1. Epithelial thickening is usually present 2. Widening of the parabasal zone; slight disorganization of parabasal zone can be seen *(Figs. 2.1.1 and 2.1.2)* 3. Intermediate and superficial layer cells with nuclear enlargement *(Fig. 2.1.3)*; occasionally with mitotic figures in the lower third *(Fig. 2.1.2)* 4. Superficial layer cells with perinuclear cytoplasmic clearing and nuclear enlargement (koilocytes) *(Figs. 2.1.1-2.1.4)* 5. Hyperchromasia; irregular nuclear membranes *(Fig. 2.1.5)*; prominent nucleoli are not typical 6. Koilocytotic atypia is often limited to a distinct focal lesion	1. Epithelium is variably thickened 2. Quiescent parabasal zone; mitotic figures are infrequent *(Fig. 2.1.6)* 3. Normal cell maturation, nuclear size decreases progressively from the parabasal layers to the epithelial surface *(Fig. 2.1.7)* 4. Cytoplasmic clearing and perinuclear "halo" in cells with normal nuclear size 5. Vesicular chromatin and prominent nucleoli can be seen, particularly in cases with intraepithelial inflammation or small hyperchromatic nuclei *(Fig. 2.1.8)* 6. Diffuse ill-defined areas with cytoplasmic clearing
Special studies	• Not particularly helpful in this differential • Ki-67 labeling is increased in parabasal intermediate layers with occasional cells labeled in superficial layers • Diffuse "block-like" expression of p16 can be seen in some lesions or patchy to negative staining	• Not particularly helpful in this differential • Ki-67 labeling is generally low, mild increase can be seen • p16 is negative or weak and focal/patchy
Treatment	None required; follow-up with repeat cervical cytology and colposcopy	None required; treatment of underlying cervicitis if present
Prognosis	Most regress spontaneously without intervention; patients with lesions harboring high-risk HPV can develop persistent infection and high-grade squamous intraepithelial lesions	Unremarkable

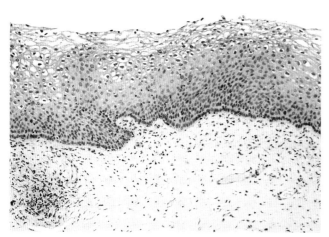

Figure 2.1.1 Low-grade squamous intraepithelial lesion. Widened parabasal zone and prominent koilocytotic atypia.

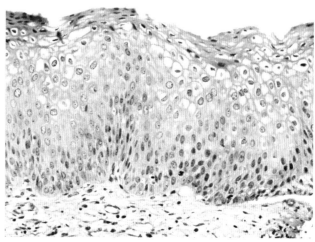

Figure 2.1.2 Low-grade squamous intraepithelial lesion. Nuclear enlargement in the intermediate layers, disorganization of the parabasal zone with occasional parabasal mitosis.

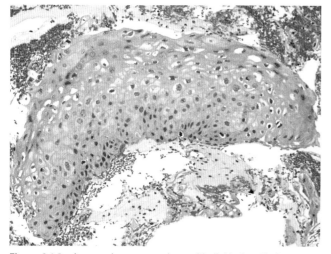

Figure 2.1.3 Low-grade squamous intraepithelial lesion. Nuclear enlargement and hyperchromasia; some cells with cytoplasmic clearing.

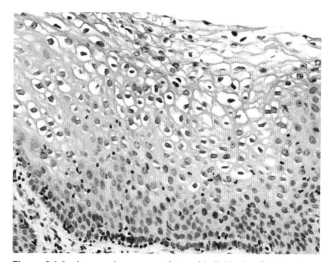

Figure 2.1.4 Low-grade squamous intraepithelial lesion. Prominent koilocytotic change.

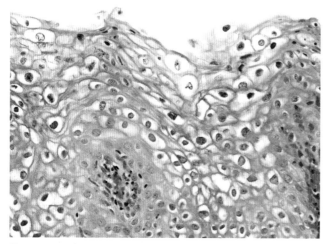

Figure 2.1.5 Low-grade squamous intraepithelial lesion, higher magnification. Nuclear enlargement, hyperchromasia, and nuclear membrane irregularities.

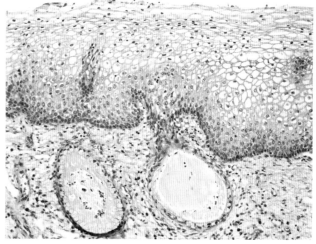

Figure 2.1.6 Nondiagnostic squamous atypia. Diffuse cytoplasmic clearing in the superficial and intermediate layers. Hyperchromasia, but no nuclear enlargement.

2 CERVIX

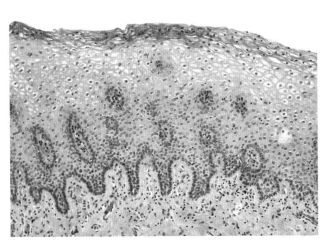

Figure 2.1.7 Nondiagnostic squamous atypia. The parabasal zone appears widened due to tangential sectioning. Mildly enlarged uniform nuclei in the intermediate layers.

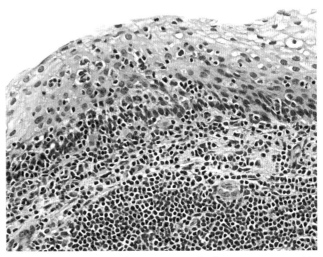

Figure 2.1.8 Nondiagnostic squamous atypia. Squamous mucosa with inflammation. Enlarged nuclei with smooth nuclear membranes and small nucleoli.

	Low-Grade Squamous Intraepithelial Lesion (LSIL)	High-Grade Squamous Intraepithelial Lesion (HSIL)
Age	Wide age range, from teenage to postmenopausal years	Wide age range, from teenage to postmenopausal years
Location	Cervix, transformation zone, ectocervix	Cervix, transformation zone, ectocervix
Symptoms	None	None
Signs	Abnormal Pap, high-risk HPV variably detected, acetowhite changes or other abnormal findings at colposcopy	Abnormal Pap, high-risk HPV usually detected, acetowhite changes or other abnormal findings at colposcopy
Etiology	HPV, low- and high-risk types	High-risk HPV, types 16 and 18 are most common
Histology	1. Preserved epithelial maturation; some expansion of parabasal zone can be seen *(Fig. 2.2.1)*, particularly with tangential sectioning *(Fig. 2.2.2)* 2. Intermediate and superficial layer cells with nuclear enlargement, hyperchromasia 3. Superficial layer cells with perinuclear cytoplasmic clearing and nuclear enlargement (koilocytes) *(Fig. 2.2.3)* 4. Enlarged hyperchromatic nuclei with irregular contours, but nucleocytoplasmic ratio is not increased *(Fig. 2.2.4)* 5. Occasionally with increased mitotic activity in the lower third of the epithelium	1. Loss of epithelial maturation except for very superficial keratinocyte layer *(Fig. 2.2.5)* 2. Expansion of immature parabasal-like cells for at least 2/3 of the epithelial thickness *(Fig. 2.2.6)* 3. "Disorganization" of parabasal zone, nuclei pointing in different directions *(Figs. 2.2.7 and 2.2.8)* 4. Enlarged hyperchromatic nuclei and scant to moderate amount of cytoplasm, increased nucleocytoplasmic ratio *(Fig. 2.2.7)* 5. Mitotic figures in the intermediate layers *(Fig. 2.2.8)*
Special studies	• Negative, patchy, or diffuse p16; diffuse "block-like" expression of p16 does not preclude diagnosis of LSIL • Ki-67 labeling is increased in parabasal intermediate layers with some cells in superficial layers labeled	• Strong, diffuse "block-like" expression of p16; rare cases can lack diffuse p16 expression • Significant increase in Ki-67 labeling throughout epithelial thickness
Treatment	None required; follow-up with repeat cervical cytology and colposcopy	Cervical excision, LEEP, or conization; close follow-up without excision can be considered in young women
Prognosis	Most regress spontaneously without intervention; patients with lesions harboring high-risk HPV can develop persistent infection and high-grade squamous intraepithelial lesions	Some cases will progress to invasive carcinoma if untreated

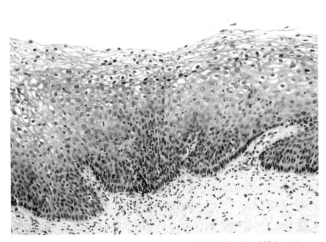

Figure 2.2.1 Low-grade squamous intraepithelial lesion. Widened parabasal zone and prominent koilocytotic atypia.

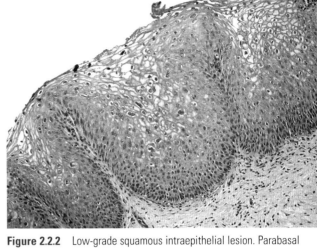

Figure 2.2.2 Low-grade squamous intraepithelial lesion. Parabasal area appears widened around stromal papillae, but the maturation is preserved, and there is prominent koilocytotic change.

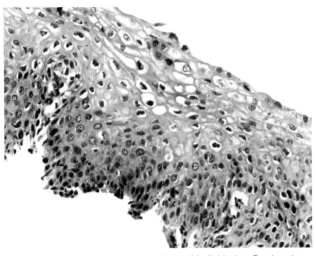

Figure 2.2.3 Low-grade squamous intraepithelial lesion. Parabasal zone shows atypia and disorganization. Maturation is preserved in the upper 2/3 of the epithelium.

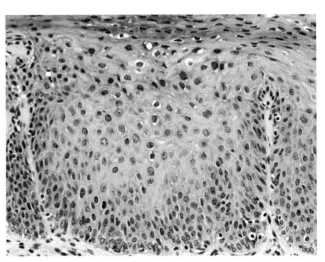

Figure 2.2.4 Low-grade squamous intraepithelial lesion. No notable koilocytosis. Nuclear enlargement in the intermediate layers. Immature cells with increased nucleocytoplasmic ratio are confined to the parabasal zone.

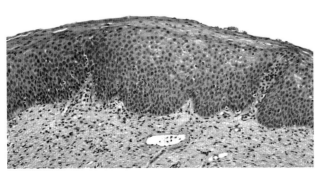

Figure 2.2.5 High-grade squamous intraepithelial lesion. Marked widening of the parabasal zone to more than 2/3 of the epithelial thickness. Preserved maturation in the very superficial epithelial layers.

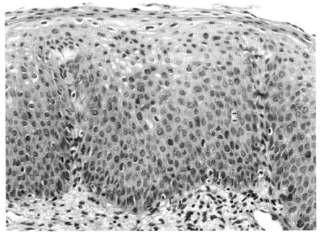

Figure 2.2.6 High-grade squamous intraepithelial lesion. Atypical parabasal-like cells extend to the intermediate layers. Mitotic figures are seen above the parabasal zone.

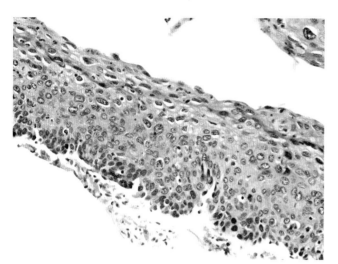

Figure 2.2.7   High-grade squamous intraepithelial lesion. Significant nuclear atypia is present throughout entire epithelial thickness, while cells retain moderate amount of eosinophilic cytoplasm.

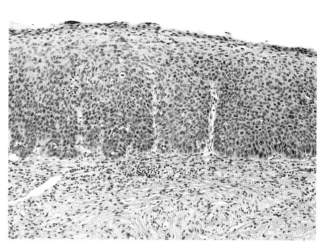

Figure 2.2.8   High-grade squamous intraepithelial lesion. Atypical immature cell proliferation with marked disorganization involving more than 2/3 of the epithelial thickness. Mitotic figures are seen in the intermediate layers.

	Papillary Immature Squamous Metaplasia (Immature Condyloma)	Papillary Squamous Cell Carcinoma
Age	22-41 y	43-80 y, most cases are in fifth to sixth decade
Location	Cervix, often proximal (high) in the endocervical canal	Cervix, vagina
Symptoms	Often asymptomatic	Vaginal bleeding, discharge, constitutional symptoms, and abdominal pain in advanced stage cases
Signs	Abnormal Pap, abnormal colposcopy findings	Abnormal Pap, abnormal colposcopy findings, cervical mass
Etiology	Most contain low-risk HPV (6 and 11 types)	High-risk HPV (type 16, most common)
Histology	1. Papillary fronds lined by immature squamous epithelium *(Figs. 2.3.1-2.3.3)* 2. No invasion into underlying cervical stroma; extension into endocervical glands can be seen 3. Some increase in nucleocytoplasmic ratio *(Fig. 2.3.3)* 4. Uniform bland nuclei; small nucleoli can be seen *(Fig. 2.3.4)* 5. Absent to rare parabasal mitoses	1. Papillary fronds lined by immature squamous epithelium *(Figs. 2.3.6 and 2.3.7)* 2. Invasion is present (unless "papillary squamous cell carcinoma *in situ*"); invasive component has typical appearance of squamous cell carcinoma. Base of the lesion must be completely examined to evaluate for the presence and depth of invasion 3. Increased nucleocytoplasmic ratio 4. Atypical nuclei with some degree of pleomorphism; hyperchromasia *(Figs. 2.3.8 and 2.3.9)* 5. Brisk mitotic activity in the upper epithelial layers *(Fig. 2.3.10)*
Special studies	• Patchy or negative p16 *(Fig. 2.3.5, **left**)* • Low to absent Ki-67 proliferative activity *(Fig. 2.3.5, **right**)* • Lack of high-risk HPV by *in situ* hybridization; low-risk HPV is detected	• Strong diffuse expression of p16 • Elevated Ki-67 proliferative activity throughout the epithelial thickness • High-risk HPV, detected by *in situ* hybridization; the assay has imperfect sensitivity, false-negative cases can be seen
Treatment	For lesions located high in the endocervical canal, excision/conization may be required for definitive diagnosis (to ensure complete removal)	Conization to evaluate the extent of the tumor/depth of invasion; subsequent treatment depending on the tumor stage including modified radical hysterectomy or chemoradiation
Prognosis	Benign, considered a variant of immature condyloma; however, a coexisting high-grade squamous intraepithelial lesions (HSIL) can be present in a proportion of cases	Stage dependent

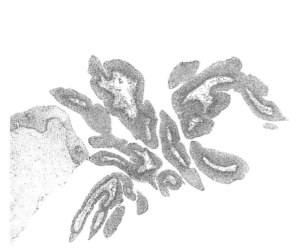

Figure 2.3.1 Papillary immature squamous metaplasia. Multiple detached papillary fragments. No extension into cervical stroma is seen in a separate fragment **(left)**.

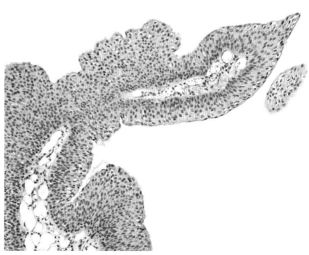

Figure 2.3.2 Papillary immature squamous metaplasia. Same case as in *Figure 2.3.1*, higher magnification. Papillae lined by immature cells.

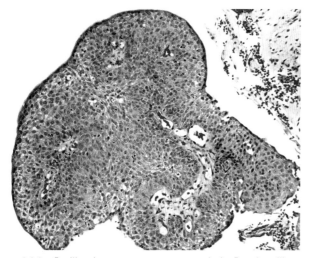

Figure 2.3.3 Papillary immature squamous metaplasia. Fused papillae lined by stratified immature epithelium.

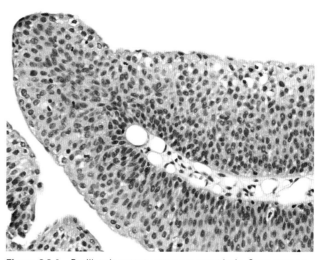

Figure 2.3.4 Papillary immature squamous metaplasia. Same case as in *Figure 2.3.1*, higher magnification. Papillary frond lined by monotonous immature cells with mild atypia; mitoses are not seen.

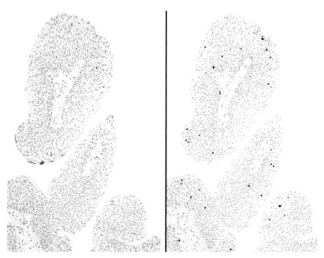

Figure 2.3.5 Papillary immature squamous metaplasia. Essentially absent expression of p16, **left**, and very low Ki-67 labeling, **right**.

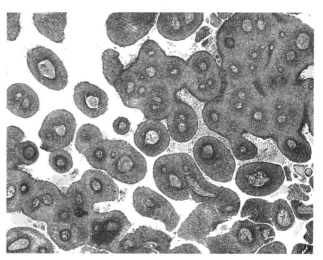

Figure 2.3.6 Papillary squamous cell carcinoma. Multiple detached and fused papillary structures.

2   CERVIX

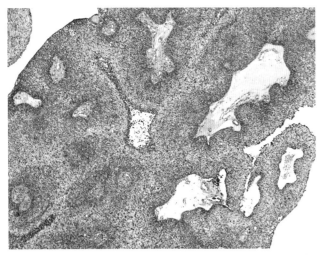

Figure 2.3.7 Papillary squamous cell carcinoma. Fused papillae lined by stratified immature epithelium.

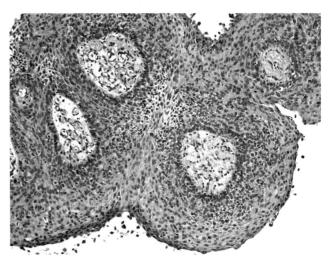

Figure 2.3.8 Papillary squamous cell carcinoma. Same case as in *Figure 2.3.6*, higher magnification. Stratified epithelium shows disorganization and brisk mitotic activity.

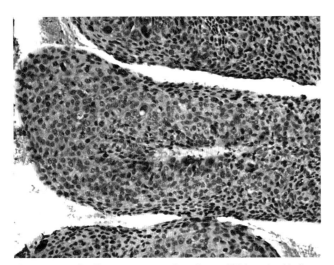

Figure 2.3.9 Papillary squamous cell carcinoma. Thickened epithelium with increased nucleocytoplasmic ratio and nuclear pleomorphism.

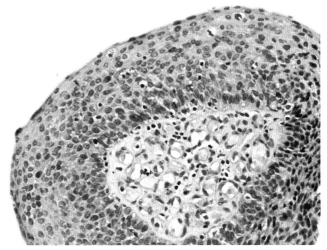

Figure 2.3.10 Papillary squamous cell carcinoma. Moderately increased nucleocytoplasmic ratio and mitotic figures in the superficial layers.

	High-Grade Squamous Intraepithelial Lesion (HSIL)	Immature Squamous Metaplasia
Age	Wide age range, from teenage to postmenopausal years	Wide age range, more common in young reproductive-age women
Location	Cervix, transformation zone, ectocervix	Cervix, transformation zone
Symptoms	Often asymptomatic	Asymptomatic or vaginal discharge
Signs	Abnormal Pap, high-risk HPV usually detected, acetowhite changes or other abnormal findings at colposcopy	Abnormal Pap usually triggers colposcopic examination and cervical biopsy; high-risk HPV may be detected coincidentally in cervical cytology specimens, abnormal findings at colposcopy may be present
Etiology	High-risk HPV, types 16 and 18 are most common	Normal evolution of the cervical transformation zone
Histology	1. Loss of epithelial maturation except for very superficial keratinocyte layers; extension into endocervical glands can occur *(Figs. 2.4.1-2.4.3)* 2. Expansion of immature parabasal-like cells for at least 2/3 of the epithelial thickness *(Fig. 2.4.2)* 3. "Disorganization" of parabasal zone, nuclei pointing in different directions 4. Enlarged hyperchromatic nuclei with nuclear membrane irregularities; increased nucleocytoplasmic ratio *(Fig. 2.4.4)* 5. Mitotic figures in the intermediate and superficial layers	1. Loss of epithelial maturation; extension into endocervical glands is common *(Figs. 2.4.5-2.4.7)* 2. Expansion of immature parabasal-like cells 3. Parabasal zone retains orderly arrangement of the nuclei *(Fig. 2.4.6)* 4. Mild nuclear enlargement; round nuclei with finely dispersed chromatin and inconspicuous nucleoli; mild increase in nucleocytoplasmic ratio *(Fig. 2.4.7)* 5. Mitotic figures can be occasionally seen in the parabasal zone
Special studies	• Strong, diffuse "block-like" expression of p16; rare cases can lack diffuse p16 expression • Significant increase in Ki-67 labeling throughout epithelial thickness	• Focal/patchy or negative staining for p16 *(Fig. 2.4.8, **left**)* • Variable Ki-67 proliferative activity, but generally it is not markedly increased *(Fig. 2.4.8, **right**)*
Treatment	Cervical excision, LEEP or conization; close follow-up without excision can be considered in young women	None needed
Prognosis	Some cases will progress to invasive carcinoma if untreated	Benign/normal variant; cervical cancer screening should continue based on other findings (previous abnormal Pap, high-risk HPV detection)

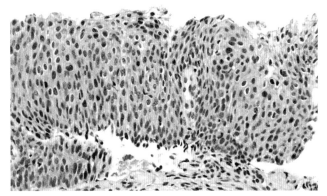

Figure 2.4.1 High-grade squamous intraepithelial lesion. Full-thickness immature cell proliferation with metaplastic-like appearance. The cells retain a moderate amount of cytoplasm. Hyperchromatic enlarged nuclei with some degree of pleomorphism.

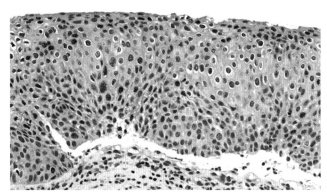

Figure 2.4.2 High-grade squamous intraepithelial lesion, metaplastic type.

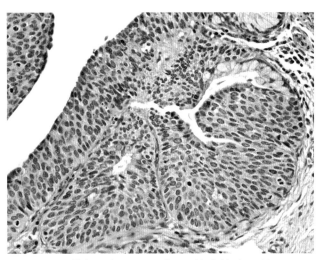

Figure 2.4.3 High-grade squamous intraepithelial lesion with endocervical gland involvement.

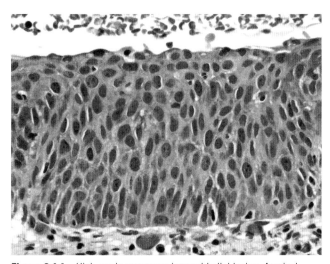

Figure 2.4.4 High-grade squamous intraepithelial lesion. Atypical nuclei with some degree of pleomorphism pointing in different directions.

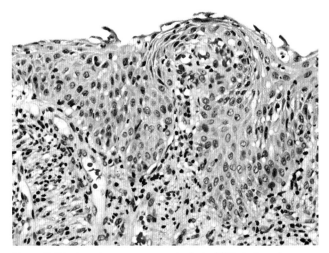

Figure 2.4.5 Immature squamous metaplasia. Mild atypia and some increase in nucleocytoplasmic ratio.

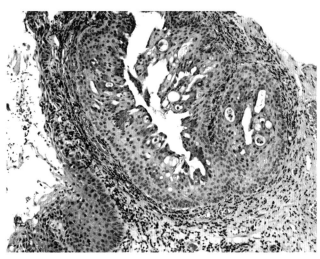

Figure 2.4.6 Immature squamous metaplasia. Endocervical gland involvement with residual endocervical glandular epithelium remaining.

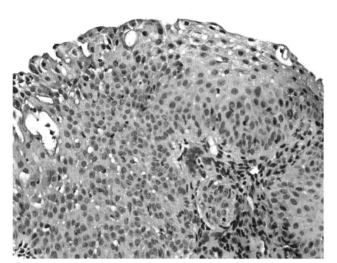

Figure 2.4.7   Immature squamous metaplasia. Thickened epithelium composed of immature cells with uniform nuclei and moderate amount of cytoplasm.

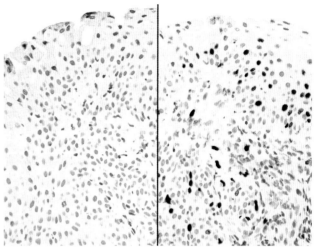

Figure 2.4.8   Immature squamous metaplasia. Same case as in *Figure 2.4.7*. Essentially absent expression of p16, **left**, and some increase in Ki-67 labeling, **right**.

	High-Grade Squamous Intraepithelial Lesion (HSIL)	Transitional Cell Metaplasia/Atrophy
Age	Wide age range, from teenage to postmenopausal years	Postmenopausal women, mean age 60-68 y
Location	Cervix, transformation zone, ectocervix, vagina	Ectocervix, transformation zone, occasionally vagina
Symptoms	Asymptomatic	Asymptomatic or vaginal discharge
Signs	Abnormal Pap, high-risk HPV usually detected, acetowhite changes or other abnormal findings at colposcopy	Abnormal Pap, high-risk HPV can be detected coincidentally, abnormal findings at colposcopy can be occasionally seen
Etiology	High-risk HPV, types 16 and 18 are most common	Unknown, related to atrophy
Histology	1. Loss of epithelial maturation except for superficial keratinocyte layers (in some cases); keratinocytes may appear "spindled" *(Figs. 2.5.1 and 2.5.2)* 2. Expansion of immature parabasal-like cells for at least 2/3 of the epithelial thickness *(Fig. 2.5.3)* 3. "Disorganization" of parabasal zone, nuclei pointing in different directions *(Fig. 2.5.4)* 4. Enlarged hyperchromatic nuclei and scant amount of cytoplasm, increased nucleocytoplasmic ratio *(Fig. 2.5.4)* 5. Mitotic figures in the intermediate and superficial layers	1. Involves full thickness of the epithelium *(Figs. 2.5.5 and 2.5.6)* 2. Immature parabasal-like cells resembling urothelium 3. Haphazard orientation of the nuclei can be seen *(Fig. 2.5.7)* 4. Mild nuclear enlargement; ovoid to spindled uniform, hyperchromatic nuclei with occasional nuclear grooves; smooth nuclear membranes *(Fig. 2.5.8)* 5. Mitotic figures are not seen
Special studies	• Strong, diffuse "block-like" expression of p16; rare cases can lack diffuse p16 expression • Significant increase in Ki-67 labeling throughout epithelial thickness	• Patchy or negative staining for p16 *(Fig. 2.5.9, **left**)* • Low to absent Ki-67 proliferative activity *(Fig. 2.5.9, **right**)*
Treatment	Cervical excision, LEEP, or conization; close follow-up without excision can be considered in young women	None needed
Prognosis	Some cases will progress to invasive carcinoma if untreated	Benign

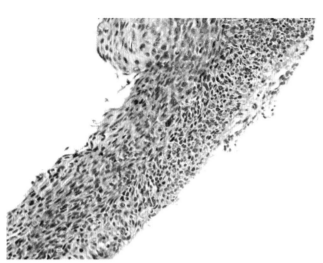

Figure 2.5.1 High-grade squamous intraepithelial lesion. Immature cells occupy entire epithelial thickness. Atypical squamous cells appear somewhat spindled. Occasional markedly enlarged nucleus is seen.

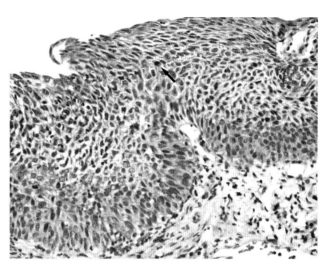

Figure 2.5.2 High-grade squamous intraepithelial lesion. Full-thickness atypical immature epithelium; occasional mitotic figure (*arrow*) in the intermediate zone.

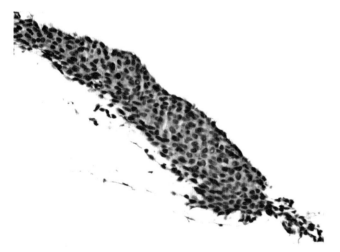

Figure 2.5.3 Attenuated high-grade squamous intraepithelial lesion in a suboptimally oriented epithelial fragment lacking stroma in an endocervical curettage.

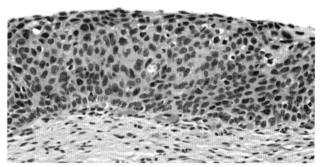

Figure 2.5.4 High-grade squamous intraepithelial lesion. Cells with atypical, hyperchromatic, and variably shaped nuclei occupy entire epithelial thickness.

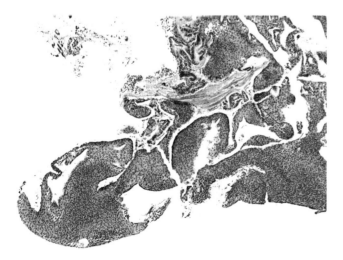

Figure 2.5.5 Transitional cell metaplasia/atrophy. Tangentially oriented cellular fragments in an endocervical curettage.

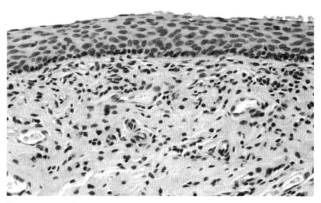

Figure 2.5.6 Transitional cell metaplasia/atrophy. Attenuated epithelium appears basophilic.

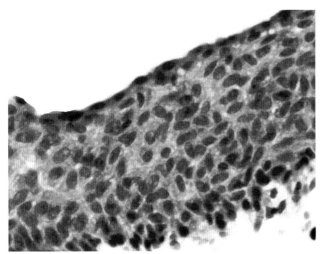

Figure 2.5.7   Transitional cell metaplasia/atrophy. Same case as in *Figure 2.5.5*, higher magnification. Disorganized mildly hyperchromatic nuclei; increased nucleocytoplasmic ratio; nuclear membranes are smooth, and chromatin is fine. Mitoses are not seen.

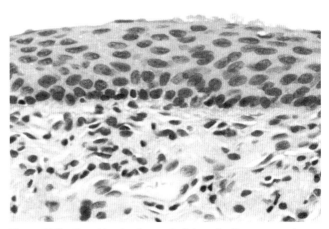

Figure 2.5.8   Transitional cell metaplasia/atrophy. Same case as in *Figure 2.5.6*, higher magnification. Mildly hyperchromatic elongated nuclei with occasional nuclear grooves.

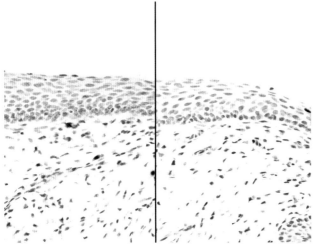

Figure 2.5.9   Transitional cell metaplasia/atrophy. Same case as in *Figure 2.5.6*. No expression of p16, **left**, and absent Ki-67 labeling, **right**.

	Attenuated High-Grade Squamous Intraepithelial Lesion (HSIL)	Atypical Immature Squamous Metaplasia
Age	Wide age range, from teenage to postmenopausal years; however, attenuated forms are more common in older women	Wide age range
Location	Cervix, transformation zone	Cervix, transformation zone
Symptoms	Often asymptomatic	Often asymptomatic
Signs	Abnormal Pap, high-risk HPV usually detected, acetowhite changes or other abnormal findings at colposcopy	Abnormal Pap, high-risk HPV may be detected, abnormal findings at colposcopy
Etiology	High-risk HPV, types 16 and 18 are most common	Not a specific biologic entity; a morphologically ambiguous lesion concerning for but not definitively diagnostic of HSIL
Histology	1. Hyperchromatic epithelial fragments; loss of epithelial maturation except for very superficial keratinocyte layers in some cases 2. Expansion of immature parabasal-like cells for at least 2/3 of the epithelial thickness *(Figs. 2.6.1 and 2.6.2)* 3. "Disorganization," nuclei pointing in different directions *(Fig. 2.6.3)* 4. Enlarged hyperchromatic nuclei with nuclear membrane irregularities; increased nucleocytoplasmic ratio *(Figs. 2.6.2 and 2.6.4)* 5. Mitotic figures in the intermediate and superficial layers	1. Loss of epithelial maturation; metaplastic-appearing epithelium 2. Expansion of immature parabasal-like cells *(Figs. 2.6.6 and 2.6.7)* 3. Some "disorganization" can be seen 4. Nuclear features are concerning for HSIL but not unequivocal *(Figs. 2.6.7 and 2.6.8)* 5. Mitotic figures in parabasal layers; no abnormal forms
Special studies	• Strong, diffuse "block-like" expression of p16 *(Fig. 2.6.5,* **left***)*; rare cases can lack diffuse p16 expression • Significant increase in Ki-67 labeling throughout epithelial thickness *(Fig. 2.6.5,* **right***)*	• Variable expression of p16 *(Fig. 2.6.9,* **left***)*; strong and diffuse expression strongly favors HSIL • Variable Ki-67 proliferative activity *(Fig. 2.6.9,* **right***)*
Treatment	Cervical excision, LEEP, or conization; close follow-up without excision can be considered in young women	Close follow-up with repeat cervical cytology and colposcopy with biopsies or cervical excision
Prognosis	Some cases will progress to invasive carcinoma if untreated	Some cases are diagnosed as HSIL in follow-up specimens

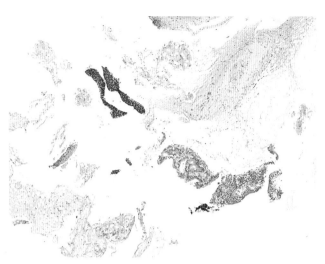

Figure 2.6.1   High-grade squamous intraepithelial lesion (HSIL). Attenuated hyperchromatic poorly oriented fragments in an endocervical curettage.

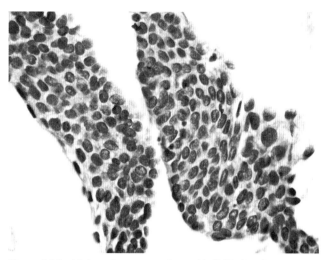

Figure 2.6.2   High-grade squamous intraepithelial lesion. Same case as in *Figure 2.6.1*, higher magnification. Full-thickness epithelial immaturity, hyperchromasia, and atypia in suboptimally oriented epithelial fragments without underlying stroma.

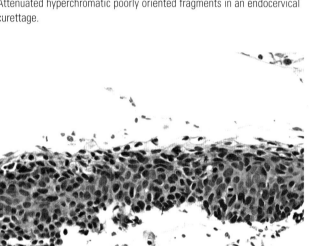

Figure 2.6.3   High-grade squamous intraepithelial lesion. Disorganized immature cell proliferation with atypia and hyperchromasia.

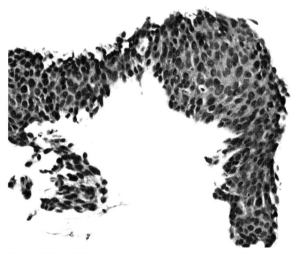

Figure 2.6.4   High-grade squamous intraepithelial lesion. Detached fragment; while the fragment is somewhat tangentially sectioned and suboptimally oriented, the degree of immaturity and atypia warrant the diagnosis of HSIL.

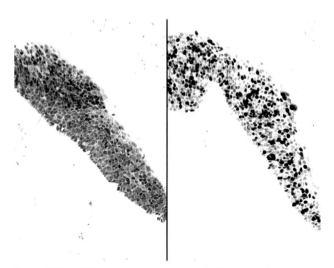

Figure 2.6.5   High-grade squamous intraepithelial lesion. Same case as in *Figure 2.6.1*. Diffuse p16 expression **(left)**; markedly increased Ki-67 labeling throughout epithelial thickness **(right)**.

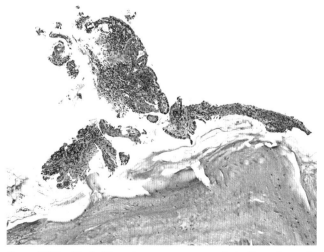

Figure 2.6.6   Atypical immature squamous metaplasia. Hyperchromatic squamous epithelial fragments in an endocervical curettage.

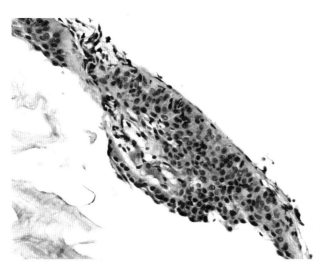

Figure 2.6.7 Atypical immature squamous metaplasia. Same case as in *Figure 2.6.6*, higher magnification. The morphologic features raise concern for HSIL.

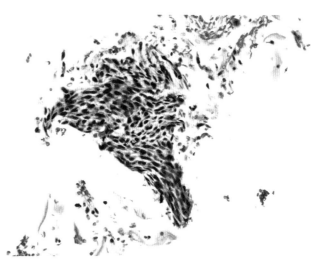

Figure 2.6.8 Atypical immature squamous metaplasia. Detached tangentially sectioned and suboptimally oriented fragment of atypical immature squamous epithelium. The fragment was depleted on the immunostained levels. HSIL cannot be excluded.

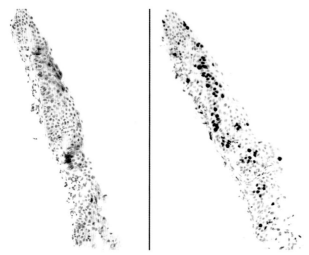

Figure 2.6.9 Atypical immature squamous metaplasia. Same case as *Figure 2.6.7*, patchy expression of p16, **left**, and some increase in Ki-67 labeling, **right** Compare to *Figure 2.6.5*.

	High-Grade Squamous Intraepithelial Lesion (HSIL) With Extension into Endocervical Glands	Superficially Invasive Squamous Cell Carcinoma
Age	Wide age range, from teenage to postmenopausal years	Most cases are between 40 and 55 y
Location	Cervix, transformation zone, ectocervix	Cervix, transformation zone
Symptoms	None	Vaginal bleeding or discharge
Signs	Abnormal Pap, high-risk HPV usually detected, acetowhite changes or other abnormal findings at colposcopy	Abnormal Pap; abnormal colposcopic findings, clinically visible cervical lesion is often not seen
Etiology	High-risk HPV, types 16 and 18 are most common	High-risk HPV, types 16 and 18 are most common
Histology	1. Surface HSIL is usually present 2. Rounded outlines of the lesional nests (Figs. 2.7.1 and 2.7.2) 3. Normal/uninvolved endocervical glands are often seen in the vicinity; partial gland involvement can be seen (Figs. 2.7.2 and 2.7.3) 4. Lesion cells within the glands with features similar to the surface lesion; some maturation can be seen in the center of the involved gland, but no paradoxical maturation at the periphery (Fig. 2.7.4) 5. Loose stroma can be seen around the glands, but no true desmoplasia	1. Background of HSIL with or without endocervical gland involvement is often seen (Figs. 2.7.5-2.7.8) 2. Irregularly shaped small nests and single cells in the stroma (Figs. 2.7.5, 2.7.6, and 2.7.8) 3. Normal endocervical glands can be seen in the vicinity 4. Paradoxical maturation can be seen (Fig. 2.7.5) 5. Stromal desmoplastic response can be seen (Fig. 2.7.5)
Special studies	Not helpful in this differential diagnosis	Not helpful in this differential diagnosis
Treatment	Cervical excision, LEEP, or conization; larger volume excision may be required to achieve negative margins in cases with extensive endocervical gland involvement	Cases of superficially invasive carcinoma without angiolymphatic invasion can be treated with cervical excision; modified radical hysterectomy +/− lymphadenectomy for early-stage cases; chemoradiation for advanced stage cases
Prognosis	Some cases will progress to invasive carcinoma if untreated	5-y survival ~95% (for superficially invasive squamous cell carcinoma, stage IA1)

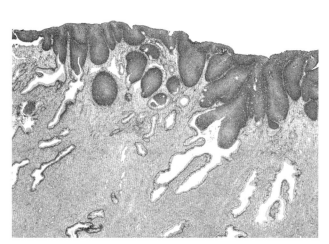

Figure 2.7.1   High-grade squamous intraepithelial lesion (HSIL) with extension into endocervical glands. Nests of lesional epithelium with rounded outlines.

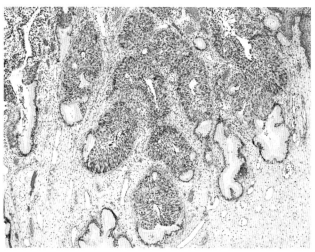

Figure 2.7.2   High-grade squamous intraepithelial lesion (HSIL) with extension into endocervical glands. Residual normal endocervical glandular epithelium is seen in the deep aspects of partially involved glands.

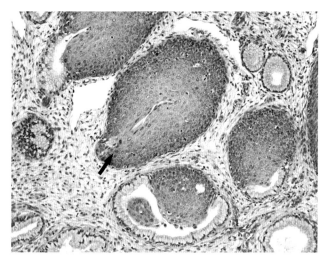

Figure 2.7.3   High-grade squamous intraepithelial lesion (HSIL) with extension into endocervical glands. Same case as in *Figure 2.7.1*, higher magnification. Nests of atypical epithelium with smooth contours. Residual glandular epithelium (*arrow*) confirms gland involvement.

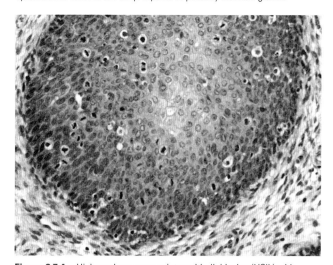

Figure 2.7.4   High-grade squamous intraepithelial lesion (HSIL) with extension into endocervical glands. Same case as in *Figure 2.7.1*, higher magnification. Atypical epithelium forming round nest with morphologic features similar to HSIL on the surface. Numerous mitotic figures are noted.

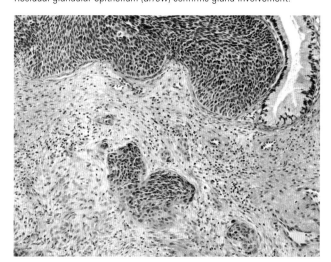

Figure 2.7.5   Superficially invasive squamous cell carcinoma. Irregular squamous epithelial nests in the stroma **(bottom)** display eosinophilic cytoplasm (paradoxical maturation). Note surrounding stromal reaction. Compare to the broad basophilic nest with smooth contour within endocervical gland **(top)**.

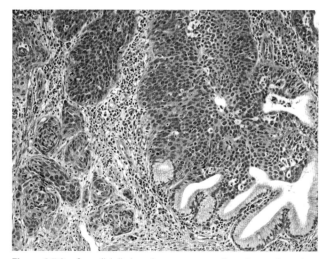

Figure 2.7.6   Superficially invasive squamous cell carcinoma. Irregular nests of carcinoma within the stroma **(left)**. Compare to HSIL involving endocervical glands **(right)**.

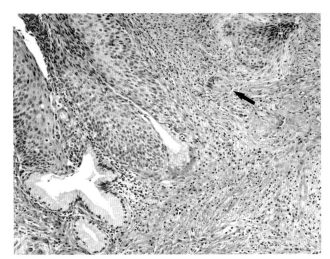

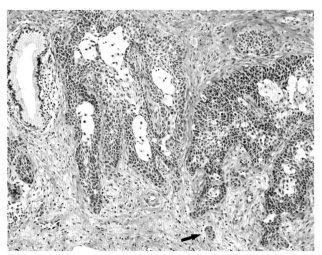

Figure 2.7.7   Superficially invasive squamous cell carcinoma. Small eosinophilic nest of carcinoma (*arrow*) with adjacent HSIL involving endocervical glands **(left)**.

Figure 2.7.8   Superficially invasive squamous cell carcinoma. Small eosinophilic nest of carcinoma (*arrow*) arising from HSIL involving endocervical glands.

	Adenoid Basal Epithelioma	High-Grade Squamous Intraepithelial Lesion (HSIL) With Extension Into Endocervical Glands
Age	Wide age range, more common in postmenopausal women, mean age 64-71 y	Wide age range, from teenage to postmenopausal years
Location	Cervix	Cervix, transformation zone
Symptoms	Asymptomatic	Asymptomatic
Signs	Abnormal Pap or an incidental finding in the hysterectomy for other indications	Abnormal Pap, abnormal findings on colposcopy
Etiology	High-risk HPV, particularly in cases associated with HSIL or squamous cell carcinoma	High-risk HPV
Histology	1. Located superficial or deep in the cervical stroma (Fig. 2.8.1) 2. Small basaloid nests with prominent peripheral palisading (Figs. 2.8.2 and 2.8.3) 3. No association with adjacent endocervical glands; loose stroma around the nests (Fig. 2.8.3) 4. Glandular/acinar differentiation is common (Fig. 2.8.4); squamous differentiation can be seen in the center of the nests 5. Uniform mildly atypical basaloid cells; cytoplasmic clearing can be seen (Figs. 2.8.3-2.8.5) 6. Mitoses are generally infrequent	1. Within the range of distribution of endocervical glands (Fig. 2.8.6) 2. The squamous nests often expand involved glands resulting in their size exceeding that of adjacent endocervical glands; smooth contours (Fig. 2.8.7) 3. Atypical stratified squamous epithelium (HSIL) similar to the lesion seen on the mucosal surface extending into preexisting endocervical gland (Fig. 2.8.8); partial gland involvement can be seen (Fig. 2.8.9) 4. Associated adjacent adenocarcinoma *in situ* can be seen; true glandular differentiation is not present 5. Cytologic atypia, enlarged hyperchromatic nuclei, eosinophilic cytoplasm (Figs. 2.8.9 and 2.8.10) 6. Often brisk mitotic activity
Special studies	Not helpful in this differential; however, some studies suggested lack of high-risk HPV and p16 expression in small isolated lesions not associated with invasive carcinoma	Not helpful in this differential
Treatment	Cervical excision to exclude other components (adenoid basal carcinoma, squamous cell carcinoma, etc.)	Cervical excision, LEEP, or conization
Prognosis	Benign; however, may be associated with HSIL or invasive carcinoma	Some cases will progress to invasive carcinoma if untreated

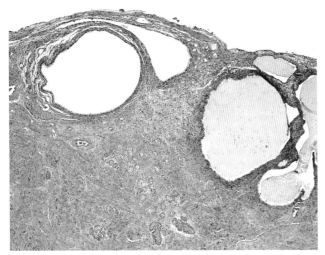

Figure 2.8.1 Adenoid basal epithelioma. Proliferation of basophilic epithelial nests in the stroma below the level of normal endocervical glands.

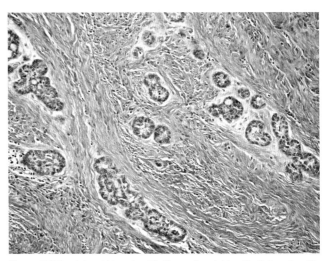

Figure 2.8.2 Adenoid basal epithelioma. Basaloid epithelial nests with peripheral palisading.

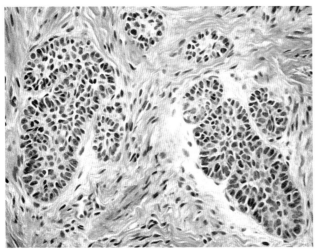

Figure 2.8.3 Adenoid basal epithelioma. Solid basaloid nests composed of uniform cells.

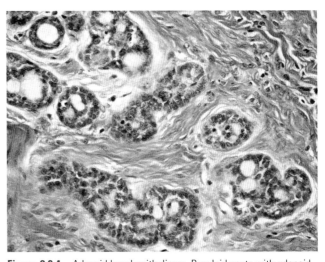

Figure 2.8.4 Adenoid basal epithelioma. Basaloid nests with adenoid cystic-like features.

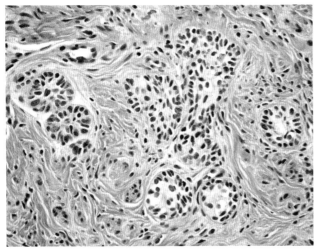

Figure 2.8.5 Adenoid basal epithelioma. Basaloid nests with cytoplasmic clearing.

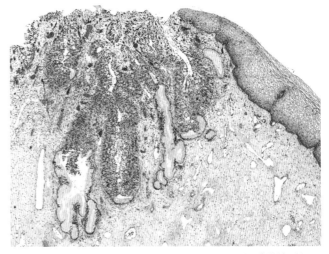

Figure 2.8.6 High-grade squamous intraepithelial lesion (HSIL) with extension into endocervical glands. Note residual endocervical glandular epithelium in the deep aspects of the glands.

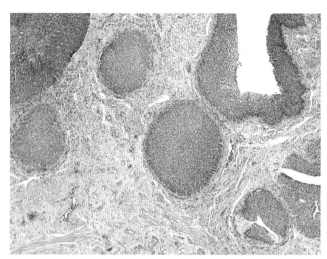

Figure 2.8.7   High-grade squamous intraepithelial lesion (HSIL) with extension into endocervical glands. Large round basophilic nests in the stroma. Residual endocervical glandular epithelium is seen **(bottom right)**.

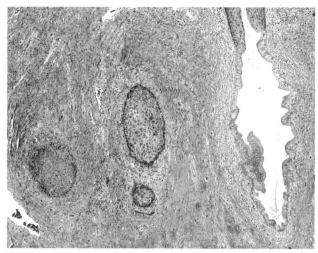

Figure 2.8.8   High-grade squamous intraepithelial lesion (HSIL) with extension into endocervical glands. Epithelial nests with smooth contours and adjacent endocervical gland.

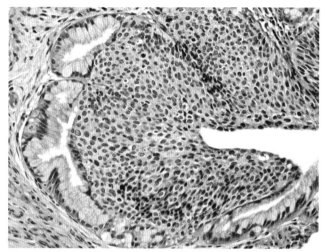

Figure 2.8.9   High-grade squamous intraepithelial lesion (HSIL) with extension into endocervical glands. Residual endocervical glandular epithelium remains at the periphery of the involved gland.

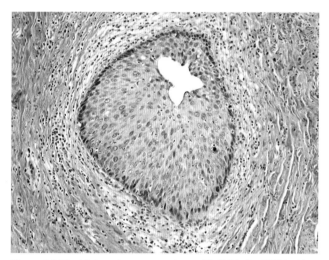

Figure 2.8.10   High-grade squamous intraepithelial lesion (HSIL) with extension into endocervical glands, higher magnification. The cells have atypical nuclei and moderate amounts of eosinophilic cytoplasm.

	High-Grade Squamous Intraepithelial Lesion (HSIL)	Stratified Mucin-Producing Intraepithelial Lesion (SMILE)
Age	Wide age range from teenage to postmenopausal years	23-57 y, mean 34 y
Location	Cervix, transformation zone	Cervix, transformation zone
Symptoms	Asymptomatic	Asymptomatic
Signs	Abnormal Pap, abnormal colposcopic findings	Abnormal Pap, abnormal colposcopic findings
Etiology	High-risk HPV	High-risk HPV, derived from the reserve cells of cervical transformation zone
Histology	1. Present on the surface or extends into endocervical glands *(Figs. 2.9.1-2.9.3)* 2. Stratified epithelium composed of immature cells with increased nucleocytoplasmic; squamous maturation can be preserved in the superficial layers 3. May undermine residual normal endocervical glandular columnar epithelium on the surface or within endocervical glands *(Figs. 2.9.1 and 2.9.3)* 4. Enlarged hyperchromatic nuclei with nuclear membrane irregularities; increased nucleocytoplasmic ratio *(Fig. 2.9.3)* 5. Mitotic figures in the intermediate and superficial layers; apoptotic bodies can be seen	1. Present on the surface or extends into endocervical glands *(Figs. 2.9.4-2.9.6)* 2. Stratified epithelium with mucin-containing columnar cells *(Figs. 2.9.6 and 2.9.7)* 3. Columnar cells with cytoplasmic mucin distributed throughout epithelial thickness *(Figs. 2.9.6 and 2.9.7)* 4. Some nuclear enlargement and atypia *(Fig. 2.9.8)* 5. Mitoses can be present, but often not frequent; apoptotic bodies can be seen
Special studies	• p63/p40 positive • Mucicarmine stain is negative; residual normal endocervical glandular cells on the surface can be positive	• p63/p40 negative, except for the basal layer in some cases • Mucicarmine stain can be used to highlight cytoplasmic mucin throughout entire epithelial thickness
Treatment	Cervical excision, LEEP, or conization; close follow-up without excision can be considered in young women	Cervical excision, conization
Prognosis	Some cases will progress to invasive carcinoma if untreated	Considered a variant of adenocarcinoma *in situ* (AIS); commonly is associated with HSIL and usual-type AIS; greater risk of coexisting invasive carcinoma than HSIL. Stratified mucin-producing carcinoma has been described

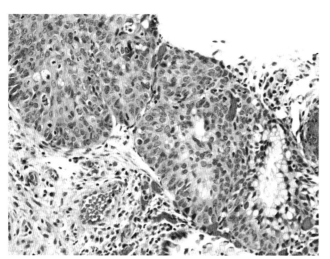

Figure 2.9.1   High-grade squamous intraepithelial lesion (HSIL). Stratified immature epithelium composed of cells with moderate amounts of eosinophilic cytoplasm. Note residual normal endocervical glandular epithelium **(right)**.

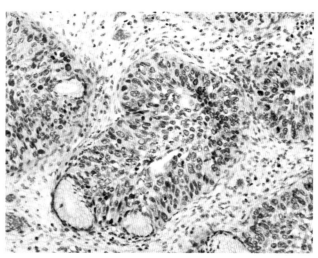

Figure 2.9.2   High-grade squamous intraepithelial lesion (HSIL) with endocervical gland involvement. Basaloid nests of lesional cells with residual glandular epithelium at the deep aspects.

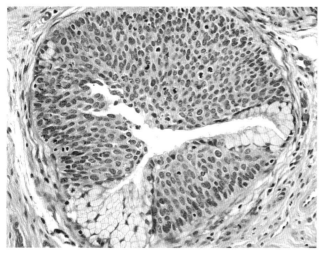

Figure 2.9.3   High-grade squamous intraepithelial lesion (HSIL) with endocervical gland involvement. Lesional cells have moderate amounts of eosinophilic cytoplasm and oval hyperchromatic nuclei.

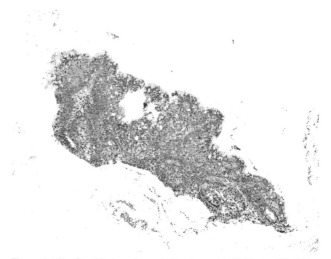

Figure 2.9.4   Stratified mucin-producing intraepithelial lesion (SMILE). Endocervical curettage; fragment of cellular mucosa at low power.

2 CERVIX

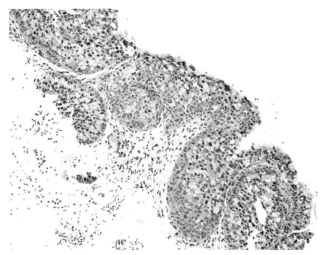

Figure 2.9.5   Stratified mucin-producing intraepithelial lesion (SMILE). Intraepithelial proliferation of cells with pale cytoplasm.

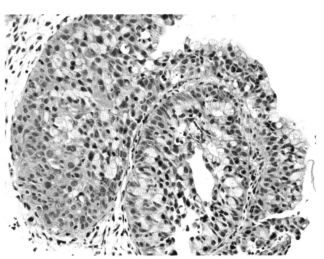

Figure 2.9.6   Stratified mucin-producing intraepithelial lesion (SMILE). Same case as in *Figure 2.9.5*, higher magnification. Cells with pale mucinous cytoplasm are present within surface epithelium and extend into endocervical gland.

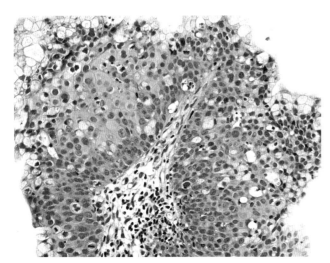

Figure 2.9.7   Stratified mucin-producing intraepithelial lesion (SMILE). Same case as in *Figure 2.9.4*, higher magnification. Lesional cells with round nuclei—some are hyperchromatic, while others have fine chromatin.

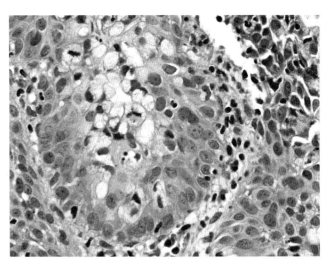

Figure 2.9.8   Stratified mucin-producing intraepithelial lesion (SMILE). Cells with mucinous cytoplasm are distributed within the stratified epithelium. Mitotic figures are seen in the **center** of the nest.

	Stratified Mucin-Producing Intraepithelial Lesion (SMILE)	Squamous Metaplasia With Overlying Mucinous Epithelium
Age	23-57 y, mean 34 y	Wide age range, more common in reproductive-age women
Location	Cervix, transformation zone	Cervix, transformation zone
Symptoms	Asymptomatic	Asymptomatic
Signs	Abnormal Pap, abnormal colposcopic findings	Abnormal Pap, abnormal colposcopic findings can lead to biopsy
Etiology	High-risk HPV, derived from the reserve cells of cervical transformation zone	Normal evolution of cervical transformation zone
Histology	1. Present on the surface or extends into endocervical glands *(Figs. 2.10.1-2.10.3)* 2. Stratified epithelium; columnar cells with cytoplasmic mucin distributed throughout entire epithelial thickness *(Fig. 2.10.3)* 3. Some nuclear enlargement and atypia *(Fig. 2.10.4)* 4. Mitoses can be present, but often not frequent; apoptotic bodies can be seen	1. Present on the surface or extends into endocervical glands *(Figs. 2.10.6 and 2.10.7)* 2. Stratified epithelium composed of immature keratinocytes with ample amount of eosinophilic cytoplasm; residual endocervical glandular epithelium is seen on the surface and within the epithelium *(Figs. 2.10.8 and 2.10.9)* 3. Round mildly enlarged centrally placed bland nuclei *(Figs. 2.10.8 and 2.10.9)* 4. Mitoses are not common, apoptotic bodies are not seen
Special studies	• p16 strong and diffuse *(Fig. 2.10.5, **left**)* • Increased Ki-67 proliferative activity *(Fig. 2.10.5, **right**)*	• p16 patchy or negative *(Fig. 2.10.10)* • Low or mildly increased Ki-67 proliferative activity, mostly in the parabasal area
Treatment	Cervical excision, conization	None needed
Prognosis	Considered a variant of adenocarcinoma *in situ* (AIS); commonly is associated with HSIL and usual-type AIS; greater risk of coexisting invasive carcinoma than HSIL. Stratified mucin-producing carcinoma has been described	Benign

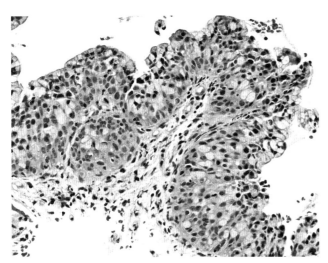

Figure 2.10.1 Stratified mucin-producing intraepithelial lesion (SMILE). Mucin-containing cells distributed throughout entire thickness of stratified epithelium.

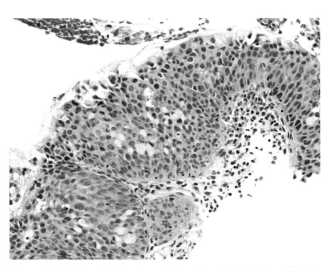

Figure 2.10.2 Stratified mucin-producing intraepithelial lesion (SMILE). Scattered cells with mucinous cytoplasm within the stratified epithelium.

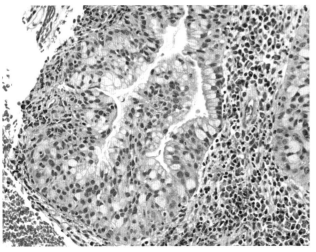

Figure 2.10.3 Stratified mucin-producing intraepithelial lesion (SMILE) involving endocervical gland.

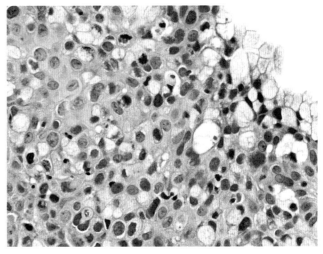

Figure 2.10.4 Stratified mucin-producing intraepithelial lesion (SMILE). Lesional cells with mucinous cytoplasm displaying predominantly round atypical nuclei with hyperchromasia or fine chromatin.

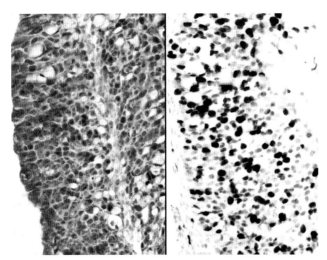

Figure 2.10.5 Stratified mucin-producing intraepithelial lesion (SMILE). Same case as in *Figure 2.10.1*. Lesional cells display diffuse expression of p16 **(left)** and elevated Ki-67 proliferative activity **(right)**.

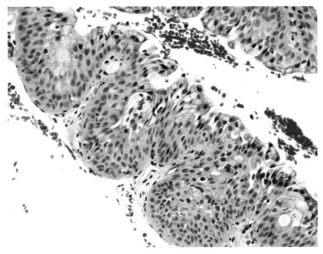

Figure 2.10.6 Squamous metaplasia with overlying mucinous epithelium. Early immature squamous metaplasia represented by proliferation of bland immature reserve layer-like cells beneath endocervical mucinous epithelium.

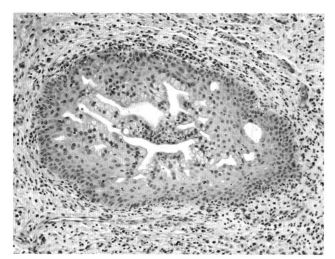

Figure 2.10.7   *Squamous metaplasia involving endocervical gland. Endocervical glandular epithelium remains in the* **center**. *Bland stratified epithelium shows some maturation toward the* **center** *of the involved gland. Note small round uniform nuclei and lack of mitoses.*

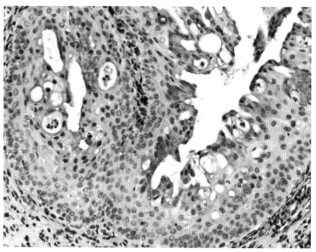

Figure 2.10.8   *Squamous metaplasia involving endocervical gland. Proliferation of bland immature keratinocytes is underlying endocervical glandular epithelium.*

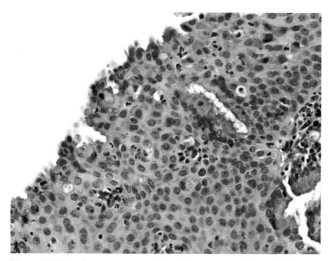

Figure 2.10.9   *Squamous metaplasia. Due to tangential sectioning and suboptimal orientation, a few endocervical cells with basophilic mucinous cytoplasm and an endocervical gland appear entrapped within immature squamous epithelium.*

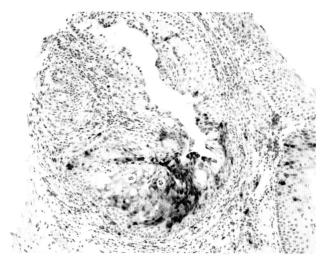

Figure 2.10.10   *Squamous metaplasia involving endocervical gland. Same case as in* Figure 2.10.9. *Patchy expression of p16.*

2 CERVIX

	Intraepithelial Spread of Bladder Urothelial Carcinoma Into the Cervix	High-Grade Squamous Intraepithelial Lesion (HSIL)
Age	Limited data, most reported cases in postmenopausal women	Wide age range, from teenage to postmenopausal years
Location	Cervix, vagina	Cervix, vagina
Symptoms	Vaginal bleeding, discharge	Often asymptomatic
Signs	History of urothelial carcinoma; often years before the diagnosis of cervical involvement; abnormal Pap	Abnormal Pap
Etiology	Risk factors include smoking, exposure to chemicals, prior radiation, prior chemotherapy with cyclophosphamide	High-risk HPV (types 16 and 18 most common)
Histology	1. Sheets and nests of epithelioid cells in the squamous mucosa; pagetoid spread *(Figs. 2.11.1 and 2.11.2)* 2. Single cell detachment and micropapillary aggregates can be seen *(Fig. 2.11.3)* 3. Hyperchromatic nuclei, apoptotic bodies, and scattered mitotic figures *(Fig. 2.11.4)*	1. Loss of epithelial maturation except for very superficial keratinocyte layers; extension into endocervical glands can occur 2. Expansion of immature parabasal-like cells for at least 2/3 of the epithelial thickness within generally intact layer of stratified squamous epithelium *(Figs. 2.11.6-2.11.8)* 3. Enlarged hyperchromatic nuclei with nuclear membrane irregularities; increased nucleocytoplasmic ratio; mitotic figures in the intermediate and superficial layers *(Figs. 2.11.7 and 2.11.8)*
Special studies	• CK20 positive • GATA-3 diffuse, moderate to strong in most cases *(Fig. 2.11.5)* • No detectable high-risk HPV by *in situ* hybridization • p16 may not be helpful in this differential as diffuse expression of p16 has been described in urothelial lesions	• CK20 negative • Weak to absent GATA-3 expression • High-risk HPV detected by *in situ* hybridization (false-negative results can be seen) • Strong and diffuse expression of p16
Treatment	Treatment for advanced stage/recurrent urothelial carcinoma	Cervical excision, LEEP, or conization
Prognosis	Multiple recurrences including distant sites are common; poor prognosis	Some cases will progress to invasive carcinoma if untreated

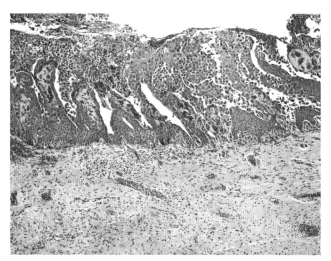

Figure 2.11.1 Intraepithelial spread of bladder urothelial carcinoma into the cervix. Disrupted epithelium with loss of cell cohesion.

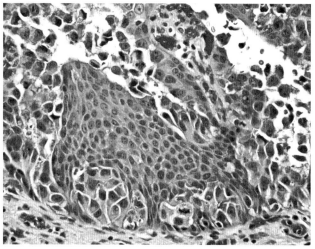

Figure 2.11.2 Intraepithelial spread of bladder urothelial carcinoma into the cervix. Same case as in *Figure 2.11.1*, higher magnification. Cell nests and individual cells with cytologic atypia within bland-appearing squamous epithelium.

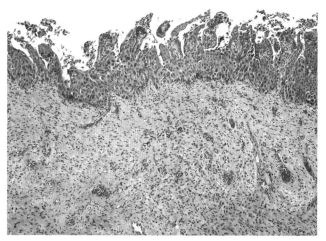

Figure 2.11.3 Intraepithelial spread of bladder urothelial carcinoma into the cervix. Epithelial disruption and pseudopapillary appearance.

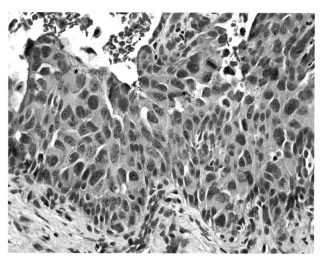

Figure 2.11.4 Intraepithelial spread of bladder urothelial carcinoma into the cervix. Same case as in *Figure 2.11.1*, higher magnification. Cells with enlarged atypical nuclei and moderate amount of eosinophilic cytoplasm can mimic HSIL. Basal layer nuclei are small and uniform. Compare to *Figure 2.11.8*.

2 CERVIX

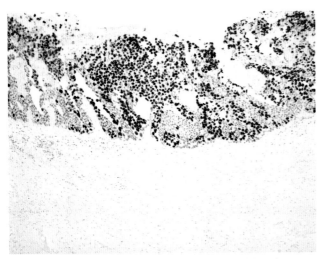

Figure 2.11.5   Intraepithelial spread of bladder urothelial carcinoma into the cervix. Same area as in *Figure 2.11.1*. Immunohistochemical stain for GATA-3 with strong nuclear labeling of urothelial cells. Background keratinocytes display weak staining.

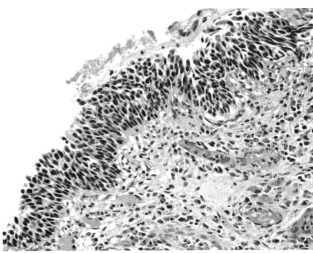

Figure 2.11.6   High-grade squamous intraepithelial lesion (HSIL). Hyperchromatic epithelium composed of uniform cell population displays some distortion on the surface.

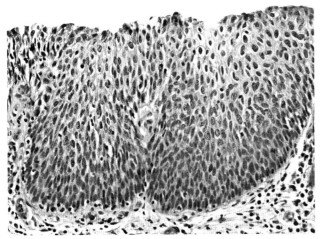

Figure 2.11.7   High-grade squamous intraepithelial lesion (HSIL). Markedly thickened atypical epithelium with immature cells occupying 2/3 of the epithelial thickness. Some epithelial maturation is preserved on the surface.

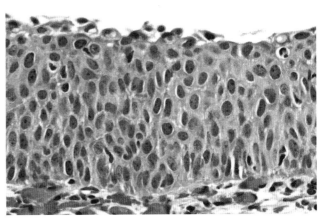

Figure 2.11.8   High-grade squamous intraepithelial lesion (HSIL). Full-thickness epithelial immaturity and atypia including basal layer.

	HPV-Related Endocervical Adenocarcinoma *In Situ*	**Tuboendometrioid Metaplasia**
Age	Reproductive-age women, median age 39 y	Reproductive-age women, occasionally postmenopausal
Location	Endocervix	Endocervix
Symptoms	Often asymptomatic, can present with vaginal bleeding or discharge	Asymptomatic
Signs	Usually microscopic, abnormal Pap/AGUS	Usually microscopic; can form small polypoid lesion
Etiology	High-risk HPV, most commonly types 16 and 18	Hormonal stimulation (pregnancy, oral contraceptives, hormone replacement therapy)
Histology	1. Hyperchromatic glands in a distribution of normal endocervical glands *(Fig. 2.12.1)* 2. Partial gland involvement with a sharp transition from lesional to normal epithelium *(Figs. 2.12.2 and 2.12.3)* 3. Variable cytoplasmic mucinous change, goblet cell differentiation can be seen *(Fig. 2.12.4)*; cilia are generally not seen 4. Hyperchromatic nuclei with pseudostratification *(Fig. 2.12.5)* 5. Frequent apoptotic bodies 6. Frequent mitotic figures, commonly in the apical portion of the cytoplasm *(Fig. 2.12.5)*	1. Hyperchromatic glands in cervical stroma in distribution of normal endocervical glands *(Fig. 2.12.6)* 2. Usually involves entire gland *(Figs. 2.12.7 and 2.12.8)* 3. Columnar cells with cell types recapitulating fallopian tube epithelium; ciliated cells *(Figs. 2.12.9 and 2.12.10)* 4. Bland nuclear features 5. Apoptotic bodies are not seen 6. Mitoses are rare
Special studies	• p16 strong, diffuse • Loss or decrease in ER and PR expression • Increased Ki-67 proliferative activity	• p16 patchy, often extensive • Generally retained ER/PR expression • Mild increase in Ki-67 labeling can be seen
Treatment	Cervical excision to achieve negative margins and rule out invasive carcinoma in women desiring preservation of fertility or simple hysterectomy	None required
Prognosis	Can progress to invasive endocervical adenocarcinoma	Benign/nonneoplastic

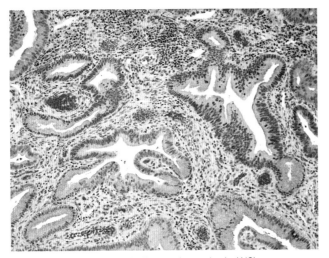

Figure 2.12.1   Endocervical adenocarcinoma *in situ* (AIS). Hyperchromatic endocervical glands within endocervical mucosa are admixed with normal glands.

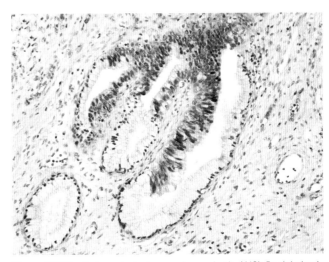

Figure 2.12.2   Endocervical adenocarcinoma *in situ* (AIS). Partial gland involvement with abrupt transition from lesional to normal epithelium. Enlarged hyperchromatic pseudostratified nuclei and occasional apoptotic bodies in AIS.

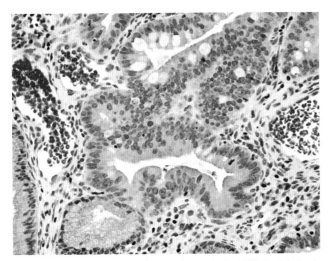

Figure 2.12.3   Endocervical adenocarcinoma *in situ* (AIS). Partial gland involvement. Remaining portion of normal gland **(lower left)** and AIS with occasional mitotic figure and focal goblet cell differentiation **(top)**.

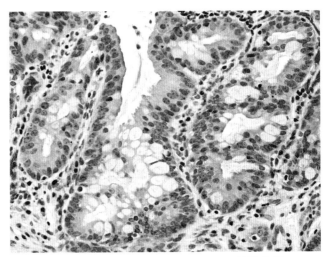

Figure 2.12.4   Endocervical adenocarcinoma *in situ* (AIS). Goblet cell differentiation. The nuclei are relatively bland with some pseudostratification.

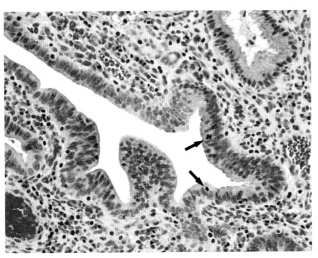

Figure 2.12.5   Endocervical adenocarcinoma *in situ* (AIS). Hyperchromatic pseudostratified nuclei with apical mitoses (*arrows*). Compare to *Figure 2.12.9*.

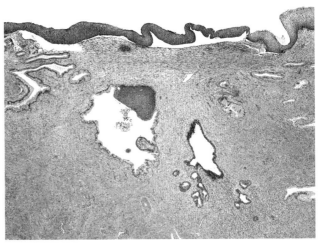

Figure 2.12.6   Tuboendometrioid metaplasia. Cervical conization with HSIL with focal endocervical gland involvement. Focus of hyperchromatic glands **(off-center to the right)**.

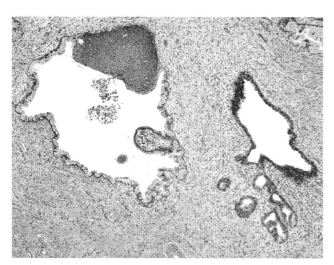

Figure 2.12.7   Tuboendometrioid metaplasia. Same case as in *Figure 2.12.6*, higher magnification. Hyperchromatic epithelium involving entire gland **(right)**. Compare to pale normal endocervical epithelium in the gland to the **left** focally involved by HSIL.

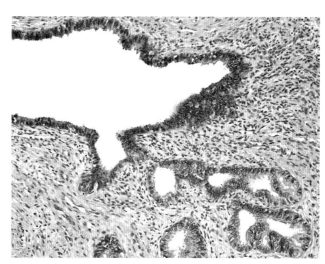

Figure 2.12.8   Tuboendometrioid metaplasia. Same case as in *Figure 2.12.1*, higher magnification.

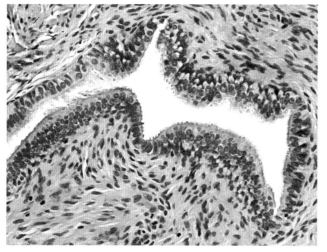

Figure 2.12.9   Tuboendometrioid metaplasia. Tall columnar epithelium is tangentially oriented in some areas creating pseudostratified appearance. Note prominent cilia and lack of mitoses.

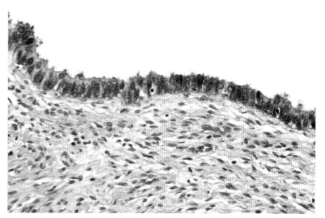

Figure 2.12.10   Tuboendometrioid metaplasia. Same case as in *Figure 2.12.8*, higher magnification. Tall columnar epithelium recapitulates cell types seen in the fallopian tube. Ciliated cells are present.

	Florid Adenocarcinoma *In Situ* (AIS, HPV-Related)	HPV-Related Invasive Well-Differentiated Adenocarcinoma of Usual Type With AIS-Like Pattern/Silva Pattern A
Age	Reproductive-age women, median age 39 y	Mean age 40-42 y
Location	Endocervix	Cervix, transformation zone, endocervical canal
Symptoms	Often asymptomatic, or vaginal bleeding, discharge	Vaginal bleeding, discharge
Signs	Usually microscopic, abnormal Pap/AGUS	Abnormal Pap, often no clinically visible lesion, or cervical mass
Etiology	High-risk HPV, most commonly types 16 and 18	High-risk HPV, adenocarcinoma *in situ* is a precursor
Histology	1. Hyperchromatic glands in a distribution of normal endocervical glands *(Figs. 2.13.1-2.13.4)* 2. Partial gland involvement with a sharp transition from lesional to normal epithelium *(Figs. 2.13.1 and 2.13.4)* 3. Normal glands and AIS rarely approach thick-walled vessels 4. Equivocal cases can be encountered *(Fig. 2.13.5)*	1. Complex glandular proliferation extending from mucosa/superficial stroma into deeper layers of cervical wall *(Fig. 2.13.6)*; background AIS can be seen *(Fig. 2.13.7)* 2. Markedly crowded glands with cribriforming in lobulated arrangement *(Figs. 2.13.7-2.13.10)*; foci of lesional glands beneath the ectocervical squamous epithelium *(Figs. 2.13.7 and 2.13.9)* 3. Neoplastic glands within near proximity of thick-walled vessels *(Fig. 2.13.11)*
Special studies	Not helpful in this differential	Not helpful in this differential
Treatment	Cervical conization to achieve negative margins and rule out invasive carcinoma in women desiring preservation of fertility or simple hysterectomy	Cervical conization with negative margins or trachelectomy in women desiring preservation of fertility, or hysterectomy +/− pelvic lymphadenectomy
Prognosis	Can recur after excision with negative margins	Recurrences are rare, but follow-up is required, particularly for cases treated with conservative excision

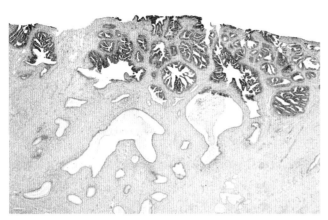

Figure 2.13.1   Florid endocervical adenocarcinoma *in situ* (AIS) involving superficial mucosa. Some glands are partially involved. The overall distribution is consistent with preexisting endocervical glands.

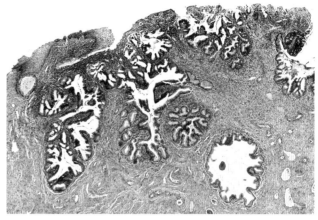

Figure 2.13.2   Florid endocervical adenocarcinoma *in situ* (AIS). Large hyperchromatic glands with intraglandular infoldings involved by AIS. Note normal endocervical gland with similar configuration **(lower right)**.

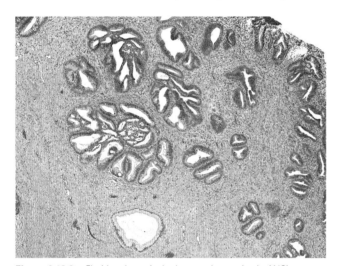

Figure 2.13.3   Florid endocervical adenocarcinoma *in situ* (AIS). Hyperchromatic glands in clusters; the gland distribution resembles that of normal endocervical glands.

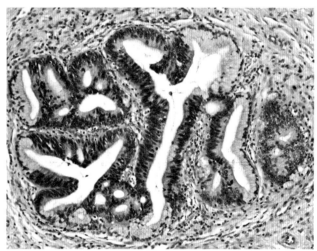

Figure 2.13.4   Florid endocervical adenocarcinoma *in situ* (AIS), higher magnification. Partial gland involvement confirms the diagnosis of AIS (absence of invasion).

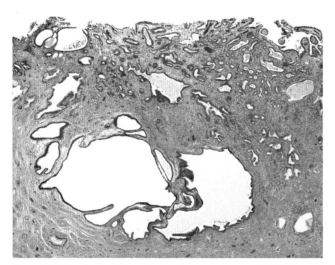

Figure 2.13.5   Equivocal case; some observers may consider this at least florid endocervical adenocarcinoma *in situ* (AIS), others would interpret it as invasive adenocarcinoma, pattern A. Extensive proliferation of hyperchromatic glands with adjacent normal endocervical glands of similar shapes and sizes. There is no unequivocal evidence of destructive stromal invasion.

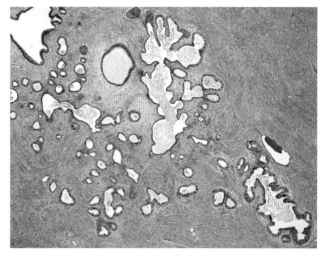

Figure 2.13.6   Invasive well-differentiated adenocarcinoma of usual type with AIS-like pattern. Simple glands extend into cervical stroma in a wedge-like focus. No normal endocervical glands are seen in the vicinity. This subtle pattern of invasion can only be appreciated at low magnification.

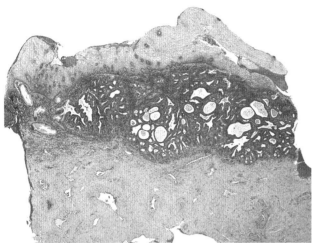

Figure 2.13.7   Invasive well-differentiated adenocarcinoma of usual type with AIS-like pattern. Lobular proliferation of complex/crowded glands beneath the ectocervical mucosa.

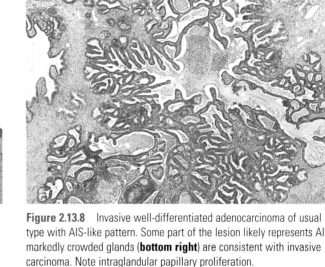

Figure 2.13.8   Invasive well-differentiated adenocarcinoma of usual type with AIS-like pattern. Some part of the lesion likely represents AIS; markedly crowded glands (**bottom right**) are consistent with invasive carcinoma. Note intraglandular papillary proliferation.

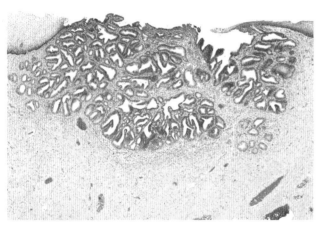

Figure 2.13.9   Invasive well-differentiated adenocarcinoma of usual type with AIS-like pattern. Disrupted ectocervical mucosa with complex proliferation of small- and medium-sized glands. The depth of proliferation, degree of glandular crowding, slight haphazard orientation of glands, variation in size and shape of the glands, and inflammatory reaction at the base of the proliferation support interpretation as invasion; however, this pattern of invasion can be associated with various levels of interobserver disagreement.

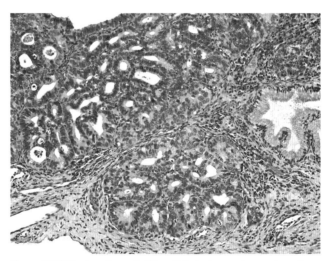

Figure 2.13.10   Invasive well-differentiated adenocarcinoma of usual type with AIS-like pattern. Crowded back-to-back glands are consistent with stromal invasion. Note size and shape of normal endocervical gland **(right)**.

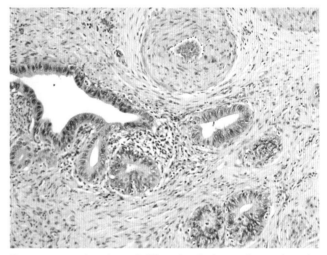

Figure 2.13.11   Invasive well-differentiated adenocarcinoma of usual type with AIS-like pattern. Simple glands without associated stromal reaction near a thick-walled vessel.

	HPV-Related Endocervical Adenocarcinoma	**Microglandular Hyperplasia**
Age	Mean age 40-42 y	Reproductive-age women
Location	Cervix, transformation zone, endocervical canal	Cervix, transformation zone, endocervix
Symptoms	Vaginal bleeding, discharge, pelvic pain	Usually asymptomatic, vaginal bleeding in cases involving endocervical polyp
Signs	Abnormal Pap, no clinically visible lesion, or cervical mass, barrel cervix	Endocervical polyp or small friable mass
Etiology	High-risk HPV, adenocarcinoma *in situ* is a precursor	Associated with progestins exposure (pregnancy or exogenous)
Histology	1. Cribriform and papillary/villoglandular proliferation *(Figs. 2.14.1-2.14.3)* 2. Adjacent HSIL or adenosquamous carcinoma components can be present 3. Columnar cells with variable amount of mucinous cytoplasm 4. Ovoid to elongated nuclei with hyperchromasia or fine chromatin; pseudostratification is common *(Figs. 2.14.4-2.14.6)* 5. Frequent mitotic figures, particularly in the apical portion of the cytoplasm *(Figs. 2.14.4 and 2.14.5)*; apoptotic bodies are seen 6. Inflammation can be present but not a constant feature; stromal desmoplasia can be seen	1. Closely packed glands in cribriform arrangement; intraglandular papillary infoldings can be seen *(Figs. 2.14.8-2.14.12)* 2. Reserve cell hyperplasia or squamous metaplasia can undermine glandular epithelium *(Fig. 2.14.8)* 3. Cuboidal to low columnar cells with cytoplasmic vacuoles *(Figs. 2.14.11 and 2.14.12)* 4. Small, uniform round to ovoid nuclei; small nucleoli can be seen 5. Mitoses are rare; cases with increased mitotic activity have been described (immunohistochemical workup is warranted in latter); apoptotic bodies are not common 6. Acute and chronic inflammatory infiltrate in the stroma and epithelium is usually present; stromal hyalinization can be seen
Special studies	• Diffuse expression of p16 *(Fig. 2.14.7,* **left***)* • Markedly increased Ki-67 proliferative activity *(Fig. 2.14.7,* **right***)* • High-risk HPV detected by *in situ* hybridization	• Patchy/focal expression of p16 • Mild increase in Ki-67 proliferative activity (positive inflammatory cells may create false impression of increased labeling) • No high-risk HPV detected by *in situ* hybridization
Treatment	Stage dependent; trachelectomy can be considered as fertility-sparing option in early stage; hysterectomy or chemotherapy and radiation therapy	Usually not required; for symptomatic cases, biopsy/polypectomy is generally curative
Prognosis	Stage dependent; recurrences can occur in stage IA1 cases treated with cold knife conization	Benign

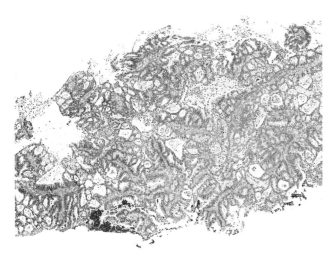

Figure 2.14.1   Endocervical adenocarcinoma. Endocervical curettage. Florid, pale epithelial proliferation with cribriform architecture.

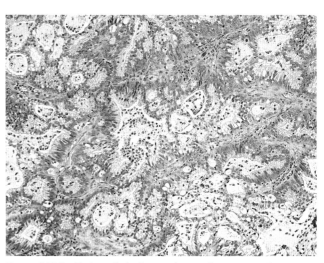

Figure 2.14.2   Endocervical adenocarcinoma. Same case as in *Figure 2.14.1*, higher magnification. Some cases can have associated inflammation.

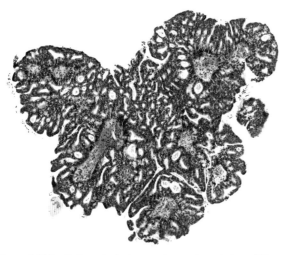

Figure 2.14.3   Endocervical adenocarcinoma. Densely basophilic fragment of glandular proliferation with cribriform architecture.

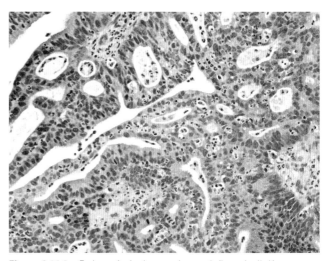

Figure 2.14.4   Endocervical adenocarcinoma. Inflamed cribriform glandular proliferation. Note mitoses and apoptotic bodies in addition to intraepithelial neutrophils.

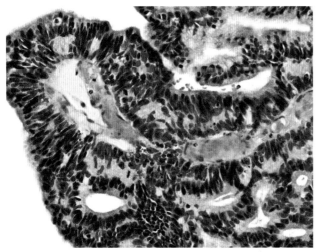

Figure 2.14.5   Endocervical adenocarcinoma. Same case as in *Figure 2.14.3*, higher magnification. Columnar cells with pseudostratified nuclei and mitotic figures.

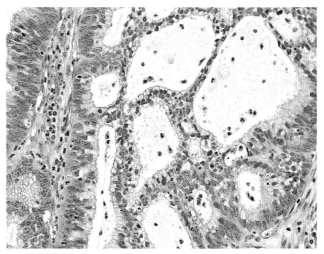

Figure 2.14.6   Endocervical adenocarcinoma. Columnar to cuboidal cells; some mucinous cytoplasm appears clear. Nuclear atypia, multiple nucleoli, and apoptotic bodies.

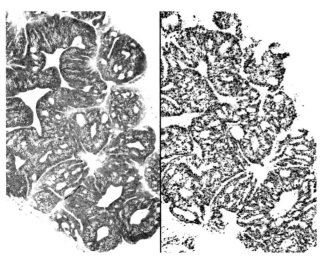

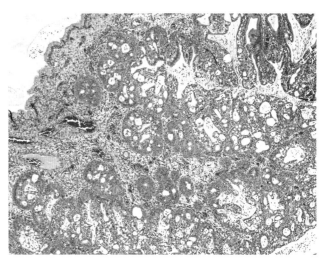

Figure 2.14.7 Endocervical adenocarcinoma. Same case as in *Figure 2.14.1*. Diffuse expression of p16 **(left)** and markedly elevated Ki-67 proliferative activity **(right)**.

Figure 2.14.8 Microglandular hyperplasia. Complex glandular proliferation with cribriform architecture and prominent reserve cell layers/early squamous metaplasia.

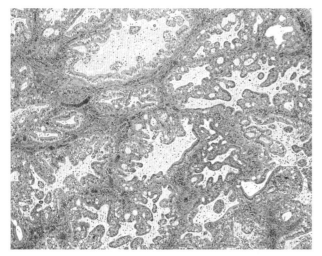

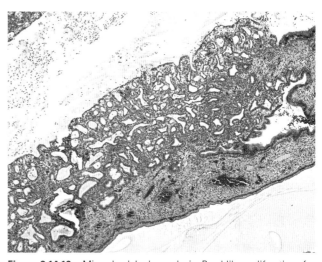

Figure 2.14.9 Microglandular hyperplasia. Endocervical polyp; crowded glands with intraluminal papillary infoldings and foci of cribriform growth.

Figure 2.14.10 Microglandular hyperplasia. Band-like proliferation of crowded small glands of varying shapes.

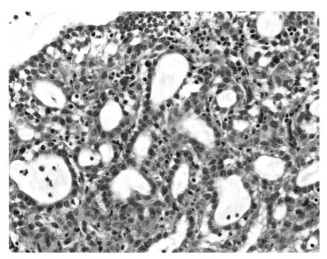

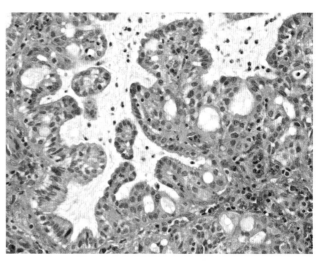

Figure 2.14.11 Microglandular hyperplasia. Same case as in *Figure 2.14.10*, higher magnification. Cuboidal cells with uniform round nuclei and vacuolated cytoplasm; mitoses are absent.

Figure 2.14.12 Microglandular hyperplasia. Same case as in *Figure 2.14.9*, higher magnification. Intraglandular papillary projections; monotonous cells with bland nuclei and lack of mitoses.

2.15

HPV-INDEPENDENT ENDOCERVICAL ADENOCARCINOMA (INCLUDING MINIMAL DEVIATION ADENOCARCINOMA/GASTRIC-TYPE ADENOCARCINOMA) VS LOBULAR ENDOCERVICAL GLANDULAR HYPERPLASIA (LEGH)

	HPV-Independent Endocervical Adenocarcinoma (Including Minimal Deviation Adenocarcinoma/Gastric-Type Adenocarcinoma)	Lobular Endocervical Glandular Hyperplasia (LEGH)
Age	Reproductive-age and postmenopausal women; mean age 50-55 y	Reproductive-age women
Location	Cervix	Cervix
Symptoms	Often asymptomatic; some present with bleeding, vaginal discharge, pain	Usually asymptomatic; vaginal discharge, bleeding can be present
Signs	None; or mass-forming lesion, barrel cervix	Often none; occasionally can present as mass-forming lesion; cystic changes on imaging
Etiology	Unknown; can be associated with Peutz-Jeghers syndrome; some cases harbor *TP53* mutations *STK11* mutations have been described	Idiopathic; can be associated with Peutz-Jeghers syndrome; LEGH has been proposed as a precursor of MDA
Histology	1. Irregular glands invade cervical stroma; lobular architecture is not seen 2. Infiltrative growth pattern *(Figs. 2.15.1 and 2.15.2)* 3. Glandular proliferation can extend into deep cervical stroma *(Fig. 2.15.3)* 4. Variably sized angulated glands *(Fig. 2.15.4)* 5. Glands can have mucinous (gastric-type) epithelium 6. Cytologic atypia is often minimal *(Fig. 2.15.5)* but usually present at least focally; nuclei are frequently slightly enlarged, round, and have pale/fine chromatin with evident nucleoli 7. Mitotic figures are uncommon but can be seen	1. Increased number of crowded endocervical glands in lobular arrangement *(Fig. 2.15.6)* 2. Lobules with rounded outlines are demarcated from the surrounding cervical stroma *(Fig. 2.15.7)* 3. Proliferation is confined to superficial and midcervical stroma 4. Variably sized glands, some cystically dilated *(Fig. 2.15.8)* 5. Glands have prominent mucinous cytoplasm or occasionally attenuated lining *(Figs. 2.15.9 and 2.15.10)* 6. Minimal or absent cytologic atypia *(Figs. 2.15.9 and 2.15.10)*; atypical forms of LEGH have been described 7. Mitotic figures are generally absent
Special studies	• Loss of PAX2 expression • Reported lack of ER and PR expression • Elevated Ki-67 labeling, may be mild • Aberrant p53 in a subset of cases	• Preserved PAX2 expression is reported • ER/PR is occasionally lost in benign endocervical glandular proliferations • No significant increase in Ki-67 labeling • No aberrant p53 patterns (wild-type pattern)
Treatment	Stage dependent; surgery, chemotherapy, and radiation therapy	None required; usually an incidental finding in the hysterectomy performed for other reasons
Prognosis	Aggressive course; pelvic and intra-abdominal recurrences are common and usually lead to death. Overall survival is <30%	Benign; some cases are associated with minimal deviation adenocarcinoma and Peutz-Jeghers syndrome

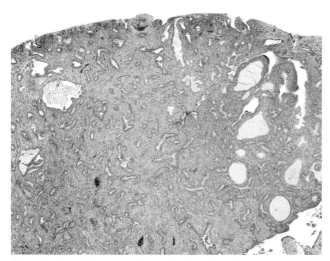

Figure 2.15.1   Adenoma malignum (minimal deviation adenocarcinoma). Diffuse infiltrative growth within superficial and deep cervical stroma.

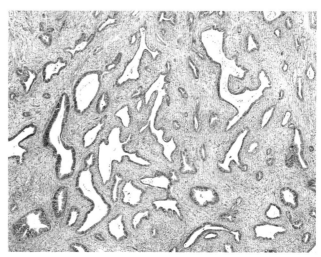

Figure 2.15.2   Adenoma malignum (minimal deviation adenocarcinoma). Irregular, angulated, and variably shaped glands infiltrating stroma. Note lack of overt stromal response.

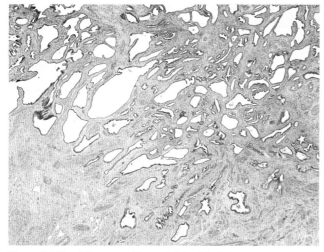

Figure 2.15.3   Adenoma malignum (minimal deviation adenocarcinoma). Deep aspect of the tumor; irregular infiltrating outline.

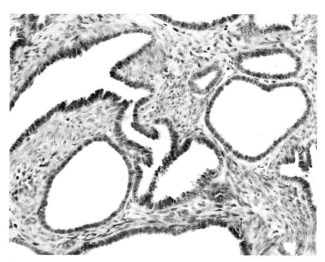

Figure 2.15.4   Adenoma malignum (minimal deviation adenocarcinoma). Same case as in *Figure 2.15.2*, higher magnification. Irregular glands lined by bland uniform nuclei.

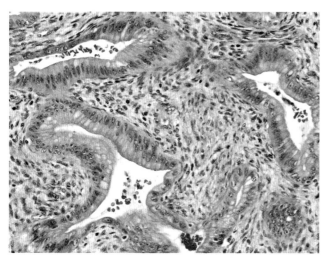

Figure 2.15.5   Adenoma malignum (minimal deviation adenocarcinoma). Same case as in *Figure 2.15.1*, higher magnification. Angulated glands lined by mildly atypical mucinous epithelium.

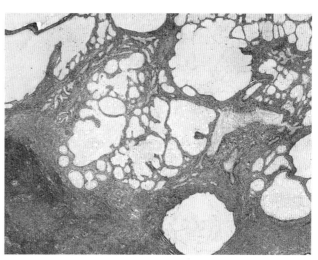

Figure 2.15.6   Lobular endocervical glandular hyperplasia. Significantly increased number of endocervical glands in lobular arrangement.

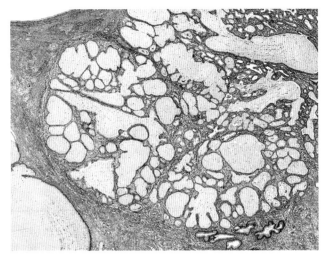

Figure 2.15.7   Lobular endocervical glandular hyperplasia. Rounded outline of the large lobule situated within superficial and midcervical stroma.

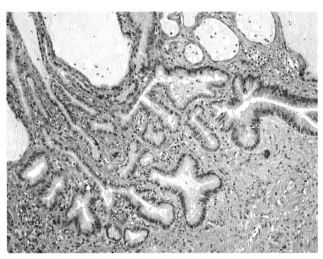

Figure 2.15.8   Lobular endocervical glandular hyperplasia. Cystically dilated and small glands within the lobule.

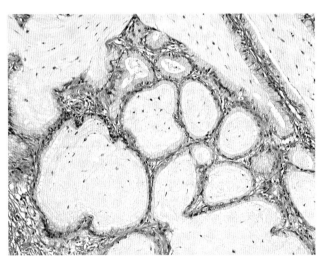

Figure 2.15.9   Lobular endocervical glandular hyperplasia. Same case as in *Figure 2.15.8*, higher magnification. Cystically dilated glands lined by attenuated bland mucinous epithelium.

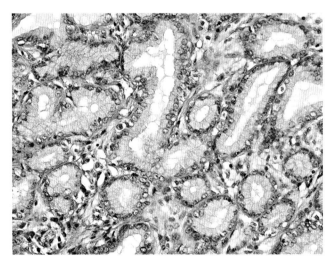

Figure 2.15.10   Lobular endocervical glandular hyperplasia. Same case as in *Figure 2.15.8*, higher magnification, different area. Small crowded glands with bland mucinous lining.

	HPV-Independent Endocervical Adenocarcinoma (Including Minimal Deviation Adenocarcinoma/Gastric-Type Adenocarcinoma)	HPV-Related Endocervical Adenocarcinoma, Mucinous Type
Age	Reproductive-age and postmenopausal women; mean age 50-55 y	Mean age 40-42 y
Location	Cervix	Cervix, transformation zone, endocervical canal
Symptoms	Often asymptomatic; some present with bleeding, vaginal discharge, pain	Vaginal bleeding, discharge, pelvic pain
Signs	None; or mass-forming lesion, barrel cervix	Abnormal Pap, no clinically visible lesion, or cervical mass, barrel cervix
Etiology	Unknown; can be associated with Peutz-Jeghers syndrome/STK11 mutations; some cases harbor TP53 mutations	High-risk HPV, adenocarcinoma *in situ* (AIS) is a precursor
Histology	1. Glandular proliferation with infiltrative growth pattern invading cervical stroma; solid growth is not typical (Figs. 2.16.1 and 2.16.2) 2. Stromal desmoplasia can be present but is often limited 3. Abundant pale or eosinophilic cytoplasm (Fig. 2.16.3) 4. Cytologic atypia is variable within and between cases (Figs. 2.16.4 and 2.16.5) 5. Nucleoli can be present (Fig. 2.16.6) 6. Mitotic figures are not very conspicuous but can be seen	1. Complex glandular proliferation with infiltrative pattern, destructive and nondestructive stromal invasion, vaguely lobulated areas and solid growth can be seen (Figs. 2.16.7-2.16.9) 2. Variable degree of stromal desmoplasia 3. Usually bluish cytoplasmic mucin in cases with mucinous differentiation (Fig. 2.16.10) 4. Generally relatively uniform cytologic features within the tumor (Fig. 2.16.11) 5. Nucleoli are not typical 6. Apical mitotic figures and apoptotic bodies are common (Fig. 2.16.12)
Special studies	• p16 is usually patchy or negative; rare cases may show overexpression • Aberrant p53 pattern in a subset of cases • Elevated Ki-67 labeling, may be mild • No HR HPV by *in situ* hybridization	• Strong and diffuse expression of p16 • Usually, no aberrant p53 (wild-type pattern) • Elevated Ki-67 labeling • HR HPV detected by *in situ* hybridization
Treatment	Stage dependent; surgery, chemotherapy, and radiation therapy	Stage dependent; trachelectomy can be considered as fertility-sparing option in early stage; hysterectomy or chemotherapy and radiation therapy
Prognosis	Aggressive course; pelvic and intra-abdominal recurrences are common and usually lead to death. Overall survival is <30%	Stage dependent; recurrences can occur in stage IA1 cases treated with cold knife conization

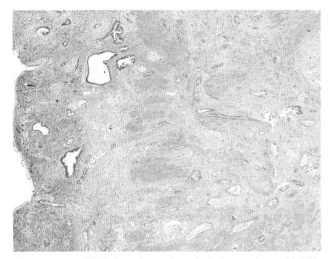

Figure 2.16.1 HPV-independent endocervical adenocarcinoma. Variably sized and shaped glands infiltrating cervical stroma.

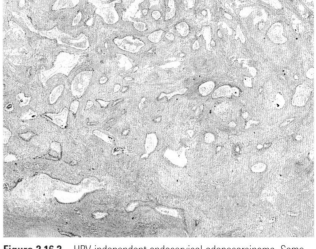

Figure 2.16.2 HPV-independent endocervical adenocarcinoma. Same case as in *Figure 2.16.1*. Deep edge of the tumor.

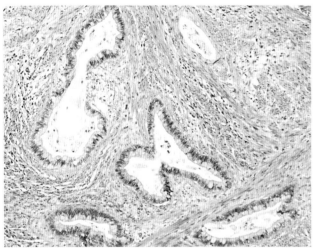

Figure 2.16.3 HPV-independent endocervical adenocarcinoma. Same case as in *Figure 2.16.1*. Irregularly shaped glands with pale/eosinophilic cytoplasm.

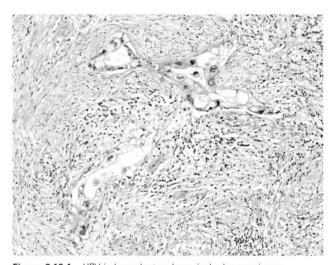

Figure 2.16.4 HPV-independent endocervical adenocarcinoma. Malignant glands with foamy cytoplasm and marked nuclear atypia.

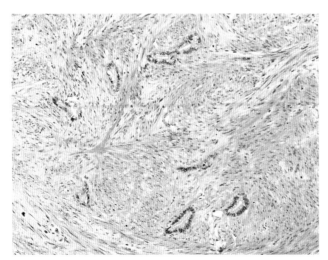

Figure 2.16.5 HPV-independent endocervical adenocarcinoma. Same case as in *Figure 2.16.4*. Some areas of tumor display glands deep in the cervical stroma with minimal atypia; note the contrast with cytologic features in *Figure 2.16.4*.

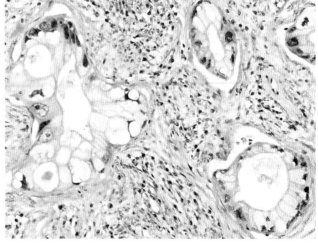

Figure 2.16.6 HPV-independent endocervical adenocarcinoma. Marked cytologic atypia, pleomorphism and notable nucleoli.

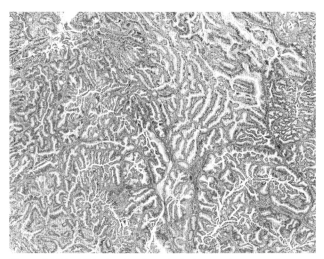

Figure 2.16.7   HPV-related endocervical adenocarcinoma, mucinous type. Densely packed glands within the stroma.

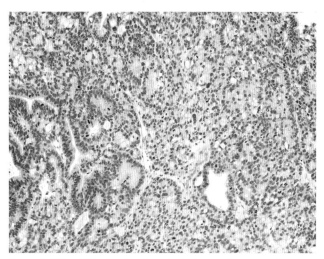

Figure 2.16.8   HPV-related endocervical adenocarcinoma, mucinous type. Solid pattern of growth with mucinous/goblet cell differentiation.

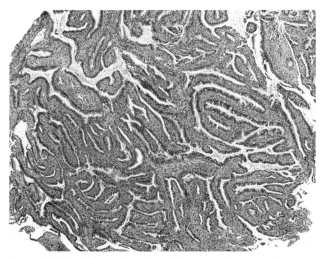

Figure 2.16.9   HPV-related endocervical adenocarcinoma, mucinous type. Maze-like, infiltrating glands.

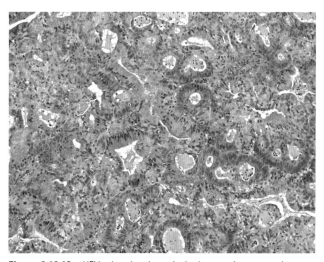

Figure 2.16.10   HPV-related endocervical adenocarcinoma, mucinous type. Complex glandular growth with cribriform arrangement and bluish cytoplasmic mucin.

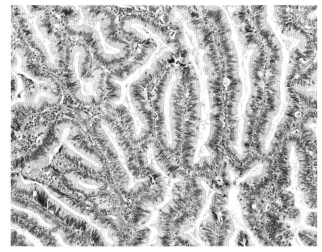

Figure 2.16.11   HPV-related endocervical adenocarcinoma, mucinous type. Same case as in *Figure 2.16.7*, higher magnification. Uniform morphologic features throughout the tumor.

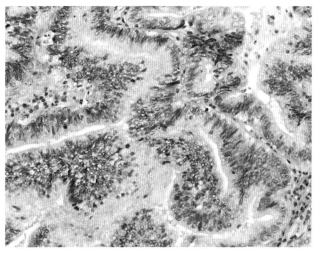

Figure 2.16.12   HPV-related endocervical adenocarcinoma, mucinous type. Mucinous glands with apical mitotic figures and occasional apoptotic bodies.

	Secondary Cervical Involvement by Endometrial Carcinoma: Cervical Stromal Invasion	Confinement to Endocervical Mucosa
Age	Same age distribution as for respective endometrial carcinoma subtypes	Same age distribution as for respective endometrial carcinoma subtypes
Location	Cervix	Cervix
Symptoms	Vaginal bleeding	Vaginal bleeding
Signs	Cervical mass in some cases, myometrial mass/lower uterine segment mass; associated with higher-grade, deep myometrial invasion, and angiolymphatic invasion	Myometrial/lower uterine segment mass
Etiology	Same as for the respective endometrial carcinoma subtypes	Same as for the respective endometrial carcinoma subtypes
Histology	1. Haphazard infiltrative growth (Figs. 2.17.1 and 2.17.2) 2. Varying depth of cervical stromal invasion including deep cervical stroma 3. Contiguous spread from deep myometrium, sparing superficial cervical wall, can be seen (Fig. 2.17.3) 4. Irregular glandular outlines, extensive papillary architecture, large areas of cribriform, and solid growth can be seen	1. Lesional glandular epithelium follows pattern of distribution of normal endocervical glands 2. Usually confined to superficial mucosa (Figs. 2.17.4 and 2.17.5) 3. Neoplastic glands are not present below the level of normal endocervical glands (Fig. 2.17.6) 4. Rounded outlines of the glands (Fig. 2.17.6); some intraglandular papillary formations or cribriforming can be seen
Special studies	Not helpful in this differential diagnosis	Not helpful in this differential diagnosis
Treatment	Addition of vaginal brachytherapy and/or pelvic radiation and chemotherapy depending on the tumor grade	Stage dependent; endocervical gland involvement doesn't alter the stage
Prognosis	The 5-y survival for women with stage II endometrial cancer is 69%	Same as for stage I endometrial carcinoma; 5-y survival is 88%

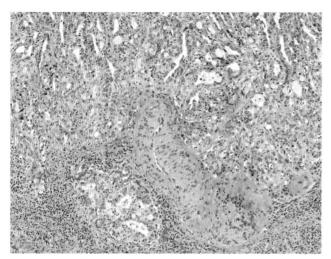

Figure 2.17.1   Secondary involvement by endometrial carcinoma: cervical stromal invasion. Markedly crowded glands invading stroma around a thick-walled vessel.

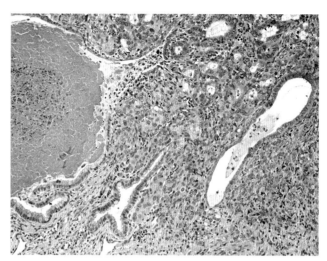

Figure 2.17.2   Secondary involvement by endometrial carcinoma: cervical stromal invasion. Small crowded glands infiltrate stroma between normal endocervical glands.

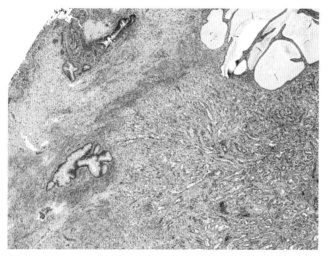

Figure 2.17.3   Secondary involvement by endometrial carcinoma: cervical stromal invasion. Invasive tumor front extends from the uterine corpus into deep cervical stroma. Superficial cervical mucosa is spared.

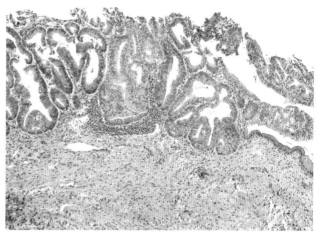

Figure 2.17.4   Secondary involvement by endometrial carcinoma: endocervical gland involvement. Rounded outlines of involved glands. Normal endocervical mucosa is focally seen on the **right**.

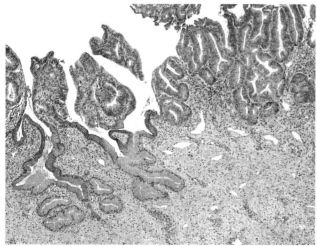

Figure 2.17.5   Secondary involvement by endometrial carcinoma: endocervical gland involvement. Superficial endocervical glandular epithelium is replaced by endometrioid carcinoma. Endocervical glands extending into superficial stroma are uninvolved.

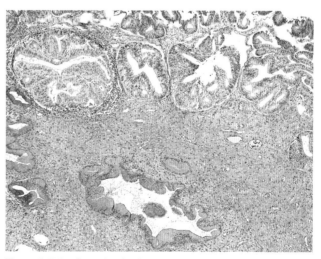

Figure 2.17.6   Secondary involvement by endometrial carcinoma: endocervical gland involvement. Rounded nests of tumor with small foci of cribriform growth within superficial endocervical mucosa.

	HPV-Related Invasive Endocervical Adenocarcinoma of Usual Type	Secondary Cervical Involvement by Endometrial Endometrioid Carcinoma, FIGO Grade 1
Age	Mean age 40-42 y	Wide age range, mean age is 63 y
Location	Cervix, transformation zone, endocervical canal	Cervical mucosa and stroma
Symptoms	Vaginal bleeding, discharge, pelvic pain	Abnormal vaginal bleeding; pelvic pain or pressure and abdominal distension in advanced cases
Signs	Abnormal Pap, no clinically visible lesion, or cervical mass, barrel cervix	Noncyclical vaginal bleeding, constitutional symptoms: obesity, diabetes, PCOS; thickened endometrial stripe or endometrial or cervical mass on MRI or sonography; abnormal Pap smear; cervical mass on examination
Etiology	High-risk HPV, adenocarcinoma *in situ* is a precursor	Unopposed estrogenic stimulation; somatic mutations in *PTEN, PIK3CA, KRAS, CTNNB1, ARID1A*; hereditary syndromes, Lynch and Cowden syndromes
Gross findings and histology	1. Cervical mass or no gross lesion 2. Complex glandular proliferation extending from mucosa/superficial stroma into deeper layers of cervical wall; background precursor lesion (AIS) can be seen *(Fig. 2.18.1)* 3. Markedly crowded glands with cribriforming in lobulated arrangement or diffuse infiltrative growth *(Figs. 2.18.2-2.18.4)* 4. Columnar cells with variable amount of mucinous cytoplasm; ovoid to elongated nuclei with hyperchromasia or fine chromatin; pseudostratification is common 5. Frequent mitotic figures, particularly in the apical portion of the cytoplasm and apoptotic bodies *(Figs. 2.18.5 and 2.18.6)*	1. Mass in the uterine corpus or lower uterine segment 2. Glandular proliferation involving endocervical mucosa and/or cervical stroma *(Figs. 2.18.7-2.18.9)*; contiguous spread from deep myometrium, sparing superficial cervical wall, can be seen 3. Variably sized/shaped glands lined by columnar cells *(Fig. 2.18.10)*; cribriform and solid growth, papillary architecture can be seen 4. Round to ovoid nuclei; pseudostratification can be seen *(Fig. 2.18.11)* 5. Mitotic activity is variable; apoptotic bodies are not common
Special studies	• Diffuse expression of p16 • Decreased or lost ER/PR expression • High-risk HPV detected by *in situ* hybridization	• Patchy/focal expression of p16 *(Fig. 2.18.12,* **left***)* • Usually strong and diffuse ER/PR expression *(Fig. 2.18.12,* **right***)* • No high-risk HPV detected by *in situ* hybridization
Treatment	Stage dependent; hysterectomy or chemotherapy and radiation therapy	Hysterectomy with bilateral salpingo-oophorectomy, pelvic and periaortic lymphadenectomy; vaginal cuff radiation +/− chemotherapy
Prognosis	Stage dependent	5-y survival for stage II tumors is 69%

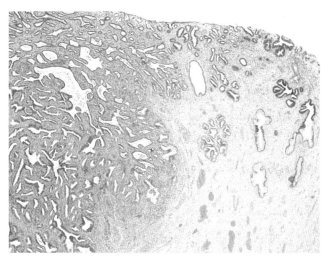

Figure 2.18.1   Invasive endocervical adenocarcinoma of usual type. Proliferation of irregular infiltrating glands extending from superficial mucosa into cervical stroma. Adenocarcinoma *in situ* is seen in the background **(right)**.

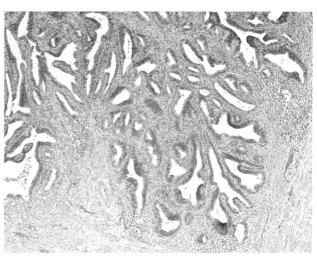

Figure 2.18.2   Invasive endocervical adenocarcinoma of usual type. Irregular angulated glands infiltrating cervical stroma.

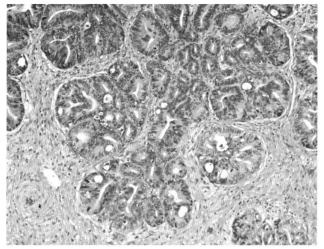

Figure 2.18.3   Invasive endocervical adenocarcinoma of usual type. Crowded glands with lobulated arrangement deep in the cervical stroma.

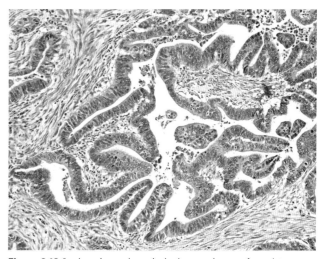

Figure 2.18.4   Invasive endocervical adenocarcinoma of usual type. Irregularly shaped glands with intraglandular papillary infoldings.

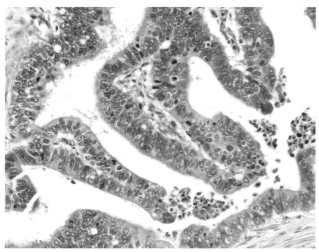

Figure 2.18.5   Invasive endocervical adenocarcinoma of usual type. Same case as in *Figure 2.18.4*, higher magnification. Note multiple mitoses.

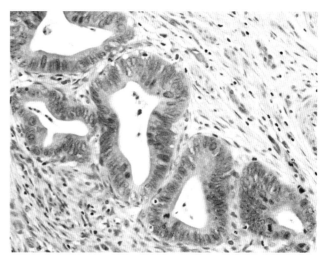

Figure 2.18.6   Invasive endocervical adenocarcinoma of usual type. Same case as in *Figure 2.18.1*, higher magnification. Irregularly shaped glands with apical mitotic figures and occasional apoptotic bodies.

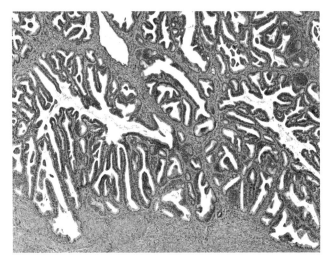

Figure 2.18.7   Secondary involvement of the cervix by endometrial endometrioid adenocarcinoma, FIGO grade 1. Irregularly shaped glands infiltrating deep cervical stroma.

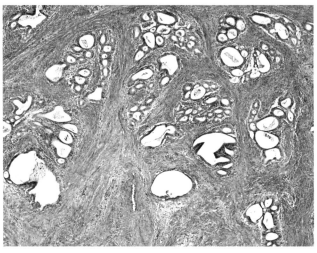

Figure 2.18.8   Secondary involvement of the cervix by endometrial endometrioid adenocarcinoma, FIGO grade 1. Tumor nests with cribriform growth deep in the cervical stroma.

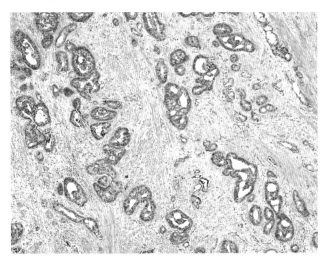

Figure 2.18.9   Secondary involvement of the cervix by endometrial endometrioid adenocarcinoma, FIGO grade 1. Small cribriform nests and individual glands.

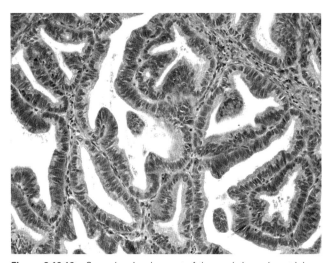

Figure 2.18.10   Secondary involvement of the cervix by endometrial endometrioid adenocarcinoma, FIGO grade 1. Same case as in *Figure 2.18.7*, higher magnification. Irregularly shaped glands lined by columnar cells; no notable mitotic activity or apoptotic bodies are seen.

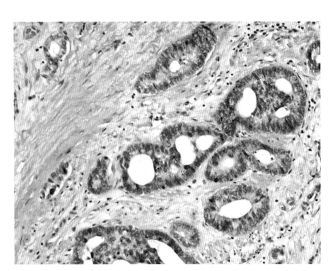

Figure 2.18.11   Secondary involvement of the cervix by endometrial endometrioid adenocarcinoma, FIGO grade 1. Same case as in *Figure 2.18.9*, higher magnification. Small glands with cribriform growth. Mitoses are lacking.

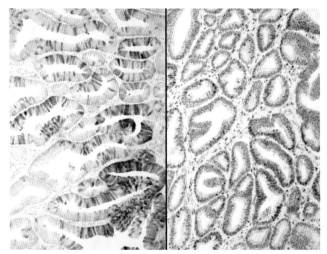

Figure 2.18.12   Secondary involvement of the cervix by endometrial endometrioid adenocarcinoma, FIGO grade 1. Same case as in *Figure 2.18.7*. Patchy expression of p16, **left**, and retained diffuse expression of ER, **right**.

	Mesonephric Hyperplasia (Hyperplastic Mesonephric Duct Remnants)	Secondary Involvement of the Cervix by Endometrial Endometrioid Adenocarcinoma
Age	Reproductive-age and postmenopausal women	Wide age range, mean age is 63 y
Location	Deep and occasionally superficial cervical stroma, lateral (9 and 3 o'clock)	Cervical mucosa and stroma
Symptoms	Asymptomatic	Abnormal vaginal bleeding; pelvic pain or pressure and abdominal distension in advanced cases
Signs	Incidental finding in the hysterectomy or large cervical conization specimens; rarely abnormal Pap	Noncyclical vaginal bleeding, constitutional symptoms: obesity, diabetes, PCOS; thickened endometrial stripe or endometrial or cervical mass on MRI or sonography; abnormal Pap smear; cervical mass on examination
Etiology	Embryonic remnants of mesonephric ducts, with subsequent hyperplasia	Unopposed estrogenic stimulation; somatic mutations in *PTEN*, *PIK3CA*, *KRAS*, *CTNNB1*, *ARID1A*; hereditary syndromes, Lynch and Cowden syndromes
Histology	1. Glandular proliferation deep in the cervical stroma; unremarkable normal endocervical mucosa *(Fig. 2.19.1)*; limited foci, usually <5 mm, are considered nonhyperplastic remnants 2. A central duct-like structure may be seen, with surrounding tubules clustered in circumscribed lobules *(Figs. 2.19.2 and 2.19.3)* 3. Cuboidal cells lining round tubules with luminal eosinophilic secretions *(Fig. 2.19.4)* 4. Round uniform nuclei with minimal if any atypia *(Fig. 2.19.5)* 5. Mitoses are rarely seen 6. No stromal response	1. Glandular proliferation involving endocervical mucosa and/or cervical stroma 2. Lack of architectural organization, diffuse infiltrative growth *(Fig. 2.19.6)* 3. Variably sized/shaped glands lined by columnar cells; cribriform and solid growth, papillary architecture can be seen *(Figs. 2.19.7 and 2.19.8)* 4. Round to ovoid enlarged atypical nuclei; pseudostratification is often seen *(Fig. 2.19.9)* 5. Mitotic activity is variable 6. Stromal response can be seen
Special studies	• Negative ER and PR • Luminal staining for CD10, positive for calretinin, strong positive for GATA-3 • Strong and diffuse expression of PAX2 • Low Ki-67 proliferative activity	• Usually strong ER/PR expression • Often negative CD10 and GATA-3 (weak focal staining is occasionally observed) • Most cases are PAX2 negative • Elevated Ki-67 proliferative activity
Treatment	None required	Hysterectomy with bilateral salpingo-oophorectomy, pelvic and periaortic lymphadenectomy; vaginal cuff radiation +/− chemotherapy
Prognosis	Benign; rarely, mesonephric carcinoma can arise in a background of mesonephric hyperplasia	5-y survival for stage II tumors is 69%

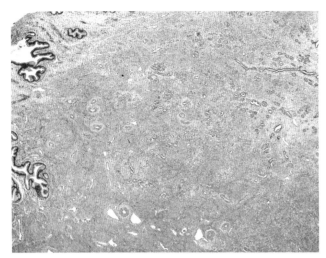

Figure 2.19.1   Mesonephric hyperplasia (hyperplastic mesonephric duct remnants). Proliferation of small glands deep in the cervical stroma. Normal endocervical glands are seen on the **left**.

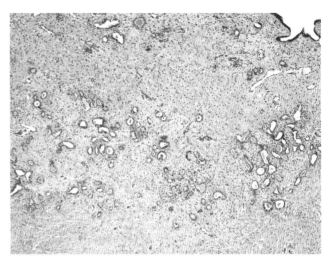

Figure 2.19.2   Mesonephric hyperplasia (hyperplastic mesonephric duct remnants). Proliferation of small glands, some of which have intraluminal eosinophilic secretions, in the cervical stroma. Note vaguely linear arrangement of this proliferation parallel to the endocervical surface.

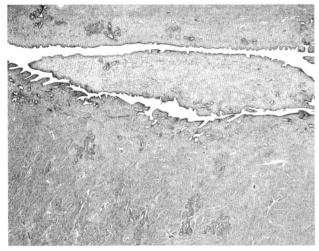

Figure 2.19.3   Mesonephric hyperplasia (hyperplastic mesonephric duct remnants). Deep lateral cervical stroma displays a central duct with small clusters/lobules of glands along the length of the duct.

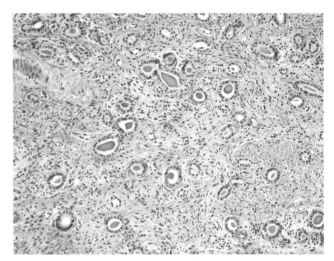

Figure 2.19.4   Mesonephric hyperplasia (hyperplastic mesonephric duct remnants). Round glands with typical dense eosinophilic secretions.

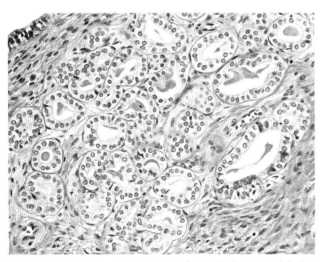

Figure 2.19.5   Mesonephric hyperplasia (hyperplastic mesonephric duct remnants). Cluster of small round and elongated glands lined by cuboidal cells with round monotonous nuclei and luminal secretions.

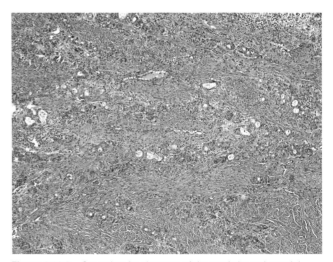

Figure 2.19.6   Secondary involvement of the cervix by endometrial endometrioid adenocarcinoma. Proliferation of small crowded glands deep in the cervical stroma.

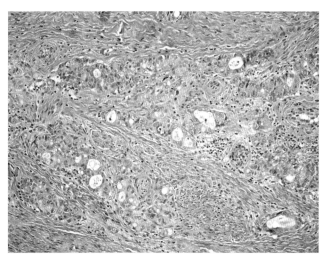

Figure 2.19.7 Secondary involvement of the cervix by endometrial endometrioid adenocarcinoma. Same case as in *Figure 2.19.6*, higher magnification. Small linear clusters of cribriform glands.

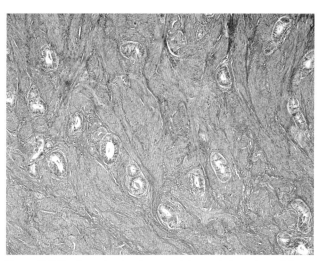

Figure 2.19.8 Secondary involvement of the cervix by endometrial endometrioid adenocarcinoma. Single-gland pattern of invasion.

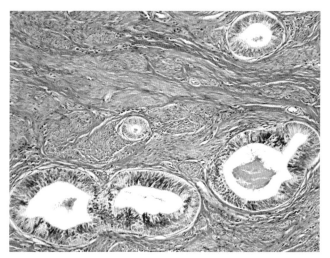

Figure 2.19.9 Secondary involvement of the cervix by endometrial endometrioid adenocarcinoma. Same case as in *Figure 2.19.8*, higher magnification. Glands are lined by columnar cells with pseudostratified nuclei; note occasional gland with luminal secretions.

	Mesonephric Hyperplasia (Hyperplastic Mesonephric Duct Remnants)	HPV-Related Invasive Endocervical Adenocarcinoma of Usual Type
Age	Reproductive-age and postmenopausal women	Mean age 40-42 y
Location	Deep and occasionally superficial cervical stroma, lateral (9 and 3 o'clock)	Cervix, transformation zone, endocervical canal
Symptoms	Asymptomatic	Vaginal bleeding, discharge, pelvic pain
Signs	Incidental finding in the hysterectomy or large cervical conization specimens; rarely abnormal Pap	Abnormal Pap, no clinically visible lesion, or cervical mass, barrel cervix
Etiology	Embryonic remnants of mesonephric ducts	High-risk HPV, adenocarcinoma *in situ* is a precursor
Histology	1. Glandular proliferation deep in the cervical stroma; can extend to superficial cervical stroma, particularly after cervical conization *(Figs. 2.20.1 and 2.20.2)* 2. Central duct-like structure can be seen; tubules and glands in vaguely circumscribed lobules *(Figs. 2.20.3 and 2.20.4)* 3. Cuboidal cells lining round tubules with luminal eosinophilic secretions 4. Round nuclei with minimal atypia *(Figs. 2.20.5 and 2.20.6)* 5. Mitoses and apoptotic bodies are rarely seen 6. No stromal response	1. Complex glandular proliferation extending from mucosa/superficial stroma into deeper layers of cervical wall; background precursor lesion (AIS) can be seen 2. Markedly crowded glands with cribriforming in lobulated arrangement or diffuse infiltrative growth *(Figs. 2.20.7 and 2.20.8)* 3. Columnar cells with variable amount of mucinous cytoplasm 4. Ovoid to elongated nuclei with hyperchromasia or fine chromatin with multiple nucleoli; pseudostratification is common *(Figs. 2.20.9 and 2.20.10)* 5. Frequent mitotic figures, particularly in the apical portion of the cytoplasm *(Figs. 2.20.9 and 2.20.10)* and apoptotic bodies 6. Stromal desmoplasia is often seen
Special studies	• Patchy expression of p16 • Luminal staining for CD10, strongly positive for GATA-3 • Strong PAX2 expression • Strong and diffuse expression of PAX8 • Low Ki-67 proliferative activity • No high-risk HPV detected by *in situ* hybridization	• Diffuse expression of p16 • Usually negative for CD10 and GATA-3 (weak focal staining is occasionally observed) • PAX2 is usually negative • Often decreased expression of PAX8 • Markedly increased Ki-67 proliferative activity • High-risk HPV detected by *in situ* hybridization
Treatment	None required	Stage dependent; hysterectomy or chemotherapy and radiation therapy
Prognosis	Benign; rarely, mesonephric carcinoma can arise in a background of mesonephric hyperplasia	Stage dependent; recurrences can occur even in stage IA1 cases treated with cold knife conization

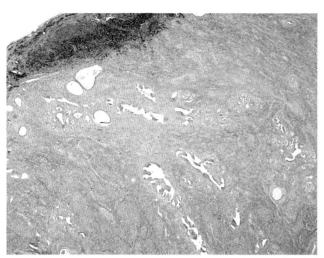

Figure 2.20.1 Mesonephric hyperplasia/remnants. Cervix with postconization changes. Glandular proliferation retaining somewhat lobulated growth extends to the superficial mucosa.

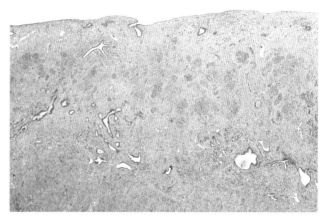

Figure 2.20.2 Mesonephric hyperplasia/remnants. Atrophic endocervical mucosa, postconization. Proliferation of small glands in linear arrangement deeper in the cervical stroma.

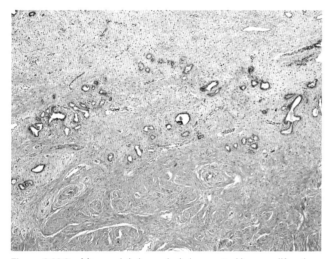

Figure 2.20.3 Mesonephric hyperplasia/remnants. Linear proliferation of small round and tubular shaped or elongated glands.

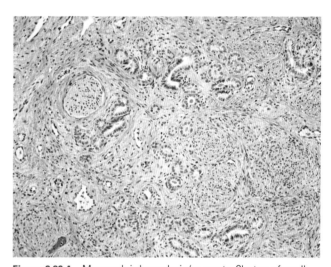

Figure 2.20.4 Mesonephric hyperplasia/remnants. Clusters of small round glands, some with luminal secretions, can be seen in the proximity of a nerve **(left)**.

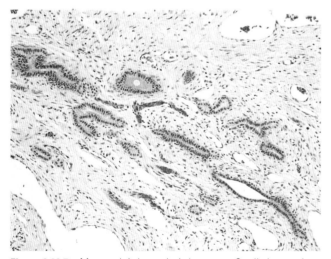

Figure 2.20.5 Mesonephric hyperplasia/remnants. Small elongated glands with bland cuboidal to low columnar lining.

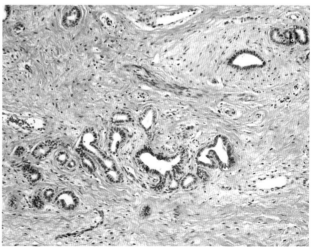

Figure 2.20.6 Mesonephric hyperplasia/remnants. Same case as in *Figure 2.20.3*, higher magnification. Bland low columnar to cuboidal cells.

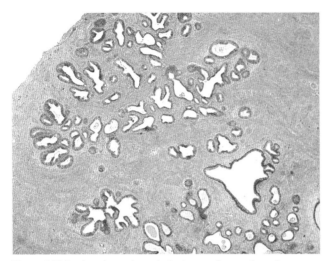

Figure 2.20.7 Invasive endocervical adenocarcinoma of usual type. Diffuse infiltrative growth; variable sized and shaped glands. This subtle pattern of invasion is best appreciated at low magnification.

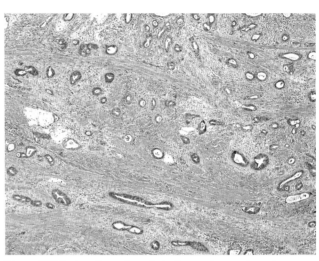

Figure 2.20.8 Invasive endocervical adenocarcinoma of usual type. Single-gland pattern of invasion.

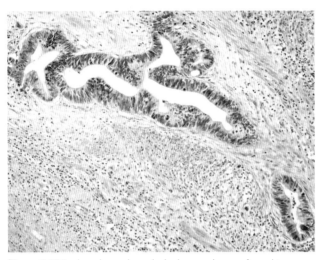

Figure 2.20.9 Invasive endocervical adenocarcinoma of usual type, high magnification. Note columnar cells with mitoses and apoptotic bodies. Stromal reaction is present.

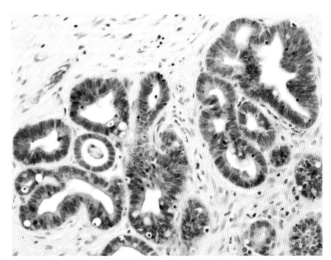

Figure 2.20.10 Invasive endocervical adenocarcinoma of usual type, high magnification. Columnar cells with hyperchromatic nuclei and apoptotic bodies.

	Secondary Cervical Involvement by Endometrial Endometrioid Carcinoma, FIGO Grade 3	Poorly Differentiated Cervical Squamous Cell Carcinoma or Adenosquamous Carcinoma
Age	57-64 y	Most cases are between 40 and 55 y
Location	Cervical mucosa and stroma	Cervix, transformation zone, endocervical canal
Symptoms	Abnormal vaginal bleeding; pelvic pain or pressure and abdominal distension in advanced cases	Vaginal bleeding, discharge, pelvic pain
Signs	Noncyclical vaginal bleeding, constitutional symptoms: obesity, diabetes, PCOS; thickened endometrial stripe or endometrial or cervical mass on MRI or sonography; abnormal Pap smear; cervical mass on examination	Abnormal Pap, no clinically visible lesion, or cervical mass, barrel cervix
Etiology	Unopposed estrogenic stimulation; somatic mutations in *PTEN, PIK3CA, KRAS, CTNNB1, ARID1A, TP53*; hereditary syndromes, Lynch and Cowden syndromes	High-risk HPV, HSIL, and adenocarcinoma *in situ* (AIS) are precursors; rarely adenosquamous carcinoma *in situ* is seen
Gross findings and histology	1. Mass in the uterine corpus or lower uterine segment 2. Neoplastic proliferation involving endocervical mucosa and/or cervical stroma; contiguous spread from deep myometrium, sparing superficial cervical wall, can be seen; no precursor lesion in the cervix 3. Solid growth with focal gland formation *(Figs. 2.21.1 and 2.21.2)*; residual glandular elements are usually present at the periphery of the tumor nests 4. Round to ovoid atypical nuclei; nuclei in squamoid-appearing areas can be relatively bland *(Figs. 2.21.3 and 2.21.4)* 5. Mitotic activity is variable	1. Cervical mass or no gross lesion 2. Complex glandular proliferation extending from mucosa/superficial stroma into deeper layers of cervical wall; background AIS or HSIL can be seen 3. Variably shaped solid nests of cells with scant to moderate amount of eosinophilic cytoplasm *(Fig. 2.21.6)* or focal glandular differentiation often within the solid areas or adjacent adenocarcinoma component (in adenosquamous carcinoma) *(Figs. 2.21.7 and 2.21.8)* 4. Significant atypia and pleomorphism in solid areas (squamous component) *(Fig. 2.21.9)* 5. Frequent mitotic figures and apoptotic bodies *(Fig. 2.21.9)*
Special studies	• Patchy/focal expression of p16 *(Fig. 2.21.5)* • Usually strong and diffuse ER/PR expression; occasionally negative • No high-risk HPV detected by *in situ* hybridization • MMR can be lost	• Diffuse expression of p16 • Decreased or lost ER/PR expression • High-risk HPV detected by *in situ* hybridization • MMR retained
Treatment	Hysterectomy with bilateral salpingo-oophorectomy, pelvic and periaortic lymphadenectomy; vaginal brachytherapy +/− pelvic radiation +/− chemotherapy	Stage dependent; hysterectomy or chemotherapy and radiation therapy
Prognosis	5-y survival for stage II tumors is 69%	Stage dependent

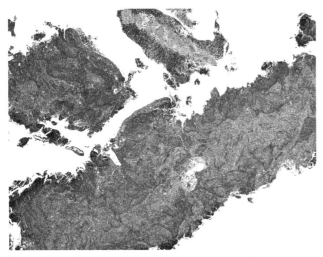

Figure 2.21.1   Secondary cervical involvement by poorly differentiated endometrial endometrioid carcinoma. Endocervical curettage with fragments of tumor mimicking infiltrative growth of cervical squamous cell carcinoma.

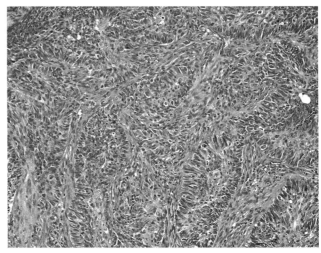

Figure 2.21.2   Secondary cervical involvement by poorly differentiated endometrial endometrioid carcinoma. Same case as in *Figure 2.21.1*, higher magnification. Islands of tumor cells with peripheral palisading.

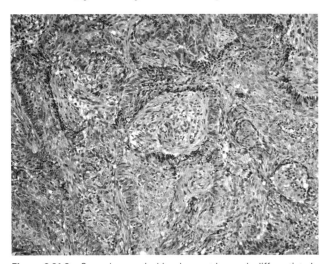

Figure 2.21.3   Secondary cervical involvement by poorly differentiated endometrial endometrioid carcinoma. Same case as in *Figure 2.21.1*. Slight squamous differentiation in the **middle** of the tumor islands.

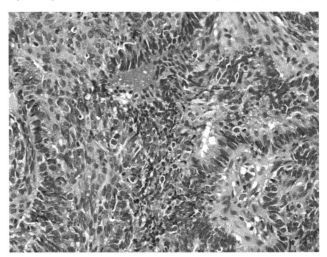

Figure 2.21.4   Secondary cervical involvement by poorly differentiated endometrial endometrioid carcinoma. Same case as in *Figure 2.21.1*, higher magnification. Cells at the periphery of the nest maintain columnar appearance. Central areas display slight squamous differentiation with more abundant eosinophilic cytoplasm and round to ovoid nuclei. Note suggestion of residual gland formation.

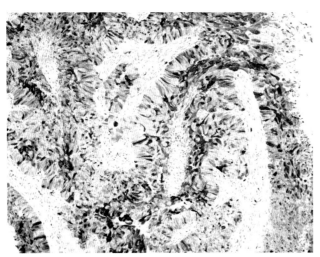

Figure 2.21.5   Secondary cervical involvement by poorly differentiated endometrial endometrioid carcinoma. Same case as in *Figure 2.21.1*. Patchy expression of p16 supports endometrial origin.

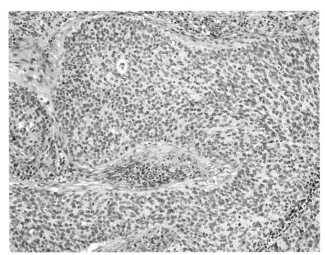

Figure 2.21.6   Poorly differentiated cervical squamous cell carcinoma. Broad nests of tumor with diffuse solid growth.

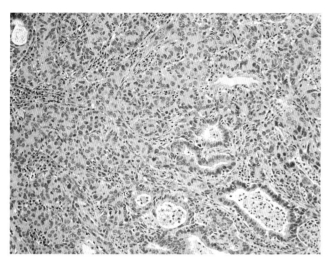

Figure 2.21.7   Cervical adenosquamous carcinoma. Diffuse solid and nested growth of squamous cell carcinoma and glandular differentiation **(lower right)**.

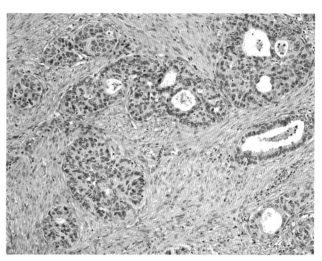

Figure 2.21.8   Cervical adenosquamous carcinoma. Nests of tumor cells with squamous and glandular features.

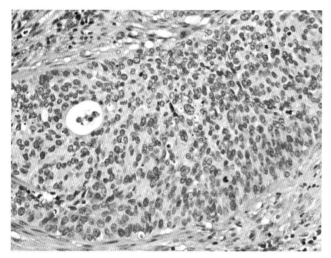

Figure 2.21.9   Poorly differentiated cervical squamous cell carcinoma. Same case as in *Figure 2.21.6*, higher magnification. Cells with eosinophilic cytoplasm and pleomorphic ovoid nuclei.

2 CERVIX

	Placental Site Nodule/Plaque	Squamous Cell Carcinoma (Well-Differentiated, Keratinizing)
Age	Reproductive years; occasionally may be seen in older women many years after pregnancy	Median age 49 y
Location	Endometrium or endocervical mucosa; occasionally seen in the fallopian tube and ovary	Cervix, transformation zone
Symptoms	No specific symptoms, occasionally associated with vaginal bleeding; usually incidental finding in endometrial or endocervical curettages	Vaginal bleeding
Signs	No specific symptoms; usually incidental finding in endometrial or endocervical curettages; does not produce a mass; placental site plaques can be >1 cm in size; abnormal Pap can be coincidental	Vaginal bleeding, abnormal Pap, cervical mass
Etiology	Chorionic-type intermediate trophoblast resulting from prior pregnancy	High-risk HPV
Histology	1. Well-circumscribed nodules or plaques *(Fig. 2.22.1)*; squamous intraepithelial lesion can be seen coincidentally 2. Single cells and clusters of lesional cells separated by abundant hyalinized stroma *(Fig. 2.22.2)*; stromal inflammation can be present in the endocervical specimens *(Fig. 2.22.3)* 3. Necrosis may be present but not very common 4. Low degree of cellularity *(Fig. 2.22.4)* 5. Epithelioid cells with enlarged and hyperchromatic but smudgy nuclei *(Fig. 2.22.5)* (atypical forms of placental site/plaque have been described) 6. Abundant eosinophilic to scant clear cytoplasm, perinuclear zone of amphophilic to basophilic cytoplasm *(Fig. 2.22.5)* 7. Mitotic figures are rare; usually absent	1. Single cells, cell clusters, and large irregularly shaped nests and sheets of tumor cells *(Figs. 2.22.7 and 2.22.8)*; high-grade squamous intraepithelial lesion (HSIL) can be seen on the surface 2. Stromal desmoplasia is common; stromal fibrosis can be seen; stromal hyalinization is not typical *(Fig. 2.22.8)* 3. Necrosis is common within the tumor nests; single intensely eosinophilic/necrotic keratinocytes are seen *(Fig. 2.22.8)* 4. High to moderate cellularity 5. Epithelioid cells with round to ovoid nuclei and atypia ranging from moderate to marked; vesicular chromatin or hyperchromasia *(Fig. 2.22.9)* 6. Areas of cells with scant cytoplasm and foci with abundant dense eosinophilic cytoplasm with evidence of keratinization *(Fig. 2.22.10)* 7. Often increased mitotic activity
Special studies	• Patchy or negative p16 *(Fig. 2.22.6,* **left***)* • HSD3B1 positive • Strong, diffuse expression of CK18 *(Fig. 2.22.6,* **right***)* • Negative or focal high molecular weight cytokeratins (CK5/6) • No detection of high-risk HPV by *in situ* hybridization	• Strong and diffuse expression of p16 • Negative or weak/focal for CK18 • Positive high molecular weight cytokeratins (CK5/6) • High-risk HPV detected by *in situ* hybridization • HSD3B1 negative

	Placental Site Nodule/Plaque	**Squamous Cell Carcinoma (Well-Differentiated, Keratinizing)**
Treatment	None for typical placental site nodule/plaque; further clinical evaluation and follow-up (if diagnosed on curettage) are warranted for atypical placental site nodule/plaque	Stage dependent; superficially invasive cases without angiolymphatic invasion can be treated with cervical excision; hysterectomy +/− lymphadenectomy for early-stage cases; chemoradiation for advanced stage cases
Prognosis	Unremarkable for typical placental site nodule/plaque; 14% of atypical placental site nodules/plaques are associated with concurrent or subsequent malignant gestational trophoblastic disease	Stage dependent; 5-y survival for stage IA is 95%-99% and declines progressively with increase in stage

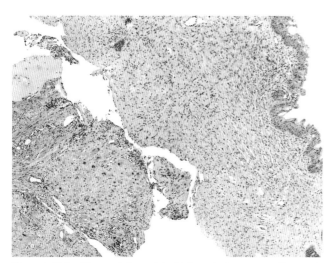

Figure 2.22.1 Placental site nodule. Endocervical curettage. Cluster of cells with abundant eosinophilic cytoplasm and dark irregular enlarged nuclei **(lower left)**. Note associated stromal hyalinization.

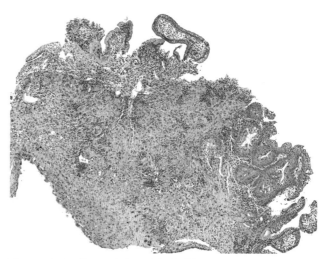

Figure 2.22.2 Placental site nodule. Proliferation of cells with abundant eosinophilic cytoplasm within endocervical stroma.

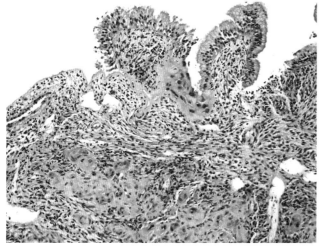

Figure 2.22.3 Placental site nodule. Same case as in *Figure 2.22.2*, higher magnification. Clusters of atypical cells with dark irregular enlarged nuclei and dense eosinophilic cytoplasm, some of which are close to the surface of endocervical mucosa.

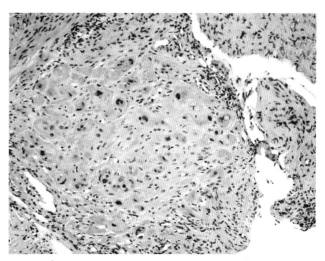

Figure 2.22.4 Placental site nodule. Same case as in *Figure 2.22.1*, higher magnification. Proliferation of cells with abundant eosinophilic cytoplasm within endocervical stroma.

2 CERVIX

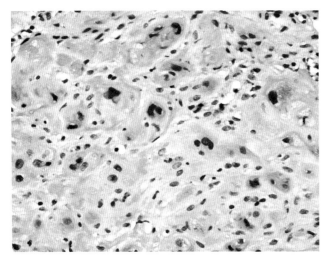

Figure 2.22.5 Placental site nodule. Same case as in *Figure 2.22.1*, higher magnification. Cells with abundant eosinophilic cytoplasm and atypical hyperchromatic nuclei. Note perinuclear areas of amphophilic cytoplasm.

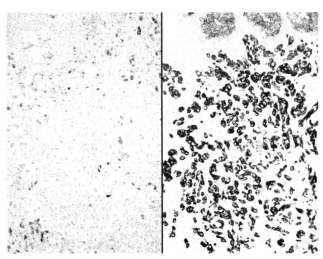

Figure 2.22.6 Placental site nodule. Same case as in *Figure 2.22.2*. Focal patchy expression of p16 **(left)** and diffuse labeling by cytokeratin 18 **(right)**.

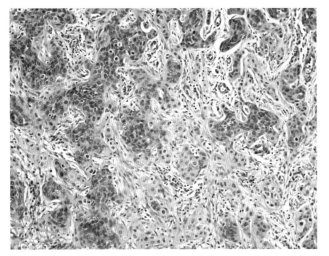

Figure 2.22.7 Squamous cell carcinoma. Irregular infiltrative tumor nests in the stroma.

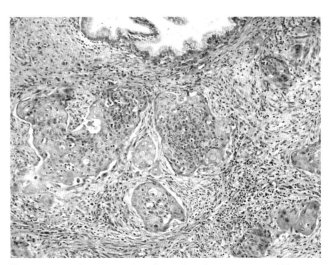

Figure 2.22.8 Squamous cell carcinoma. Invasive tumor nests within reactive stroma; cells with cytoplasmic keratinization (paradoxical maturation) at the periphery of the nests and more immature cells in the **center**.

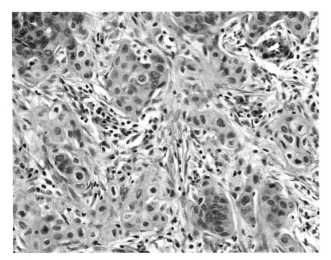

Figure 2.22.9 Squamous cell carcinoma. Same case as in *Figure 2.22.7*, higher magnification. Cells with moderately atypical, relatively uniform round to ovoid nuclei, some with scant amount of cytoplasm, others with more abundant eosinophilic cytoplasm.

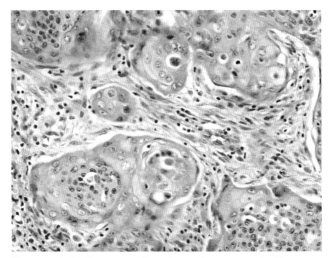

Figure 2.22.10 Squamous cell carcinoma. Same case as in *Figure 2.22.8*, higher magnification. Cells with dense pink-orange cytoplasm indicating keratinization. Note dyskeratotic cells.

	Squamous Cell Carcinoma	Neuroendocrine Carcinoma
Age	Most cases are between 40 and 55 y	Wide age range; most cases are between 36 and 42 y
Location	Cervix, transformation zone	Cervix, transformation zone
Symptoms	Abnormal Pap smear, vaginal bleeding, or discharge	Abnormal Pap smear; vaginal bleeding; paraneoplastic syndrome
Signs	Abnormal colposcopic findings, cervical mass	Abnormal colposcopic findings, cervical mass, barrel cervix
Etiology	High-risk HPV, types 16 and 18 cause majority of cases	High-risk HPV causes majority of cases
Histology	1. Sheets, nests, and single tumor cells (*Figs. 2.23.1 and 2.23.2*) 2. Central necrosis within large nests can be present but not a constant feature (*Fig. 2.23.3*) 3. Cases with basaloid morphology can display peripheral palisading 4. Squamous differentiation, dense eosinophilic cytoplasm; keratinization can be present (*Figs. 2.23.4 and 2.23.5*) 5. Hyperchromatic nuclei or coarse chromatin; multinucleation can be seen; multiple nucleoli may be present but generally not prominent (*Fig. 2.23.6*) 6. Apoptotic bodies can be present but not a constant feature 7. Variable mitotic activity 8. Intraepithelial component (HSIL) can be found on the surface; can coexist with endocervical adenocarcinoma	1. Nested, insular, trabecular, or diffuse growth (*Figs. 2.23.7 and 2.23.8*) 2. Prominent necrosis (geographic in large cell variant) 3. Prominent peripheral palisading (large cell variant) (*Fig. 2.23.9*) 4. Small cell variant: uniform cells, scant amount of cytoplasm, prominent crush artifact; large cell variant: abundant eosinophilic or amphophilic cytoplasm 5. Small cell variant: hyperchromasia, finely dispersed chromatin ("salt and pepper"), nuclear molding (*Fig. 2.23.10*); large cell variant: vesicular nuclei with prominent nucleoli and marked pleomorphism (*Fig. 2.23.11*) 6. Numerous apoptotic bodies (small cell variant) 7. Brisk mitotic activity 8. Often coexist with endocervical adenocarcinoma (*in situ* or invasive) (*Fig. 2.23.7*)
Special studies	• Negative or very focal expression of neuroendocrine markers (chromogranin, synaptophysin, INSM1) • Positive for p40, p63 (*Fig. 2.23.2,* **inset**)	• Positive neuroendocrine markers (chromogranin, synaptophysin, CD56, INSM1); rarely, small cell carcinomas can be negative (*Fig. 2.23.12,* **far left**, chromogranin; second from left CD56) • Most cases negative for p40, p63, CK5/6; positive for low molecular weight keratins (*Fig. 2.23.12,* **far right**, p40; second from right, CK5/6) • Can be TTF-1 positive (small cell variant)

	Squamous Cell Carcinoma	**Neuroendocrine Carcinoma**
Treatment	Stage dependent; superficially invasive cases without angiolymphatic invasion can be treated with cervical excision; radical hysterectomy +/− lymphadenectomy for early-stage cases; chemoradiation for advanced stage cases	Hysterectomy +/− lymphadenectomy for early-stage cases; chemoradiation for advanced stage cases
Prognosis	Stage dependent, 5-y survival for stage IA is 95%-99% and declines progressively with increase in stage	Poor outcome for all stages

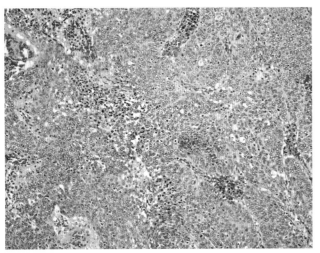

Figure 2.23.1   Squamous cell carcinoma. Diffuse sheets of tumor cells.

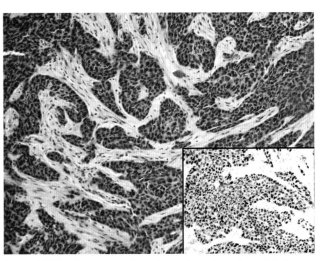

Figure 2.23.2   Squamous cell carcinoma. Irregular and angulated basophilic nests and islands of tumor cells. Immunohistochemical stain for p40 is strongly positive **(inset)**.

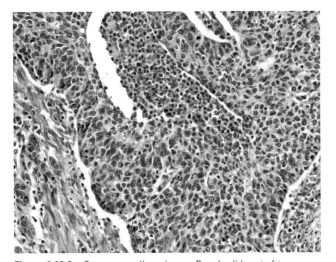

Figure 2.23.3   Squamous cell carcinoma. Broad solid nest of tumor cells with central necrosis.

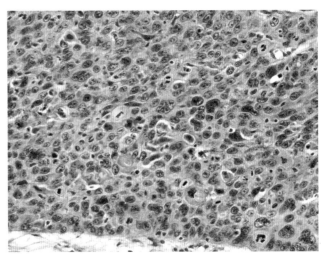

Figure 2.23.4   Squamous cell carcinoma. Diffuse sheet of atypical cells with markedly pleomorphic nuclei and moderate amount of eosinophilic cytoplasm. Note densely eosinophilic dyskeratotic cells and a few mitotic figures.

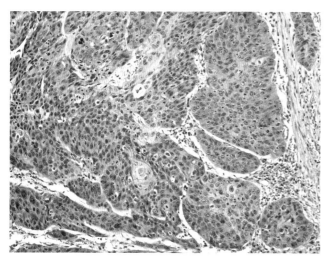

Figure 2.23.5   Squamous cell carcinoma. Infiltrating nests of tumor cells. Note squamous differentiation and a focus of keratinization.

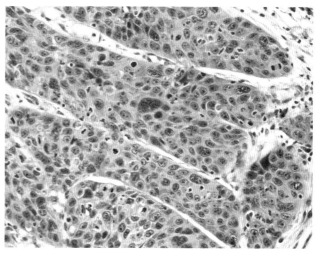

Figure 2.23.6   Squamous cell carcinoma. Atypical cells with markedly pleomorphic nuclei with multiple nucleoli.

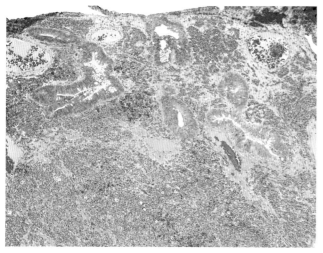

Figure 2.23.7   Neuroendocrine carcinoma, small cell variant. Diffuse sheets of basophilic cells. Note endocervical adenocarcinoma component close to the surface.

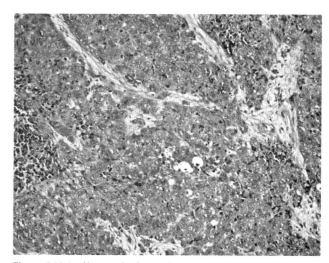

Figure 2.23.8   Neuroendocrine carcinoma, large cell variant. Tumor nests composed of cells with eosinophilic cytoplasm and large nuclei.

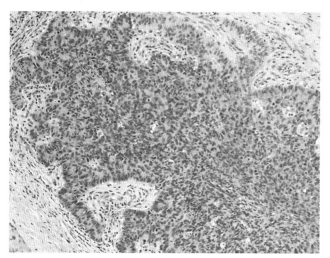

Figure 2.23.9   Neuroendocrine carcinoma, large cell variant. Insular growth pattern and rosette-like structures; note peripheral palisading.

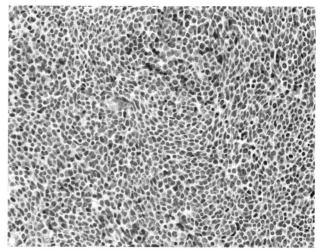

Figure 2.23.10   Neuroendocrine carcinoma, small cell variant. Same case as in *Figure 2.23.7*, higher magnification. Monotonous tumor cells with nuclear molding.

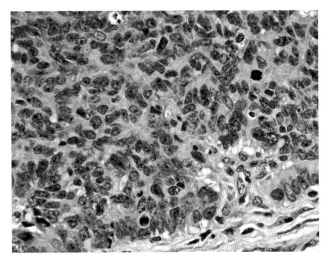

Figure 2.23.11   Neuroendocrine carcinoma, large cell variant. Same case as in *Figure 2.23.9*, higher magnification. Markedly atypical enlarged nuclei with coarse chromatin and occasional prominent nucleoli.

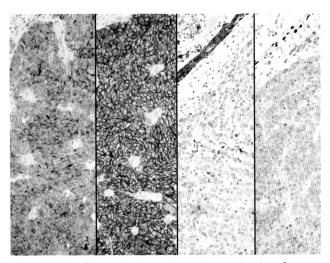

Figure 2.23.12   Neuroendocrine carcinoma, large cell variant. Same case as in *Figure 2.23.9*. Immunohistochemical stains diffusely positive for chromogranin **(far left)** and CD56 **(second from the left)** and negative for p40 **(far right)** and CK5/6 **(second from the right)**. Note attenuated cervical squamous epithelium serving as internal positive control for p40 and CK5/6.

	Embryonal Rhabdomyosarcoma, Botryoid Type	Inflamed Benign Endocervical Polyp
Age	Classically in infants and young girls; also in adults, mean age 44 y	Adults, most common in fourth to sixth decades; rare in children and adolescents
Location	Cervix, vagina (in pediatric cases), endometrium	Cervix, transformation zone, endocervix
Symptoms	Vaginal bleeding	Asymptomatic, or postcoital bleeding, vaginal discharge
Signs	Cervical polyp/mass protruding through the cervical os	Usually small polypoid growth, giant forms have been described, usually solitary
Etiology	Derived from myogenic progenitor cells; mutations in RAS signaling pathway. Somatic and germline mutations in *DICER1* (DICER syndrome) are seen in a subset	Often seen in multigravida
Histology	1. Cambium layer: hypercellular stroma beneath the surface epithelium *(Figs. 2.24.1 and 2.24.2)* 2. Edematous hypocellular stroma with hypercellular foci *(Fig. 2.24.3)* 3. Packets of dense cellularity composed of atypical immature cells with scant cytoplasm and apoptotic bodies *(Fig. 2.24.4)*; strap cells and cross-striations are seen in a proportion of cases *(Fig. 2.24.5)* 4. Frequent mitoses in hypercellular foci 5. Heterologous elements (cartilage) are common	1. Surface erosion with granulation tissue-like stromal change and inflammation in subepithelial zone *(Figs. 2.24.7-2.24.9)* 2. Dense or edematous stroma with clusters of thick-walled vessels *(Fig. 2.24.8)* 3. Variably distributed mixed inflammatory cell infiltrate; no morphologic features of skeletal muscle are seen *(Fig. 2.24.10)* 4. Mitoses are not seen 5. Cartilaginous elements are not seen
Special studies	• Positive desmin, muscle-specific actin, myogenin, MYOD1 *(Fig. 2.24.6)* • Hypercellular areas negative for CD45 • Increased Ki-67 labeling in hypercellular/primitive myxoid areas • Loss of ER/PR in hypercellular areas	• Negative myogenin, MYOD1; desmin and actin expression can be seen in the stroma *(Fig. 2.24.11)* • Cellular infiltrate CD45 positive • Ki-67 labeling can be present in inflammatory cells • ER/PR expression in hypercellular areas
Treatment	Surgery, multiagent chemotherapy	Biopsy usually removes entire lesion and is generally curative
Prognosis	70%-90% 5-y survival in children; poor prognosis in adults with <30% 5-y survival reported in some series, although the data are limited	Benign

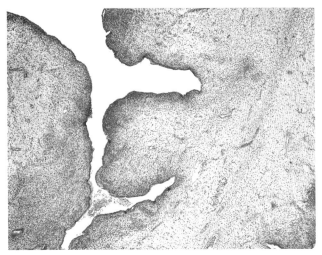

Figure 2.24.1   Embryonal rhabdomyosarcoma, botryoid type. Polypoid lesion with edematous stroma and hypercellular zone beneath the surface epithelium (cambium layer).

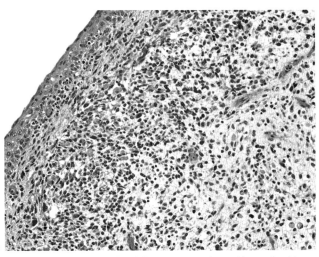

Figure 2.24.2   Embryonal rhabdomyosarcoma, botryoid type. Cambium layer, higher magnification.

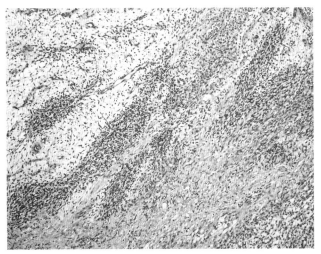

Figure 2.24.3   Embryonal rhabdomyosarcoma, botryoid type. Edematous stroma with zones of hypercellularity.

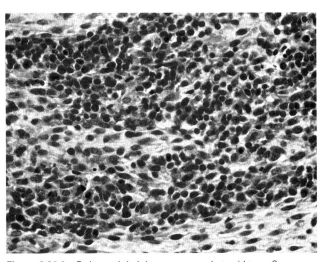

Figure 2.24.4   Embryonal rhabdomyosarcoma, botryoid type. Same case as in *Figure 2.24.3*, higher magnification. Hypercellular area composed of immature hyperchromatic cells with frequent mitoses.

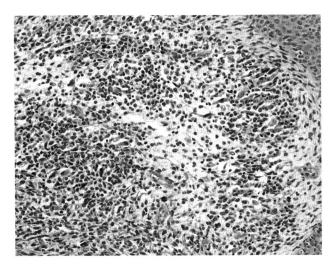

Figure 2.24.5   Embryonal rhabdomyosarcoma, botryoid type. Note the presence of scattered rhabdomyoblasts.

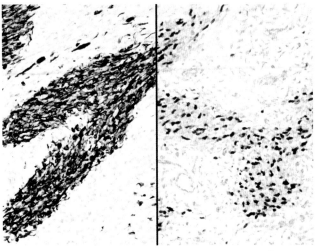

Figure 2.24.6   Embryonal rhabdomyosarcoma, botryoid type. Same case as in *Figure 2.24.3*. Tumor cells are positive for desmin **(left)** and myogenin **(right)**.

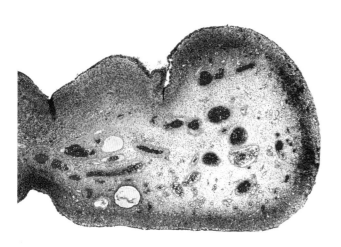

Figure 2.24.7   Endocervical polyp with surface inflammation. Central core with dilated vessels.

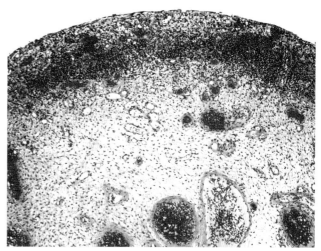

Figure 2.24.8   Endocervical polyp with surface inflammation. Same case as in *Figure 2.24.7*, higher magnification. Zone of dense surface and laminar subsurface inflammation can mimic a cambium layer.

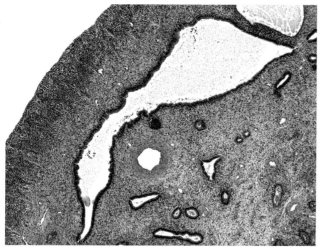

Figure 2.24.9   Endocervical polyp with dilated glands and stromal inflammation. Thick-walled vessels in the **center**.

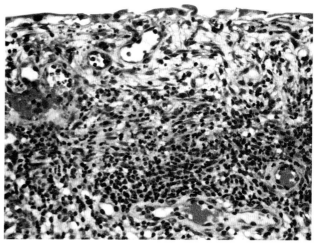

Figure 2.24.10   Endocervical polyp with surface inflammation. Same case as in *Figure 2.24.7*, higher magnification. Mixed inflammatory infiltrate beneath the attenuated and focally eroded surface epithelium.

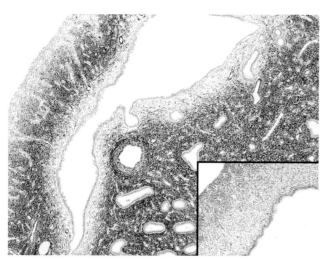

Figure 2.24.11   Endocervical polyp with surface inflammation. Same case as in *Figure 2.24.9*. Polyp stroma is positive for desmin, but subepithelial zone mimicking a cambium layer is negative; no expression of myogenin is seen **(inset)**.

	NTRK-Rearranged Spindle Cell Neoplasm/Sarcoma	Inflammatory Myofibroblastic Tumor
Age	Median age: 31 y	Usually, premenopausal women
Location	Cervix	Uterus, cervix
Symptoms	Vaginal bleeding, cervical mass	Abnormal vaginal bleeding or pelvic pain/pressure
Signs	Cervical mass	Pelvic mass; gross mass within the myometrium, lower uterine segment, or cervix
Etiology	Rearrangement of NTRK1, NTRK2, and NTRK3 with various fusion partners leading to overexpression of Trk. NTRK1-TPM3 fusion is the most common, often occurring with CDKN2A deletion	Similar to its nongynecologic counterpart, associated with rearrangements of the ALK gene; other rearrangements, such as ROS1 or RET, may be seen as well as rarely NTRK3 rearrangements (described in nongynecologic sites)
Histology	1. Infiltrative borders *(Fig. 2.25.1)* 2. A fascicular, storiform, or patternless arrangement of fibroblast-like spindle cells *(Figs. 2.25.2 and 2.25.3)* 3. Spindle cells with eosinophilic cytoplasm and some nuclear atypia *(Figs. 2.25.4 and 2.25.5)* 4. Hyalinization of tumor vessels; staghorn vascular pattern may be seen *(Figs. 2.25.6 and 2.25.7)* 5. Variable mitotic activity *(Fig. 2.25.8)* 6. Lymphocytic infiltrate can be present but is not a constant feature 7. No lymphovascular space invasion (limited data) 8. Necrosis may be present	1. Borders may be smooth or infiltrative 2. Predominantly myxoid pattern (with fasciitis-like appearance) with minor fascicular component (with leiomyoma-like appearance); generally, myxoid areas are hypocellular *(Figs. 2.25.9 and 2.25.10)* 3. Spindle- to stellate-shaped myofibroblastic cells with pale eosinophilic cytoplasm; usually bland nuclei with evenly dispersed chromatin but may be vesicular with prominent nucleoli *(Figs. 2.25.11 and 2.25.12)* 4. Generally, no distinct vascular patterns 5. Variable mitotic activity, but mitotic index is typically low 6. Edematous background with lymphocytes and plasma cells 7. No lymphovascular space invasion 8. Necrosis usually absent but has been described in a small subset of cases with aggressive behavior
Special studies	• ALK IHC/FISH: negative • Desmin: negative • CD34, S100: positive • ER/PR: usually negative • Pan-Trk IHC: positive	• ALK (IHC): positive in most cases; ALK rearrangement (FISH) in most cases • Smooth muscle actin/desmin: variably positive • S100: negative • ER/PR: variably positive • Pan-Trk IHC: can be positive
Treatment	Resection; targeted TRK inhibitor for unresectable or recurrent tumors	Myomectomy (resection) or hysterectomy; targeted TK-inhibitors (crizotinib) can be considered in aggressive cases with proven ALK fusions
Prognosis	Is considered tumor of low malignant potential; metastases and aggressive clinical course has been described in rare cases	Benign in most cases, but a small subset may exhibit aggressive behavior (histologic criteria for malignancy based on limited data) recurrences can occur; metastases are rare

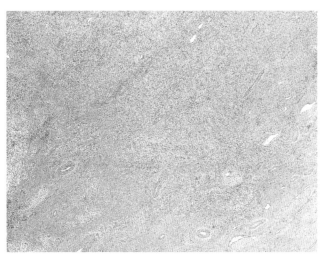

Figure 2.25.1   NTRK-rearranged spindle cell neoplasm/sarcoma. Infiltrative tumor border deep in the cervical stroma.

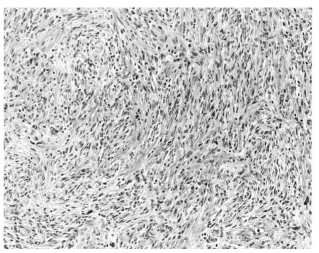

Figure 2.25.2   NTRK-rearranged spindle cell neoplasm/sarcoma. Spindle cell neoplasm with vaguely fascicular growth.

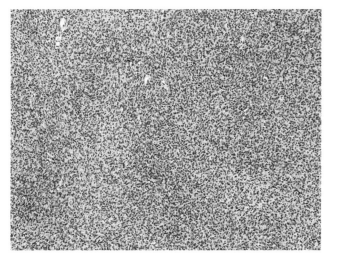

Figure 2.25.3   NTRK-rearranged spindle cell neoplasm/sarcoma. Densely cellular neoplasm with spindled to epithelioid features.

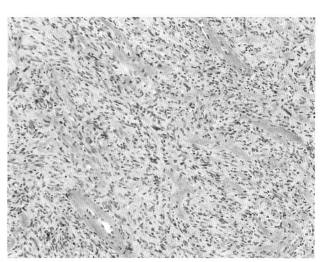

Figure 2.25.4   NTRK-rearranged spindle cell neoplasm/sarcoma. Spindle cells with eosinophilic cytoplasm with mild nuclear atypia.

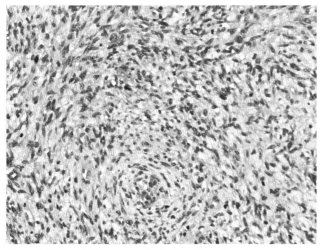

Figure 2.25.5   NTRK-rearranged spindle cell neoplasm/sarcoma. Haphazardly arranged spindle cells with moderate atypia.

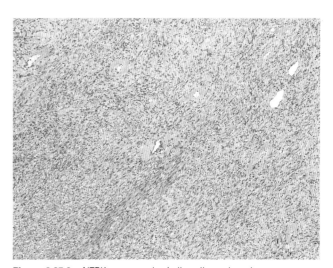

Figure 2.25.6   NTRK-rearranged spindle cell neoplasm/sarcoma. Spindle cell tumor with hyalinized vessels.

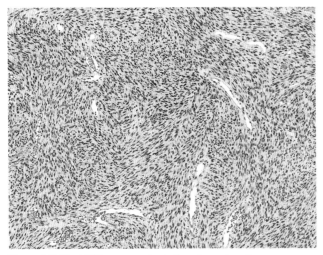

Figure 2.25.7   NTRK-rearranged spindle cell neoplasm/sarcoma. Fascicles of spindle cells and vaguely staghorn vessels.

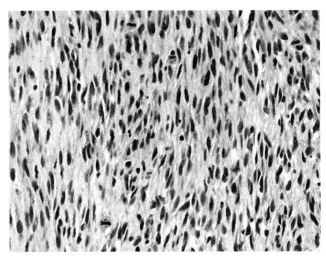

Figure 2.25.8   NTRK-rearranged spindle cell neoplasm/sarcoma. Spindle cell neoplasm with moderate atypia and frequent mitotic figures.

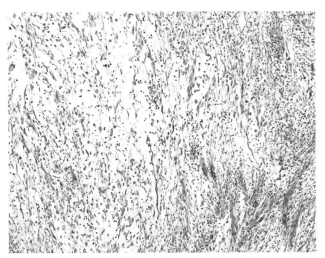

Figure 2.25.9   Inflammatory myofibroblastic tumor. Myxoid, hypocellular spindle cell neoplasm with notable inflammatory infiltrate.

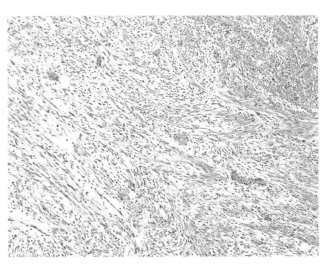

Figure 2.25.10   Inflammatory myofibroblastic tumor. Areas of the tumor with leiomyoma-like appearance adjacent to the hypocellular areas.

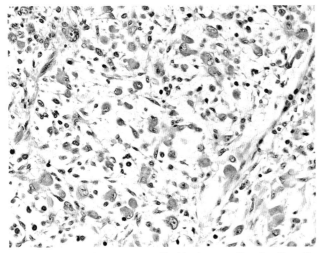

Figure 2.25.11   Inflammatory myofibroblastic tumor. Ganglion-like cells with eosinophilic cytoplasm.

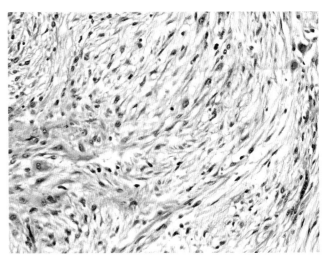

Figure 2.25.12   Inflammatory myofibroblastic tumor. Spindle- to stellate-shaped cells with pale eosinophilic cytoplasm.

SUGGESTED READINGS

2.1 and 2.2

Darragh TM, Colgan TJ, Thomas Cox J, et al. The lower anogenital squamous terminology standardization project for HPV-associated lesions: background and consensus recommendations from the college of American Pathologists and the American Society for Colposcopy and Cervical Pathology. *Int J Gynecol Pathol.* 2013;32:76-115.

Keating JT, Ince T, Crum CP. Surrogate biomarkers of HPV infection in cervical neoplasia screening and diagnosis. *Adv Anat Pathol.* 2001;8:83-92.

McCluggage WG. Premalignant lesions of the lower female genital tract: cervix, vagina and vulva. *Pathology.* 2013;45:214-228.

Resnick M, Lester S, Tate JE, et al. Viral and histopathologic correlates of MN and MIB-1 expression in cervical intraepithelial neoplasia. *Hum Pathol.* 1996;27:234-239.

Tumors of the cervix. In: Kurman RJ, Ronnett BM, Sherman ME, Wilkinson EJ, eds. *Atlas of Tumor Pathology, 4th series, fasc 13. Tumors of the Cervix, Vagina, and Vulva.* Armed Forces Institute of Pathology; 2010:68-105.

Wright TC, Ronnett BM, Kurman RJ, et al. Precancerous lesions of the cervix. In: Kurman RJ, Ellenson LH, Ronnett BM, eds. *Blaustein's Pathology of the Female Genital Tract.* 6th ed. Springer; 2011:208-225.

2.3

Brinck U, Jakob C, Bau O, et al. Papillary squamous cell carcinoma of the uterine cervix: report of three cases and a review of its classification. *Int J Gynecol Pathol.* 2000;19:231-235.

Hong SA, Yoo SH, Choi J, et al. a review and update on papillary immature metaplasia of the uterine cervix: a distinct subset of low-grade squamous intraepithelial lesion, proposing a possible cell of origin. *Arch Pathol Lab Med.* 2018;142(8):973-981.

Kang GH, Min K, Shim YH, et al. Papillary immature metaplasia of the uterine cervix: a report of 5 cases with an emphasis on the differential diagnosis from reactive squamous metaplasia, high-grade squamous intraepithelial lesion and papillary squamous cell carcinoma. *J Korean Med Sci.* 2001;16:762-768.

Randall ME, Andersen WA, Mills SE, et al. Papillary squamous cell carcinoma of the uterine cervix: a clinicopathologic study of nine cases. *Int J Gynecol Pathol.* 1986;5:1-10.

Trivijitsilp P, Mosher R, Sheets EE, et al. Papillary immature metaplasia (immature condyloma) of the cervix: a clinicopathologic analysis and comparison with papillary squamous carcinoma. *Hum Pathol.* 1998;29:641-648.

Ward BE, Saleh AM, Williams JV, et al. Papillary immature metaplasia of the cervix: a distinct subset of exophytic cervical condyloma associated with HPV-6/11 nucleic acids. *Mod Pathol.* 1992;5:391-395.

2.4-2.6

Crum CP, Egawa K, Fu YS, et al. Atypical immature metaplasia (AIM). A subset of human papilloma virus infection of the cervix. *Cancer.* 1983;51:2214-2219.

Egan AJ, Russell P. Transitional (urothelial) cell metaplasia of the uterine cervix: morphological assessment of 31 cases. *Int J Gynecol Pathol.* 1997;16:89-98.

Geng L, Connolly DC, Isacson C, et al. Atypical immature metaplasia (AIM) of the cervix: is it related to high-grade squamous intraepithelial lesion (HSIL)? *Hum Pathol.* 1999;30:345-351.

Kong CS, Balzer BL, Troxell ML, et al. P16ink4a immunohistochemistry is superior to HPV in situ hybridization for the detection of high-risk HPV in atypical squamous metaplasia. *Am J Surg Pathol.* 2007;31:33-43.

Park JJ, Genest DR, Sun D, et al. Atypical immature metaplastic-like proliferations of the cervix: diagnostic reproducibility and viral (HPV) correlates. *Hum Pathol.* 1999;30:1161-1165.

Regauer S, Reich O. Ck17 and p16 expression patterns distinguish (atypical) immature squamous metaplasia from high-grade cervical intraepithelial neoplasia (CIN III). *Histopathology.* 2007;50:629-635.

Reich O, Regauer S. Thin HSIL of the cervix: detecting a variant of high-grade squamous intraepithelial lesions with a p16INK4a antibody. *Int J Gynecol Pathol.* 2017;36(1):71-75.

Skapa P, Robova H, Rob L, et al. P16(ink4a) immunoprofiles of squamous lesions of the uterine cervix—implications for the reclassification of atypical immature squamous metaplasia. *Pathol Oncol Res.* 2013;19:707-714.

Stoler MH, Wright TC Jr, Ferenczy A, et al. Routine use of adjunctive p16 immunohistochemistry improves diagnostic agreement of cervical biopsy interpretation: results from the CERTAIN study. *Am J Surg Pathol.* 2018;42(8):1001-1009.

Weir MM, Bell DA, Young RH. Transitional cell metaplasia of the uterine cervix and vagina: an underrecognized lesion that may be confused with high-grade dysplasia. A report of 59 cases. *Am J Surg Pathol.* 1997;21:510-517.

2.7

Darragh TM, Colgan TJ, Thomas Cox J, et al. The lower anogenital squamous terminology standardization project for HPV-associated lesions: background and consensus recommendations from the college of American Pathologists and the American Society for Colposcopy and Cervical Pathology. *Int J Gynecol Pathol.* 2013;32:76-115.

Tumors of the cervix. In: Kurman RJ, Ronnett BM, Sherman ME, Wilkinson EJ, eds. *Atlas of Tumor Pathology, 4th series, fasc 13. Tumors of the Cervix, Vagina, and Vulva.* Armed Forces Institute of Pathology; 2010:105-121.

Witkiewicz AK, Wright TC, Ferenczy A, et al. Carcinoma and other tumors of the cervix. In: Kurman RJ, Ellenson LH, Ronnett BM, eds. *Blaustein's Pathology of the Female Genital Tract.* 6th ed. Springer; 2011:254-261.

2.8

Brainard JA, Hart WR. Adenoid basal epitheliomas of the uterine cervix: a reevaluation of distinctive cervical basaloid lesions currently classified as adenoid basal carcinoma and adenoid basal hyperplasia. *Am J Surg Pathol.* 1998;22:965-975.

2 CERVIX

Goyal A, Wang Z, Przybycin CG, et al. Application of p16 immuno-histochemistry and RNA in situ hybridization in the classification of adenoid basal tumors of the cervix. *Int J Gynecol Pathol.* 2016;35:82-91.

Hart WR. Symposium part II: special types of adenocarcinoma of the uterine cervix. *Int J Gynecol Pathol.* 2002;21:327-346.

Parwani AV, Smith Sehdev AE, Kurman RJ, et al. Cervical adenoid basal tumors comprised of adenoid basal epithelioma associated with various types of invasive carcinoma: clinicopathologic features, human papillomavirus DNA detection, and p16 expression. *Hum Pathol.* 2005;36:82-90.

Russell MJ, Fadare O. Adenoid basal lesions of the uterine cervix: evolving terminology and clinicopathological concepts. *Diagn Pathol.* 2006;1:18.

2.9 and 2.10

Boyle DP, McCluggage WG. Stratified mucin-producing intraepithelial lesion (SMILE): report of a case series with associated pathological findings. *Histopathology.* 2015;66:658-663.

Lastra RR, Park KJ, Schoolmeester JK. Invasive stratified mucin-producing carcinoma and stratified mucin-producing intraepithelial lesion (smile): 15 cases presenting a spectrum of cervical neoplasia with description of a distinctive variant of invasive adenocarcinoma. *Am J Surg Pathol.* 2016;40:262-269.

Park JJ, Sun D, Quade BJ, et al. Stratified mucin-producing intraepithelial lesions of the cervix: adenosquamous or columnar cell neoplasia? *Am J Surg Pathol.* 2000;24:1414-1419.

2.11

Chang A, Amin A, Gabrielson E, et al. Utility of GATA3 immunohistochemistry in differentiating urothelial carcinoma from prostate adenocarcinoma and squamous cell carcinomas of the uterine cervix, anus, and lung. *Am J Surg Pathol.* 2012;36:1472-1476.

Chen ME, Pisters LL, Malpica A, et al. Risk of urethral, vaginal and cervical involvement in patients undergoing radical cystectomy for bladder cancer: results of a contemporary cystectomy series from M.D. Anderson Cancer Center. *J Urol.* 1997;157:2120-2123.

Gailey MP, Bellizzi AM. Immunohistochemistry for the novel markers glypican 3, pax8, and p40 (ΔNp63) in squamous cell and urothelial carcinoma. *Am J Clin Pathol.* 2013;140:872-880.

Miettinen M, McCue PA, Sarlomo-Rikala M, et al. GATA3: a multispecific but potentially useful marker in surgical pathology: a systematic analysis of 2500 epithelial and nonepithelial tumors. *Am J Surg Pathol.* 2014;38(1):13-22.

Reyes MC, Park KJ, Lin O, et al. Urothelial carcinoma involving the gynecologic tract: a morphologic and immunohistochemical study of 6 cases. *Am J Surg Pathol.* 2012;36:1058-1065.

Schwartz LE, Khani F, Bishop JA, et al. Carcinoma of the uterine cervix involving the genitourinary tract: a potential diagnostic dilemma. *Am J Surg Pathol.* 2016;40:27-35.

2.12 and 2.14

Abi-Raad R, Alomari A, Hui P, et al. Mitotically active microglandular hyperplasia of the cervix: a case series with implications for the differential diagnosis. *Int J Gynecol Pathol.* 2014;33:524-530.

Biscotti CV, Hart WR. Apoptotic bodies: a consistent morphologic feature of endocervical adenocarcinoma in situ. *Am J Surg Pathol.* 1998;22:434-439.

Cameron RI, Maxwell P, Jenkins D, et al. Immunohistochemical staining with mib1, bcl2 and p16 assists in the distinction of cervical glandular intraepithelial neoplasia from tubo-endometrial metaplasia, endometriosis and microglandular hyperplasia. *Histopathology.* 2002;41:313-321.

Heller DS, Nguyen L, Goldsmith LT. Association of cervical microglandular hyperplasia with exogenous progestin exposure. *J Low Genit Tract Dis.* 2016;20:162-164.

Moritani S, Ioffe OB, Sagae S, et al. Mitotic activity and apoptosis in endocervical glandular lesions. *Int J Gynecol Pathol.* 2002;21:125-133.

Nucci MR. Pseudoneoplastic glandular lesions of the uterine cervix: a selective review. *Int J Gynecol Pathol.* 2014;33:330-338.

O'Neill CJ, McCluggage WG. P16 expression in the female genital tract and its value in diagnosis. *Adv Anat Pathol.* 2006;13:8-15.

Young RH, Scully RE. Atypical forms of microglandular hyperplasia of the cervix simulating carcinoma. A report of five cases and review of the literature. *Am J Surg Pathol.* 1989;13:50-56.

2.13, 2.15, and 2.16

Alvarado-Cabrero I, Parra-Herran C, Stolnicu S, et al. The Silva pattern-based classification for HPV-associated invasive endocervical adenocarcinoma and the distinction between in situ and invasive adenocarcinoma: relevant issues and recommendations from the International Society of Gynecological Pathologists. *Int J Gynecol Pathol.* 2021;40(Suppl 1):S48-S65.

Diaz De Vivar A, Roma AA, Park KJ, et al. Invasive endocervical adenocarcinoma: proposal for a new pattern-based classification system with significant clinical implications: a multi-institutional study. *Int J Gynecol Pathol.* 2013;32:592-601.

Garg S, Nagaria TS, Clarke B, et al. Molecular characterization of gastric-type endocervical adenocarcinoma using next-generation sequencing. *Mod Pathol.* 2019;32(12):1823-1833.

Hart WR. Symposium part II: special types of adenocarcinoma of the uterine cervix. *Int J Gynecol Pathol.* 2002;21:327-346.

Jones MA, Young RH, Scully RE. Diffuse laminar endocervical glandular hyperplasia. A benign lesion often confused with adenoma malignum (minimal deviation adenocarcinoma). *Am J Surg Pathol.* 1991;15:1123-1129.

Jones MA, Young RH. Endocervical type a (noncystic) tunnel clusters with cytologic atypia. A report of 14 cases. *Am J Surg Pathol.* 1996;20:1312-1318.

Lu S, Shen D, Zhao Y, Kang N, et al. Primary endocervical gastric-type adenocarcinoma: a clinicopathologic and immunohistochemical analysis of 23 cases. *Diagn Pathol.* 2019;14(1):72.

Maruyama R, Nagaoka S, Terao K, et al. Diffuse laminar endocervical glandular hyperplasia. *Pathol Int.* 1995;45:283-286.

Nucci MR, Clement PB, Young RH. Lobular endocervical glandular hyperplasia, not otherwise specified: a clinicopathologic analysis of thirteen cases of a distinctive pseudoneoplastic lesion and comparison with fourteen cases of adenoma malignum. *Am J Surg Pathol.* 1999;23:886-891.

Nucci MR. Pseudoneoplastic glandular lesions of the uterine cervix: a selective review. *Int J Gynecol Pathol.* 2014;33:330-338.

Park E, Kim SW, Kim S, et al. Genetic characteristics of gastric-type mucinous carcinoma of the uterine cervix. *Mod Pathol.* 2021;34(3):637-646.

Parra-Herran C, Taljaard M, Djordjevic B, et al. Pattern-based classification of invasive endocervical adenocarcinoma, depth of invasion measurement and distinction from adenocarcinoma in situ: interobserver variation among gynecologic pathologists. *Mod Pathol.* 2016;29(8):879-992.

Pirog EC, Park KJ, Kiyokawa T, et al. Gastric-type adenocarcinoma of the cervix: tumor with wide range of histologic appearances. *Adv Anat Pathol.* 2019;26(1):1-12.

Roma AA. Patterns of invasion of cervical adenocarcinoma as predicators of outcome. *Adv Anat Pathol.* 2015;22:345-354.

Rutgers JK, Roma AA, Park KJ, et al. Pattern classification of endocervical adenocarcinoma: reproducibility and review of criteria. *Mod Pathol.* 2016;29(9):1083-1094.

Turashvili G, Morency EG, Kracun M, et al. Morphologic features of gastric-type cervical adenocarcinoma in small surgical and cytology specimens. *Int J Gynecol Pathol.* 2019;38(3):263-275.

Wheeler DT, Kurman RJ. The relationship of glands to thick-wall blood vessels as a marker of invasion in endocervical adenocarcinoma. *Int J Gynecol Pathol.* 2005;24:125-130.

Zaino RJ. Glandular lesions of the uterine cervix. *Mod Pathol.* 2000;13:261-274.

Zaino RJ. Symposium part I: adenocarcinoma in situ, glandular dysplasia, and early invasive adenocarcinoma of the uterine cervix. *Int J Gynecol Pathol.* 2002;21:314-326.

2.17

Tambouret R, Clement PB, Young RH. Endometrial endometrioid adenocarcinoma with a deceptive pattern of spread to the uterine cervix: a manifestation of stage IIb endometrial carcinoma liable to be misinterpreted as an independent carcinoma or a benign lesion. *Am J Surg Pathol.* 2003;27:1080-1088.

Witkiewicz AK, Wright TC, Ferenczy A, et al. Carcinoma and other tumors of the cervix. In: Kurman RJ, Ellenson LH, Ronnett BM, eds. *Blaustein's Pathology of the Female Genital Tract.* 6th ed. Springer; 2011:273-280.

Zaino RJ, Abendroth C, Yemelyanova A, et al. Endocervical involvement in endometrial adenocarcinoma is not prognostically significant and the pathologic assessment of the pattern of involvement is not reproducible. *Gynecol Oncol.* 2013;128:83-87.

2.18 and 2.21

Ansari-Lari MA, Staebler A, Zaino RJ, et al. Distinction of endocervical and endometrial adenocarcinomas: immunohistochemical p16 expression correlated with human papillomavirus (HPV) DNA detection. *Am J Surg Pathol.* 2004;28:160-167.

O'Neill CJ, McCluggage WG. P16 expression in the female genital tract and its value in diagnosis. *Adv Anat Pathol.* 2006;13:8-15.

Staebler A, Sherman ME, Zaino RJ, et al. Hormone receptor immunohistochemistry and human papillomavirus in situ hybridization are useful for distinguishing endocervical and endometrial adenocarcinomas. *Am J Surg Pathol.* 2002;26:998-1006.

Yemelyanova A, Ji H, Shih Ie M, et al. Utility of p16 expression for distinction of uterine serous carcinomas from endometrial endometrioid and endocervical adenocarcinomas: immunohistochemical analysis of 201 cases. *Am J Surg Pathol.* 2009;33:1504-1514.

2.19 and 2.20

Ferry JA, Scully RE. Mesonephric remnants, hyperplasia, and neoplasia in the uterine cervix. A study of 49 cases. *Am J Surg Pathol.* 1990;14:1100-1111.

Howitt BE, Emori MM, Drapkin R, et al. Gata3 is a sensitive and specific marker of benign and malignant mesonephric lesions in the lower female genital tract. *Am J Surg Pathol.* 2015;39:1411-1419.

McCluggage WG, Oliva E, Herrington CS, et al. CD10 and calretinin staining of endocervical glandular lesions, endocervical stroma and endometrioid adenocarcinomas of the uterine corpus: CD10 positivity is characteristic of, but not specific for, mesonephric lesions and is not specific for endometrial stroma. *Histopathology.* 2003;43:144-150.

Nucci MR. Pseudoneoplastic glandular lesions of the uterine cervix: a selective review. *Int J Gynecol Pathol.* 2014;33:330-338.

Rabban JT, McAlhany S, Lerwill MF, et al. Pax2 distinguishes benign mesonephric and mullerian glandular lesions of the cervix from endocervical adenocarcinoma, including minimal deviation adenocarcinoma. *Am J Surg Pathol.* 2010;34:137-146.

Roma AA, Goyal A, Yang B. Differential expression patterns of GATA3 in uterine mesonephric and nonmesonephric lesions. *Int J Gynecol Pathol.* 2015;34:480-486.

Seidman JD, Tavassoli FA. Mesonephric hyperplasia of the uterine cervix: a clinicopathologic study of 51 cases. *Int J Gynecol Pathol.* 1995;14:293-299.

2.22

Huettner PC, Gersell DJ. Placental site nodule: a clinicopathologic study of 38 cases. *Int J Gynecol Pathol.* 1994;13:191-198.

Kalhor N, Ramirez PT, Deavers MT, et al. Immunohistochemical studies of trophoblastic tumors. *Am J Surg Pathol.* 2009;33:633-638.

Mao TL, Kurman RJ, Jeng YM, et al. HSD3B1 as a novel trophoblast-associated marker that assists in the differential diagnosis of trophoblastic tumors and tumorlike lesions. *Am J Surg Pathol.* 2008;32(2):236-242.

Mao TL, Seidman JD, Kurman RJ, et al. Cyclin E and p16 immunoreactivity in epithelioid trophoblastic tumor—an aid in differential diagnosis. *Am J Surg Pathol.* 2006;30:1105-1110.

Shih IM, Kurman RJ. The pathology of intermediate trophoblastic tumors and tumor-like lesions. *Int J Gynecol Pathol.* 2001;20:31-47.

Shih IM, Seidman JD, Kurman RJ. Placental site nodule and characterization of distinctive types of intermediate trophoblast. *Hum Pathol.* 1999;30:687-694.

Young RH, Kurman RJ, Scully RE. Placental site nodules and plaques. A clinicopathologic analysis of 20 cases. *Am J Surg Pathol.* 1990;14:1001-1009.

2.23

Albores-Saavedra J, Martinez-Benitez B, Luevano E. Small cell carcinomas and large cell neuroendocrine carcinomas of the endometrium and cervix: polypoid tumors and those arising in polyps may have a favorable prognosis. *Int J Gynecol Pathol.* 2008;27:333-339.

Eichhorn JH, Young RH. Neuroendocrine tumors of the genital tract. *Am J Clin Pathol.* 2001;115(suppl):S94-S112.

Ganesan R, Hirschowitz L, Dawson P, et al. Neuroendocrine carcinoma of the cervix: review of a series of cases and correlation with outcome. *Int J Surg Pathol.* 2016;24(6):490-496.

Gardner GJ, Reidy-Lagunes D, Gehrig PA. Neuroendocrine tumors of the gynecologic tract: a society of gynecologic oncology (SGO) clinical document. *Gynecol Oncol.* 2011;122:190-198.

Houghton O, McCluggage WG. The expression and diagnostic utility of p63 in the female genital tract. *Adv Anat Pathol.* 2009;16:316-321.

McCluggage WG, Kennedy K, Busam KJ. An immunohistochemical study of cervical neuroendocrine carcinomas: neoplasms that are commonly TTF1 positive and which may express CK20 and p63. *Am J Surg Pathol.* 2010;34:525-532.

Rouzbahman M, Clarke B. Neuroendocrine tumors of the gynecologic tract: select topics. *Semin Diagn Pathol.* 2013;30:224-233.

Ting CH, Wang TY, Wu PS. Insulinoma-associated Protein 1 expression and its diagnostic significance in female genital tract neuroendocrine carcinomas. *Int J Gynecol Pathol.* 2021;40(5):452-459.

Xing D, Zheng G, Schoolmeester JK, et al. Next-generation sequencing reveals recurrent somatic mutations in small cell neuroendocrine carcinoma of the uterine cervix. *Am J Surg Pathol.* 2018;42(6):750-760.

2.24

Amesse LS, Taneja A, Broxson E, et al. Protruding giant cervical polyp in a young adolescent with a previous rhabdomyosarcoma. *J Pediatr Adolesc Gynecol.* 2002;15:271-277.

Bernal KL, Fahmy L, Remmenga S, et al. Embryonal rhabdomyosarcoma (sarcoma botryoides) of the cervix presenting as a cervical polyp treated with fertility-sparing surgery and adjuvant chemotherapy. *Gynecol Oncol.* 2004;95:243-246.

Daya DA, Scully RE. Sarcoma botryoides of the uterine cervix in young women: a clinicopathological study of 13 cases. *Gynecol Oncol.* 1988;29:290-304.

de Kock L, Yoon JY, Apellaniz-Ruiz M, et al. Significantly greater prevalence of DICER1 alterations in uterine embryonal rhabdomyosarcoma compared to adenosarcoma. *Mod Pathol.* 2020;33(6):1207-1219.

Dehner LP, Jarzembowski JA, Hill DA. Embryonal rhabdomyosarcoma of the uterine cervix: a report of 14 cases and a discussion of its unusual clinicopathological associations. *Mod Pathol.* 2012;25:602-614.

Doros L, Yang J, Dehner L, et al. DICER1 mutations in embryonal rhabdomyosarcomas from children with and without familial PPB-tumor predisposition syndrome. *Pediatr Blood Cancer.* 2012;59(3):558-560.

Ferguson SE, Gerald W, Barakat RR, et al. Clinicopathologic features of rhabdomyosarcoma of gynecologic origin in adults. *Am J Surg Pathol.* 2007;31:382-389.

Khalil AM, Azar GB, Kaspar HG, et al. Giant cervical polyp. A case report. *J Reprod Med.* 1996;41:619-621.

Kommoss FKF, Stichel D, Mora J, et al. Clinicopathologic and molecular analysis of embryonal rhabdomyosarcoma of the genitourinary tract: evidence for a distinct DICER1-associated subgroup. *Mod Pathol.* 2021;34(8):1558-1569.

Li RF, Gupta M, McCluggage WG, et al. Embryonal rhabdomyosarcoma (botryoid type) of the uterine corpus and cervix in adult women: report of a case series and review of the literature. *Am J Surg Pathol.* 2013;37:344-355.

Lippert LJ, Richart RM, Ferenczy A. Giant benign endocervical polyp: report of a case. *Am J Obstet Gynecol.* 1974;118:1140-1141.

Shern JF, Chen L, Chmielecki J, et al. Comprehensive genomic analysis of rhabdomyosarcoma reveals a landscape of alterations affecting a common genetic axis in fusion-positive and fusion-negative tumors. *Cancer Discov.* 2014;4(2):216-231.

Yoon JY, Apellaniz-Ruiz M, Chong AL, et al. The value of DICER1 mutation analysis in "subtle" diagnostically challenging embryonal rhabdomyosarcomas of the uterine cervix. *Int J Gynecol Pathol.* 2021;40(5):435-440.

2.25

Bennett JA, Croce S, Pesci A, et al. Inflammatory myofibroblastic tumor of the uterus: an immunohistochemical study of 23 cases. *Am J Surg Pathol.* 2020;44(11):1441-1449.

Bennett JA, Nardi V, Rouzbahman M, et al. Inflammatory myofibroblastic tumor of the uterus: a clinicopathological, immunohistochemical, and molecular analysis of 13 cases highlighting their broad morphologic spectrum. *Mod Pathol.* 2017;30(10):1489-1503.

Chiang S, Cotzia P, Hyman DM, et al. NTRK fusions define a novel uterine sarcoma subtype with features of fibrosarcoma. *Am J Surg Pathol.* 2018;42(6):791-798.

Chiang S. S100 and Pan-Trk staining to report NTRK fusion-positive uterine sarcoma: proceedings of the ISGyP Companion Society Session at the 2020 USCAP Annual Meeting. *Int J Gynecol Pathol.* 2021;40(1):24-27.

Croce S, Hostein I, Longacre TA, et al. Uterine and vaginal sarcomas resembling fibrosarcoma: a clinicopathological and molecular analysis of 13 cases showing common NTRK-rearrangements and the description of a COL1A1-PDGFB fusion novel to uterine neoplasms. *Mod Pathol.* 2019;32(7):1008-1022.

Croce S, Hostein I, McCluggage WG. NTRK and other recently described kinase fusion positive uterine sarcomas: a review of a group of rare neoplasms. *Genes Chromosomes Cancer.* 2021;60(3):147-159.

Demetri GD, Antonescu CR, Bjerkehagen B, et al. Diagnosis and management of tropomyosin receptor kinase (TRK) fusion sarcomas: expert recommendations from the World Sarcoma Network. *Ann Oncol.* 2020;31(11):1506-1517.

Hechtman JF, Benayed R, Hyman DM, et al. Pan-Trk immunohistochemistry is an efficient and reliable screen for the detection of NTRK fusions. *Am J Surg Pathol.* 2017;41(11):1547-1551.

Hechtman JF, Benayed R, Hyman DM, et al. Pan-Trk immunohistochemistry is an efficient and reliable screen for the detection of NTRK fusions. *Am J Surg Pathol.* 2017;41(11):1547-1551.

Mandato VD, Valli R, Mastrofilippo V, et al. Uterine inflammatory myofibroblastic tumor: more common than expected: case report and review. *Medicine (Baltimore).* 2017;96(48):e8974.

Parra-Herran C, Quick CM, Howitt BE, et al. Inflammatory myofibroblastic tumor of the uterus: clinical and pathologic review of 10 cases including a subset with aggressive clinical course. *Am J Surg Pathol.* 2015;39(2):157-168.

Rabban JT, Devine WP, Sangoi AR, et al. NTRK fusion cervical sarcoma: a report of three cases, emphasising morphological and immunohistochemical distinction from other uterine sarcomas, including adenosarcoma. *Histopathology.* 2020;77(1):100-111.

Rabban JT, Zaloudek CJ, Shekitka KM, et al. Inflammatory myofibroblastic tumor of the uterus: a clinicopathologic study of 6 cases emphasizing distinction from aggressive mesenchymal tumors. *Am J Surg Pathol.* 2005;29(10):1348-1355.

Yamamoto H, Nozaki Y, Kohashi K, et al. Diagnostic utility of pan-Trk immunohistochemistry for inflammatory myofibroblastic tumours. *Histopathology.* 2020;76(5):774-778.

2 CERVIX

3

Uterine Corpus (Epithelial Lesions)

	Menstrual Endometrium	Anovulation-Related Endometrial Stromal Breakdown/Dysfunctional Uterine Bleeding
Age	Reproductive-age women	Reproductive-age women; when related to true anovulation, is more common in perimenopause
Location	Endometrium	Endometrium
Symptoms	Cyclical vaginal bleeding	Irregular vaginal bleeding, often mid cycle
Signs	Vaginal bleeding	Vaginal bleeding; mildly increased endometrial thickness/stripe (<10 mm)
Etiology	Normal/physiologic	Anovulatory cycle, failed follicle, absence of progression to luteal phase, PCOS; occasionally coagulopathy
Histology	1. Markedly fragmented endometrium with loss of normal architecture; extensive hemorrhage; diffuse stromal breakdown, aggregates of condensed predecidual cells admixed with blood and inflammatory cells, including numerous neutrophils *(Figs. 3.1.1-3.1.3)* 2. Fragmented endometrial glands with secretory exhaustion forming cords *(Fig .3.1.4)* 3. Sheets of syncytial metaplasia 4. Extensive fibrin is often present	1. Variably fragmented sample with subcapsular stromal condensation (early stromal breakdown) or hyperchromatic stromal balls *(Figs. 3.1.5-3.1.7)* 2. Endometrial glands with features of interval, proliferative (often disordered) or early secretory endometrium *(Figs. 3.1.5-3.1.7)* 3. Epithelial metaplastic changes (eosinophilic, papillary, syncytial, tubal metaplasia) can be seen *(Fig. 3.1.8)* 4. Fibrin thrombi in the stroma in cases of prolonged bleeding *(Fig. 3.1.6)*
Special studies	None helpful in this differential	None helpful in this differential
Treatment	None indicated	Management of the underlying cause; hormonal therapy with cyclic estrogens/progestins
Prognosis	Unremarkable	Benign, but can affect fertility. Unopposed estrogenic stimulation is a risk factor for development of endometrial hyperplasia/carcinoma; resampling should be considered if the symptoms persist

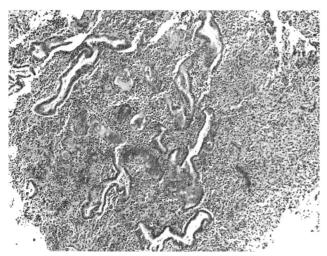

Figure 3.1.1 Menstrual endometrium. Markedly disrupted endometrium with loss of normal architecture and extensive stromal hemorrhage.

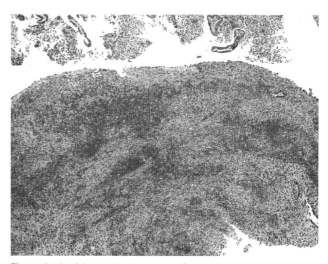

Figure 3.1.2 Menstrual endometrium. Stromal hemorrhage and diffuse stromal breakdown.

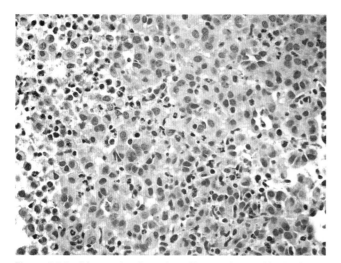

Figure 3.1.3 Menstrual endometrium. Clusters of predecidualized stromal cells with inflammatory cells including numerous neutrophils.

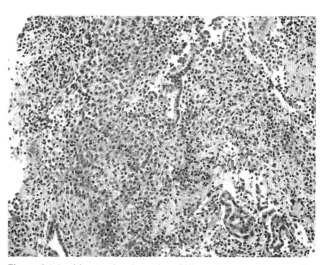

Figure 3.1.4 Menstrual endometrium. Diffuse stromal breakdown with fragmented late secretory glands.

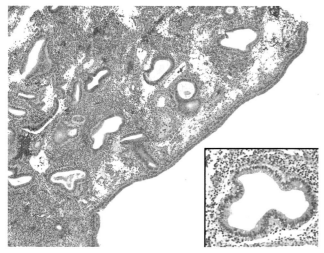

Figure 3.1.5 Interval endometrium with early stromal breakdown. **Inset**, higher magnification, some glands with subnuclear vacuoles indicating developing secretory changes.

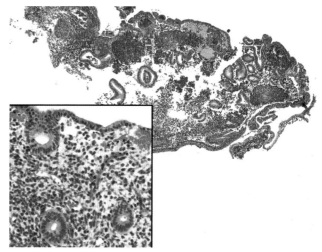

Figure 3.1.6 Proliferative endometrium with stromal breakdown (stromal balls) and fibrin underneath the endometrial surface epithelium. **Inset**, higher magnification, background endometrium with proliferative glands with mitoses.

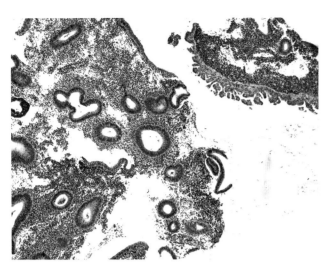 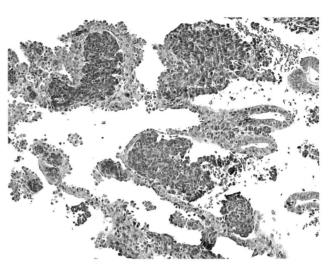

Figure 3.1.7   Disordered proliferative endometrium with early stromal collapse. Condensed subsurface stroma and surface epithelial metaplastic changes (fragment, **upper right**).

Figure 3.1.8   Endometrial stromal breakdown. Stromal balls surrounded by epithelium with prominent eosinophilic metaplastic changes.

	Artifactual Glandular Crowding	Endometrial Hyperplasia
Age	Any age, more common in reproductive years	Reproductive years and postmenopausal
Location	Endometrium	Endometrium
Symptoms	Abnormal vaginal bleeding is usually an indication for endometrial biopsy	Abnormal vaginal bleeding
Signs	No specific signs	Constitutional symptoms: obesity, diabetes, PCOS; thickened endometrial stripe on sonography
Etiology	N/A	Unopposed estrogenic stimulation; somatic mutations in *PTEN, KRAS, CTNNB1*; hereditary syndromes, Lynch and Cowden syndromes
Histology	1. Distorted tissue with "glandular molding," "telescoping," and tearing of the stroma around the glands *(Figs. 3.2.1-3.2.3)* 2. Endometrial stromal breakdown and associated tissue fragmentation *(Fig. 3.2.4)* 3. Squamous morular metaplasia is very uncommon 4. Endometrial glands without cytologic atypia, similar to the background noncrowded endometrium *(Fig. 3.2.5)* 5. Epithelial metaplastic changes can be present	1. Glandular crowding in the relatively intact fragments of endometrium; dilated glands of different sizes, complex, irregular glandular outlines *(Figs. 3.2.6 and 3.2.7)* 2. Endometrial stromal breakdown can be present, but tissue fragmentation should not interfere with the assessment of architecture 3. Squamous metaplasia can be present *(Fig. 3.2.8)* 4. Cytologic atypia can be present 5. Epithelial metaplastic changes can be present
Special studies	Not helpful in this differential	Not helpful in this differential
Treatment	None	Hormonal treatment (progestins) or hysterectomy in cases of atypical hyperplasia (if fertility preservation is not desired)
Prognosis	No prognostic significance; however, endometrial sampling should be repeated, if symptoms persist	Dependent on the presence or absence of cytologic atypia; cases of complex atypical hyperplasia have up to 40% chance of coexisting endometrial carcinoma

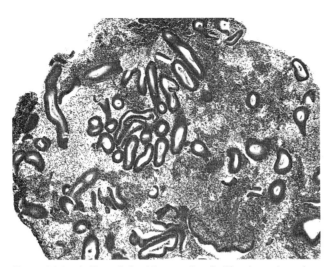

Figure 3.2.1   Artifactual glandular crowding. Proliferative endometrium with small tubular glands. Gland-to-stroma ratio appears increased due to stromal disruption.

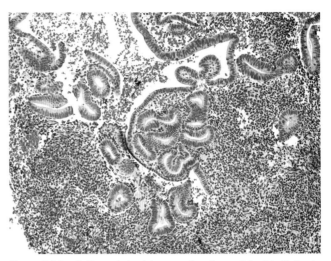

Figure 3.2.2   Artifactual glandular crowding. Focus of "molded" glands beneath the endometrial surface (**center**) due to stromal disruption, note extravasated blood.

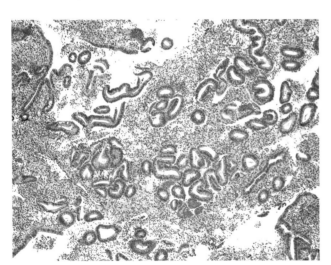

Figure 3.2.3   Artifactual glandular crowding. Proliferative endometrium. Stromal disruption creates a few foci with increased gland-to-stroma ratio. Glands are small and retain tubular shapes.

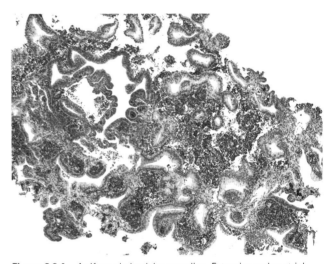

Figure 3.2.4   Artifactual glandular crowding. Extensive endometrial stromal breakdown; stromal balls and prominent epithelial metaplastic changes. A few glands appear back to back due to stromal collapse.

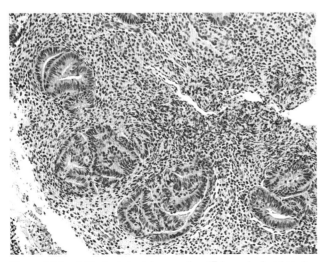

Figure 3.2.5   Artifactual glandular crowding. "Telescoping" and crush, common artifacts seen in endometrial biopsies with tissue distortion.

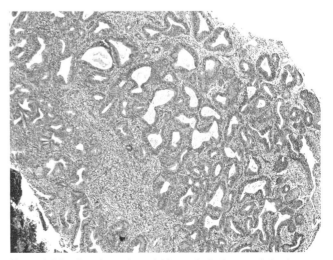

Figure 3.2.6   Complex endometrial hyperplasia. Increased gland-to-stroma ratio. Endometrial glands of different shapes and sizes.

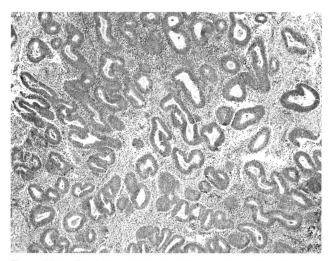

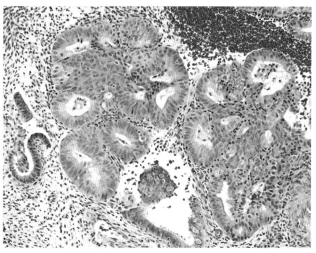

Figure 3.2.7   Simple hyperplasia. Despite some stromal disruption, most of the stroma is intact. Glands are crowded and irregularly shaped; some are cystically dilated.

Figure 3.2.8   Foci of complex hyperplasia with squamous metaplasia.

	Complex Atypical Hyperplasia	Complex Hyperplasia Without Atypia (+/− Metaplastic Changes)
Age	Wide age range; mean age is 53 y	Wide age range, most commonly in perimenopause
Location	Endometrium	Endometrium
Symptoms	Abnormal vaginal bleeding	Abnormal vaginal bleeding
Signs	Noncyclical vaginal bleeding, constitutional symptoms: obesity, diabetes, PCOS; thickened endometrial stripe on sonography	Noncyclical vaginal bleeding, constitutional symptoms: obesity, diabetes, PCOS; thickened endometrial stripe on sonography
Etiology	Unopposed estrogenic stimulation; somatic mutations in *PTEN, KRAS, CTNNB1*; hereditary syndromes, Lynch and Cowden syndromes	Unopposed estrogenic stimulation
Histology	1. Glands of atypical hyperplasia appear pale compared to the nonhyperplastic/nonatypical endometrial glands (if present) *(Fig. 3.3.1)* 2. Enlarged rounded vesicular nuclei; stratification and loss of polarity *(Fig. 3.3.2)* 3. Nucleoli often inconspicuous *(Fig. 3.3.3)* but occasionally may be evident 4. In presence of metaplastic change (particularly tubal/ciliated), may see nuclear rounding, nuclear enlargement, stratification, vesicular nuclei with nucleoli *(Fig. 3.3.4)*	1. Basophilic-appearing endometrial glands at low magnification *(Fig. 3.3.1)* 2. Hyperchromatic elongated nuclei, oriented perpendicular to the basement membrane *(Fig. 3.3.2)* 3. Nucleoli are not seen (unless superimposed metaplastic changes are present) 4. In presence of metaplastic changes (particularly tubal/ciliated change), evaluation of atypia can be difficult; nuclear rounding, some enlargement, and occasional nucleoli are often seen; however, chromatin is evenly distributed *(Figs. 3.3.5 and 3.3.6)*
Special studies	Not helpful in this differential diagnosis	Not helpful in this differential diagnosis
Treatment	Hysterectomy or progestins therapy if fertility preservation is desired	Progestins therapy to control bleeding; additional endometrial sampling in follow-up to exclude atypical hyperplasia
Prognosis	Significant percent (20%-40%) of uteri with complex atypical hyperplasia diagnosed on preoperative biopsy, demonstrate carcinoma in the hysterectomy specimen	Very small chance (1%-3%) of progression to carcinoma; however, repeat endometrial sampling is recommended for follow-up, particularly if symptoms persist

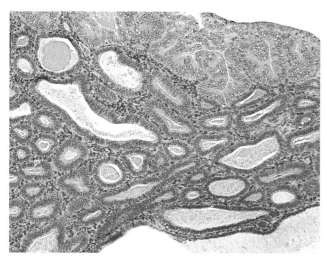

Figure 3.3.1   Focal complex atypical hyperplasia **(top)** in a background of complex hyperplasia without atypia. Atypical glands appear pale compared to darker more basophilic glands without atypia.

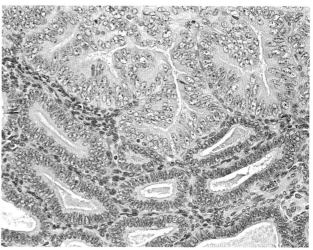

Figure 3.3.2   Focal complex atypical hyperplasia **(top)** in a background of complex hyperplasia without atypia. Same case as in *Figure 3.3.1*, higher magnification. Atypical glands **(top)** with nuclear enlargement, rounding, stratification, vesicular chromatin, and nucleoli. Compare with more elongated basophilic nuclei, aligned perpendicular to the basement membrane in glands without atypia **(bottom)**.

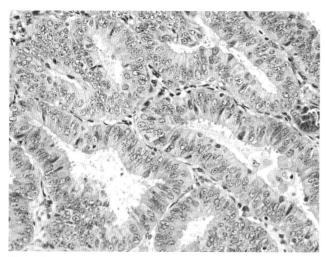

Figure 3.3.3   Complex atypical hyperplasia. Back-to-back glands with enlarged round nuclei with stratification and occasional nucleoli.

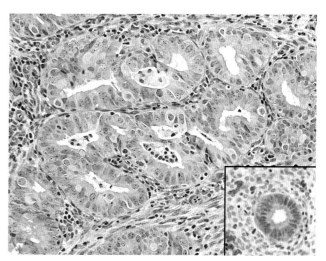

Figure 3.3.4   Complex atypical hyperplasia with superimposed tubal metaplastic changes. Nuclear enlargement and inconspicuous, often multiple nucleoli. Compare to normal proliferative endometrial gland from the background endometrium **(inset)**.

3   UTERINE CORPUS
(EPITHELIAL LESIONS)

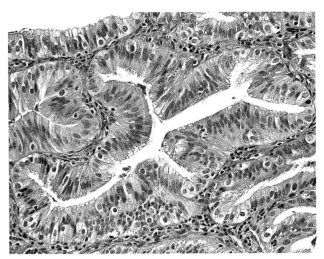

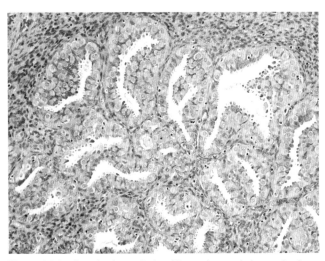

Figure 3.3.5   Complex hyperplasia with tubal metaplastic changes. Evaluation of atypia is difficult in this setting. No definite atypia identified.

Figure 3.3.6   Complex hyperplasia with prominent tubal metaplastic changes. Evaluation of atypia is difficult in this setting. No definite atypia identified.

	Endometrial Hyperplasia/Carcinoma With Secretory Differentiation	Secretory Endometrium
Age	Broad age range, from third decade to postmenopause	Reproductive-age women
Location	Endometrium	Endometrium
Symptoms	Abnormal vaginal bleeding	Abnormal vaginal bleeding
Signs	Constitutional symptoms, obesity, diabetes mellitus, polycystic ovarian syndrome, estrogen-producing ovarian tumors	Menometrorrhagia is usually an indication for an endometrial biopsy
Etiology	Unopposed estrogenic stimulation. Somatic mutations in *PTEN, PIK3CA, ARID1A,* and *KRAS*. Lynch syndrome (germline mutations in mismatch repair genes) and Cowden syndrome (germline mutation in *PTEN*)	Physiologic change; menometrorrhagia can be caused by ovarian cycle disturbances, submucosal leiomyomas, etc.
Histology	1. Distinct areas of crowded glands with divergent appearance compared to background endometrium 2. Architectural disorder: the long axes of the glands pointing in different directions; budding, branching glands, and staghorn-shaped *(Figs. 3.4.1 and 3.4.2)* glands 3. Crowded hyperplastic glands without secretory changes can be present *(Fig. 3.4.3)*; cribriform or confluent glands in cases of carcinoma 4. Nuclear features divergent from the background endometrial glands; cytologic atypia in cases of atypical hyperplasia and carcinoma *(Fig. 3.4.4)* 5. Mitotic figures can be seen but often rare	1. Diffusely crowded endometrial glands with relatively uniform glandular and stromal changes of secretory phase *(Fig. 3.4.5)* 2. Crowded irregular glands with long axis parallel to each other *(Fig. 3.4.6)* 3. Occasional noncrowded inactive glands without secretory changes (basalis) can be seen 4. Small, uniform, bland-appearing nuclei *(Fig. 3.4.7)* 5. Mitotic figures are rare (usually absent)
Special studies	• None helpful in this differential • Ki 67 has been suggested by some; increased proliferative activity in glands	• None helpful in this differential • Ki 67 has been suggested by some; low proliferative activity in glands *(Fig. 3.4.5,* **inset**)
Treatment	Repeat sampling during the first part of the menstrual cycle can be recommended for further evaluation and determination of presence of cytologic atypia	In cases with concern for underlying endometrial hyperplasia, repeat biopsy during the first part of the menstrual cycle should be recommended; treatment of an underlying condition
Prognosis	Increased risk of concurrent endometrial carcinoma, if cytologic atypia is present	Unremarkable; related to an underlying condition

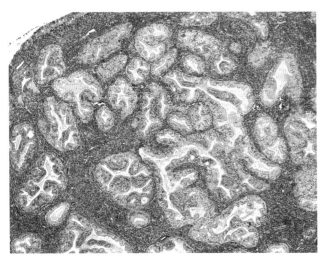

Figure 3.4.1 Complex hyperplasia with secretory changes. Haphazardly arranged irregularly shaped glands of varying sizes.

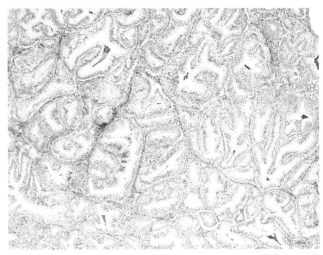

Figure 3.4.2 Complex hyperplasia with extensive secretory changes. Markedly crowded endometrial glands with irregular shapes.

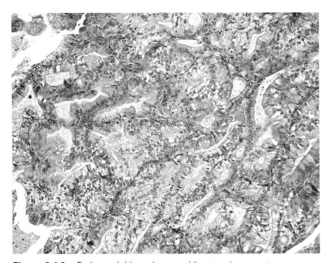

Figure 3.4.3 Endometrioid carcinoma with extensive secretory changes. Confluent endometrial glands. Range of early (sub- and supranuclear vacuoles) to midsecretory changes.

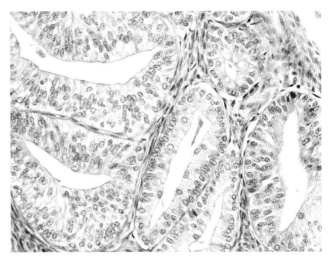

Figure 3.4.4 Complex atypical hyperplasia with extensive secretory changes. Same case as in *Figure 3.4.2*, higher magnification. Nuclei with vesicular chromatin and some stratification. Occasional nucleoli are seen.

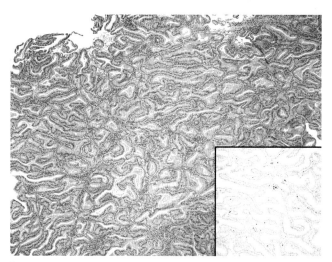

Figure 3.4.5   Secretory endometrium. Crowded endometrial glands without significant variation in size and shape. Ki 67 proliferative activity is essentially zero **(inset)**.

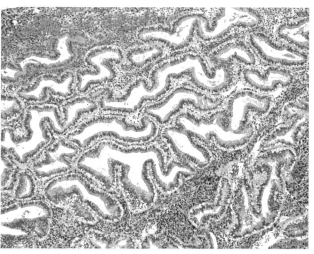

Figure 3.4.6   Early secretory endometrium. Irregular crowded endometrial glands with long axis parallel to each other. Note uniform subnuclear vacuoles reflecting early secretory phase.

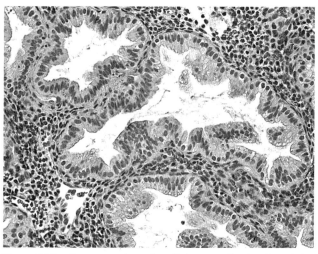

Figure 3.4.7   Secretory endometrium. Higher magnification, irregularly shaped glands in predecidualized stroma with small round basally placed nuclei.

	Endometrial Hyperplasia/Carcinoma With Progestin Treatment Effect	Secretory/Gestational Endometrium
Age	Premenopausal women, occasional postmenopausal	Reproductive-age women
Location	Endometrium	Endometrium
Symptoms	N/A, follow-up endometrial sampling	Abnormal vaginal bleeding
Signs	History of prior endometrial hyperplasia/carcinoma, ongoing treatment with progestins; constitutional symptoms, obesity, diabetes mellitus, polycystic ovarian syndrome, estrogen-producing ovarian tumors	Menometrorrhagia is usually an indication for an endometrial biopsy; spontaneous (or rarely elective) abortion, positive urine/serum β-hCG
Etiology	Unopposed estrogenic stimulation. Somatic mutations in *PTEN, PIK3CA, ARID1A*, and *KRAS*. Lynch syndrome (germline mutations in mismatch repair genes) and Cowden syndrome (germline mutation in *PTEN*)	Physiologic change; menometrorrhagia can be caused by ovarian cycle disturbances, submucosal leiomyomas, etc.; gestation, spontaneous abortion
Histology	1. Areas of extensively decidualized endometrial stroma with rare inactive glands are usually seen (resembling decidua/gestational endometrium) *(Fig. 3.5.1)* 2. Varying amount of glandular proliferation; glands of varying sizes, dilated irregular glands as well as small glands *(Fig. 3.5.2)* 3. Glandular proliferation with cribriform, papillary, and solid growth; squamous differentiation is often prominent *(Figs. 3.5.2-3.5.5)* 4. Small round nuclei with smudged chromatin or persistent cytologic atypia 5. Mitotic figures are rare	1. Diffusely crowded endometrial glands with relatively uniform glandular and stromal changes of secretory phase; occasional noncrowded inactive glands without secretory changes (basalis) can be seen *(Fig. 3.5.6)*; areas of decidua (if gestational endometrium) 2. Relatively uniformly sized glands 3. Crowded irregular glands with long axis parallel to each other *(Fig. 3.5.7)*; or hypersecretory glands (if gestational endometrium); solid growth, papillary architecture and squamous differentiation are not seen 4. Small, uniform, bland-appearing nuclei 5. Mitotic figures are rare (usually absent) Also see *Figures 3.4.5-3.4.7*
Special studies	None helpful in this differential	None helpful in this differential
Treatment	Continued progestin therapy or hysterectomy	In cases with negative urine/serum β-hCG and with concern for underlying endometrial hyperplasia, repeat biopsy during the first part of the menstrual cycle should be recommended; treatment of an underlying condition
Prognosis	Complete resolution of carcinoma/hyperplasia is seen in a proportion of patients (up to 40%)	Unremarkable; related to an underlying condition

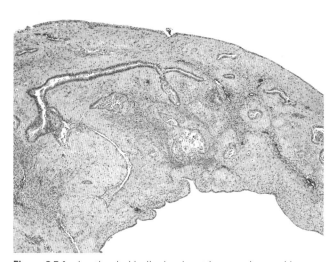

Figure 3.5.1 Inactive decidualized endometrium, consistent with exogenous progestin therapy effect with focal residual glandular proliferation.

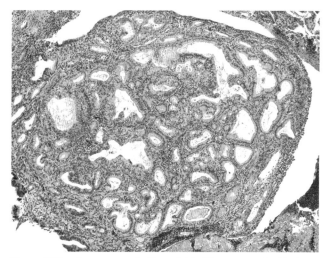

Figure 3.5.2 Same case as in *Figure 3.5.1*, different area. Residual endometrial hyperplasia. Complex back-to-back glands of different sizes and shapes.

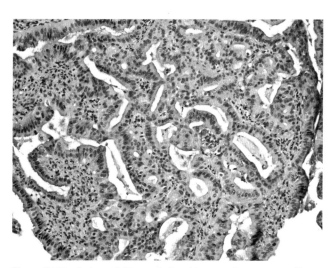

Figure 3.5.3 Endometrial hyperplasia with progestin treatment effect. Irregular, merging glands with luminal secretions.

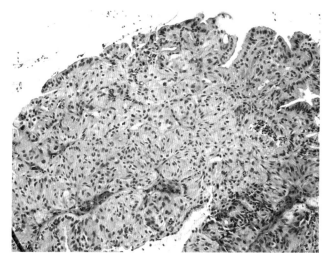

Figure 3.5.4 Focus of residual endometrioid carcinoma with progestin treatment effect. Glandular proliferation appears solid, but nuclei are bland and small. Such solid growth associated with therapy does not warrant elevation of FIGO grade.

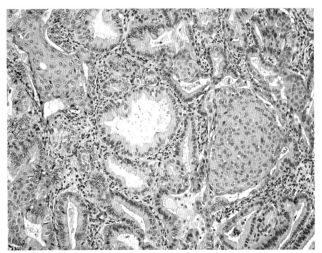

Figure 3.5.5   Endometrial hyperplasia with progestin treatment effect. Crowded glands with secretory changes and foci of squamous differentiation. Note small basally placed nuclei in the glandular epithelium.

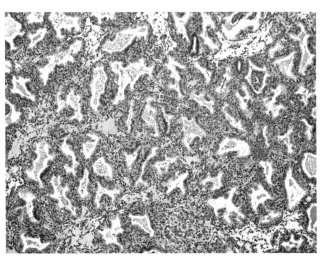

Figure 3.5.6   Secretory endometrium. Crowded endometrial glands without significant variation in size and shape. A few small inactive glands are present for comparison **(upper right)**.

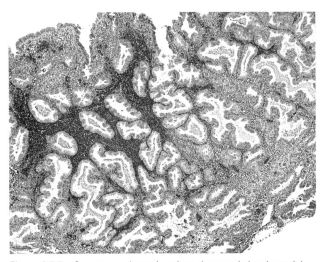

Figure 3.5.7   Secretory endometrium. Irregular crowded endometrial glands with long axis parallel to each other. Predecidualized stroma synchronous with the glandular changes of mid to late secretory phase.

	Complex Atypical Hyperplasia	FIGO Grade 1 Endometrioid Carcinoma
Age	Wide age range; mean age is 53 y	Wide age range; mean age is 63 y
Location	Endometrium	Endometrium
Symptoms	Abnormal vaginal bleeding	Abnormal vaginal bleeding; pelvic pain or pressure and abdominal distension in advanced cases
Signs	Noncyclical vaginal bleeding, constitutional symptoms: obesity, diabetes, PCOS; thickened endometrial stripe on sonography	Noncyclical vaginal bleeding, constitutional symptoms: obesity, diabetes, PCOS; thickened endometrial stripe or endometrial mass on MRI or sonography; abnormal Pap smear
Etiology	Unopposed estrogenic stimulation; somatic mutations in *PTEN, KRAS, CTNNB1*; hereditary syndromes, Lynch and Cowden syndromes	Unopposed estrogenic stimulation; somatic mutations in *PTEN, PIK3CA, KRAS, CTNNB1, ARID1A*; hereditary syndromes, Lynch and Cowden syndromes
Histology	1. Crowded back-to-back glands surrounded by stroma *(Fig. 3.6.1)* 2. Small foci of cribriforming (<2 mm) can be seen *(Fig. 3.6.2)* 3. Normal-appearing endometrial stroma can appear compressed between crowded glands 4. No extensive papillary architecture with true fibrovascular cores; intraglandular infoldings can be present 5. Fragments of crowded glands with rounded outlines	1. Confluent glands without intervening stroma *(Fig. 3.6.3)* 2. Cribriform growth >2 mm *(Fig. 3.6.4)* 3. Altered desmoplastic inflamed stroma (this criterion cannot be used in a polyp) *(Fig. 3.6.5)* 4. Complex papillary architecture 5. Long anastomosing fragments of glandular epithelium without intervening stroma, forming papillary structures (in biopsy/curettage) *(Fig. 3.6.6)*
Special studies	Not helpful in this differential diagnosis	Not helpful in this differential diagnosis
Treatment	Hysterectomy or progestin therapy if fertility preservation is desired	Hysterectomy with bilateral salpingo-oophorectomy, +/− pelvic and periaortic lymphadenectomy. Progestin therapy can be considered for fertility preservation (tumors limited to endometrium on MRI or transvaginal ultrasound and in the absence of suspicious/metastatic disease on imaging)
Prognosis	Significant percent (20%-40%) of uteri with complex atypical hyperplasia (diagnosed on preoperative biopsy) demonstrate carcinoma in the hysterectomy specimen	Stage dependent; 5-y survival for stage IA tumors is 95%

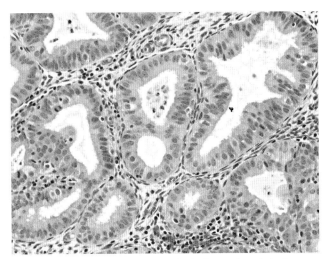

Figure 3.6.1   Complex atypical hyperplasia. Focus of nearly back-to-back glands with some shape irregularity, surrounded by nearly normal endometrial stroma.

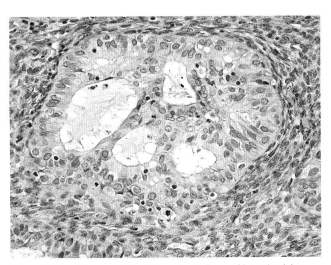

Figure 3.6.2   Complex atypical hyperplasia. Focus of intraglandular cribriforming (<1 mm).

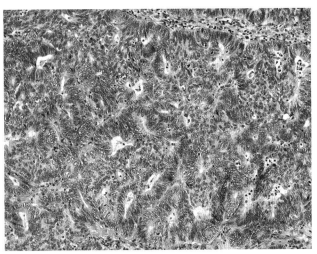

Figure 3.6.3   Endometrioid carcinoma, FIGO grade 1. Glandular confluence without intervening stroma.

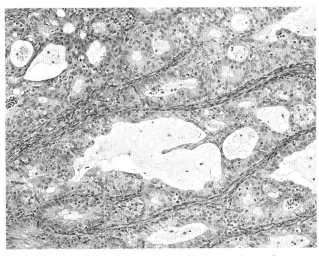

Figure 3.6.4   Endometrioid carcinoma, FIGO grade 1. Areas of cribriform growth (>2 mm).

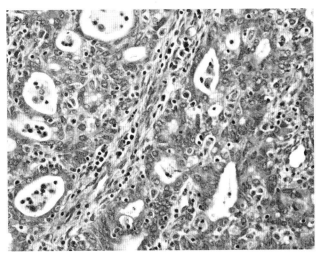

Figure 3.6.5   Endometrioid carcinoma, FIGO grade 1. Altered, fibroblastic stroma with inflammation; small glands with some confluence.

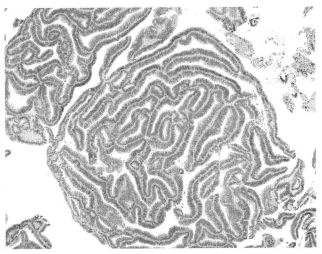

Figure 3.6.6   Endometrioid carcinoma, FIGO grade 1; endometrial curettage specimen, long interconnected fragments of glandular epithelium, forming papillary structures.

3.7

FRAGMENTS OF FIGO GRADE 1 ENDOMETRIOID CARCINOMA WITH METAPLASTIC-LIKE DIFFERENTIATION VS BENIGN ENDOMETRIAL TISSUE WITH METAPLASTIC CHANGES IN BIOPSY/CURETTAGE SPECIMENS

	Fragments of FIGO Grade 1 Endometrioid Carcinoma With Metaplastic-like Differentiation in Biopsy/Curettage	Benign Endometrial Tissue With Metaplastic Changes
Age	Wide age range; mean age is 63 y	Usually in reproductive-age women, occasionally, in postmenopausal
Location	Endometrium	Endometrium
Symptoms	Abnormal vaginal bleeding; pelvic pain or pressure and abdominal distension in advanced cases	Abnormal vaginal bleeding
Signs	Noncyclical vaginal bleeding, constitutional symptoms: obesity, diabetes, PCOS; thickened endometrial stripe or endometrial mass on MRI or sonography; abnormal Pap smear	Abnormal vaginal bleeding
Etiology	Unopposed estrogenic stimulation; somatic mutations in *PTEN, PIK3CA, KRAS, CTNNB1, ARID1A*; hereditary syndromes, Lynch and Cowden syndromes	Related to relative excess of estrogens; often associated with endometrial stromal breakdown; can be related to IUD
Histology	1. Confluent glands without intervening stroma (*Figs. 3.7.1 and 3.7.2*); cribriform growth 2. Altered desmoplastic inflamed stroma (this criterion cannot be used in a polyp) 3. Complex papillary architecture (*Figs. 3.7.3 and 3.7.4*) 4. Cytologic atypia, usually mild (*Fig. 3.7.5*) 5. Mitotic figures can be seen, but not a constant feature	1. Often involves surface endometrium (*Fig. 3.7.6*); no true glandular confluence; tangentially oriented sheets of metaplastic epithelium can mimic cribriform growth, but usually not very extensive (*Figs. 3.7.7 and 3.7.8*) 2. Stromal breakdown is often seen; no stromal desmoplasia (*Figs. 3.7.6 and 3.7.9*) 3. Small areas with papillary-like growths lacking well-developed fibrovascular cores (*Fig. 3.7.10*) 4. Mild cytologic atypia can be seen (*Fig. 3.7.10*) 5. Mitotic figures are rare
Special studies	Not helpful in this differential diagnosis	Not helpful in this differential diagnosis
Treatment	Hysterectomy with bilateral salpingo-oophorectomy, +/− pelvic and periaortic lymphadenectomy. Progestin therapy can be considered for fertility preservation (tumors limited to endometrium on MRI or transvaginal ultrasound and in the absence of suspicious/metastatic disease on imaging)	None required; treatment of underlying causes if needed
Prognosis	Stage dependent; 5-y survival for stage IA tumors is 95%	Benign; however, if symptoms persist, repeat endometrial sampling is recommended to exclude underlying neoplastic process

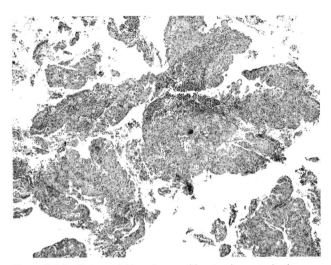

Figure 3.7.1 Endometrioid carcinoma with extensive metaplastic changes. Confluent epithelial proliferation with some cribriform formations. Associated inflammation is commonly seen.

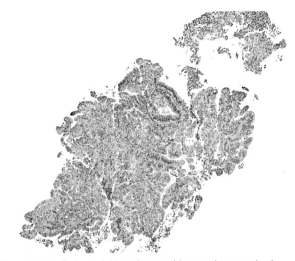

Figure 3.7.2 Endometrioid carcinoma with extensive metaplastic changes and secretory changes.

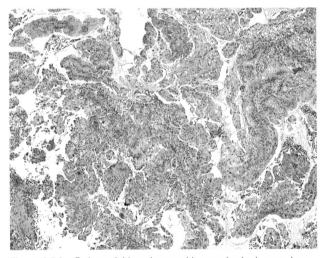

Figure 3.7.3 Endometrioid carcinoma with metaplastic changes. Long papillary structures with well-developed fibrovascular cores.

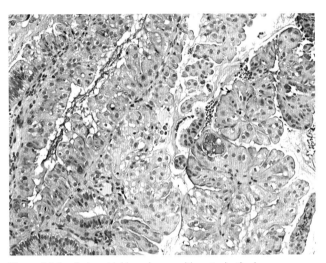

Figure 3.7.4 Endometrioid carcinoma with metaplastic changes. Same case as in *Figure 3.7.3*, higher magnification. Papillae are lined by epithelium with abundant eosinophilic and vacuolated cytoplasm. The nuclei are small and bland.

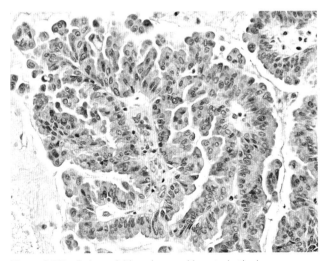

Figure 3.7.5 Endometrioid carcinoma with metaplastic changes. Prominent papillary architecture with mucinous differentiation. Detached cell clusters. Mildly atypical vesicular nuclei.

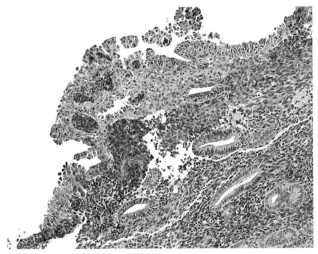

Figure 3.7.6 Proliferative endometrium with focal endometrial stromal breakdown. Surface epithelium overlying collapsed subepithelial stroma displays prominent eosinophilic and papillary metaplastic change. Detached papillary clusters can be seen.

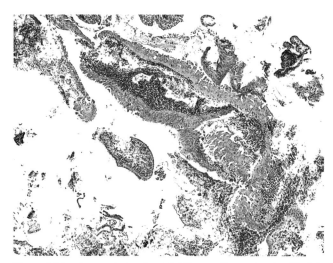

Figure 3.7.7   Fragmented endometrial tissue with prominent epithelial metaplastic changes.

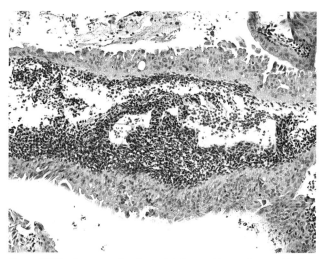

Figure 3.7.8   Fragmented endometrial tissue with prominent epithelial metaplastic changes. Same case as in *Figure 3.7.7*, higher magnification. Surface epithelium uniformly thickened and eosinophilic.

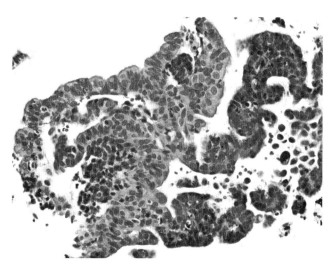

Figure 3.7.9   Endometrial stromal breakdown and associated surface epithelial metaplastic changes. The nuclei can appear stratified. Note cilia on the surface.

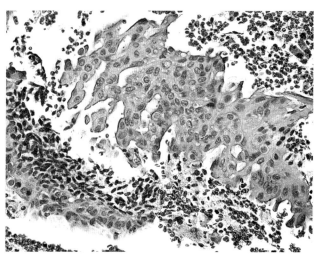

Figure 3.7.10   Fragmented endometrial tissue with prominent epithelial metaplastic changes. Same case as in *Figure 3.7.7*, higher magnification. Detached tangentially oriented fragment of eosinophilic epithelium may mimic papillary structure. Note lack of fibrovascular core. The nuclei are relatively uniform and mildly atypical.

	FIGO Grade 1 Endometrioid Carcinoma With Prominent Squamous Differentiation	FIGO Grade 2 Endometrioid Carcinoma
Age	Wide age span from third decade to late postmenopause; most cases are between 55 and 65 y	Wide age span from third decade to late postmenopause; most cases are between 55 and 65 y
Location	Endometrium	Endometrium
Symptoms	Vaginal bleeding	Vaginal bleeding
Signs	Abnormal uterine or postmenopausal bleeding; constitutional symptoms, obesity, diabetes mellitus, polycystic ovarian syndrome, estrogen producing ovarian tumors	Abnormal uterine or postmenopausal bleeding; constitutional symptoms, obesity, diabetes mellitus, polycystic ovarian syndrome, estrogen-producing ovarian tumors
Etiology	Unopposed estrogenic stimulation. Somatic mutations in *PTEN*, *PIK3CA*, *ARID1A*, and *KRAS* Lynch syndrome (germline mutations in mismatch repair genes) and Cowden syndrome (germline mutation in *PTEN*)	Unopposed estrogenic stimulation. Somatic mutations in *PTEN*, *PIK3CA*, *ARID1A*, and *KRAS* Lynch syndrome (germline mutations in mismatch repair genes) and Cowden syndrome (germline mutation in *PTEN*)
Histology	1. Solid (squamous)-appearing areas are tinctorially different from the glandular areas, usually more eosinophilic or pale *(Figs. 3.8.1 and 3.8.2)* 2. Squamous areas are usually surrounded by glandular areas 3. Cells in the squamous areas have moderate to abundant eosinophilic cytoplasm; well-defined cell membranes can be seen *(Fig. 3.8.3)* 4. N:C ratio is not significantly increased 5. Nuclei in squamous areas are bland and uniform, often smaller and less atypical than those in glandular areas *(Fig. 3.8.4)* 6. Keratinization *(Fig. 3.8.3)* can be seen	1. No difference in staining between solid and glandular areas *(Fig. 3.8.5)* 2. Solid areas variably distributed, often at the edges of the tumor nests 3. The amount and quality of the cytoplasm is similar between solid and glandular areas; cell borders are indiscernible *(Fig. 3.8.6)* 4. N:C ratio can be increased 5. Nuclear features are similar in solid and glandular areas *(Fig. 3.8.7)* 6. Keratinization is absent in nonsquamous solid areas
Special studies	Positive p63 staining in squamous areas (suggested by some experts)	Negative p63 staining in solid nonsquamous areas (suggested by some experts)
Treatment	Hysterectomy with bilateral salpingo-oophorectomy, +/− pelvic and periaortic lymphadenectomy. Conservative management with progestins can be considered for fertility preservation (tumors limited to endometrium on MRI or transvaginal ultrasound and in the absence of suspicious/metastatic disease on imaging); otherwise stage dependent (see FIGO grade 2 endometrioid carcinoma)	Hysterectomy with bilateral salpingo-oophorectomy, +/− pelvic and periaortic lymphadenectomy Stage IA tumors are generally cured by surgery alone; adjuvant vaginal brachytherapy for stage IB, +/− pelvic RT for cases with adverse risk factors; stages III and IV, chemotherapy +/− RT and vaginal brachytherapy
Prognosis	Stage dependent	Stage dependent

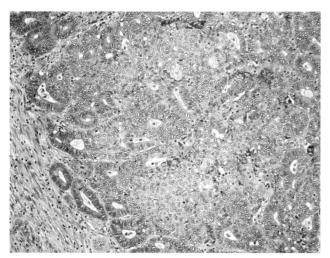

Figure 3.8.1   Endometrioid carcinoma, FIGO grade 1 with squamous differentiation. Squamous areas **(center)** appear pale compared to more basophilic glandular areas at the periphery.

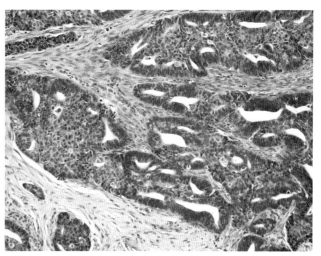

Figure 3.8.2   Endometrioid carcinoma, FIGO grade 1 with squamous differentiation. Squamous areas occupying centers of the tumor nests are eosinophilic compared to more basophilic glands at the periphery.

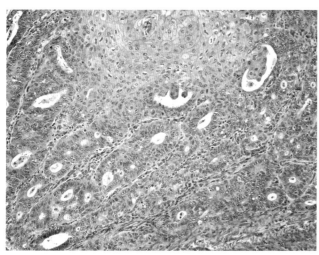

Figure 3.8.3   Endometrioid carcinoma, FIGO grade 1 with squamous differentiation. Pale squamous area **(top)** has eosinophilic focus of keratinization. The cells in squamous areas have abundant cytoplasm and defined cell borders.

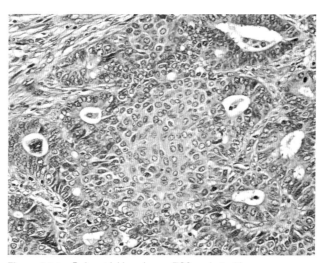

Figure 3.8.4   Endometrioid carcinoma, FIGO grade 1 with squamous differentiation. Higher magnification, squamous cells in the center with abundant pale pink cytoplasm and elongated nuclei with occasional grooves. Glandular cells forming glands are columnar with rounded vesicular nuclei.

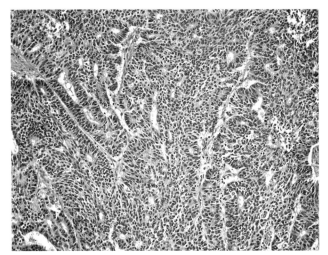

Figure 3.8.5 Endometrioid carcinoma, FIGO grade 2. Solid and glandular areas have similar tinctorial properties at low power.

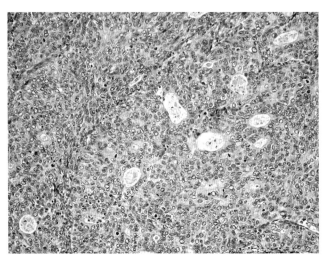

Figure 3.8.6 Endometrioid carcinoma, FIGO grade 2. Predominantly solid growth in this area with occasional glands with round lumina. The cells occupying solid areas and lining glandular spaces are identical.

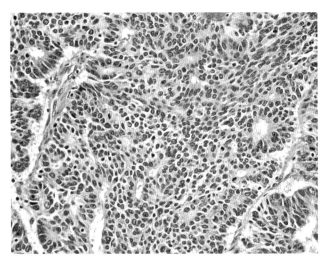

Figure 3.8.7 Endometrioid carcinoma, FIGO grade 2. Same case as in *Figure 3.8.5*, higher magnification. Tumor cell nuclei are similar in solid and gland-forming areas.

	Endometrioid Carcinoma With Papillary Architecture	Serous Carcinoma
Age	Wide age range, from third decade into late postmenopause; mean age 63 y	Postmenopausal; mean age in late 60s
Location	Endometrium	Endometrium
Symptoms	Vaginal bleeding, discharge	Postmenopausal bleeding; pelvic pain, abdominal distension in advanced cases
Signs	Constitutional symptoms, obesity, diabetes mellitus, polycystic ovarian syndrome, estrogen-producing ovarian tumors	Often present with subclinical advanced-stage disease
Etiology	Unopposed estrogenic stimulation. Somatic mutations in *PTEN, PIK3CA, ARID1A*, and *KRAS* Lynch syndrome (germline mutations in mismatch repair genes) and Cowden syndrome (germline mutation in *PTEN*)	Somatic *TP53* mutation is nearly ubiquitous. Often associated with extensive copy number changes. A subset of cases has *ERBB2*/HER2 overexpression/amplification *PIK3CA, FBXW7, PPP2R1A* mutations in a subset of cases May be associated with *BRCA1/2* mutations and manifest a defect in homologous recombination repair (HRD)
Histology	1. Background of endometrial hyperplasia 2. Papillary structures with smooth apical epithelial surfaces *(Figs. 3.9.1 and 3.9.2)* 3. Squamous differentiation and/or metaplastic features (mucinous, tubal, etc.) can be present *(Fig. 3.9.3)* 4. Low to intermediate cytologic grade *(Fig. 3.9.4)*; vesicular chromatin; uniform small nucleoli; mitotic figures are infrequent 5. Relatively clean background	1. Background of atrophic endometrium, serous intraepithelial carcinoma; often involves endometrial polyp 2. Irregular scalloped outlines of the papillae *(Figs. 3.9.5 and 3.9.6)* 3. Squamous, mucinous differentiation is typically absent 4. High cytologic grade; brisk mitotic activity *(Fig. 3.9.7)* 5. Debris in the background can be seen *(Fig. 3.9.5)*
Special studies	• Weak focal expression of p53 (wild-type pattern) • Patchy expression of p16 • Positive ER and PR • Loss of PTEN can be seen in some cases • Loss of MMR in a subset of cases	• Strong, diffuse, or completely absent expression of p53 • Strong, diffuse expression of p16 • Often diminished or lost expression of ER and PR • PTEN retained • MMR expression retained

	Endometrioid Carcinoma With Papillary Architecture	**Serous Carcinoma**
Treatment	Hysterectomy and bilateral salpingo-oophorectomy +/− lymphadenectomy; adjuvant chemotherapy +/− radiotherapy depending on tumor stage	Hysterectomy and bilateral salpingo-oophorectomy, lymphadenectomy, peritoneal sampling; +/− adjuvant chemotherapy, +/− radiotherapy
Prognosis	Prognosis is dependent on tumor stage, grade, and patients' age. Survival is not compromised in low-grade tumors, stage IA	Significantly worse prognosis compared to endometrioid carcinoma; reported 5-y survival for all stages 38%; 5-y survival for stage I carcinoma is 53%-57%

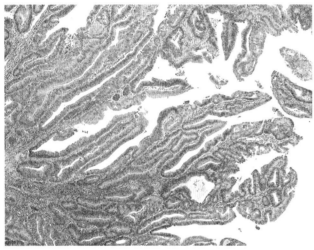

Figure 3.9.1   Endometrioid carcinoma, FIGO grade 1 with papillary/villoglandular architecture. Papillary structures have smooth outlines.

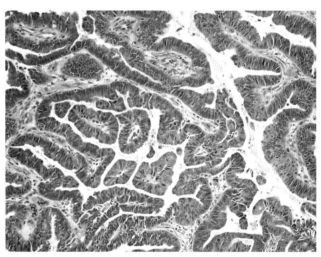

Figure 3.9.2   Endometrioid carcinoma, FIGO grade 1 with papillary architecture. Papillary structures with slightly irregular contours. The luminal borders are relatively smooth.

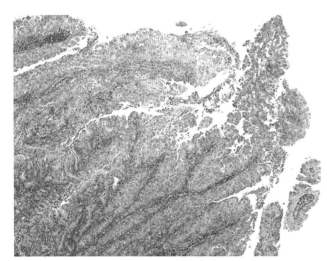

Figure 3.9.3   Endometrioid carcinoma, FIGO grade 1 with papillary architecture and extensive surface metaplastic-like differentiation (squamous and eosinophilic).

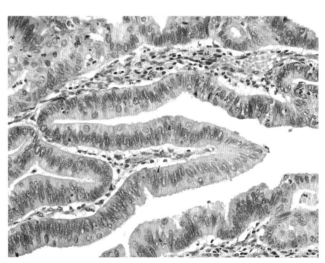

Figure 3.9.4   Endometrioid carcinoma, FIGO grade 1 with papillary/villoglandular architecture. Same case as in *Figure 3.9.1*, higher magnification. Papillae are lined by columnar cells with basally placed elongated nuclei arranged perpendicular to the basement membrane. Cytologic atypia is mild.

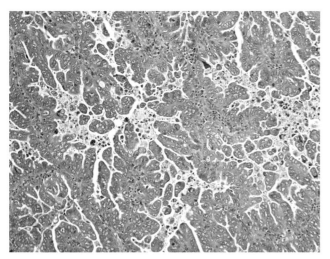

Figure 3.9.5   Serous carcinoma. Markedly irregular luminal borders with detached cell clusters. Note debris in the background.

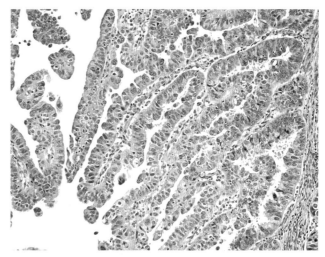

Figure 3.9.6   Serous carcinoma. Irregular, scalloped luminal borders; occasional detached cell clusters.

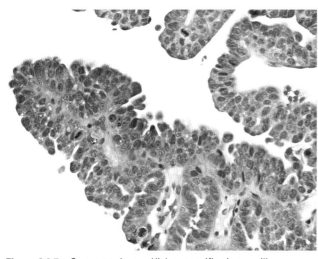

Figure 3.9.7   Serous carcinoma. Higher magnification, papillary structure with irregular border lined by atypical cells with pleomorphic nuclei and occasional prominent nucleoli. Mitoses are frequent.

3   UTERINE CORPUS (EPITHELIAL LESIONS)

	Endometrioid Carcinoma With Small Nonvillous Papillae	Serous Carcinoma
Age	Wide age range; mean age 63 y (same as for typical endometrial endometrioid carcinoma)	Postmenopausal; mean age in late 60s
Location	Endometrium	Endometrium
Symptoms	Vaginal bleeding, discharge	Postmenopausal bleeding; pelvic pain, abdominal distension in advanced cases
Signs	Constitutional symptoms, obesity, diabetes mellitus, polycystic ovarian syndrome, estrogen-producing ovarian tumors	Often present with subclinical advanced-stage disease
Etiology	Unopposed estrogenic stimulation. Somatic mutations in *PTEN*, *PIK3CA*, *ARID1A*, and *KRAS* Lynch syndrome (germline mutations in mismatch repair genes) and Cowden syndrome (germline mutation in *PTEN*)	Somatic *TP53* mutation is nearly ubiquitous. Often associated with extensive copy number changes. A subset of cases has *ERBB2*/HER2 overexpression/amplification *PIK3CA*, *FBXW7*, *PPP2R1A* mutations in a subset of cases May be associated with *BRCA1/2* mutations and manifest a defect in homologous recombination repair (HRD)
Histology	1. Background of endometrial hyperplasia and areas of typical endometrioid carcinoma can be present 2. Often no glandular confluence 3. Small intraglandular or surface papillae consist of buds of cells with metaplastic-like changes *(Figs. 3.10.1-3.10.3)* 4. Low cytologic grade, mildly enlarged round nuclei with small nucleoli; low nucleocytoplasmic ratio *(Fig. 3.10.4)* 5. Mitotic figures are infrequent 6. Relatively clean background, mucin can be seen	1. Background of atrophic endometrium, serous intraepithelial carcinoma; often involves endometrial polyp; other patterns of serous carcinoma (papillary, glandular) can be present 2. Often no glandular confluence 3. Prominent intraglandular papillary infoldings *(Fig. 3.10.6)* 4. High cytologic grade, enlarged hyperchromatic or vesicular nuclei, high nucleocytoplasmic ratio *(Fig. 3.10.7)* 5. Brisk mitotic activity 6. Debris in the background
Special studies	• Weak focal expression of p53 (wild-type pattern) *(Fig. 3.10.5, **left**)* • Patchy expression of p16 *(Fig. 3.10.5, **right**)* • Positive ER and PR, although can be diminished in metaplastic-appearing papillae • Loss of PTEN • Loss of MMR in a subset of endometrioid carcinoma cases, in general	• Strong, diffuse, or completely absent expression of p53 *(Fig. 3.10.8, **left**)* • Strong, diffuse expression of p16 *(Fig. 3.10.8, **right**)* • Often diminished or lost expression of ER and PR • PTEN retained • MMR expression retained

	Endometrioid Carcinoma With Small Nonvillous Papillae	**Serous Carcinoma**
Treatment	Same as typical endometrioid carcinoma. See Section 3.9	See Section 3.9
Prognosis	Same as typical endometrioid carcinoma. See Section 3.9	See Section 3.9

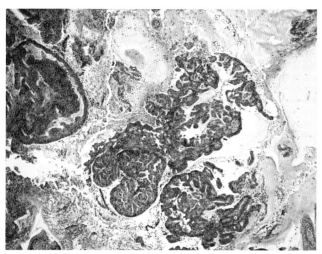

Figure 3.10.1   Endometrioid carcinoma with small nonvillous papillae. Endometrial curettage, glandular proliferation with busy papillary architecture.

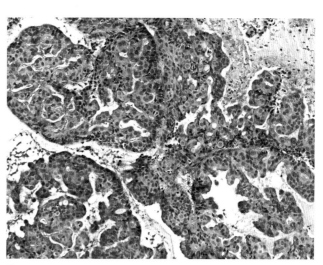

Figure 3.10.2   Endometrioid carcinoma with small nonvillous papillae. Same case as in *Figure 3.10.1*, higher magnification, tightly packed intraglandular epithelial infoldings.

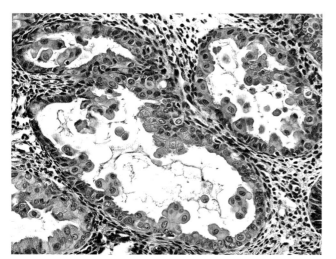

Figure 3.10.3   Endometrioid carcinoma with small nonvillous papillae. Associated endometrial hyperplasia displays dilated glands with intraglandular papillary tufts and detached cell clusters.

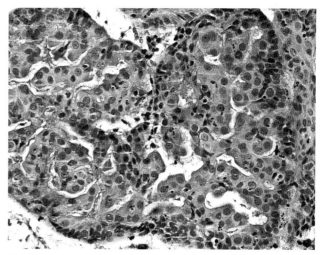

Figure 3.10.4   Endometrioid carcinoma with small nonvillous papillae. Same case as in *Figure 3.10.2*, higher magnification, intraglandular papillary infoldings composed of cells with abundant eosinophilic cytoplasm and round bland nuclei. Cells have metaplastic-like appearance.

3 UTERINE CORPUS (EPITHELIAL LESIONS)

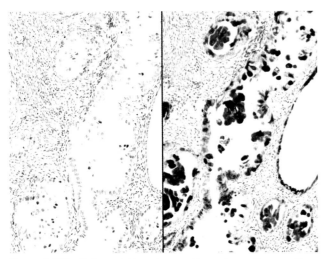

Figure 3.10.5   Endometrioid carcinoma with small non-villous papillae. Weak and focal expression of p53 (wild-type pattern) **(left)** and focally strong, but patchy expression of p16 **(right)**.

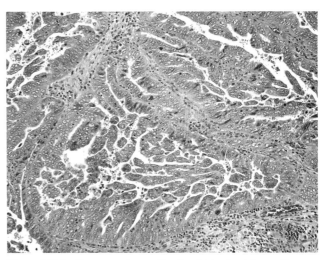

Figure 3.10.6   Serous carcinoma. Prominent intraglandular papillary infoldings; round and elongated detached intraluminal cell clusters.

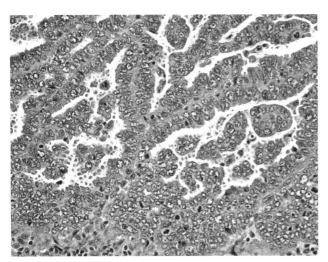

Figure 3.10.7   Serous carcinoma. Higher magnification, markedly atypical cells with vesicular pleomorphic nuclei with nucleoli. Numerous mitoses.

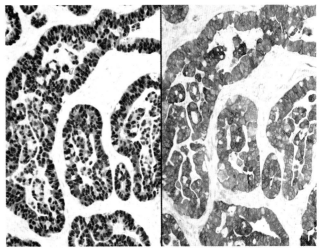

Figure 3.10.8   Serous carcinoma. Strong and diffuse expression of both p53 **(left)** and p16 **(right)**.

	Endometrioid Carcinoma	Serous Carcinoma With Glandular Architecture
Age	Wide age range, from third decade into late postmenopause; mean age 63 y	Postmenopausal; mean age in late 60s
Location	Endometrium	Endometrium
Symptoms	Vaginal bleeding, discharge	Postmenopausal bleeding
Signs	Constitutional symptoms, obesity, diabetes mellitus, polycystic ovarian syndrome, estrogen-producing ovarian tumors	Often presents with subclinical advanced-stage disease
Etiology	Unopposed estrogenic stimulation. Somatic mutations in *PTEN, PIK3CA, ARID1A, KRAS,* and *TP53* Lynch syndrome (germline mutations in mismatch repair genes) and Cowden syndrome (germline mutation in *PTEN*)	Somatic *TP53* mutation is nearly ubiquitous. Often associated with extensive copy number changes. A subset of cases has *ERBB2*/HER2 overexpression/amplification *PIK3CA, FBXW7, PPP2R1A* mutations seen in a subset of cases May be associated with *BRCA1/2* mutations and manifest a defect in homologous recombination repair (HRD)
Histology	1. Background of endometrial hyperplasia 2. Squamous differentiation or metaplastic features (mucinous, tubal, etc.) can be present 3. Smooth luminal borders; small round glands present in some areas; solid growth can be seen in higher-grade tumors *(Figs. 3.11.1 and 3.11.2)* 4. Low to intermediate cytologic grade; rare cases with high-grade cytologic features; vesicular chromatin; uniform small nucleoli *(Fig. 3.11.3)* 5. Mitotic figures are infrequent 6. Relatively clean background	1. Background of atrophic endometrium, serous intraepithelial carcinoma; often involves endometrial polyp 2. Squamous, mucinous differentiation is typically absent 3. Elongated glands with irregular scalloped luminal borders; or small slit-like spaces; solid growth is not common but can be seen *(Figs. 3.11.4-3.11.7, 3.11.9)* 4. High cytologic grade; vesicular or smudged chromatin; multiple red nucleoli can be seen *(Figs. 3.11.8 and 3.11.10)* 5. Brisk mitotic activity 6. Debris in the background
Special studies	• Weak focal expression of p53 (wild-type pattern) • Patchy expression of p16 *(Fig. 3.11.2,* **inset***)* • Positive ER and PR • Loss of PTEN can be seen in some cases • Loss of MMR in a subset of cases	• Strong, diffuse, or completely absent expression of p53 *(Fig. 3.11.11,* **left***)* • Strong, diffuse expression of p16 *(Fig. 3.11.11,* **right***)* • Often diminished or lost expression of ER and PR • PTEN retained • MMR expression retained

	Endometrioid Carcinoma	**Serous Carcinoma With Glandular Architecture**
Treatment	Same as typical endometrioid carcinoma. See Section 3.9	See Section 3.9
Prognosis	Same as typical endometrioid carcinoma; dependent on grade, stage, and presence of risk factors. See Section 3.9	See Section 3.9

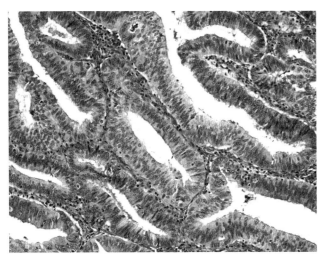

Figure 3.11.1   Endometrioid carcinoma. Elongated hyperchromatic glands with smooth luminal borders.

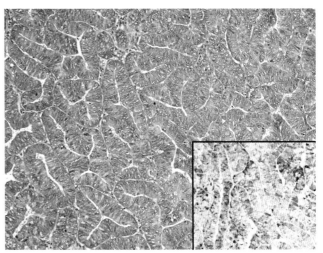

Figure 3.11.2   Endometrioid carcinoma. Densely packed glands with compressed slit-like lumina; however, luminal borders are smooth. Patchy expression of p16 **(inset)**.

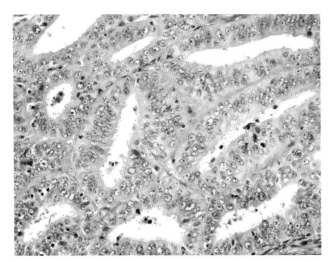

Figure 3.11.3   Endometrioid carcinoma. Glandular growth and diffuse moderate to marked cytologic atypia warrant diagnosis of FIGO grade 2 carcinoma. Immunohistochemistry should be performed to exclude glandular variant of serous carcinoma. Compare to *Figure 3.11.6.*

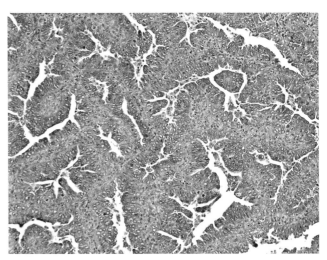

Figure 3.11.4   Serous carcinoma. Irregularly shaped large glands with slit-like scalloped luminal borders.

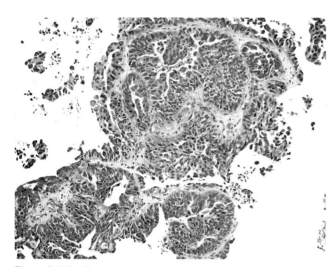

Figure 3.11.5   Serous carcinoma. Endometrial biopsy, fragment of intact hyperchromatic glands with scalloped lumina.

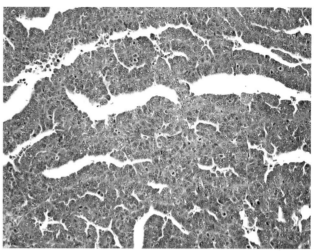

Figure 3.11.6   Serous carcinoma. Elongated hyperchromatic glands with mildly irregular luminal borders lined by high-grade cells may mimic FIGO grade 2 endometrioid carcinoma (upgraded based on cytologic atypia). Immunohistochemistry (not shown) supports the diagnosis of serous carcinoma.

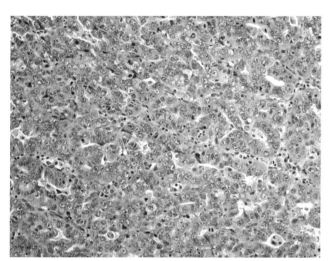

Figure 3.11.7   Serous carcinoma. Densely packed glands with compressed slit like lumina with some irregularity to luminal outlines. Cytologically, high-grade nuclei with pleomorphism and nucleoli. Compare to *Figure 3.11.2*. Immunohistochemistry is confirmatory of serous carcinoma (not shown).

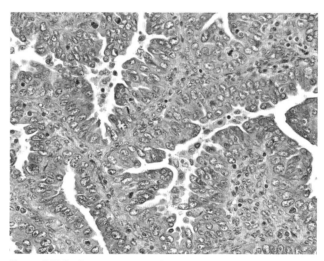

Figure 3.11.8   Serous carcinoma. Same case as in *Figure 3.11.4*, higher magnification. Cytologically, high-grade cell lining irregular glands. Note nuclear pleomorphism and frequent mitoses.

3   UTERINE CORPUS (EPITHELIAL LESIONS)

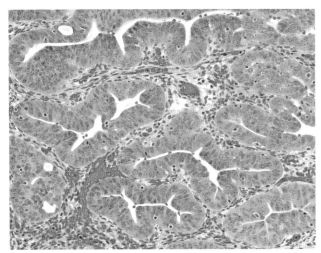

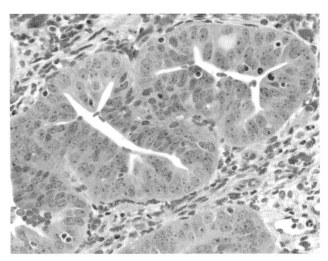

Figure 3.11.9 Serous carcinoma. Glandular pattern. The luminal borders are relatively smooth with minimal scalloping. This variant may mimic endometrioid carcinoma. Immunohistochemistry (not shown) is typical of serous carcinoma.

Figure 3.11.10 Serous carcinoma. Same case as in *Figure 3.11.9*. High-grade nuclei with prominent nucleoli and occasional mitotic figures.

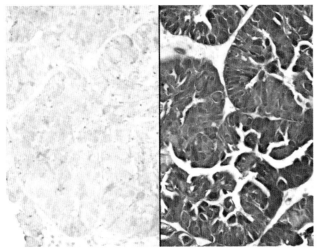

Figure 3.11.11 Serous carcinoma. Less common pattern of p53 staining associated with mutant *TP53* gene, complete lack of expression, "null phenotype" **(left)** and strong and diffuse expression of p16 **(right)**.

	Serous Endometrial Intraepithelial Carcinoma	Benign Endometrial Tissue With Reactive/Degenerative Atypia
Age	Postmenopausal women, older than 60 y; some series reported wider age range 44-93, median age 68 y	Usually in postmenopausal women
Location	Endometrium	Endometrium
Symptoms	Vaginal bleeding	Vaginal bleeding
Signs	Postmenopausal bleeding	Postmenopausal bleeding
Etiology	*TP53* mutation	Unknown; considered degenerative change
Histology	1. Background atrophic endometrium; often involves surfaces of endometrial polyp *(Fig. 3.12.1)* 2. Single layer of markedly atypical columnar cells; pseudostratification can be seen *(Figs. 3.12.2 and 3.12.3)* 3. Increased nucleocytoplasmic ratio 4. Enlarged vesicular nuclei with nucleoli or hyperchromasia *(Figs. 3.12.2 and 3.12.3)*	1. Background atrophic or inactive endometrium; no strong association with endometrial polyp 2. Strips of epithelium with eosinophilic cytoplasm and enlarged hyperchromatic nuclei *(Fig. 3.12.4)* 3. Nucleocytoplasmic ratio is not significantly increased; ample amount of cytoplasm *(Figs. 3.12.4,* **right** *and 3.12.5)* 4. Enlarged hyperchromatic nuclei typically with smudged chromatin; nucleoli can be occasionally seen *(Figs. 3.12.4,* **right** *and 3.12.5)*
Special studies	• Strong diffuse or completely absent expression of p53 • Markedly increased Ki 67 proliferative activity • Diffuse expression of p16 • Immunoprofile is identical to endometrial serous carcinoma (**see** *Fig. 3.10.8*)	• Focal, generally weak expression of p53; occasional strongly staining nuclei can be seen *(Fig. 3.12.6,* **left***)* • Low to absent Ki 67 proliferative activity *(Fig. 3.12.6,* **center***)* • Usually patchy expression of p16; extensive p16 expression can be seen in cases with prominent metaplastic changes *(Fig. 3.12.6,* **right***)*
Treatment	Hysterectomy, bilateral salpingo-oophorectomy with staging (lymph node dissection and peritoneal sampling)	None required; if symptoms persist, repeat sampling should be considered
Prognosis	Precursor of endometrial serous carcinoma; cases with intraepithelial carcinoma only, occasionally present with peritoneal disease; when diagnosed on a biopsy/curettage, should be considered "at least" serous intraepithelial carcinoma until complete evaluation of endometrium in the hysterectomy to ensure lack of invasion	Unremarkable

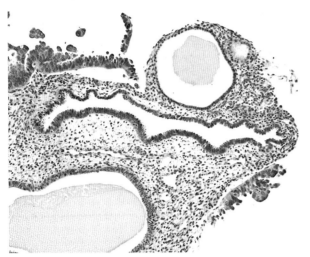

Figure 3.12.1   Serous intraepithelial carcinoma (endometrial intraepithelial carcinoma, EIC). Strips of hyperchromatic epithelium lining surface of the atrophic endometrium.

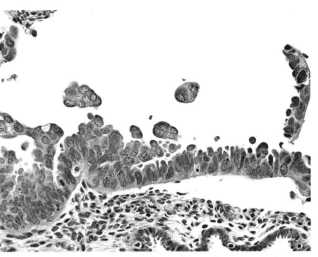

Figure 3.12.2   Serous intraepithelial carcinoma. Same case as in *Figure 3.12.1*, higher magnification. Strip of atypical epithelium with irregular luminal surface and detached cell clusters. The cells have pleomorphic nuclei; occasional prominent nucleoli are seen.

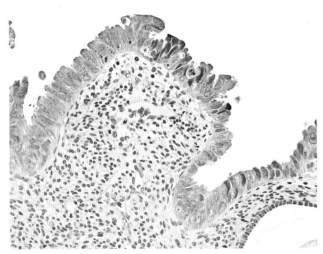

Figure 3.12.3   Serous intraepithelial carcinoma involving surface of the endometrial polyp. Tall columnar markedly atypical cells; compare and contrast with atrophic endometrial gland, **lower right**.

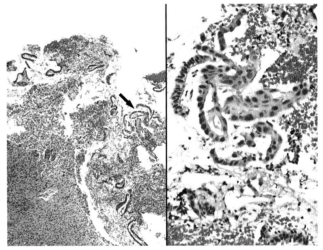

Figure 3.12.4   Endometrium with reactive/degenerative atypia. Low magnification **(left)**, superficial strips of atrophic endometrium and fragment of stroma suggestive of a polyp. Higher magnification **(right)** of same focus highlighted with the *arrow* on the left; strips of epithelium with eosinophilic cytoplasm and enlarged nuclei with smudged chromatin.

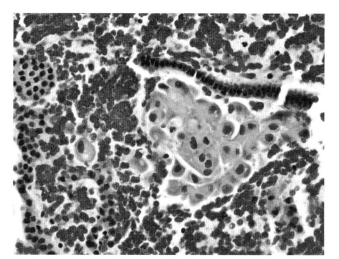

Figure 3.12.5 Endometrium with reactive/degenerative atypia. High magnification, large cells with metaplastic-like appearance and abundant eosinophilic cytoplasm (eosinophilic metaplasia) and detached superficial strips of atrophic endometrium.

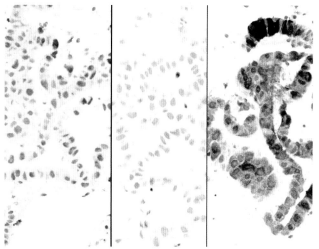

Figure 3.12.6 Endometrium with reactive/degenerative atypia. Weak and focal staining for p53 **(left)**, virtually absent Ki 67 proliferative activity **(center)**, and extensive expression of p16 **(right)** can be observed in epithelium with superimposed metaplastic changes, which can be problematic in a limited sample. Immunohistochemical findings should be interpreted as a panel and in context of morphology.

	High-Grade Neuroendocrine Carcinoma	Endometrioid Carcinoma, FIGO Grade 3
Age	Peri- or postmenopausal	Postmenopausal, occasionally perimenopausal
Location	Endometrium; can occur elsewhere in the gynecologic tract	Endometrium; can occur elsewhere in the gynecologic tract
Symptoms	Abnormal vaginal bleeding, paraneoplastic syndrome (rare)	Abnormal vaginal bleeding
Signs	Uterine enlargement or pelvic mass; endometrial mass on imaging	Uterine enlargement or pelvic mass; endometrial mass on imaging
Etiology	Unknown; may develop as a component of mixed endometrial carcinoma	May represent progression from lower-grade endometrioid carcinoma
Histology	1. Diffuse solid, insular, or trabecular patterns (or combination) *(Figs. 3.13.1-3.13.3)* 2. Separate component of endometrial carcinoma (endometrioid, serous type, or carcinosarcoma) can be present 3. Rosette-like structures can be present 4. Squamous differentiation within neuroendocrine component is not typical (can be seen in the coexisting endometrioid carcinoma component, if present) 5. Small cell neuroendocrine carcinoma: oval or spindled cells, scant cytoplasm, evenly dispersed chromatin ("salt and pepper") or hyperchromasia, nuclear molding *(Fig. 3.13.4)*. Large cell neuroendocrine carcinoma: polygonal cells, moderate amount of eosinophilic or amphophilic cytoplasm, round vesicular nuclei with prominent nucleoli *(Fig. 3.13.5)* 6. Brisk mitotic activity and apoptotic bodies 7. Necrosis is common	1. Diffuse solid growth; nested growth can be seen 2. Solid areas intermixed with foci of retained glandular differentiation *(Fig. 3.13.7)* 3. Glands and/or papillary structures can be seen, pseudorosettes not seen 4. Squamous differentiation can be seen *(Fig. 3.13.7)* 5. Cohesive cell growth; cells cytologically similar in glandular and solid areas; oval cells with moderate amount of cytoplasm and elongated to round nuclei, prominent nucleoli can be seen *(Figs. 3.13.8 and 3.13.9)* 6. Mitotic activity can be increased; apoptotic bodies can be seen, but not a constant feature 7. Necrosis can be present
Special studies	• Positive chromogranin, synaptophysin, INSM1; CD56 (extensive strong expression of at least 2 markers) *(Fig. 3.13.6)* • Variable expression of PAX8, cytokeratins, often minimal; ER and PR can be lost	• Negative chromogranin, synaptophysin, INSM1; CD56, less specific and can be expressed • Positive PAX8, cytokeratins, ER, PR (usually diffuse)
Treatment	Hysterectomy, bilateral salpingo-oophorectomy, and staging; chemotherapy +/− radiation therapy (alternative chemo regimens have been recommended)	Hysterectomy, bilateral salpingo-oophorectomy, adjuvant therapy is stage dependent
Prognosis	Poor; often advanced stage at presentation; however, favorable outcome has been reported in tumors confined to endometrial polyp	5-y survival: 30%-75%; dependent on stage and other risk factors

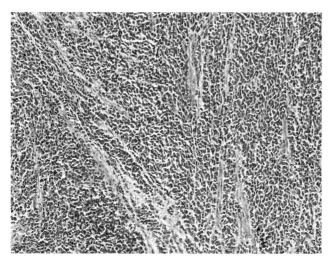

Figure 3.13.1 High-grade neuroendocrine carcinoma, small cell variant. Diffuse and corded growth patterns.

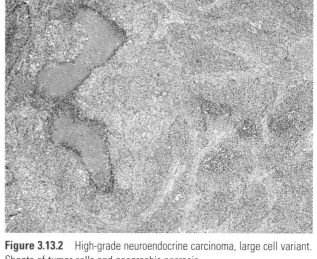

Figure 3.13.2 High-grade neuroendocrine carcinoma, large cell variant. Sheets of tumor cells and geographic necrosis.

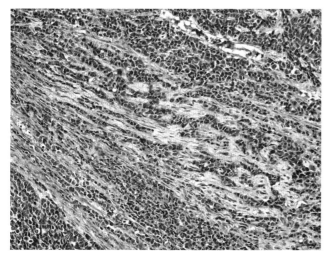

Figure 3.13.3 High-grade neuroendocrine carcinoma. Trabecular growth pattern.

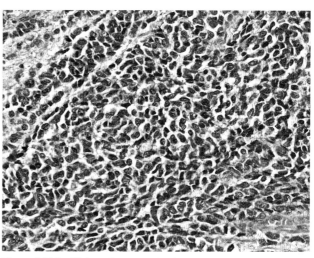

Figure 3.13.4 High-grade neuroendocrine carcinoma, small cell variant. Same case as in *Figure 3.13.1*, higher magnification. Basophilic cells with scant cytoplasm and hyperchromatic nuclei.

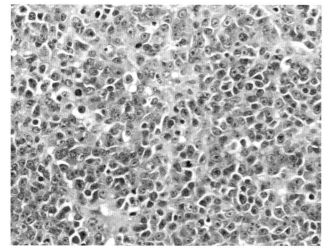

Figure 3.13.5 High-grade neuroendocrine carcinoma, large cell variant, high magnification. Polygonal cells with amphophilic cytoplasm and large vesicular nuclei with prominent red nucleoli. Frequent mitoses.

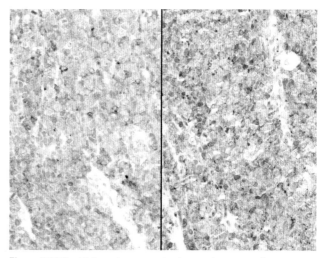

Figure 3.13.6 High-grade neuroendocrine carcinoma, small cell variant. Same case as in *Figure 3.13.1*. Diffuse expression of chromogranin **(left)** and synaptophysin **(right)**.

3 UTERINE CORPUS (EPITHELIAL LESIONS)

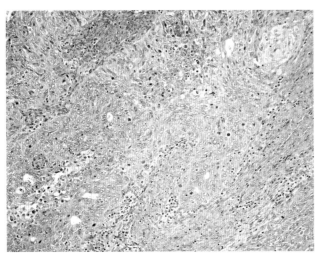

Figure 3.13.7   Endometrioid carcinoma, FIGO grade 3. Solid tumor with focal gland formation. Focus of squamous differentiation **(upper right)**.

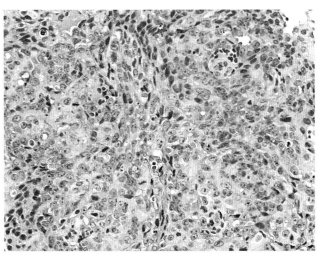

Figure 3.13.8   Endometrioid carcinoma, FIGO grade 3. Higher magnification, nests of cells with oval to round nuclei; nucleoli are inconspicuous and occasionally multiple.

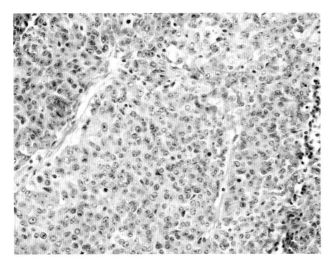

Figure 3.13.9   Endometrioid carcinoma, FIGO grade 3. Same case as in *Figure 3.13.7*, different area, higher magnification. Solid sheets of cells with pale pink cytoplasm and round nuclei with nucleoli. Immunohistochemical workup is warranted to exclude neuroendocrine carcinoma. Compare with *Figure 3.13.5*.

	Endometrioid Carcinoma With Clear Cells	Clear Cell Carcinoma
Age	Wide age range, from third decade into late postmenopause	Postmenopausal; mean age at diagnosis in late seventh decade
Location	Endometrium	Endometrium, including lower uterine segment; may occur elsewhere in the gynecologic tract
Symptoms	Abnormal vaginal bleeding, discharge	Abnormal vaginal bleeding, discharge
Signs	Endometrial mass; Constitutional symptoms, obesity, diabetes mellitus, polycystic ovarian syndrome, estrogen-producing ovarian tumors	Endometrial mass No strong association with obesity and diabetes
Etiology	Unopposed estrogenic stimulation. Somatic mutations in *PTEN, PIK3CA, ARID1A, KRAS*, and *TP53* Lynch syndrome (germline mutations in mismatch repair genes) and Cowden syndrome (germline mutation in *PTEN*)	Somatic mutations in *PTEN, TP53, ARID1A, PIK3CA*, and *KRAS*; Lynch syndrome (germline mutations in mismatch repair genes)
Histology	1. Background endometrium with complex atypical hyperplasia 2. Glandular or solid growth patterns, areas with typical morphology of endometrioid carcinoma without clear cell (secretory) change *(Fig. 3.14.1)* 3. Stromal hyalinization is not typical; inflamed desmoplastic "altered" stroma can be seen 4. Glandular structures with smooth luminal borders and secretory changes *(Fig. 3.14.2)* 5. Columnar cells with cytoplasmic clearing (subnuclear and supranuclear cytoplasmic vacuoles) *(Fig. 3.14.3)* 6. Areas of squamous differentiation with or without cytoplasmic clearing *(Fig. 3.14.4)* 7. Areas with clear cytoplasm merge with glands with more typical endometrioid appearance *(Fig. 3.14.5)* 8. Low-grade uniform nuclei; nucleoli can be present, but generally not very prominent	1. Background of inactive to atrophic or occasionally proliferative endometrium; some describe intraepithelial clear cell carcinoma as a precursor lesion 2. Combination of glandular, papillary (+/− ring-like structures), tubulocystic, and solid patterns *(Figs. 3.14.6-3.14.8)* 3. Hyalinized stroma in areas with papillary architecture *(Fig. 3.14.8)* 4. Irregular scalloped luminal borders with detached tumor cells in the gland lumina 5. Cuboidal cells often with eosinophilic cytoplasm and prominent hobnail change *(Fig. 3.14.9)* 6. Solid growth can be present, but squamous differentiation is absent 7. Distinct areas of cells with clear cytoplasm and areas with endometrioid appearance, in cases of mixed epithelial-type carcinoma 8. Relatively monotonous and yet atypical high-grade nuclei; occasionally significant nuclear pleomorphism, hyperchromasia, or smooth chromatin and prominent nucleoli *(Fig. 3.14.10)*
Special studies	• Often not helpful in this differential as markers are not very sensitive/specific (HNF1β and Napsin A expression can be seen in either entity) • Usually no abnormal p53 expression (scattered weakly positive cells)	• Often not helpful in this differential as markers are not very sensitive/specific (HNF1β and Napsin A expression can be seen in either entity) • Strong and diffuse or completely absent expression of p53 is seen in a proportion of cases

	Endometrioid Carcinoma With Clear Cells	Clear Cell Carcinoma
	• Retained expression of ER and PR (expression can be decreased in areas with extensive metaplastic changes)	• Loss of ER expression in some cases
Treatment	Hysterectomy and bilateral salpingo-oophorectomy, lymphadenectomy; adjuvant chemotherapy +/− radiotherapy depending on tumor stage	Hysterectomy with bilateral salpingo-oophorectomy and staging with or without adjuvant chemotherapy +/− radiotherapy depending on tumor stage
Prognosis	Tumor stage, grade, and patients' age are considered prognostic factors	Prognosis is stage dependent; however, 5-y survival is <50% regardless of stage. In some series, clear cell carcinoma is reported to be resistant to adjuvant chemotherapy
	Survival is not compromised in low-grade tumors, stage IA	

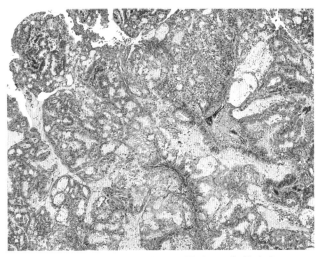

Figure 3.14.1   Endometrioid carcinoma with clear cells. Foci of tumor with clear cytoplasm (see *Fig. 3.14.5*); other areas with typical endometrioid carcinoma appearance without clear cell (secretory) change.

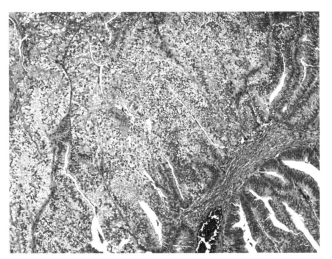

Figure 3.14.2   Endometrioid carcinoma with clear cells. Extensive secretory changes with pseudosolid appearance merging with glandular foci with typical hyperchromatic columnar epithelium **(lower right)**.

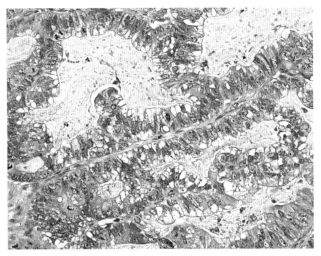

Figure 3.14.3   Endometrioid carcinoma with clear cells. Endometrial carcinoma glands with sub- and supranuclear vacuoles, resembling secretory changes. Vesicular nuclei are located in the midportion of columnar cells. Mitoses are seen.

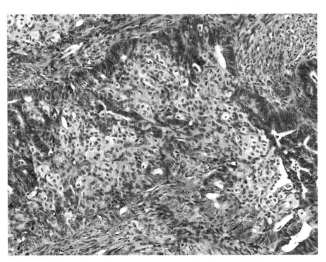

Figure 3.14.4   Endometrioid carcinoma with clear cells. Areas of squamous differentiation in the middle of tumor nests display cytoplasmic clearing. Surrounding endometrial carcinoma glands have typical endometrioid morphology.

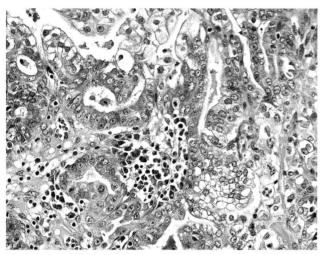

Figure 3.14.5 Endometrioid carcinoma with clear cells. Same case as in *Figure 3.14.1*, higher magnification. Foci of epithelium with cytoplasmic clearing merge with columnar glands with metaplastic-like appearance.

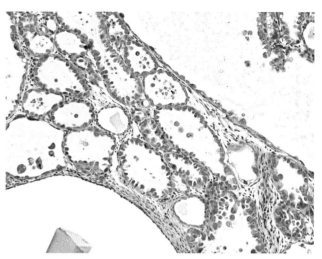

Figure 3.14.6 Clear cell carcinoma. Tubulocystic pattern. Dilated gland lined by single layer of cells with prominent hobnail change.

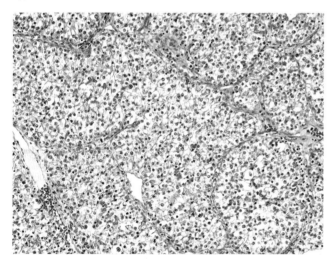

Figure 3.14.7 Clear cell carcinoma. Solid pattern. Sheets of cells with clear cytoplasm and round uniform nuclei.

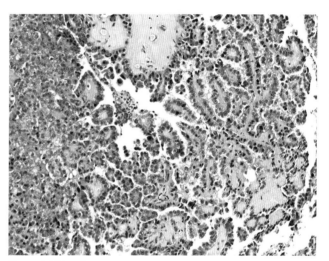

Figure 3.14.8 Clear cell carcinoma. Papillary pattern. Fibrovascular cores with prominent hyalinization.

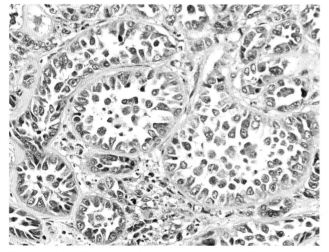

Figure 3.14.9 Clear cell carcinoma. Glandular pattern. Glands are lined by cells with vesicular pleomorphic nuclei and hobnail cells; detached cells in the lumen. Stroma surrounding the glands is focally hyalinized.

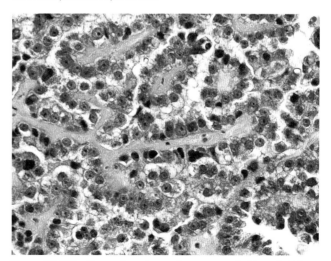

Figure 3.14.10 Clear cell carcinoma. Same case as in *Figure 3.14.8*, higher magnification. Cells lining hyalinized papillae have relatively uniform round nuclei with prominent nucleoli.

	Arias-Stella Reaction	Clear Cell Carcinoma
Age	Usually reproductive age; may occur in postmenopausal years for patients taking progesterone	Postmenopausal
Location	Usually endometrium; may occur in the endocervix	Endometrium, including lower uterine segment; may occur elsewhere in the gynecologic tract
Symptoms	Depends on clinical indications for biopsy/curettage; incidental finding, usually associated with pregnancy	Abnormal vaginal bleeding
Signs	Depends on clinical indications for biopsy/curettage	Pelvic mass in some advanced-stage cases; polypoid mass may be present at hysteroscopy or in gross specimen
Etiology	Progesterone-induced pseudoneoplastic atypia; associated with pregnancy or hormonal therapy (progestins)	Somatic mutations in *PTEN*, *TP53*, *ARID1A*, *PIK3CA*, and *KRAS*; Lynch syndrome (germline mutations in mismatch repair genes)
Histology	1. Background endometrium shows either gestational or progestin changes *(Fig. 3.15.1)* 2. No admixture of glandular, papillary, tubulocystic, and solid architectural patterns; no "ring-like" structures; intraglandular tufting can occur *(Fig. 3.15.2)* 3. Endometrial glands lined by enlarged cells with abundant clear or eosinophilic cytoplasm 4. Hobnail shapes can be seen; no admixture of columnar, low cuboidal, and flat cells *(Fig. 3.15.3)* 5. Nuclei are enlarged 6. Nuclei are smudgy or vesicular; intranuclear inclusions may be present; nucleoli are not a typical feature *(Figs. 3.15.4 and 3.15.5)* 7. Usually no mitotic activity, but some cases can have rare mitotic figures 8. No hyaline globules 9. No hyalinized stroma	1. No gestational or progestin changes in background endometrium 2. Usual admixed architectural patterns: glandular, papillary, tubulocystic, and solid; "ring-like" structures and detached epithelial tufts can be seen *(Figs. 3.15.6-3.15.8)* 3. Tumor cells are of variable size (usually medium sized) and include abundant clear or eosinophilic cytoplasm *(Fig. 3.15.9)* 4. Admixture of cell types: hobnail, columnar, low cuboidal, and flat *(Fig. 3.15.10)* 5. Variable nuclear size, but most are medium sized 6. Nuclei tend to be round with either vesicular chromatin or hyperchromasia; no intranuclear inclusions; nucleoli are typically small to medium sized and centrally located *(Fig. 3.15.9)* 7. Variable mitotic index although often low 8. Hyaline globules can be seen 9. Hyalinized stroma (especially within stromal cores of small papillae) may be present
Special studies	Immunohistochemistry not of significant help for this differential diagnosis although Ki-67 index in Arias-Stella reaction is either 0% or extremely low	Immunohistochemistry not of significant help for this differential diagnosis; however, clear cell carcinoma tends to have a higher Ki-67 index

	Arias-Stella Reaction	**Clear Cell Carcinoma**
Treatment	None	Dependent on stage and other risk factors; may include hysterectomy with bilateral salpingo-oophorectomy and surgical staging, chemotherapy, and/or radiation therapy
Prognosis	No prognostic significance	5-y survival ranges from <50% to 63%; dependent on stage and other risk factors

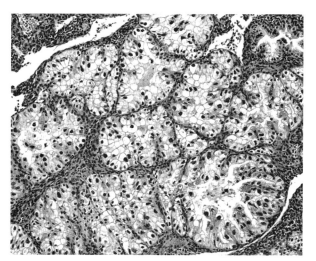

Figure 3.15.1 Arias-Stella reaction in a background of hypersecretory gestational endometrium. There is glandular crowding and cytoplasmic clearing, which can simulate clear cell carcinoma at low- and high-power magnifications.

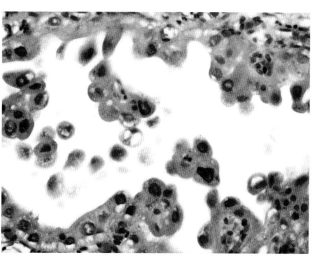

Figure 3.15.2 Arias-Stella reaction with intraglandular tufting.

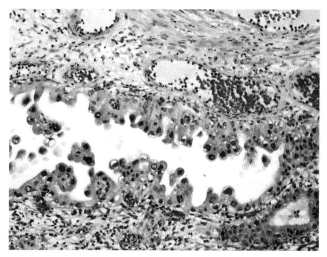

Figure 3.15.3 Arias-Stella reaction with hobnail cells.

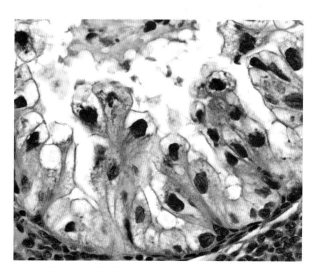

Figure 3.15.4 Arias-Stella reaction with clear cytoplasm, large nuclei, and smudgy chromatin.

3 UTERINE CORPUS (EPITHELIAL LESIONS)

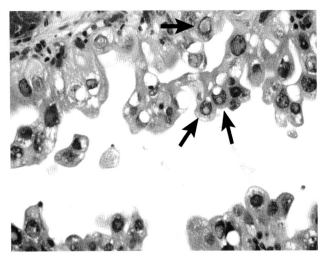

Figure 3.15.5   Arias-Stella reaction with intranuclear inclusions (*arrows*).

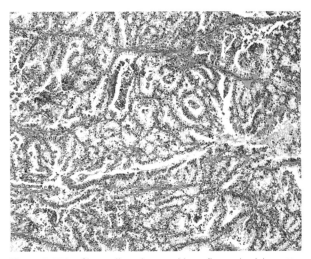

Figure 3.15.6   Clear cell carcinoma with confluent glandular pattern.

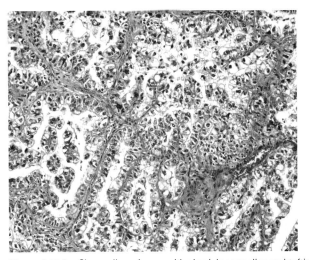

Figure 3.15.7   Clear cell carcinoma with glandular crowding and tufting mimicking hypersecretory gestational endometrium.

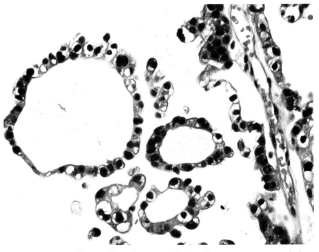

Figure 3.15.8   Clear cell carcinoma with ring-like structures, consisting of round papillae without significant epithelial stratification or stromal cores.

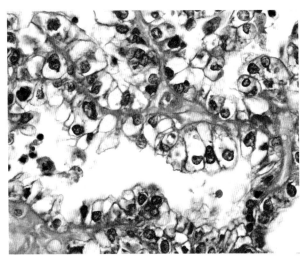

Figure 3.15.9   Clear cell carcinoma showing polygonal cells with abundant clear cytoplasm. The nuclei are relatively uniform with only mild variation in size and shape. They are medium sized and round and mostly have slightly pale chromatin with small to medium-sized central nucleoli.

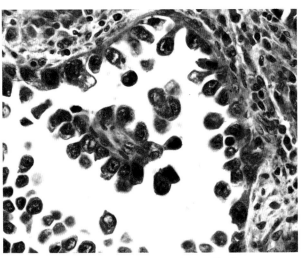

Figure 3.15.10   Clear cell carcinoma with hobnail cells.

	Corded and Hyalinized Pattern of Endometrioid Carcinoma	**MMMT**
Age	25-83 y (mean, 52)	Postmenopausal
Location	Endometrium; similar patterns can be seen in ovarian endometrioid carcinomas	Endometrium; can occur elsewhere in the gynecologic tract
Symptoms	Expected to be similar to usual-type endometrioid carcinomas: abnormal vaginal bleeding	Abnormal vaginal bleeding
Signs	Expected to be similar to usual-type endometrioid carcinomas: pelvic mass in some advanced-stage cases; polypoid mass may be present at hysteroscopy or in gross specimen	Uterine enlargement or pelvic mass; polypoid mass may be present at hysteroscopy or in gross specimen
Etiology	Variant pattern of endometrioid carcinoma; expected to usually lack *TP53* mutations; however, rare cases with *TP53* mutations have been described. Some cases harbor *CTNNB1* mutations	The sarcoma component is clonally related to the carcinoma component and believed to arise from the latter; *TP53* mutations common
Histology	1. Variable proportions of usual-type endometrioid and corded and hyalinized carcinoma components; the latter components are present within stroma producing a biphasic appearance; no sarcoma component present 2. One component exhibits glandular differentiation similar to other usual-type endometrioid carcinomas, including occasional squamous and other metaplastic-like differentiation *(Fig. 3.16.1)* 3. The other component without glandular differentiation is characterized by cords, hyalinized stroma, and some degree of spindle cell differentiation; these components can be misclassified as sarcoma; the cytologic features resemble those in the glandular components *(Figs. 3.16.2-3.16.7)* 4. Cytologic features of both components are typically low grade; occasionally, high-grade cytologic features can be seen in glandular component. Formal FIGO grading criteria not established or validated for this variant 5. Low mitotic index	1. Intimate admixture of carcinoma and sarcoma components *(Fig. 3.16.8)* 2. Carcinoma component is typically serous, endometrioid, or unclassified; other histologic types of carcinoma can occur *(Fig. 3.16.9)* 3. Sarcoma component may be unclassified or of a specific type (eg, rhabdomyosarcoma, chondrosarcoma, etc.) *(Fig. 3.16.10)* 4. Cytologic features of both components are typically high grade 5. High mitotic index in both components
Special studies	• p53: no abnormal expression pattern • p16: diffuse expression not expected (limited data) • Nuclear beta-catenin staining is seen in some cases	• p53: often abnormal expression pattern (complete absence of expression or diffuse staining) in both carcinoma (serous) and sarcoma components • p16: often diffuse expression in both components

	Corded and Hyalinized Pattern of Endometrioid Carcinoma	MMMT
	• Cytokeratin expression variable in corded and hyalinized components but can occasionally be negative • Desmin and myogenin expression not expected (limited data) • Ki 67: expected to be low to intermediate	• Cytokeratin expression tends to be lost in sarcoma component but can be positive • Desmin and myogenin positive in specific sarcoma components (leiomyosarcoma and rhabdomyosarcoma) • Ki 67 index: high
Treatment	Dependent on grade, stage, and other risk factors; may include observation, hormonal therapy, hysterectomy with bilateral salpingo-oophorectomy, surgical staging, chemotherapy, and/or radiation therapy	Dependent on stage and other risk factors; may include hysterectomy with bilateral salpingo-oophorectomy and surgical staging, chemotherapy, and/or radiation therapy
Prognosis	Based on limited data, 83% disease-free survival at 2.9 y (mean follow-up interval); dependent on stage and other risk factors. Cases harboring CTNNB1 mutations may have different prognosis	5-y survival: 30%-40%; dependent on stage and other risk factors

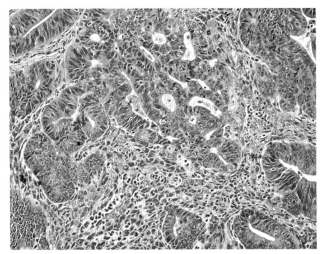

Figure 3.16.1   Corded and hyalinized pattern of endometrioid carcinoma. The top center of the photograph shows the cribriform architecture of usual-type endometrioid carcinomas. Below and to the left of this focus are corded areas of the carcinoma within stroma mimicking malignant mixed müllerian tumor (MMMT; carcinosarcoma).

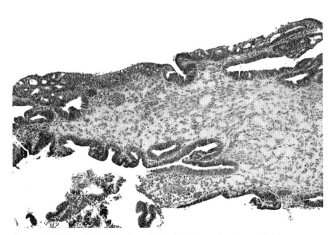

Figure 3.16.2   Corded and hyalinized pattern of endometrioid carcinoma. Corded and hyalinized patterns are present within stroma.

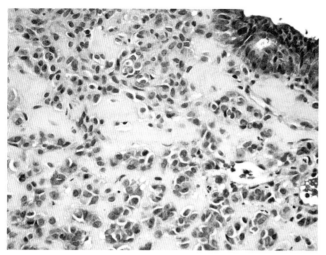

Figure 3.16.3 Corded and hyalinized pattern of endometrioid carcinoma. Same case as *Figure 3.16.2*.

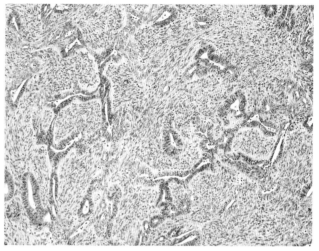

Figure 3.16.4 Corded and hyalinized pattern of endometrioid carcinoma. Intimate admixture of spindle cell stroma and glands simulating malignant mixed müllerian tumor (MMMT; carcinosarcoma).

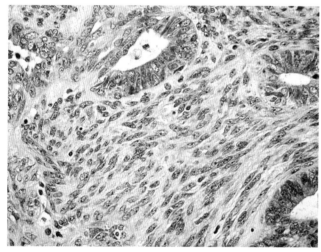

Figure 3.16.5 Corded and hyalinized pattern of endometrioid carcinoma. Same case as *Figure 3.16.4*. Note the similarity of nuclei between the glands and spindle cells within stroma.

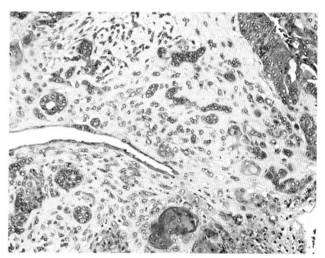

Figure 3.16.6 Corded and hyalinized pattern of endometrioid carcinoma. The stroma is slightly myxoid rather than overtly hyalinized. The appearance with the corded pattern can falsely suggest a chondrosarcomatous component of malignant mixed müllerian tumor (MMMT; carcinosarcoma).

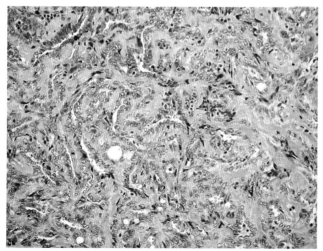

Figure 3.16.7 Corded and hyalinized pattern of endometrioid carcinoma. The corded component appears to merge with the glandular component. The nuclei of both components are similar.

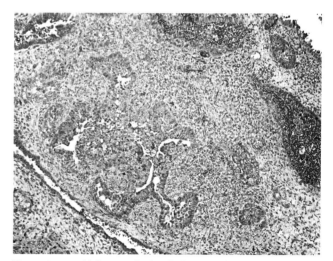

Figure 3.16.8 Malignant mixed müllerian tumor (MMMT; carcinosarcoma) with biphasic appearance consisting of intimate admixture of carcinoma and sarcoma components.

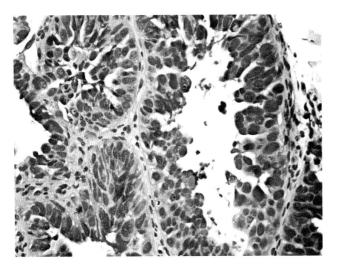

Figure 3.16.9   Malignant mixed müllerian tumor (MMMT; carcinosarcoma) with epithelial component composed of serous carcinoma.

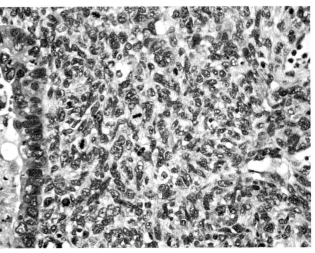

Figure 3.16.10   Malignant mixed müllerian tumor (MMMT; carcinosarcoma) showing sarcoma component containing atypical spindle cells with mitotic activity. The carcinoma component is present at the left side of the photograph.

3.17

HIGH-GRADE ENDOMETRIAL CARCINOMA (FIGO GRADE 3 ENDOMETRIOID CARCINOMA/SEROUS CARCINOMA) VS MALIGNANT MIXED MÜLLERIAN TUMOR (MMMT; CARCINOSARCOMA)

	High-Grade Endometrial Carcinoma (FIGO Grade 3 Endometrioid Carcinoma/Serous Carcinoma)	MMMT
Age	Postmenopausal	Postmenopausal
Location	Endometrium; can occur elsewhere in the gynecologic tract	Endometrium; can occur elsewhere in the gynecologic tract
Symptoms	Abnormal vaginal bleeding	Abnormal vaginal bleeding
Signs	Uterine enlargement or pelvic mass; polypoid mass may be present at hysteroscopy or in gross specimen	Uterine enlargement or pelvic mass; polypoid mass may be present at hysteroscopy or in gross specimen
Etiology	FIGO grade 3 endometrioid carcinoma represents progression from lower-grade endometrioid carcinoma; serous carcinoma evolves from intraepithelial serous carcinoma	The sarcoma component is clonally related to the carcinoma component and believed to arise from the latter; *TP53* mutations common
Histology	1. Monophasic tumor 2. Usual architectural features of serous or FIGO grade 3 endometrioid carcinoma *(Figs. 3.17.1 and 3.17.2)* 3. No sarcoma component; occasionally, stroma may be cellular, can have mitotic figures, or may exhibit reactive/reparative atypical changes (and/or solid patterns of carcinoma), resulting in misclassification as sarcoma *(Figs. 3.17.3 and 3.17.4)* 4. Cytologic features of carcinoma typically high grade (usually, serous > endometrioid) *(Fig. 3.17.5)* 5. High mitotic index in carcinoma	1. Biphasic appearance with intimate admixture of carcinoma and sarcoma components *(Figs. 3.17.6 and 3.17.7)* 2. Carcinoma component is typically serous, endometrioid, or unclassified; other histologic types of carcinoma can occur *(Fig. 3.17.8)* 3. Sarcoma component may be unclassified or of a specific type (eg, rhabdomyosarcoma, chondrosarcoma, etc.) *(Fig. 3.17.9)* 4. Cytologic features of both components are typically high grade *(Fig. 3.17.10)* 5. High mitotic index in both components
Special studies	• p53: abnormal expression pattern (complete absence of expression or diffuse staining) in serous carcinoma; a subset of high-grade endometrioid carcinomas can exhibit abnormal p53 expression; stroma should not have abnormal p53 pattern • p16: diffuse expression in serous carcinoma; nondiffuse expression in high-grade endometrioid carcinoma; stroma should not have diffuse pattern • Stroma should be cytokeratin (−) • Desmin and myogenin typically negative in stroma • Ki 67 index: high in carcinoma, not elevated in stroma	• p53: often abnormal expression pattern (complete absence of expression or diffuse staining) in both carcinoma (serous) and sarcoma components • p16: often diffuse expression in both components • Cytokeratin expression tends to be lost in sarcoma component but can be positive • Desmin and myogenin positive in specific sarcoma components (leiomyosarcoma and rhabdomyosarcoma) • Ki 67 index: high in both carcinoma and sarcoma components

	High-Grade Endometrial Carcinoma (FIGO Grade 3 Endometrioid Carcinoma/Serous Carcinoma)	MMMT
Treatment	Dependent on histologic type, stage, and other risk factors; may include observation, hysterectomy with bilateral salpingo-oophorectomy and surgical staging, chemotherapy, and/or radiation therapy	Dependent on stage and other risk factors; may include hysterectomy with bilateral salpingo-oophorectomy and surgical staging, chemotherapy, and/or radiation therapy
Prognosis	5-y survival: 36%-75%; dependent on histologic type, stage, and other risk factors	5-y survival: 30%-40%; dependent on stage and other risk factors

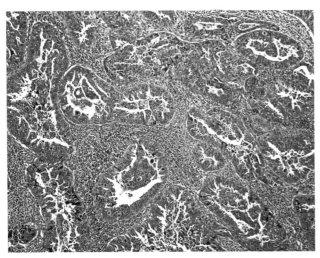

Figure 3.17.1   Serous carcinoma with glandular architecture; however, the epithelial component of malignant mixed müllerian tumor (MMMT; carcinosarcoma) can be identical. The stroma is cellular due to inflammation, but no sarcomatous elements are present.

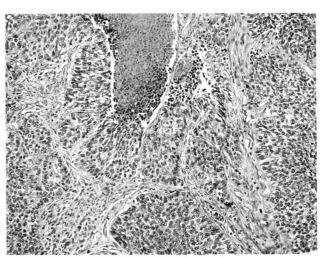

Figure 3.17.2   FIGO grade 3 endometrioid carcinoma showing cellular solid nests with central necrosis. The epithelial component of malignant mixed müllerian tumor (MMMT; carcinosarcoma) can be identical, but there is no sarcomatous component.

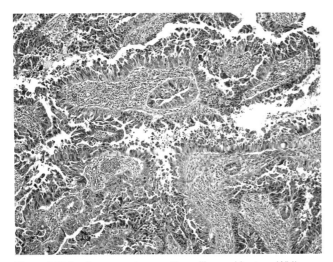

Figure 3.17.3   Serous carcinoma with papillary architecture. While sarcomatous stroma is not present, the amount of inflammation and cellularity of the stroma at this magnification can resemble malignant mixed müllerian tumor (MMMT; carcinosarcoma).

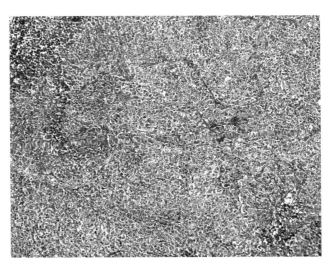

Figure 3.17.4   FIGO grade 3 endometrioid carcinoma with solid diffuse sheets of tumor that can mimic the sarcoma component of malignant mixed müllerian tumor (MMMT; carcinosarcoma).

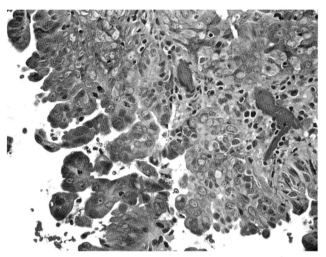

Figure 3.17.5   Serous carcinoma with usual cytologic features; however, the epithelial component of malignant mixed müllerian tumor (MMMT; carcinosarcoma) can be identical.

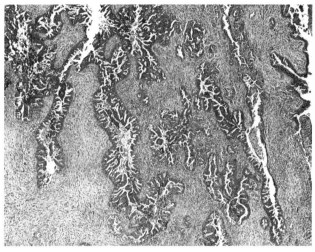

Figure 3.17.6   Malignant mixed müllerian tumor (MMMT; carcinosarcoma) with intimate admixture of carcinoma and sarcoma components.

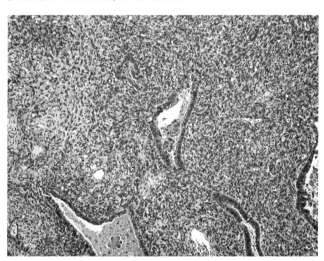

Figure 3.17.7   Malignant mixed müllerian tumor (MMMT; carcinosarcoma) with intimate admixture of carcinoma and sarcoma components.

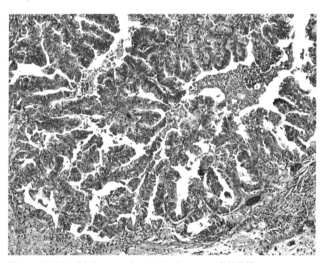

Figure 3.17.8   Malignant mixed müllerian tumor (MMMT; carcinosarcoma) showing carcinoma component with complex papillary architecture, which potentially can be misclassified as pure carcinoma if the sarcoma component is not present in a biopsy/curettage specimen.

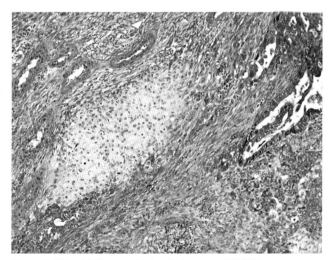

Figure 3.17.9   Malignant mixed müllerian tumor (MMMT; carcinosarcoma) with chondrosarcomatous focus.

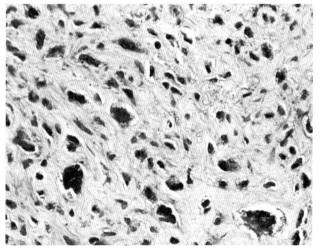

Figure 3.17.10   Malignant mixed müllerian tumor (MMMT; carcinosarcoma) showing sarcoma component with high-grade nuclei.

3   UTERINE CORPUS (EPITHELIAL LESIONS)

	Dedifferentiated Carcinoma	High-Grade Endometrial Carcinoma
Age	51-55 y (median)	Postmenopausal
Location	Endometrium; can occur in the ovary	Endometrium; can occur elsewhere in the gynecologic tract
Symptoms	Abnormal vaginal bleeding/pelvic pain	Abnormal vaginal bleeding
Signs	Expected to be similar to other high-grade endometrial carcinomas; polypoid mass may be present at hysteroscopy or in gross specimen	Uterine enlargement or pelvic mass; polypoid mass may be present at hysteroscopy or in gross specimen
Etiology	Appear to represent evolution/dedifferentiation from low-grade endometrioid carcinoma component. From one-half to two-thirds of cases are mismatch repair deficient/microsatellite instability-high. Mutations in PI3K pathway are prevalent. Dedifferentiation is associated with inactivation of core SWI/SNF complex proteins	FIGO grade 3 endometrioid carcinoma represents progression from lower-grade endometrioid carcinoma; the sarcoma component is clonally related to the carcinoma component and believed to arise from the latter for MMMT
Histology	1. Glandular (low-grade endometrioid carcinoma) and solid (undifferentiated carcinoma) components (glandular and solid components may be synchronous, or solid component may develop as recurrence subsequent to pure glandular component); often with abrupt transition between both components *(Fig. 3.18.1)* 2. Component of low-grade endometrioid carcinoma shows typical architectural and cytologic features with usual glandular pattern, FIGO grade 1 or 2 (+/− squamous differentiation) *(Fig. 3.18.2)*	1. Biphasic appearance with intimate admixture of carcinoma and sarcoma components in MMMT *(Fig. 3.18.6)*; glandular and solid components in FIGO grade 3 endometrioid carcinoma *(Fig. 3.18.7)* 2. Glandular (carcinoma) component shows typical architectural and cytologic features of serous, endometrioid, or unclassified carcinoma in MMMT (other histologic types of carcinoma can occur); typical architectural and cytologic features of FIGO grade 3 endometrioid carcinoma with usual glandular pattern (+/− squamous differentiation); cytologic features show greater nuclear atypia than the low-grade endometrioid carcinoma component of dedifferentiated carcinoma
	3. Solid component shows diffuse sheets without gland formation or nested growth pattern *(Fig. 3.18.3)*; round tumor cells with discohesive appearance cytologically similar to lymphoma (rhabdoid features may be seen) *(Fig. 3.18.4)*; cytologic features in solid component show greater nuclear atypia and mitotic activity than glandular component; no sarcomatous elements or spindle cell differentiation, but myxoid stroma occasionally can be seen 4. Necrosis may be present (common in undifferentiated component) *(Fig. 3.18.5)*	3. Solid component shows typical architectural and cytologic features of sarcoma (homologous or heterologous) in MMMT *(Fig. 3.18.8)*; usual nonsquamous pattern in FIGO grade 3 endometrioid carcinoma with cohesive tumor cells *(Fig. 3.18.9)* and cytologic similarity between glandular and solid components (solid component may have sheets or nested growth pattern) 4. Necrosis may be present *(Fig. 3.18.10)*

	Dedifferentiated Carcinoma	High-Grade Endometrial Carcinoma
Special studies	• Cytokeratin: often markedly diminished (and can be completely negative) in undifferentiated carcinoma component • PAX8: may be negative in undifferentiated component • Loss of E-cadherin in some cases • Loss of BRG1, SMARCA2, and INI1 in some cases	• Cytokeratin: diffuse expression in carcinoma components of FIGO grade 3 endometrioid carcinoma and MMMT • PAX8: positive in carcinoma component of MMMT, negative in sarcoma component; positive in FIGO grade 3 endometrioid carcinoma
Treatment	Dependent on stage and other risk factors; may include hysterectomy with bilateral salpingo-oophorectomy and surgical staging, chemotherapy, and/or radiation therapy	Dependent on histologic type, stage, and other risk factors; may include observation, hysterectomy with bilateral salpingo-oophorectomy and surgical staging, chemotherapy, and/or radiation therapy
Prognosis	29%-59% survival at 7-9 mo (median follow-up interval)	5-y survival: 30%-75%; dependent on histologic type, stage, and other risk factors

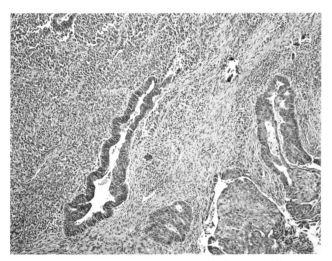

Figure 3.18.1   Dedifferentiated carcinoma with abrupt transition between low-grade endometrioid carcinoma (**center**) and undifferentiated carcinoma (**left**).

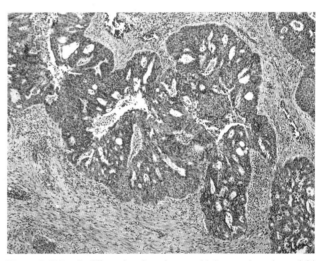

Figure 3.18.2   Dedifferentiated carcinoma with low-grade endometrioid carcinoma component.

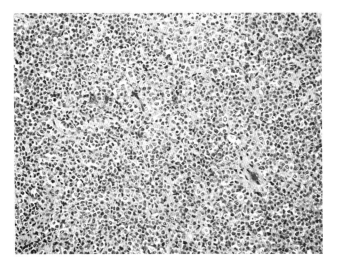

Figure 3.18.3 Dedifferentiated carcinoma with sheets of undifferentiated carcinoma.

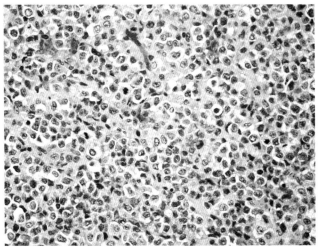

Figure 3.18.4 Dedifferentiated carcinoma with undifferentiated carcinoma component. The latter is discohesive and resembles lymphoma. The cells are round, atypical, and mitotically active and have high nuclear-to-cytoplasmic ratios.

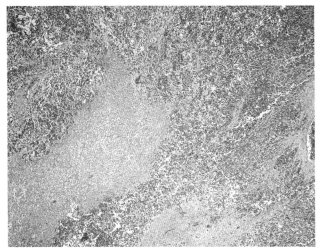

Figure 3.18.5 Dedifferentiated carcinoma with sheets of necrosis in the component of undifferentiated carcinoma.

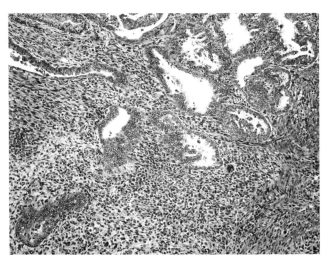

Figure 3.18.6 Malignant mixed müllerian tumor (MMMT; carcinosarcoma) with intimate admixture of carcinoma and sarcoma components.

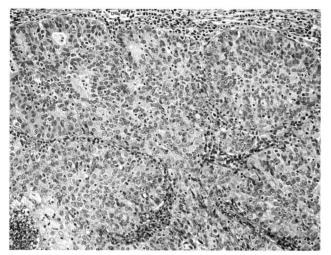

Figure 3.18.7   FIGO grade 3 endometrioid carcinoma showing solid component with focal glandular differentiation (**upper left**).

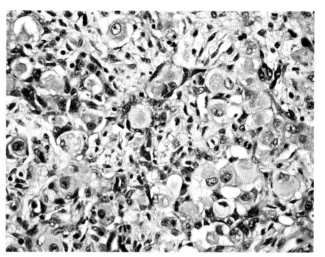

Figure 3.18.8   Malignant mixed müllerian tumor (MMMT; carcinosarcoma) with rhabdomyosarcoma component.

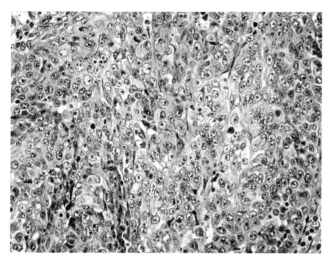

Figure 3.18.9   FIGO grade 3 endometrioid carcinoma with solid sheets of tumor. The cells are cohesive in contrast to the discohesive nature in dedifferentiated carcinoma.

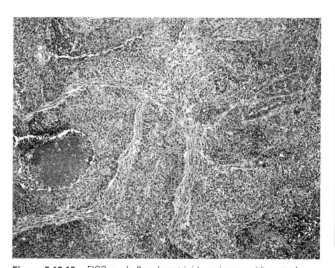

Figure 3.18.10   FIGO grade 3 endometrioid carcinoma with central necrosis within cellular solid nests. In contrast, dedifferentiated carcinoma has diffuse sheets of necrosis.

	Mesonephric/Mesonephric-Like Adenocarcinoma	Endometrioid Carcinoma
Age	Variable, ranging from pre- to postmenopausal	59-63 y (mean)
Location	Endometrium; more common location is the cervix	Endometrium; may occur elsewhere in the gynecologic tract
Symptoms	Limited data, but include abnormal vaginal bleeding and lower abdominal pain	Abnormal vaginal bleeding
Signs	Limited data, but expected findings similar to other endometrial carcinomas	Pelvic mass in some advanced-stage cases; polypoid mass may be present at hysteroscopy or in gross specimen
Etiology	Unknown; may represent origin from mesonephric remnants/hyperplasia in the upper cervix (with predominant development of carcinoma in uterine corpus), in which cervical primary origin was not recognized	Estrogen-driven pathogenesis with hyperplasia evolving to carcinoma
Histology	1. Mixture of architectural patterns: tubular, glandular, solid, spindle, retiform, papillary, and glomeruloid; tubular profiles tend to be smaller than glands in most endometrioid carcinomas *(Figs. 3.19.1-3.19.4)*; the overall histologic appearance can resemble female adnexal tumor of wolffian origin (FATWO) in the broad ligament (see Section 7.10)	1. Predominantly glandular patterns *(Fig. 3.19.8)*, but papillary and solid architecture may be seen
	2. Cells often low cuboidal, but columnar shapes may be seen *(Figs. 3.19.5 and 3.19.6)*	2. Cells often columnar *(Fig. 3.19.9)*
	3. Epithelium often single layer without stratification	3. Pseudostratified epithelium
	4. Lacks squamous differentiation and other metaplastic-like cell types	4. Squamous differentiation and other metaplastic-like cell types may be present *(Fig. 3.19.10)*
	5. High nuclear-to-cytoplasmic ratio with frequent blue appearance at low-power magnification	5. Variable nuclear-to-cytoplasmic ratio but can have more cytoplasm than usually seen in mesonephric adenocarcinomas
	6. Nuclei round to oval with hyperchromasia	6. Nuclei often oval to columnar but can be round; variable chromatin appearance
	7. Variable mitotic activity	7. Variable mitotic activity
	8. Background of hyperplasia not expected	8. Background of hyperplasia may be present
Special studies	• GATA-3 (+) • ER/PR (−) • CD10 usually has luminal edge staining pattern *(Fig. 3.19.7)* • TTF1 (+)	• GATA-3 (−) • ER/PR (+) • CD10 often lacks luminal edge staining pattern • TTF1 is generally negative

	Mesonephric/Mesonephric-Like Adenocarcinoma	**Endometrioid Carcinoma**
Treatment	Unclear as this histologic type in the endometrium is rare; probably managed with at least surgery, depending on stage and other risk factors	Dependent on grade, stage, and other risk factors; may include observation, hormonal therapy, hysterectomy with bilateral salpingo-oophorectomy, surgical staging, chemotherapy, and/or radiation therapy
Prognosis	Based on limited data, appear to behave more aggressively than endometrioid carcinoma	Dependent on grade, stage, and other risk factors

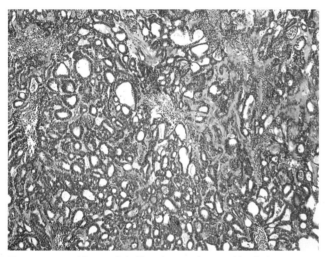

Figure 3.19.1   Mesonephric-like adenocarcinoma with tubular pattern.

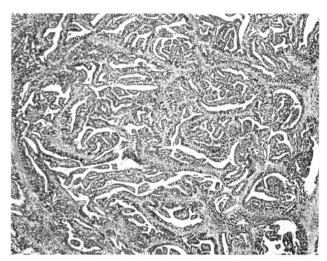

Figure 3.19.2   Mesonephric-like adenocarcinoma with retiform/papillary pattern.

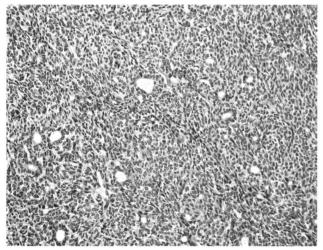

Figure 3.19.3   Mesonephric-like adenocarcinoma with solid pattern. Tubules are focally present.

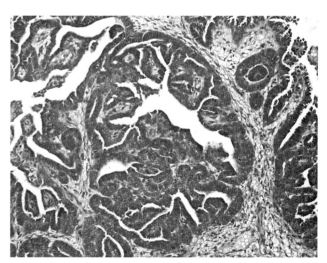

Figure 3.19.4   Mesonephric-like adenocarcinoma with glomeruloid pattern.

3 UTERINE CORPUS (EPITHELIAL LESIONS)

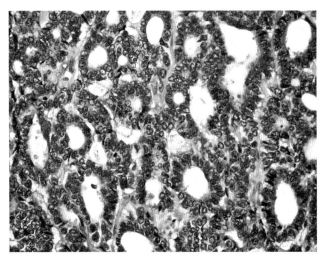

Figure 3.19.5 Mesonephric-like adenocarcinoma. Tubules are lined by a single nonstratified layer of low cuboidal cells with round nuclei and high nuclear-to-cytoplasmic ratios.

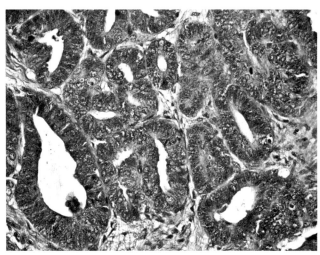

Figure 3.19.6 Mesonephric-like adenocarcinoma. Some glands are lined by a single layer of low cuboidal cells, while others contain columnar cells with pseudostratification. The nuclear-to-cytoplasmic ratios are high. These features can simulate an endometrioid carcinoma.

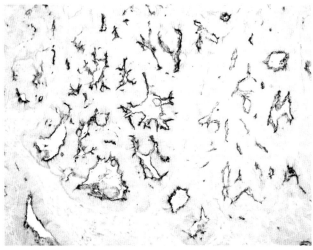

Figure 3.19.7 Mesonephric-like adenocarcinoma. CD10 immunostain with luminal edge staining pattern.

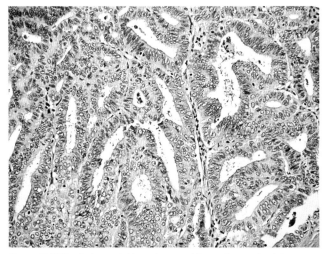

Figure 3.19.8 Endometrioid carcinoma with usual-type glandular pattern.

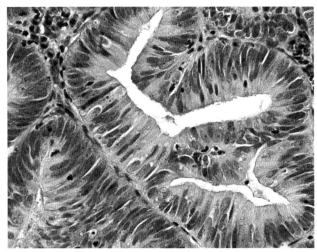

Figure 3.19.9 Endometrioid carcinoma with columnar cells. The nuclei are more oval, nuclear-to-cytoplasmic ratios are not as high, and chromatin is not as coarse compared with mesonephric adenocarcinoma.

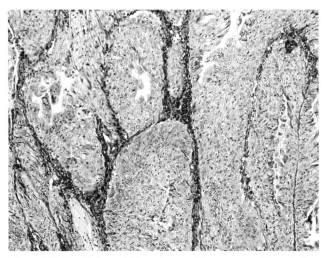

Figure 3.19.10 Endometrioid carcinoma with squamous differentiation.

3.20

ENDOMETRIAL CARCINOMA INVOLVING IRREGULAR ENDOMETRIAL-MYOMETRIAL JUNCTION VS ENDOMETRIAL CARCINOMA WITH SUPERFICIAL MYOINVASION

	Endometrial Carcinoma Involving Irregular Endometrial-Myometrial Junction	Endometrial Carcinoma With Superficial Myoinvasion
Age	59-63 y (mean)	59-63 y (mean)
Location	Endometrium	Endometrium
Symptoms	Abnormal vaginal bleeding	Abnormal vaginal bleeding
Signs	Polypoid mass may be present at hysteroscopy or in gross specimen	Polypoid mass may be present at hysteroscopy or in gross specimen
Etiology	Endometrioid carcinoma involves irregular endometrial-myometrial junction mimicking myometrial invasion; this differential diagnosis pertains to endometrioid histologic type	Endometrial carcinoma invades the myometrium; this differential diagnosis pertains to endometrioid histologic type
Histology	1. Carcinoma involves the endometrial-myometrial junction; the junction can be irregular *(Figs. 3.20.1 and 3.20.2)*	1. Carcinoma can be confined to the endometrial-myometrial junction in some areas, while myoinvasion may be present elsewhere
	2. No marked crowding of nests with haphazard arrangement in the myometrium at the irregular endometrial-myometrial junction	2. Marked crowding of nests with haphazard arrangement may be seen in the myometrium at the endometrial-myometrial junction *(Fig. 3.20.7)*
	3. Nests of carcinoma in the myometrium at the endometrial-myometrial junction are round with smooth contours *(Fig. 3.20.3)*	3. Nests of carcinoma in the myometrium at the endometrial-myometrial junction can be round with smooth contours but may show irregular outlines
	4. No MELF (microcystic, elongated, and fragmented) glandular pattern in the myometrium at the endometrial-myometrial junction	4. MELF (microcystic, elongated, and fragmented) glandular pattern may be present in the myometrium at the endometrial-myometrial junction (glands show flat and thin epithelium with eosinophilic cytoplasm, producing a microcystic appearance) *(Figs. 3.20.8 and 3.20.9)*
	5. Associated endometrial stroma or benign glands within the focus involved by carcinoma (particularly at the periphery) may be present *(Figs. 3.20.4-3.20.6)* (benign glands occasionally can be present within the superficial myometrium without evident associated stroma [*Fig. 3.20.1*])	5. No associated endometrial stroma or benign glands within the focus of question
	6. Mild inflammation can be present adjacent to carcinoma involving the endometrial-myometrial junction	6. Marked associated inflammatory response may be present in the foci of question
	7. No associated altered stroma	7. Associated altered stromal response with fibromyxoid change, edema, or desmoplasia may be present *(Figs. 3.20.8 and 3.20.9)*
Special studies	Immunohistochemistry of no help for this differential diagnosis	Immunohistochemistry of no help for this differential diagnosis

	Endometrial Carcinoma Involving Irregular Endometrial-Myometrial Junction	**Endometrial Carcinoma With Superficial Myoinvasion**
Treatment	Dependent on grade and other risk factors; may include observation, hysterectomy with bilateral salpingo-oophorectomy, and/or radiation therapy	Dependent on grade and other risk factors; may include observation, hysterectomy with bilateral salpingo-oophorectomy, and/or radiation therapy
Prognosis	Dependent on grade and other risk factors; however, cases without myometrial invasion have a better prognosis than those with myometrial invasion	Dependent on grade and other risk factors

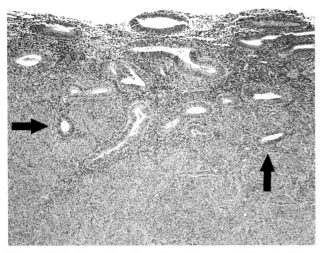

Figure 3.20.1   Normal irregular endometrial-myometrial junction. Note that some glands (*arrows*) can be found in the myometrium without obvious surrounding endometrial stroma.

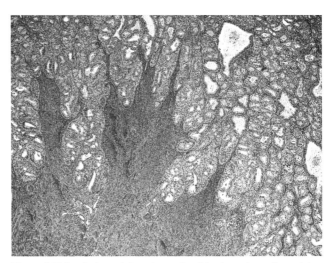

Figure 3.20.2   Endometrial carcinoma involving irregular endometrial-myometrial junction.

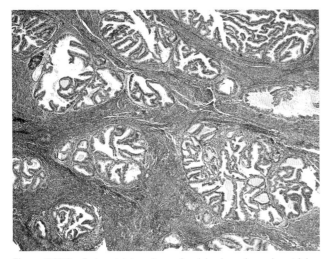

Figure 3.20.3   Endometrial carcinoma involving irregular endometrial-myometrial junction. Note the smooth borders of the round groups of glands.

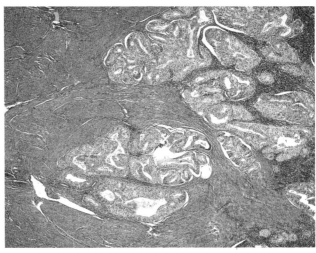

Figure 3.20.4   Endometrial carcinoma involving irregular endometrial-myometrial junction. The endometrial-myometrial junction is on the right-hand side of the photograph.

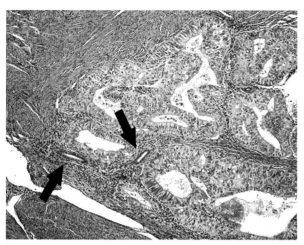

Figure 3.20.5 Endometrial carcinoma involving irregular endometrial-myometrial junction. Same focus from the lower left portion of *Figure 3.20.4*. Note the benign glands (*arrows*) at the interface between the tumor and myometrium.

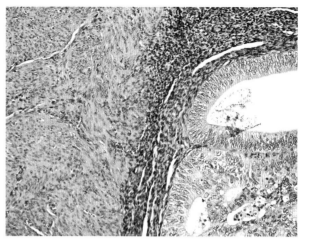

Figure 3.20.6 Endometrial carcinoma involving irregular endometrial-myometrial junction. An intervening band of endometrial stroma is in between the myometrium and carcinoma.

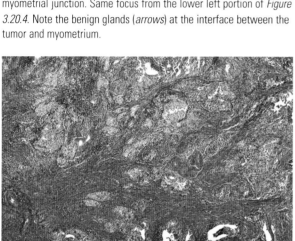

Figure 3.20.7 Endometrial carcinoma with superficial myoinvasion. The glands are too crowded and haphazardly arranged for confinement to an irregular endometrial-myometrial junction.

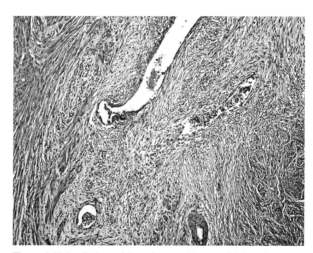

Figure 3.20.8 Endometrial carcinoma with superficial myoinvasion exhibiting MELF (microcystic, elongated, and fragmented) pattern. At low-power magnification, the smaller microcystic and elongated glands at the **lower left and center** right may not be readily obvious as being invasive. The myometrium surrounding the glands is altered.

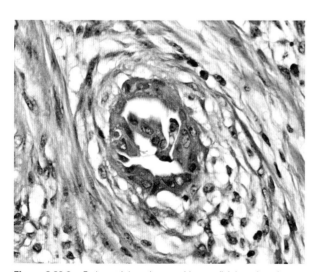

Figure 3.20.9 Endometrial carcinoma with superficial myoinvasion exhibiting MELF (microcystic, elongated, and fragmented) pattern. The gland is lined by a flat and deceptively bland layer with abundant eosinophilic cytoplasm. The surrounding myometrium is slightly loose and edematous.

	Endometrial Carcinoma With Involvement of Adenomyosis	Endometrial Carcinoma With Myoinvasion
Age	59-63 y (mean)	59-63 y (mean)
Location	Endometrium	Endometrium
Symptoms	Abnormal vaginal bleeding	Abnormal vaginal bleeding
Signs	Polypoid mass may be present at hysteroscopy or in gross specimen	Polypoid mass may be present at hysteroscopy or in gross specimen
Etiology	Endometrioid carcinoma extends into adenomyosis, which can simulate myometrial invasion; this differential diagnosis pertains to endometrioid histologic type	Endometrial carcinoma invades the myometrium; this differential diagnosis pertains to endometrioid histologic type
Histology	1. Background of uninvolved adenomyosis elsewhere *(Fig. 3.21.1, also Figs. 4.8.7)*	1. Background of adenomyosis elsewhere usually not present but occasionally can be seen
	2. Carcinoma involves adenomyosis; extension into adenomyosis can be deep and florid *(Fig. 3.21.2)*; pattern of extension of carcinoma into adenomyosis can sometimes have the appearance of elongated tracts/diverticula traveling in and out of the plane of section when foci are oriented longitudinally *(Figs. 3.21.2 and 3.21.3)*	2. Carcinoma sometimes can be confined to adenomyosis in some areas, while myoinvasion may be present elsewhere
	3. No marked crowding of foci of question within the myometrium; no haphazard arrangement of foci of question within the myometrium	3. Marked crowding of foci of question within the myometrium may be seen; haphazard arrangement of foci of question within the myometrium may be seen *(Figs. 3.21.7-3.21.9)*
	4. Nests of carcinoma in foci of question are round with smooth contours *(Figs. 3.21.2 and 3.21.4)*	4. Nests of carcinoma in foci of question can be round with smooth contours but may show irregular outlines
	5. No MELF (microcystic, elongated, and fragmented) glandular pattern in carcinoma in foci of question	5. MELF (microcystic, elongated, and fragmented) glandular pattern may be present in carcinoma in foci of question (glands show flat and thin epithelium with eosinophilic cytoplasm, producing a microcystic appearance) *(Fig. 3.21.10)*
	6. Associated endometrial stroma or benign glands within the focus involved by carcinoma (particularly at the periphery) may be present (benign glands occasionally can be present within the myometrium without evident associated stroma) *(Figs. 3.21.4-3.21.6)*	6. No associated endometrial stroma or benign glands within the focus of question
	7. Mild inflammation can be present adjacent to carcinoma involving the foci of question	7. Marked associated inflammatory response may be present in the foci of question *(Fig. 3.21.8)*
	8. No associated altered stroma	8. Associated altered stromal response with fibromyxoid change, edema, or desmoplasia may be present *(Fig. 3.21.10)*

	Endometrial Carcinoma With Involvement of Adenomyosis	Endometrial Carcinoma With Myoinvasion
Special studies	Immunohistochemistry of no help for this differential diagnosis	Immunohistochemistry of no help for this differential diagnosis
Treatment	Dependent on grade and other risk factors; may include observation, hysterectomy with bilateral salpingo-oophorectomy, and/or radiation therapy	Dependent on grade and other risk factors; may include observation, hysterectomy with bilateral salpingo-oophorectomy, and/or radiation therapy
Prognosis	Dependent on grade and other risk factors; however, cases without myometrial invasion have a better prognosis than do those with myometrial invasion	Dependent on stage, grade, and other risk factors

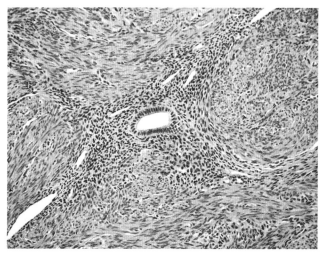

Figure 3.21.1 Adenomyosis.

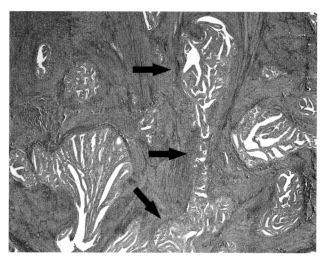

Figure 3.21.2 Endometrial carcinoma extends into multiple foci of adenomyosis. Note the smooth borders of the round groups of glands within the myometrium. Also, the extension of carcinoma in some foci is distributed along elongated tracts of adenomyosis (*arrows*).

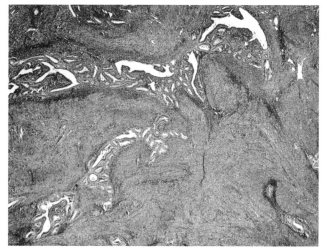

Figure 3.21.3 Endometrial hyperplasia with extension into elongated tracts of adenomyosis.

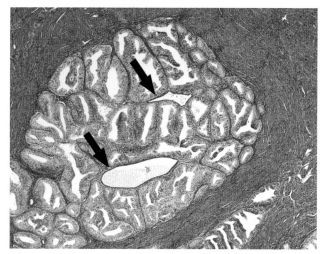

Figure 3.21.4 Endometrial carcinoma with involvement of adenomyosis. Note the smooth borders of the round group of glands within the myometrium. In addition, benign glands (*arrows*) are present within carcinoma.

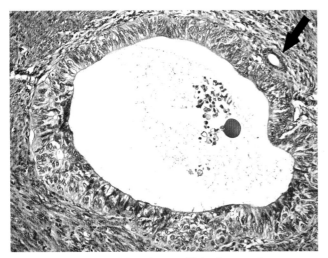

Figure 3.21.5   Endometrial carcinoma with involvement of adenomyosis. A benign gland (*arrow*) is adjacent to carcinoma.

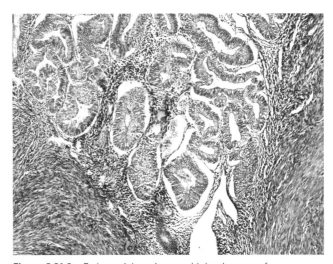

Figure 3.21.6   Endometrial carcinoma with involvement of adenomyosis. An intervening band of endometrial stroma is in between the myometrium and carcinoma.

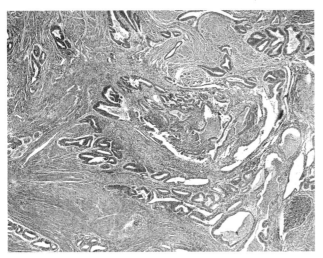

Figure 3.21.7   Endometrial carcinoma with destructive myoinvasion.

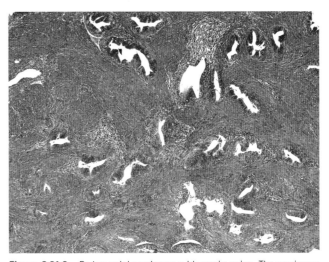

Figure 3.21.8   Endometrial carcinoma with myoinvasion. The carcinoma glands are too crowded and haphazard for confinement to adenomyosis, and an associated inflammatory response is present.

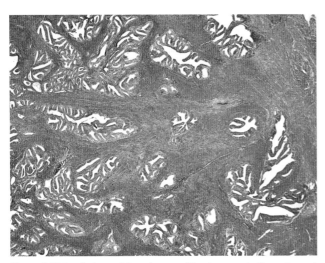

Figure 3.21.9   Endometrial carcinoma with adenomyosis-like pattern of myoinvasion. The carcinoma glands are too crowded and haphazard for confinement to adenomyosis.

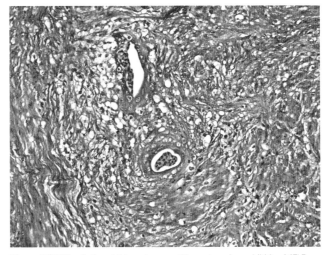

Figure 3.21.10   Endometrial carcinoma with myoinvasion exhibiting MELF (microcystic, elongated, and fragmented) pattern. The glands are lined by flat and deceptively bland layers with abundant eosinophilic cytoplasm. The surrounding myometrium is slightly myxoid with a mild inflammatory response.

	Endometrial Carcinoma With Vascular Pseudoinvasion	Endometrial Carcinoma With True LVSI
Age	Postmenopausal	Postmenopausal
Location	Endometrium	Endometrium
Symptoms	Abnormal vaginal bleeding	Abnormal vaginal bleeding
Signs	Pelvic mass in some advanced-stage cases; polypoid mass may be present at hysteroscopy or in gross specimen	Pelvic mass in some advanced-stage cases; polypoid mass may be present at hysteroscopy or in gross specimen
Etiology	Artifactual displacement of tumor into lymph-vascular spaces, which occurs more frequently in robotic-assisted laparoscopic hysterectomies compared with abdominal hysterectomies, presumably due to mechanical displacement of tumor from increased uterine pressure created by the intrauterine manipulator (may also be related to the presence of exophytic tumors within the endometrial cavity and contamination of cutting field during gross examination of specimen); this phenomenon can occur with all histologic types	Endometrial carcinoma invades lymph-vascular spaces; true LVSI can occur with all histologic types; assessment of LVSI in the uterus likely has suboptimal interobserver reproducibility (for cases falling short of an unequivocal diagnosis, terminology such as "equivocal for LVSI," "suspicious for LVSI," or "concerning for LVSI" may be useful depending on the level of concern)
Histology	1. No true LVSI 2. Detached small clusters of tumor cells within large thick-walled vessels (particularly in the outer half of the myometrium) 3. Disaggregated tumor cells (+/− admixed inflammation or stromal tissue) within lymph-vascular spaces (Figs. 3.22.1 and 3.22.2) 4. Tumor within lymph-vascular spaces immediately adjacent to invasive tumor with retraction artifact (Fig. 3.22.3) 5. Detached clusters of tumor cells within artifactual myometrial clefts (Fig. 3.22.4) 6. High volume of tumor within lymph-vascular spaces in setting of low-grade/low-stage tumor may be seen 7. No attachment of tumor to endothelial lining within lymph-vascular spaces 8. Tumor does not conform to shape of lymph-vascular space	1. LVSI is present in ~10% of endometrioid carcinomas but more frequent in aggressive histologic types 2. Tumor can be within small and large vessels 3. No disaggregated tumor cells within lymph-vascular spaces 4. No tumor within lymph-vascular spaces immediately adjacent to invasive tumor with retraction artifact 5. Detached clusters of tumor cells within artifactual myometrial clefts may or may not occur (vascular pseudoinvasion and true LVSI can occur simultaneously) 6. High volume of tumor within lymph-vascular spaces may occur in setting of high-grade/high-stage tumor 7. Attachment of tumor to endothelial lining within lymph-vascular spaces (Fig. 3.22.6) 8. Tumor conforms to shape of lymph-vascular space (Fig. 3.22.7)

	Endometrial Carcinoma With Vascular Pseudoinvasion	Endometrial Carcinoma With True LVSI
	9. No tumor cell clusters that are cohesive with smooth borders in lymph-vascular spaces *(Fig. 3.22.5)* 10. Tumor cells within lymph-vascular space do not show change in cytologic morphology with more eosinophilic cytoplasm 11. No tumor within lymph-vascular spaces adjacent to large vessels 12. No perivascular inflammation in the myometrium	9. Clusters of tumor cells within lymph-vascular spaces are cohesive and have smooth borders *(Fig. 3.22.7)* 10. Tumor cells within lymph-vascular space can show change in cytologic morphology with more eosinophilic cytoplasm (occasionally, may have histiocyte-like appearance) *(Fig. 3.22.8)* 11. Tumor within lymph-vascular spaces adjacent to large vessels *(Fig. 3.22.9)* 12. Perivascular inflammation in the myometrium *(Fig. 3.22.10)*
Special studies	Immunohistochemistry of no help for this differential diagnosis (if the differential diagnosis concerns whether or not the focus of concern is within a lymph-vascular space, then markers such as CD31 can help; however, the differential diagnosis discussed in this section pertains specifically to cases where the focus of concern is within a lymph-vascular space but that the question relates to whether it is true LVSI vs carcinoma that has been artifactually displaced into a lymph-vascular space)	Immunohistochemistry of no help for this differential diagnosis
Treatment	Dependent on histologic type/grade and other risk factors; may include observation, hysterectomy with bilateral salpingo-oophorectomy, surgical staging, chemotherapy, and/or radiation therapy; no specific treatment for this finding	True LVSI is considered a risk factor that can influence treatment decisions; may include observation, hysterectomy with bilateral salpingo-oophorectomy, surgical staging, chemotherapy, and/or radiation therapy
Prognosis	Vascular pseudoinvasion is not known to be of prognostic significance	Presence of true LVSI and its extent (focal vs extensive [≥5 vessels]) have prognostic significance for low-stage tumors

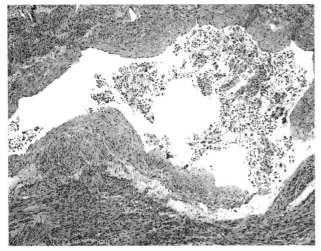

Figure 3.22.1   Vascular pseudoinvasion. Disaggregated tumor is present within a lymph-vascular space.

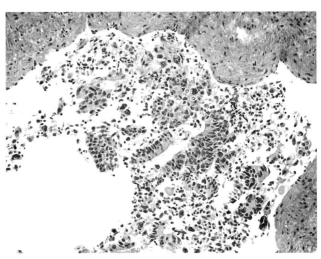

Figure 3.22.2   Vascular pseudoinvasion. Higher-power magnification of *Figure 3.22.1.*

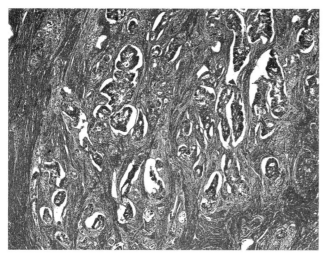

Figure 3.22.3   Myoinvasive endometrial carcinoma with stromal retraction artifact. This pattern of stromal retraction artifact can simulate extensive lymph-vascular space invasion at low-power magnification.

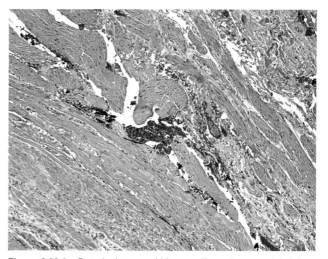

Figure 3.22.4   Detached tumor within an artifactual myometrial cleft.

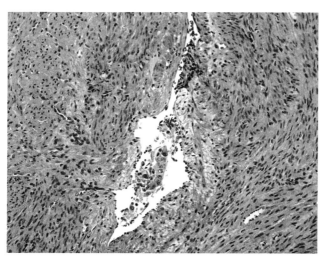

Figure 3.22.5   Vascular pseudoinvasion. The tumor cluster is small, does not have smooth borders, and does not conform to the shape of the lymph-vascular space.

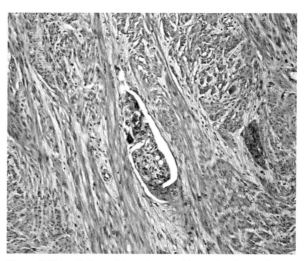

Figure 3.22.6   Endometrial carcinoma with true lymph-vascular space invasion showing attachment to the endothelium.

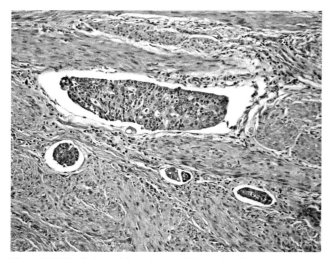

Figure 3.22.7   Endometrial carcinoma with true lymph-vascular space invasion. The tumor clusters are cohesive, have smooth borders, and conform to the shape of the lymph-vascular spaces.

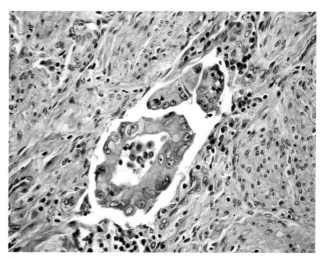

Figure 3.22.8   Endometrial carcinoma with true lymph-vascular space invasion. The tumor cluster shows cytologic alterations with metaplastic-like features and abundant eosinophilic cytoplasm.

3 UTERINE CORPUS (EPITHELIAL LESIONS)

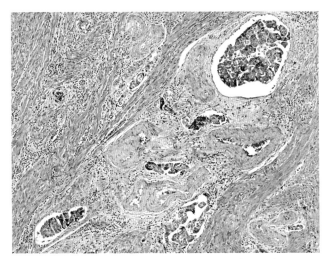

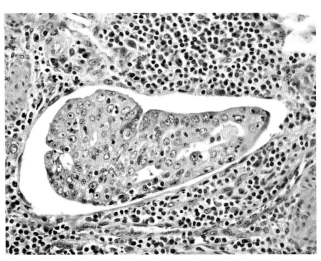

Figure 3.22.9 Endometrial carcinoma with true lymph-vascular space invasion. Tumor is present within lymph-vascular spaces adjacent to large thick-walled vessels.

Figure 3.22.10 Endometrial carcinoma with true lymph-vascular space invasion showing perivascular inflammation.

	Minute and Detached Fragments of Ovarian/Tubal High-Grade Serous Carcinoma in Uterine Biopsy/Curettage	Primary Endometrial Serous Carcinoma
Age	Peri- or postmenopausal (uncommonly premenopausal)	Postmenopausal
Location	Fragments of ovarian/tubal carcinoma in endometrial specimen	Endometrium
Symptoms	Abnormal vaginal bleeding	Abnormal vaginal bleeding
Signs	No endometrial mass at hysteroscopy or in gross specimen; ovarian/tubal mass may not be detected clinically; may be incidentally detected in Pap smear or ECC	Polypoid mass may be present at hysteroscopy or in gross specimen
Etiology	Primary origin in the ovary/fallopian tube; initially detected in endometrial or endocervical biopsy/curettage via transtubal spread; potential for misclassification as endometrial primary	Primary origin in the endometrium
Histology	1. Detached and minute clusters, small papillae, and/or individual cells; usually scanty amount of tumor (Figs. 3.23.1-3.23.5) 2. +/− irregular surface contours, +/− hobnail cells 3. Round to columnar cells with high nuclear-to-cytoplasmic ratios 4. Round to oval nuclei with marked atypia (Fig. 3.23.6) 5. High mitotic index 6. Background intact endometrium without intraepithelial or invasive serous carcinoma; background proliferative (or weakly proliferative) endometrium can be seen 7. +/− psammoma bodies	1. If sample is adequate, tumor is typically intact with papillary and/or glandular architecture and fragments are large; often abundant amount of tumor (Figs. 3.23.7 and 3.23.8) 2. +/− irregular surface contours, +/− hobnail cells 3. Round to columnar cells with high nuclear-to-cytoplasmic ratios 4. Round to oval nuclei with marked atypia (Fig. 3.23.9) 5. High mitotic index 6. Background intact and atrophic endometrium with intraepithelial and/or invasive serous carcinoma (Fig. 3.23.10) 7. +/− psammoma bodies
Special studies	WT-1 usually positive with diffuse pattern	WT-1 usually negative; small subset of cases can be positive
Treatment	Hysterectomy with bilateral salpingo-oophorectomy, surgical staging, and chemotherapy	Dependent on stage and other risk factors; may include observation, hysterectomy with bilateral salpingo-oophorectomy and surgical staging, chemotherapy, and/or radiation therapy
Prognosis	5-y survival: ~30%	5-y survival: 36%-53% (dependent on stage and other risk factors)

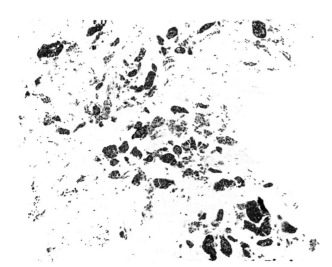

Figure 3.23.1   Fragments of tubal high-grade serous carcinoma with detached small papillae in an endocervical curettage.

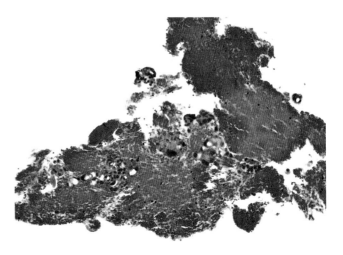

Figure 3.23.2   Fragments of ovarian high-grade serous carcinoma in a hysteroscopic myomectomy. Detached small papillae can be present within blood and may be overlooked at low-power magnification if one only assesses portions of the specimen devoid of blood.

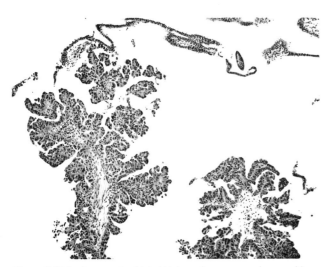

Figure 3.23.3   Fragments of tubal high-grade serous carcinoma with medium-sized papillae in an endometrial biopsy.

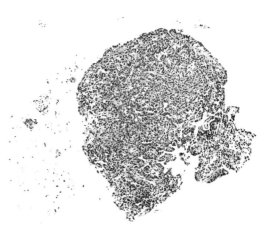

Figure 3.23.4   Fragment of tubal high-grade serous carcinoma with glandular architecture in an endocervical curettage.

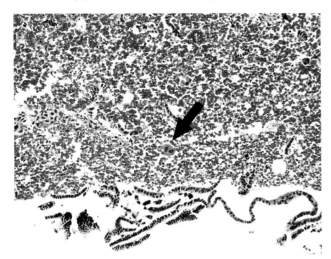

Figure 3.23.5   Scant and minute cluster of ovarian high-grade serous carcinoma (*arrow*) in an endometrial biopsy. Strips of atrophic endometrium are seen at the lower part of the image.

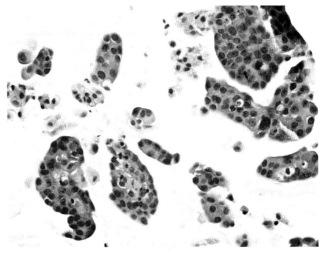

Figure 3.23.6   Fragments of tubal high-grade serous carcinoma in an endocervical curettage (same case as *Fig. 3.23.1*). Notable atypia is present.

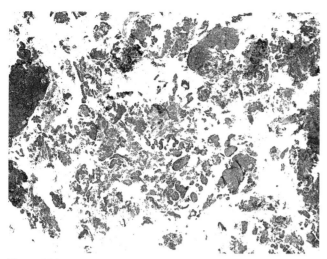

Figure 3.23.7 Primary endometrial serous carcinoma with abundant tumor in an endometrial biopsy.

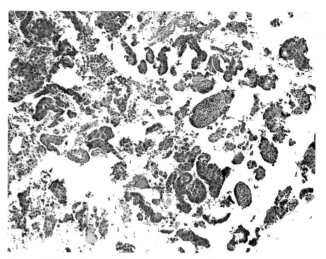

Figure 3.23.8 Primary endometrial serous carcinoma with detached small papillae (same case as *Fig. 3.23.7*).

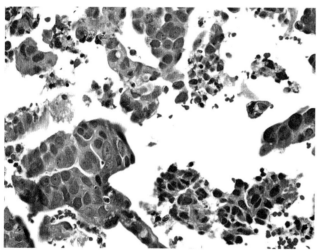

Figure 3.23.9 Primary endometrial serous carcinoma with typical cytologic features, which may be identical to those of tumors of tubal/ovarian origin.

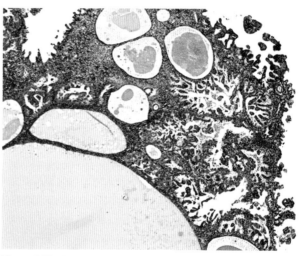

Figure 3.23.10 Primary endometrial serous carcinoma arising within an endometrial polyp.

	Metastatic Nongynecologic Carcinoma With Glandular Pattern Involving Endometrium	Endometrial Endometrioid Carcinoma
Age	34-88 y (mean, 60)	59-63 y (mean)
Location	Metastatic nongynecologic primary involving the endometrium	Endometrium; may occur elsewhere in the gynecologic tract
Symptoms	Abnormal vaginal bleeding; primary tumor may be occult	Abnormal vaginal bleeding
Signs	May be incidental finding in endometrial specimen	Pelvic mass in some advanced-stage cases; polypoid mass may be present at hysteroscopy or in gross specimen
Etiology	Metastatic nongynecologic primary involving the endometrium via direct extension or hematogenous or lymphatic routes; most common primary sites: breast, colorectal, pancreaticobiliary, and stomach (regardless of histologic pattern)	Estrogen-driven pathogenesis with hyperplasia evolving to primary endometrial carcinoma
Histology	1. Absence of hyperplasia in background endometrium 2. Distribution of disease preferentially involving the outer half of the myometrium/serosa (Fig. 3.24.1); involvement of the endometrium may show expansion of stromal compartment with tumor growing between normal endometrial glands (Figs. 3.24.2 and 3.24.3); endometrial involvement (without associated myometrial/serosal involvement) can be seen uncommonly 3. Absence of squamous differentiation or other metaplastic-like features 4. May have endometrioid-like appearance (Fig. 3.24.4) 5. May have dirty necrosis with garland pattern (colorectal) 6. +/− tumor within lymph-vascular spaces within the endometrial stroma and/or myometrium (Fig. 3.24.5)	1. +/− hyperplasia in background endometrium (Fig. 3.24.8) 2. Distribution of disease preferentially involving the endometrium only or inner half of the myometrium (both inner and outer halves may be involved) 3. +/− squamous metaplasia or other metaplastic-like features (Fig. 3.24.9) 4. Typical endometrioid appearance (Fig. 3.24.10) 5. Necrosis may be present in high-grade tumors 6. Lymph-vascular space invasion in the myometrium (if present)
Special studies	• PAX8 (−) (Fig. 3.24.6) • ER/PR (−) (except for breast) (Fig. 3.24.7) • CK7: dependent on primary site • CK20: dependent on primary site	• PAX8 (+) • ER/PR (+) • CK7 diffuse (+) • CK20 (−) or focal/patchy
Treatment	Dependent on primary site	Dependent on grade, stage, and other risk factors; may include observation, hormonal therapy, hysterectomy with bilateral salpingo-oophorectomy, surgical staging, chemotherapy, and/or radiation therapy
Prognosis	Poor	5-y survival: 83%; dependent on stage, grade, and other risk factors

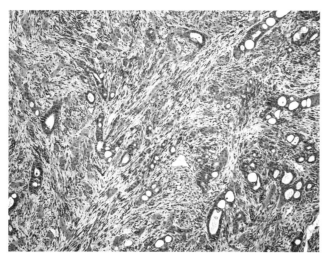

Figure 3.24.1   Metastatic nongynecologic (small bowel) carcinoma involving the myometrium with a pattern that can simulate myometrial invasion by endometrial carcinoma.

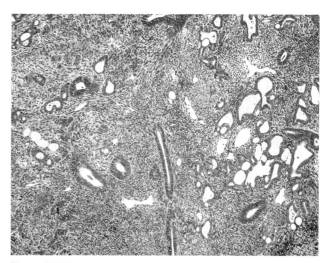

Figure 3.24.2   Metastatic nongynecologic (small bowel) carcinoma involving the endometrium with growth in between normal endometrial glands.

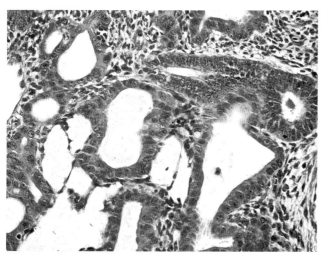

Figure 3.24.3   Metastatic nongynecologic (small bowel) carcinoma involving the endometrium. Note the normal endometrial gland (**right center**).

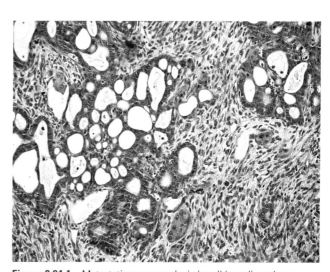

Figure 3.24.4   Metastatic nongynecologic (small bowel) carcinoma involving the endometrium with a cribriform pattern, which can mimic an endometrial endometrioid carcinoma.

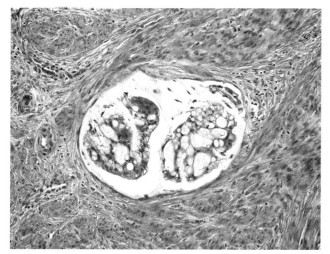

Figure 3.24.5   Metastatic nongynecologic (small bowel) carcinoma involving the myometrium with lymph-vascular space invasion and goblet cell differentiation.

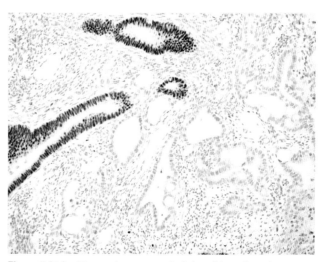

Figure 3.24.6   Metastatic nongynecologic (small bowel) carcinoma involving the endometrium. PAX8 immunostain is positive in normal endometrial glands and negative in tumor.

3   UTERINE CORPUS (EPITHELIAL LESIONS)

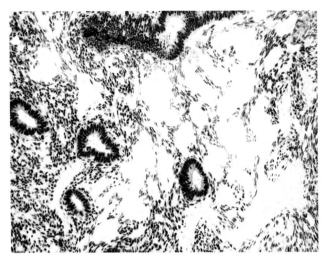

Figure 3.24.7   Metastatic nongynecologic (small bowel) carcinoma involving the endometrium. PR immunostain is positive in normal endometrial glands and stroma and negative in tumor.

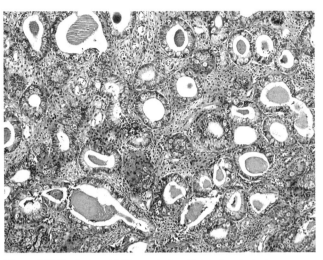

Figure 3.24.8   Endometrial hyperplasia with tubal metaplasia.

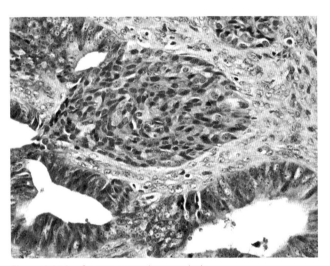

Figure 3.24.9   Squamous morular metaplasia.

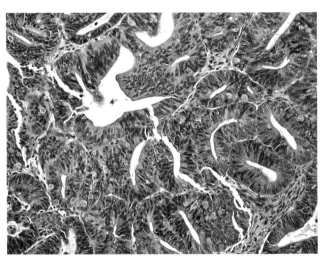

Figure 3.24.10   Endometrial endometrioid carcinoma with usual-type glandular pattern.

3.25

SECONDARY UTERINE CORPUS INVOLVEMENT BY CERVICAL POORLY DIFFERENTIATED SQUAMOUS CELL CARCINOMA VS PRIMARY ENDOMETRIAL FIGO GRADE 3 ENDOMETRIOID CARCINOMA

	Secondary Uterine Corpus Involvement by Cervical Poorly Differentiated Squamous Cell Carcinoma	Primary Endometrial FIGO Grade 3 Endometrioid Carcinoma
Age	55 y (median age)	57-64 y (mean/median)
Location	Cervix	Endometrium; may occur elsewhere in the gynecologic tract
Symptoms	Can be asymptomatic for small tumors; abnormal vaginal bleeding	Abnormal vaginal bleeding
Signs	Gross mass may be evident; may have prior abnormal Pap smear or cervical biopsy; HPV (+) testing on liquid-based Pap smear	Pelvic mass in some advanced-stage cases; polypoid mass may be present at hysteroscopy or in gross specimen
Etiology	Primary origin in the cervix (HPV related) with HSIL as precursor; tumor can extend into uterine corpus (occurs in 22% of cases) simulating a primary endometrial FIGO grade 3 endometrioid carcinoma	Primary origin in the endometrium, with FIGO grade 3 endometrioid carcinoma representing progression from lower-grade endometrioid carcinoma of the endometrium
Histology	1. Solid architecture, +/− papillary growth; solid areas may appear basaloid when squamous differentiation is not obvious *(Fig. 3.25.1)* 2. Round to irregular nests without glandular spaces 3. Squamous differentiation may be present, +/− keratinization *(Fig. 3.25.2)* 4. Central necrosis may be present within round basaloid nests *(Fig. 3.25.3)*; peripheral palisading may be present *(Fig. 3.25.4)*; oval cells/spindle cell differentiation may be present within basaloid nests 5. HSIL may be present in the cervix or extend into the endometrium *(Fig. 3.25.5)* 6. No endometrial hyperplasia	1. Solid architecture with glandular component, +/− papillary growth; solid areas usually basaloid appearing 2. Round to irregular nests; may have glandular spaces in solid component *(Fig. 3.25.8)*; glandular component will be present in nonsolid areas *(Fig. 3.25.9)* 3. Squamous differentiation may be present, usually no keratinization; squamous differentiation usually more immature appearing than in squamous cell carcinoma 4. Central necrosis may be present within round basaloid nests *(Fig. 3.25.10)*; peripheral palisading may be present; oval cells/spindle cell differentiation may be present within basaloid nests when exhibiting immature squamous differentiation 5. No HSIL in the cervix or endometrium 6. Endometrial hyperplasia may be present
Special studies	• p16: diffuse expression *(Fig. 3.25.6)* • HPV *in situ* hybridization (+) *(Fig. 3.25.7)*	• p16: nondiffuse expression • HPV *in situ* hybridization: not detectable
Treatment	Stage dependent: may include hysterectomy, chemotherapy, and/or radiation therapy	Dependent on stage and other risk factors; hysterectomy with bilateral salpingo-oophorectomy and surgical staging; may include observation, chemotherapy, and/or radiation therapy
Prognosis	5-y survival (cervical carcinomas in general): 90%-95% (stage I) and <50% (stage II+), respectively; corpus involvement may be associated with worse prognosis	5-y survival: 45%-75% (dependent on stage and other risk factors)

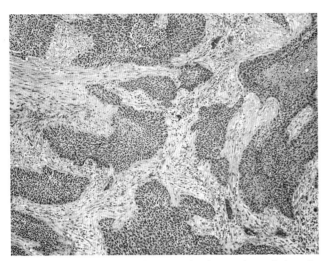

Figure 3.25.1   Secondary uterine corpus involvement by cervical poorly differentiated squamous cell carcinoma showing solid, basaloid, round, and irregular nests with haphazard arrangements and desmoplasia.

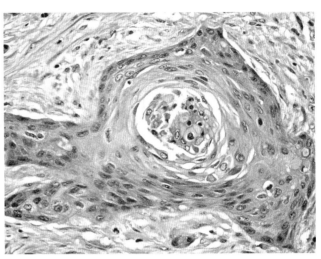

Figure 3.25.2   Secondary uterine corpus involvement by cervical poorly differentiated squamous cell carcinoma with mature squamous differentiation.

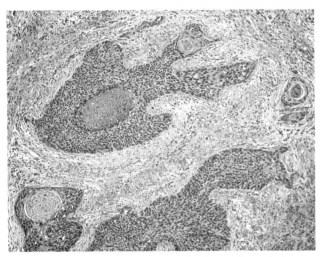

Figure 3.25.3   Secondary uterine corpus involvement by cervical poorly differentiated squamous cell carcinoma. Note the presence of central necrosis within basaloid nests, which can simulate FIGO grade 3 endometrioid carcinoma.

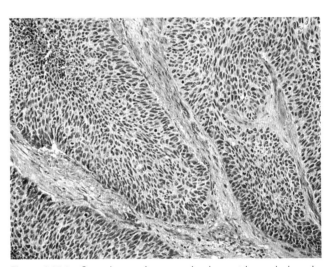

Figure 3.25.4   Secondary uterine corpus involvement by cervical poorly differentiated squamous cell carcinoma with peripheral palisading similar to FIGO grade 3 endometrioid carcinoma.

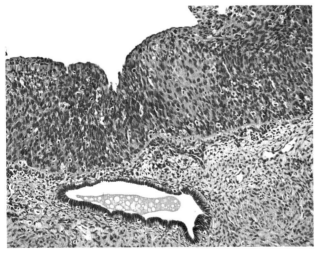

Figure 3.25.5   Secondary uterine corpus involvement with cervical HSIL colonizing the endometrium. Note the underlying benign endometrial gland.

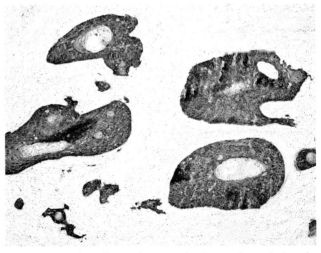

Figure 3.25.6   Secondary uterine corpus involvement by cervical poorly differentiated squamous cell carcinoma with p16 immunostain showing diffuse expression.

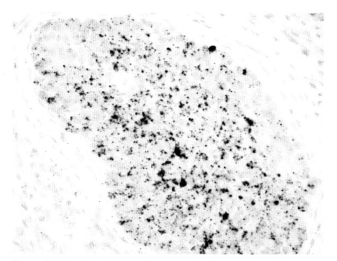

Figure 3.25.7 Secondary uterine corpus involvement by cervical poorly differentiated squamous cell carcinoma with HPV 16 *in situ* hybridization showing punctate nuclear signals.

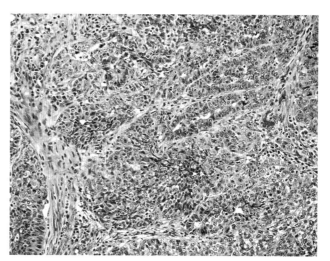

Figure 3.25.8 Primary endometrial FIGO grade 3 endometrioid carcinoma with subtle glandular spaces within solid component.

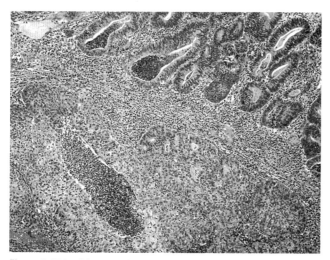

Figure 3.25.9 Primary endometrial FIGO grade 3 endometrioid carcinoma with obvious glandular component.

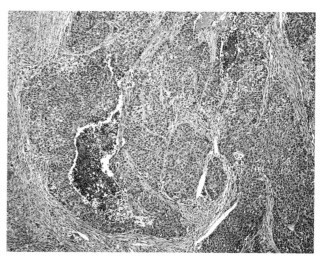

Figure 3.25.10 Primary endometrial FIGO grade 3 endometrioid carcinoma with solid basaloid nests containing central necrosis. Although this pattern is characteristic of FIGO grade 3 endometrioid carcinoma, it can overlap with cervical poorly differentiated squamous cell carcinoma.

3 UTERINE CORPUS (EPITHELIAL LESIONS)

3.26

ENDOMETRIAL BIOPSY/CURETTAGE: SECONDARY ENDOMETRIAL INVOLVEMENT BY ENDOCERVICAL WELL-DIFFERENTIATED ADENOCARCINOMA OF USUAL TYPE VS PRIMARY ENDOMETRIAL FIGO GRADE 1 ENDOMETRIOID CARCINOMA

	Endometrial Biopsy/Curettage: Secondary Endometrial Involvement by Endocervical Well-Differentiated Adenocarcinoma of Usual Type	Primary Endometrial FIGO Grade 1 Endometrioid Carcinoma
Age	Most cases in fifth to sixth decades; can be seen in third decade	Wide age range, from third decade into late postmenopause; mean age at diagnosis in mid seventh decade
Location	Endometrium and endocervix	Endometrium, secondary extension to endocervix can be seen
Symptoms	Abnormal vaginal bleeding; often asymptomatic	Vaginal bleeding, discharge
Signs	Abnormal Pap smear results, cervical mass, or incidental finding on endometrial biopsy for evaluation of bleeding or infertility	Constitutional symptoms, obesity, diabetes mellitus, polycystic ovarian syndrome, estrogen producing ovarian tumors
Etiology	High-risk HPV infection; most commonly implicated viral types HPV 16, HPV 18, HPV 45, and HPV 33	Unopposed estrogenic stimulation. Somatic mutations in *PTEN*, *PIK3CA*, *ARID1A*, and *KRAS* Lynch syndrome (germline mutations in mismatch repair genes) and Cowden syndrome (germline mutation in *PTEN*)
Histology	1. Neoplastic epithelium "colonizes" the surface of normal endometrium *(Figs. 3.26.1 and 3.26.2)*; or detached fragments of complex glandular proliferation *(Fig. 3.26.3)* 2. Mucinous differentiation is common *(Fig. 3.26.4)*; goblet cell differentiation can be present 3. No squamous differentiation (unless an adenosquamous carcinoma); metaplastic features are infrequent 4. Columnar cells with hyperchromatic elongated nuclei 5. Frequent apoptotic bodies and mitotic figures, typically in the apical portion of the cytoplasm, so-called floating mitosis *(Figs. 3.26.5 and 3.26.6)*	1. Surface-only involvement is not typical of endometrioid carcinoma; fragments of complex confluent glandular and papillary proliferation *(Fig. 3.26.8)*; complex atypical hyperplasia can be present in the background 2. Mucinous differentiation can be seen, but goblet cells are not typical 3. Squamous differentiation is common; metaplastic (tubal) features can be seen 4. Cuboidal to columnar cells with hyperchromatic or vesicular elongated to round nuclei *(Fig. 3.26.9)*; may have nucleoli 5. Apoptotic bodies can be occasionally seen, but not prominent; mitoses are generally infrequent
Special studies	• Strong and diffuse expression of p16 *(Fig. 3.26.7, **left**)* • Decreased or lost ER and PR expression *(Fig. 3.26.7, **right**)* • Positive *in situ* hybridization for high-risk HPV	• Patchy, focal expression of p16 *(Fig. 3.26.10, **left**)* • Retained expression of ER and PR *(Fig. 3.26.10, **right**)* • No detectable HPV by *in situ* hybridization

	Endometrial Biopsy/Curettage: Secondary Endometrial Involvement by Endocervical Well-Differentiated Adenocarcinoma of Usual Type	**Primary Endometrial FIGO Grade 1 Endometrioid Carcinoma**
Treatment	Staging with cervical excision and imaging studies; further treatment is stage dependent and includes modified radical hysterectomy with lymph node dissection or primary chemotherapy and radiation therapy in advanced-stage cases	Hysterectomy with or without lymphadenectomy depending on the depth of myometrial invasion. Conservative management with progestins is an option in patients desiring preservation of fertility after thorough clinical workup to ensure low stage
Prognosis	Hysterectomy can be curative in cases with superficially invasive carcinoma; prognosis is variable in advanced-stage tumors	Hysterectomy is generally curative in cases with <50% of myometrial invasion

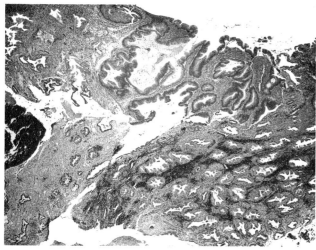

Figure 3.26.1   Endocervical adenocarcinoma with endometrial extension. Neoplastic epithelium colonizes endometrial surface and extends into endometrial glands **(top)**; background endometrium is secretory **(lower right)**.

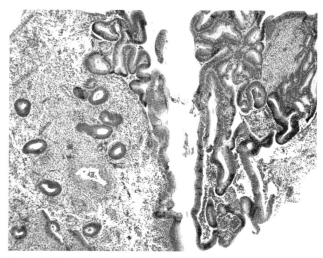

Figure 3.26.2   Endocervical adenocarcinoma with endometrial extension. Neoplastic epithelium colonizes endometrial surface **(center)**; the underlying endometrium is proliferative. Folded long strips of lesional epithelium **(right)** may mimic endometrial carcinoma.

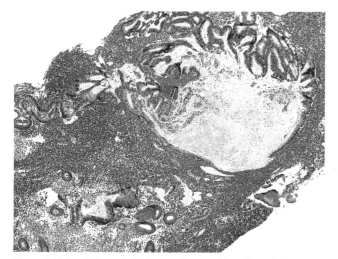

Figure 3.26.3   Endocervical adenocarcinoma with endometrial extension. Focus of complex glandular proliferation may be misinterpreted as primary endometrial process.

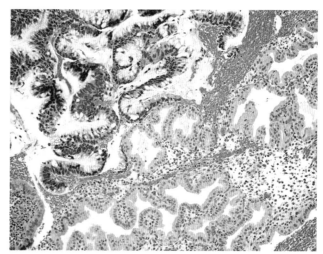

Figure 3.26.4   Endocervical adenocarcinoma with endometrial extension. Detached fragments of neoplastic epithelium with mucinous and goblet cell differentiation **(upper left)** in contrast with secretory endometrium **(lower right)**.

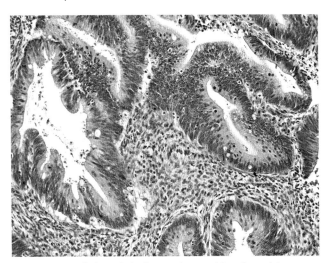

Figure 3.26.5   Endocervical adenocarcinoma with endometrial extension. Same case as in *Figure 3.26.1*, higher magnification. Hyperchromatic epithelium composed of tall columnar cells with apical mucinous cytoplasm. Frequent apoptotic bodies and apical mitoses.

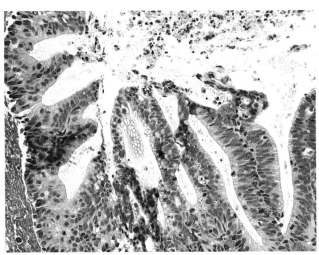

Figure 3.26.6   Endocervical adenocarcinoma with endometrial extension. Same case as in *Figure 3.26.3*, higher magnification. Epithelium with hybrid endometrioid and mucinous appearance. Frequent apoptotic bodies.

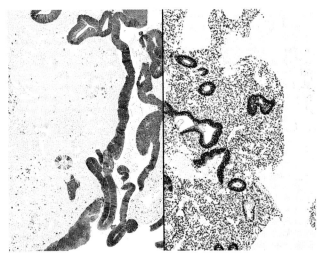

Figure 3.26.7   Endocervical adenocarcinoma with endometrial extension. Same case as in *Figure 3.26.2*. Diffuse expression of p16 **(left)** in the neoplastic epithelium that "colonizes" endometrial surface; proliferative endometrial glands below are essentially negative. **Right**: complete absence of PR expression in neoplastic endocervical epithelium and diffuse expression in endometrial glands.

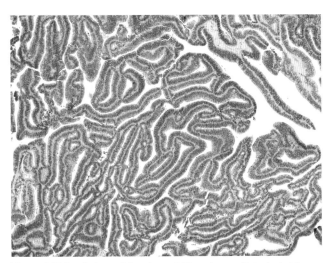

Figure 3.26.8   Endometrial endometrioid carcinoma. Detached strips of carcinoma in the curettage. Endocervical adenocarcinoma can be considered based on morphologic features: papillary/villoglandular architecture, tall hyperchromatic epithelium, or lack of endometrial hyperplasia or squamous differentiation.

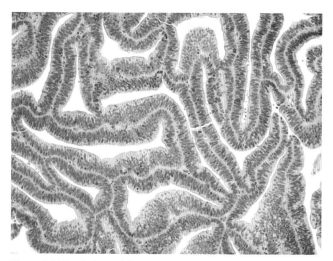

Figure 3.26.9 Endometrial endometrioid carcinoma. Detached strips of carcinoma in the curettage. Same case as in *Figure 3.26.8*, higher magnification. Note absence of mitotic figures and apoptotic bodies.

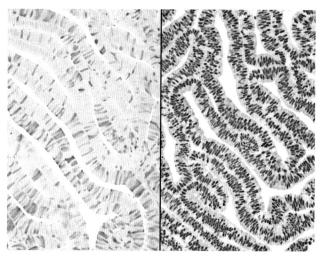

Figure 3.26.10 Endometrial endometrioid carcinoma. Patchy expression of p16 **(left)** and diffuse expression of PR **(right)**; ER showed similar diffuse expression (not shown).

	Endocervical Microglandular Hyperplasia (MGH) in Biopsy/Curettage Specimens	Microglandular Hyperplasia (MGH)-Like Endometrial Carcinoma in Biopsy/Curettage Specimens
Age	Reproductive-age women	Wide age range; mean age is 63 y
Location	Cervix, transformation zone, endocervix	Endometrium
Symptoms	Usually asymptomatic, vaginal bleeding in cases involving endocervical polyp	Abnormal vaginal bleeding; pelvic pain or pressure and abdominal distension in advanced cases
Signs	Endocervical polyp or small friable mass	Noncyclical vaginal bleeding, constitutional symptoms: obesity, diabetes, PCOS; thickened endometrial stripe or endometrial mass on MRI or sonography; abnormal Pap smear
Etiology	Associated with progestin exposure (pregnancy or exogenous)	Unopposed estrogenic stimulation; somatic mutations in *PTEN, PIK3CA, KRAS, CTNNB1, ARID1A*; hereditary syndromes, Lynch and Cowden syndromes
Histology	1. Closely packed glands, some in cribriform arrangement *(Figs. 3.27.1 and 3.27.2)* 2. Reserve cell layer or squamous metaplasia can undermine glandular epithelium *(Figs. 3.27.3 and 3.27.4)* 3. Cuboidal to low columnar cells; extensive vacuolation caused by cystic dilatation of intracellular spaces *(Fig. 3.27.5)*. Intracellular mucin is usually absent 4. Small, uniform round to ovoid nuclei; small nucleoli can be seen *(Figs. 3.27.4 and 3.27.5)* 5. Mitoses are rare; cases with increased mitotic activity have been described 6. Acute and chronic inflammatory infiltrate with frequent plasma cells in the stroma and epithelium is usually present *(Fig. 3.27.5)*; stromal hyalinization or edema can be seen	1. Confluent glands without intervening stroma; cribriform growth *(Figs. 3.27.6 and 3.27.7)* 2. Lack of reserve cell layer *(Figs. 3.27.8 and 3.27.9)*. Squamous metaplasia may be seen, often in the middle of the epithelial nests rather than undermining glandular epithelium 3. Cytoplasmic vacuolation may be seen in cases with secretory differentiation *(Figs. 3.27.9 and 3.27.10)*. Intracellular mucin can be seen in cases with mucinous differentiation 4. Cytologic atypia, often mild *(Figs. 3.27.9 and 3.27.10)* 5. Mitotic figures can be seen, but not a constant feature 6. Acute and chronic inflammation can be present, but not a constant feature *(Fig. 3.27.8)*
Special studies	• Not particularly helpful in this differential diagnosis • P40/p63 immunohistochemical stain may be considered to highlight reserve cell layer undermining columnar epithelium *(Fig. 3.27.1, **inset**)*	• Not particularly helpful in this differential diagnosis • P40/p63 immunohistochemical stain may label scattered tumor cell but not in the linear fashion surrounding epithelial nests

	Endocervical Microglandular Hyperplasia (MGH) in Biopsy/Curettage Specimens	Microglandular Hyperplasia (MGH)-Like Endometrial Carcinoma in Biopsy/Curettage Specimens
Treatment	Usually not required; for symptomatic cases, biopsy/polypectomy is generally curative	Hysterectomy with bilateral salpingo-oophorectomy, +/− pelvic and periaortic lymphadenectomy. Progestin therapy can be considered for fertility preservation (tumors limited to endometrium on MRI or transvaginal ultrasound and in the absence of suspicious/metastatic disease on imaging)
Prognosis	Benign	Stage dependent; 5-y survival for stage IA tumors is 95%

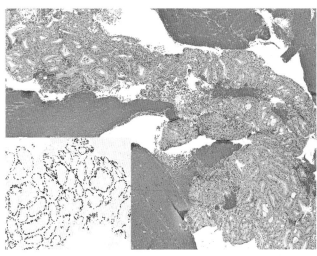

Figure 3.27.1   Microglandular hyperplasia. Fragments of complex glandular proliferation with focal cribriform growth. P40 immunostain highlights reserve cell layer **(inset)**.

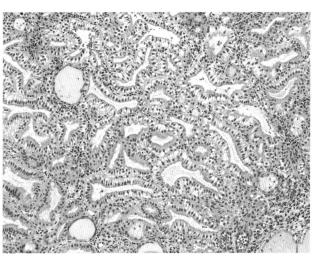

Figure 3.27.2   Microglandular hyperplasia. Back-to-back glands with prominent vacuolation.

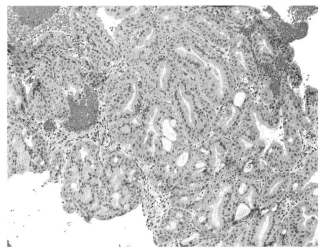

Figure 3.27.3   Microglandular hyperplasia. Same case as in *Figure 3.27.1*. Fragments of cribriform glandular proliferation with notable reserve cell layer typical of cervical transformation zone tissue.

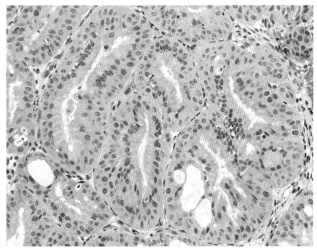

Figure 3.27.4   Microglandular hyperplasia. Same case as in *Figure 3.27.1*. Columnar cell with bland nuclei with occasional nucleoli forming gland lumina; outer reserve cell layer.

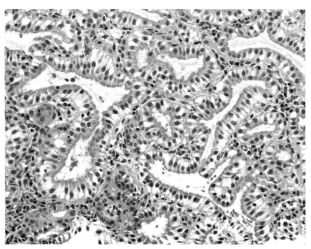

Figure 3.27.5   Microglandular hyperplasia. Same case as in *Figure 3.27.2*. Columnar cell with notable intercellular vacuoles. Note stromal inflammation with plasma cells.

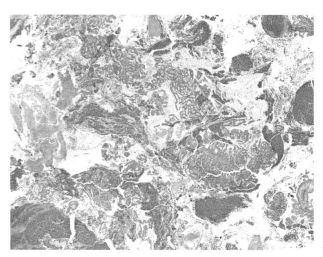

Figure 3.27.6   Endometrial endometrioid carcinoma. Fragmented complex glandular proliferation in the curettage specimen.

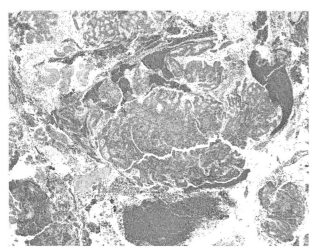

Figure 3.27.7   Endometrial endometrioid carcinoma. Same case as in *Figure 3.27.6*. Fragments of glandular proliferation with papillary architecture and focal cribriform growth.

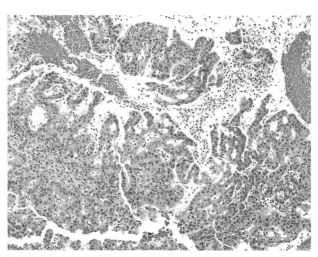

Figure 3.27.8   Endometrial endometrioid carcinoma. Same case as in *Figure 3.27.6*. Complex glandular proliferation with bland cytologic features. Acute inflammation in the lesional epithelium.

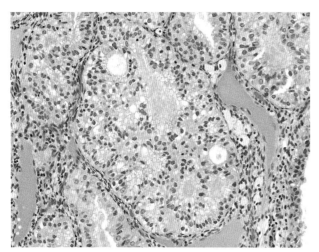

Figure 3.27.9   Endometrial endometrioid carcinoma with secretory differentiation. Cribriform growth and prominent cytoplasmic vacuolation. Note absence of reserve cell layer/squamous differentiation.

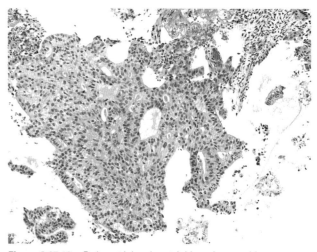

Figure 3.27.10   Endometrial endometrioid carcinoma with secretory differentiation. Detached fragment of confluent glandular proliferation with some secretory changes.

SUGGESTED READINGS

3.1 and 3.2

Huang EC, Mutter GL, Crum CP, et al. Clinical outcome in diagnostically ambiguous foci of 'gland crowding' in the endometrium. *Mod Pathol.* 2010;23:1486-1491.

Lastra RR, McCluggage WG, Ellenson LH. Benign diseases of the endometrium. In: Kurman RJ, Ellenson LH, Ronnett BM, eds. *Blaustein's Pathology of the Female Genital Tract.* 7th ed Springer; 2019:383-394.

3.3

Ellenson LH, Ronnett BM, Kurman RJ. Precursor lesions of endometrial carcinoma. In: Kurman RJ, Ellenson LH, Ronnett BM, eds. *Blaustein's Pathology of the Female Genital Tract.* 7th ed.. Springer; 2019:439-472.

3.4

Gurda GT, Baras AS, Kurman RJ. Ki-67 index as an ancillary tool in the differential diagnosis of proliferative endometrial lesions with secretory change. *Int J Gynecol Pathol.* 2014;33:114-119.

Lastra RR, McCluggage WG, Ellenson LH. Benign diseases of the Endometrium. In: Kurman RJ, Ellenson LH, Ronnett BM, eds. *Blaustein's Pathology of the Female Genital Tract.* 7th ed. Springer; 2019:380-383, 498-500.

Tobon H, Watkins GJ. Secretory adenocarcinoma of the endometrium. *Int J Gynecol Pathol.* 1985;4:328-335.

Truskinovsky AM, Lifschitz-Mercer B, Czernobilsky B. Hyperplasia and carcinoma in secretory endometrium: a diagnostic challenge. *Int J Gynecol Pathol.* 2014;33:107-113.

3.5

Gunderson CC, Dutta S, Fader AN, et al. Pathologic features associated with resolution of complex atypical hyperplasia and grade 1 endometrial adenocarcinoma after progestin therapy. *Gynecol Oncol.* 2014;132:33-37.

Lastra RR, McCluggage WG, Ellenson LH. Benign diseases of the endometrium. In: Kurman RJ, Ellenson LH, Ronnett BM, eds. *Blaustein's Pathology of the Female Genital Tract.* 7th ed. Springer; 2019:380-383, 458.

Wheeler DT, Bristow RE, Kurman RJ. Histologic alterations in endometrial hyperplasia and well-differentiated carcinoma treated with progestins. *Am J Surg Pathol.* 2007;31:988-998.

3.6

Kendall BS, Ronnett BM, Isacson C, et al. Reproducibility of the diagnosis of endometrial hyperplasia, atypical hyperplasia, and well-differentiated carcinoma. *Am J Surg Pathol.* 1998;22:1012-1019.

Kurman RJ, Norris HJ. Evaluation of criteria for distinguishing atypical endometrial hyperplasia from well-differentiated carcinoma. *Cancer.* 1982;49:2547-2559.

Longacre TA, Chung MH, Jensen DN, et al. Proposed criteria for the diagnosis of well-differentiated endometrial carcinoma. A diagnostic test for myoinvasion. *Am J Surg Pathol.* 1995;19:371-406.

Mazur MT. Endometrial hyperplasia/adenocarcinoma. A conventional approach. *Ann Diagn Pathol.* 2005;9:174-181.

McKenney JK, Longacre TA. Low-grade endometrial adenocarcinoma: a diagnostic algorithm for distinguishing atypical endometrial hyperplasia and other benign (and malignant) mimics. *Adv Anat Pathol.* 2009;16:1-22.

3.7

Clement PB, Young RH. Endometrioid carcinoma of the uterine corpus: a review of its pathology with emphasis on recent advances and problematic aspects. *Adv Anat Pathol.* 2002;9:145-184.

Hendrickson MR, Kempson RL. Endometrial epithelial metaplasias: proliferations frequently misdiagnosed as adenocarcinoma. Report of 89 cases and proposed classification. *Am J Surg Pathol.* 1980;4:525-542.

Jacques SM, Qureshi F, Lawrence WD. Surface epithelial changes in endometrial adenocarcinoma: diagnostic pitfalls in curettage specimens. *Int J Gynecol Pathol.* 1995;14:191-197.

Lehman MB, Hart WR. Simple and complex hyperplastic papillary proliferations of the endometrium: a clinicopathologic study of nine cases of apparently localized papillary lesions with fibrovascular stromal cores and epithelial metaplasia. *Am J Surg Pathol.* 2001;25:1347-1354.

McCluggage WG, McBride HA. Papillary syncytial metaplasia associated with endometrial breakdown exhibits an immunophenotype that overlaps with uterine serous carcinoma. *Int J Gynecol Pathol.* 2012;31:206-210.

Nicolae A, Preda O, Nogales FF. Endometrial metaplasias and reactive changes: a spectrum of altered differentiation. *J Clin Pathol.* 2011;64:97-106.

Shah SS, Mazur MT. Endometrial eosinophilic syncytial change related to breakdown: immunohistochemical evidence suggests a regressive process. *Int J Gynecol Pathol.* 2008;27:534-538.

Zaman SS, Mazur MT. Endometrial papillary syncytial change. A nonspecific alteration associated with active breakdown. *Am J Clin Pathol.* 1993;99:741-745.

3.8

Blanco LZ Jr, Heagley DE, Lee JC, et al. Immunohistochemical characterization of squamous differentiation and morular metaplasia in uterine endometrioid adenocarcinoma. *Int J Gynecol Pathol.* 2013;32:283-292.

Zaino RJ, Kurman RJ. Squamous differentiation in carcinoma of the endometrium: a critical appraisal of adenoacanthoma and adenosquamous carcinoma. *Semin Diagn Pathol.* 1988;5:154-171.

3 UTERINE CORPUS (EPITHELIAL LESIONS)

Zaino RJ, Kurman R, Herbold D, et al. The significance of squamous differentiation in endometrial carcinoma. Data from a gynecologic oncology group study. *Cancer.* 1991;68:2293-2302.

3.9-3.11

Bartosch C, Manuel Lopes J, Oliva E. Endometrial carcinomas: a review emphasizing overlapping and distinctive morphological and immunohistochemical features. *Adv Anat Pathol.* 2011;18:415-437.

Clement PB, Young RH. Non-endometrioid carcinomas of the uterine corpus: a review of their pathology with emphasis on recent advances and problematic aspects. *Adv Anat Pathol.* 2004;11:117-142.

Cosgrove CM, Tritchler DL, Cohn DE, et al. An NRG Oncology/GOG study of molecular classification for risk prediction in endometrioid endometrial cancer. *Gynecol Oncol.* 2018;148(1):174-180.

Fadare O, Brooks AS, Martel M. A 54-year-old woman with menorrhagia. Mixed mucinous and endometrioid carcinoma with small nonvillous papillae. *Arch Pathol Lab Med.* 2006;130:400-402.

Gatius S, Matias-Guiu X. Practical issues in the diagnosis of serous carcinoma of the endometrium. *Mod Pathol.* 2016;29(suppl 1): S45-S58.

León-Castillo A, de Boer SM, Powell ME, et al.; TransPORTEC consortium. Molecular classification of the PORTEC-3 trial for high-risk endometrial cancer: impact on prognosis and benefit from adjuvant therapy. *J Clin Oncol.* 2020;38(29):3388-3397.

Murray SK, Young RH, Scully RE. Uterine endometrioid carcinoma with small nonvillous papillae: an analysis of 26 cases of a favorable-prognosis tumor to be distinguished from serous carcinoma. *Int J Surg Pathol.* 2000;8:279-289.

Talhouk A, McConechy M, Leung S. et al. A clinically applicable molecular-based classification for endometrial cancers. *Br J Cancer.* 2015;113:299-310.

Yemelyanova A, Ji H, Shih Ie M, et al. Utility of p16 expression for distinction of uterine serous carcinomas from endometrial endometrioid and endocervical adenocarcinomas: immunohistochemical analysis of 201 cases. *Am J Surg Pathol.* 2009;33:1504-1514.

Zaino RJ, Kurman RJ, Brunetto VL, et al. Villoglandular adenocarcinoma of the endometrium: a clinicopathologic study of 61 cases. A gynecologic oncology group study. *Am J Surg Pathol.* 1998;22:1379-1385.

3.12

Ambros RA, Sherman ME, Zahn CM, et al. Endometrial intraepithelial carcinoma: a distinctive lesion specifically associated with tumors displaying serous differentiation. *Hum Pathol.* 1995;26:1260-1267.

Baergen RN, Warren CD, Isacson C, et al. Early uterine serous carcinoma: clonal origin of extrauterine disease. *Int J Gynecol Pathol.* 2001;20:214-219.

Sherman ME, Bur ME, Kurman RJ. P53 in endometrial cancer and its putative precursors: evidence for diverse pathways of tumorigenesis. *Hum Pathol.* 1995;26:1268-1274.

Simon RA, Peng SL, Liu F, et al. Tubal metaplasia of the endometrium with cytologic atypia: analysis of p53, Ki-67, TERT, and long-term follow-up. *Mod Pathol.* 2011;24:1254-1261.

Soslow RA, Pirog E, Isacson C. Endometrial intraepithelial carcinoma with associated peritoneal carcinomatosis. *Am J Surg Pathol.* 2000;24:726-732.

Wheeler DT, Bell KA, Kurman RJ, et al. Minimal uterine serous carcinoma: diagnosis and clinicopathologic correlation. *Am J Surg Pathol.* 2000;24:797-806.

3.13

Albores-Saavedra J, Martinez-Benitez B, Luevano E. Small cell carcinomas and large cell neuroendocrine carcinomas of the endometrium and cervix: polypoid tumors and those arising in polyps may have a favorable prognosis. *Int J Gynecol Pathol.* 2008;27:333-339.

Bartosch C, Manuel Lopes J, Oliva E. Endometrial carcinomas: a review emphasizing overlapping and distinctive morphological and immunohistochemical features. *Adv Anat Pathol.* 2011;18:415-437.

Bosse T, Nout RA, McAlpine JN, et al. Molecular classification of grade 3 endometrioid endometrial cancers identifies distinct prognostic subgroups. *Am J Surg Pathol.* 2018;42(5):561-568.

Eichhorn JH, Young RH. Neuroendocrine tumors of the genital tract. *Am J Clin Pathol.* 2001;115(suppl):S94-S112.

Gardner GJ, Reidy-Lagunes D, Gehrig PA. Neuroendocrine tumors of the gynecologic tract: a society of gynecologic oncology (SGO) clinical document. *Gynecol Oncol.* 2011;122:190-198.

Howitt BE, Dong F, Vivero M, et al. Molecular characterization of neuroendocrine carcinomas of the endometrium: representation in all 4 TCGA groups. *Am J Surg Pathol.* 2020;44(11):1541-1548.

Huntsman DG, Clement PB, Gilks CB, et al. Small-cell carcinoma of the endometrium. A clinicopathological study of sixteen cases. *Am J Surg Pathol.* 1994;18:364-375.

Joehlin-Price A, Van Ziffle J, Hills NK, et al. Molecularly classified uterine FIGO Grade 3 endometrioid carcinomas show distinctive clinical outcomes but overlapping morphologic features. *Am J Surg Pathol.* 2021;45(3):421-429.

Kuji S, Watanabe R, Sato Y, et al. A new marker, insulinoma-associated protein 1 (INSM1), for high-grade neuroendocrine carcinoma of the uterine cervix: analysis of 37 cases. *Gynecol Oncol.* 2017;144(2):384-390.

Mulvany NJ, Allen DG. Combined large cell neuroendocrine and endometrioid carcinoma of the endometrium. *Int J Gynecol Pathol.* 2008;27:49-57.

Pocrnich CE, Ramalingam P, Euscher ED, et al. Neuroendocrine carcinoma of the endometrium: a clinicopathologic study of 25 cases. *Am J Surg Pathol.* 2016;40:577-586.

Posligua L, Malpica A, Liu J, et al. Combined large cell neuroendocrine carcinoma and papillary serous carcinoma of the endometrium with pagetoid spread. *Arch Pathol Lab Med.* 2008;132:1821-1824.

Rouzbahman M, Clarke B. Neuroendocrine tumors of the gynecologic tract: select topics. *Semin Diagn Pathol.* 2013;30: 224-233.

3.14 and 3.15

An HJ, Logani S, Isacson C, et al. Molecular characterization of uterine clear cell carcinoma. *Mod Pathol.* 2004;17:530-537.

Arias-Stella J. The Arias-Stella reaction: facts and fancies four decades after. *Adv Anat Pathol.* 2002;9:12-23.

Arias-Stella J Jr, Arias-Velasquez A, Arias-Stella J. Normal and abnormal mitoses in the atypical endometrial change associated with chorionic tissue effect [corrected]. *Am J Surg Pathol.* 1994;18:694-701.

Bartosch C, Manuel Lopes J, Oliva E. Endometrial carcinomas: a review emphasizing overlapping and distinctive morphological and immunohistochemical features. *Adv Anat Pathol.* 2011;18:415-437.

Clement PB, Young RH. Non-endometrioid carcinomas of the uterine corpus: a review of their pathology with emphasis on recent advances and problematic aspects. *Adv Anat Pathol.* 2004;11:117-142.

Fadare O, Desouki MM, Gwin K, et al. Frequent expression of napsin a in clear cell carcinoma of the endometrium: potential diagnostic utility. *Am J Surg Pathol.* 2014;38:189-196.

Fadare O, Parkash V, Dupont WD, et al. The diagnosis of endometrial carcinomas with clear cells by gynecologic pathologists: an assessment of interobserver variability and associated morphologic features. *Am J Surg Pathol.* 2012;36:1107-1118.

Fadare O, Zheng W, Crispens MA, et al. Morphologic and other clinicopathologic features of endometrial clear cell carcinoma: a comprehensive analysis of 50 rigorously classified cases. *Am J Cancer Res.* 2013;3:70-95.

Huettner PC, Gersell DJ. Arias-Stella reaction in nonpregnant women: a clinicopathologic study of nine cases. *Int J Gynecol Pathol.* 1994;13:241-247.

Silva EG, Young RH. Endometrioid neoplasms with clear cells: a report of 21 cases in which the alteration is not of typical secretory type. *Am J Surg Pathol.* 2007;31:1203-1208.

Vang R, Barner R, Wheeler DT, et al. Immunohistochemical staining for Ki-67 and p53 helps distinguish Arias-Stella reaction from high-grade endometrial carcinoma, including clear cell carcinoma. *Int J Gynecol Pathol.* 2004;23:223-233.

3.16

Buza N, Tavassoli FA. Comparative analysis of P16 and P53 expression in uterine malignant mixed mullerian tumors. *Int J Gynecol Pathol.* 2009;28:514-521.

Ladwig NR, Umetsu SE, Zaloudek C, Rabban J, Garg K. Corded and Hyalinized Endometrioid Adenocarcinoma (CHEC) of the uterine corpus are characterized by CTNNB1 mutations and can show adverse clinical outcomes. *Int J Gynecol Pathol.* 2021;40(2):103-115.

Murray SK, Clement PB, Young RH. Endometrioid carcinomas of the uterine corpus with sex cord-like formations, hyalinization, and other unusual morphologic features: a report of 31 cases of a neoplasm that may be confused with carcinosarcoma and other uterine neoplasms. *Am J Surg Pathol.* 2005;29:157-166.

Safdar NS, Thompson EF, Gilks CB, et al. Corded and hyalinized and spindled endometrioid endometrial carcinoma: a clinicopathologic and molecular analysis of 9 tumors based on the TCGA classifier. *Am J Surg Pathol.* 2021;45(8):1038-1046.

3.17 and 3.18

Buza N, Tavassoli FA. Comparative analysis of P16 and P53 expression in uterine malignant mixed mullerian tumors. *Int J Gynecol Pathol.* 2009;28:514-521.

Holmes BJ, Gown AM, Vang R, et al. PAX8 expression in uterine malignant mesodermal mixed tumor (carcinosarcoma). *Int J Gynecol Pathol.* 2014;33:425-431.

Köbel M, Hoang LN, Tessier-Cloutier B, et al. Undifferentiated endometrial carcinomas show frequent loss of core switch/sucrose nonfermentable complex proteins. *Am J Surg Pathol.* 2018;42(1):76-83.

Kihara A, Amano Y, Matsubara D, et al. BRG1, INI1, and ARID1B deficiency in endometrial carcinoma: a clinicopathologic and immunohistochemical analysis of a large series from a single institution. *Am J Surg Pathol.* 2020;44(12):1712-1724.

Murali R, Davidson B, Fadare O, et al. High-grade endometrial carcinomas: morphologic and immunohistochemical features, diagnostic challenges and recommendations. *Int J Gynecol Pathol.* 2019;38:S40-S63.

Silva EG, Deavers MT, Bodurka DC, et al. Association of low-grade endometrioid carcinoma of the uterus and ovary with undifferentiated carcinoma: a new type of dedifferentiated carcinoma? *Int J Gynecol Pathol.* 2006;25:52-58.

Tafe LJ, Garg K, Chew I, et al. Endometrial and ovarian carcinomas with undifferentiated components: clinically aggressive and frequently underrecognized neoplasms. *Mod Pathol.* 2010;23:781-789.

Yemelyanova A, Gown AM, Wu LS, et al. PAX8 expression in uterine adenocarcinomas and mesonephric proliferations. *Int J Gynecol Pathol.* 2014;33:492-499.

3.19

Clement PB, Young RH, Keh P, et al. Malignant mesonephric neoplasms of the uterine cervix. A report of eight cases, including four with a malignant spindle cell component. *Am J Surg Pathol.* 1995;19:1158-1171.

Euscher ED, Bassett R, Duose DY, et al. Mesonephric-like carcinoma of the endometrium: a subset of endometrial carcinoma with an aggressive behavior. *Am J Surg Pathol.* 2020;44(4):429-443.

Howitt BE, Emori MM, Drapkin R, et al. GATA3 is a sensitive and specific marker of benign and malignant mesonephric lesions in the lower female genital tract. *Am J Surg Pathol.* 2015;39(10):1411-1419.

Kolin DL, Costigan DC, Dong F, et al. A combined morphologic and molecular approach to retrospectively identify KRAS-mutated mesonephric-like adenocarcinomas of the endometrium. *Am J Surg Pathol.* 2019;43(3):389-398.

Mirkovic J, McFarland M, Garcia E, et al. Targeted genomic profiling reveals recurrent KRAS mutations in mesonephric-like adenocarcinomas of the female genital tract. *Am J Surg Pathol.* 2018;42(2):227-233.

Ordi J, Nogales FF, Palacin A, et al. Mesonephric adenocarcinoma of the uterine corpus: CD10 expression as evidence of mesonephric differentiation. *Am J Surg Pathol.* 2001;25:1540-1545.

Pors J, Cheng A, Leo JM, et al. Comparison of GATA3, TTF1, CD10, and calretinin in identifying mesonephric and mesonephric-like carcinomas of the gynecologic tract. *Am J Surg Pathol.* 2018;42(12):1596-1606.

Pors J, Segura S, Chiu DS, et al. Clinicopathologic characteristics of mesonephric adenocarcinomas and mesonephric-like adenocarcinomas in the gynecologic tract: a multi-institutional study. *Am J Surg Pathol.* 2021;45(4):498-506.

Silver SA, Devouassoux-Shisheboran M, Mezzetti TP, et al. Mesonephric adenocarcinomas of the uterine cervix: a study of 11 cases with immunohistochemical findings. *Am J Surg Pathol.* 2001,25.379-387.

Wani Y, Notohara K, Tsukayama C. Mesonephric adenocarcinoma of the uterine corpus: a case report and review of the literature. *Int J Gynecol Pathol.* 2008;27:346-352.

3.20 and 3.21

Ali A, Black D, Soslow RA. Difficulties in assessing the depth of myometrial invasion in endometrial carcinoma. *Int J Gynecol Pathol.* 2007;26:115-123.

Hanley KZ, Dustin SM, Stoler MH, et al. The significance of tumor involved adenomyosis in otherwise low-stage endometrioid adenocarcinoma. *Int J Gynecol Pathol.* 2010;29:445-451.

Jacques SM, Lawrence WD. Endometrial adenocarcinoma with variable-level myometrial involvement limited to adenomyosis: a clinicopathologic study of 23 cases. *Gynecol Oncol.* 1990;37:401-407.

Joehlin-Price AS, McHugh KE, Stephens JA, et al. The Microcystic, Elongated, and Fragmented (MELF) pattern of invasion: a single institution report of 464 consecutive FIGO grade 1 endometrial endometrioid adenocarcinomas. *Am J Surg Pathol.* 2017;41(1):49-55.

Kihara A, Yoshida H, Watanabe R, et al. Clinicopathologic association and prognostic value of Microcystic, Elongated, and Fragmented (MELF) pattern in endometrial endometrioid carcinoma. *Am J Surg Pathol.* 2017;41(7):896-905.

Murray SK, Young RH, Scully RE. Unusual epithelial and stromal changes in myoinvasive endometrioid adenocarcinoma: a study of their frequency, associated diagnostic problems, and prognostic significance. *Int J Gynecol Pathol.* 2003;22:324-333.

Quick CM, May T, Horowitz NS, et al. Low-grade, low-stage endometrioid endometrial adenocarcinoma: a clinicopathologic analysis of 324 cases focusing on frequency and pattern of myoinvasion. *Int J Gynecol Pathol.* 2012;31:337-343.

3.22

Bosse T, Peters EE, Creutzberg CL et al. Substantial lymph-vascular space invasion (LVSI) is a significant risk factor for recurrence in endometrial cancer—a pooled analysis of PORTEC 1 and 2 trials. *Eur J Cancer.* 2015;51(13):1742-1750.

Folkins AK, Nevadunsky NS, Saleemuddin A, et al. Evaluation of vascular space involvement in endometrial adenocarcinomas: laparoscopic vs abdominal hysterectomies. *Mod Pathol.* 2010;23:1073-1079.

Kitahara S, Walsh C, Frumovitz M, et al. Vascular pseudoinvasion in laparoscopic hysterectomy specimens for endometrial carcinoma: a grossing artifact? *Am J Surg Pathol.* 2009;33:298 303.

Krizova A, Clarke BA, Bernardini MQ, et al. Histologic artifacts in abdominal, vaginal, laparoscopic, and robotic hysterectomy specimens: a blinded, retrospective review. *Am J Surg Pathol.* 2011;35:115-126.

Logani S, Herdman AV, Little JV, et al. Vascular "pseudo invasion" in laparoscopic hysterectomy specimens: a diagnostic pitfall. *Am J Surg Pathol.* 2008;32:560-565.

McKenney JK, Kong CS, Longacre TA. Endometrial adenocarcinoma associated with subtle lymph-vascular space invasion and lymph node metastasis: a histologic pattern mimicking intravascular and sinusoidal histiocytes. *Int J Gynecol Pathol.* 2005;24:73-78.

Peters EEM, Bartosch C, McCluggage WG, et al. Reproducibility of lymphovascular space invasion (LVSI) assessment in endometrial cancer. *Histopathology.* 2019;75(1):128-136.

Peters, EEM, León-Castillo A, Smit VTHBM, et al. Defining substantial lymphovascular space invasion in endometrial cancer. *Int J Gynecol Pathol.* 2022;41(3):220-226.

3.23

Bagby C, Ronnett BM, Yemelyanova A, et al. Clinically occult tubal and ovarian high-grade serous carcinomas presenting in uterine samples: diagnostic pitfalls and clues to improve recognition of tumor origin. *Int J Gynecol Pathol.* 2013;32:433-443.

3.24

Kumar NB, Hart WR. Metastases to the uterine corpus from extragenital cancers. A clinicopathologic study of 63 cases. *Cancer.* 1982;50:2163-2169.

Mazur MI, Hsueh S, Gersell DJ. Metastases to the female genital tract. Analysis of 325 cases. *Cancer.* 1984;53:1978-1984.

3.25

Noguchi H, Shiozawa I, Kitahara T, et al. Uterine body invasion of carcinoma of the uterine cervix as seen from surgical specimens. *Gynecol Oncol.* 1988;30:173-182.

Reyes C, Murali R, Park KJ. Secondary involvement of the adnexa and uterine corpus by carcinomas of the uterine cervix: a detailed morphologic description. *Int J Gynecol Pathol.* 2015;34:551-563.

3.26

Ansari-Lari MA, Staebler A, Zaino RJ, et al. Distinction of endocervical and endometrial adenocarcinomas: immunohistochemical p16 expression correlated with human papillomavirus (hpv) DNA detection. *Am J Surg Pathol.* 2004;28:160-167.

Reyes C, Murali R, Park KJ. Secondary involvement of the adnexa and uterine corpus by carcinomas of the uterine cervix: a detailed morphologic description. *Int J Gynecol Pathol.* 2015;34:551-563.

Staebler A, Sherman ME, Zaino RJ, et al. Hormone receptor immunohistochemistry and human papillomavirus in situ hybridization are useful for distinguishing endocervical and endometrial adenocarcinomas. *Am J Surg Pathol.* 2002;26:998-1006.

Yemelyanova A, Vang R, Seidman JD, et al. Endocervical adenocarcinomas with prominent endometrial or endomyometrial involvement simulating primary endometrial carcinomas: utility of HPV DNA detection and immunohistochemical expression of p16 and hormone receptors to confirm the cervical origin of the corpus tumor. *Am J Surg Pathol.* 2009;33:914-924.

Yemelyanova A, Ji H, Shih Ie M, et al. Utility of p16 expression for distinction of uterine serous carcinomas from endometrial endometrioid and endocervical adenocarcinomas: immunohistochemical analysis of 201 cases. *Am J Surg Pathol.* 2009;33:1504-1514.

3.27

Abi-Raad R, Alomari A, Hui P, et al. Mitotically active microglandular hyperplasia of the cervix: a case series with implications for the differential diagnosis. *Int J Gynecol Pathol.* 2014;33:524-530.

Chekmareva M, Ellenson LH, Pirog EC. Immunohistochemical differences between mucinous and microglandular adenocarcinomas of the endometrium and benign endocervical epithelium. *Int J Gynecol Pathol.* 2008;27(4):547-554.

Houghton O, McCluggage WG. The expression and diagnostic utility of p63 in the female genital tract. *Adv Anat Pathol.* 2009;16(5):316-321.

Nucci MR. Pseudoneoplastic glandular lesions of the uterine cervix: a selective review. *Int J Gynecol Pathol.* 2014;33:330-338.

Wright TC, Ronnett BM. Benign diseases of the cervix. In: Kurman RJ, Ellenson LH, Ronnett BM, eds. *Blaustein's Pathology of the Female Genital Tract.* 7th ed. Springer; 2019:219-222.

3 UTERINE CORPUS (EPITHELIAL LESIONS)

4

Uterine Corpus (Pure Mesenchymal and Mixed Epithelial-Mesenchymal Lesions)

	Atypical Leiomyoma	Leiomyosarcoma
Age	43–45 y (mean)	Usually, >50 y
Location	Uterus	Uterus
Symptoms	Asymptomatic, menorrhagia, or pelvic pain/pressure	Abnormal vaginal bleeding and/or pelvic pain; clinical features can overlap with those of leiomyoma
Signs	May have enlarged uterus on clinical examination; gross mass within the myometrium	Pelvic mass; gross mass within the myometrium; clinical features can overlap with those of leiomyoma
Etiology	Pathogenesis unclear; *MED12* mutations in majority; *HMGA2* or *HMGA1* fusions in a subset; another subset of cases can have somatic or germline fumarate hydratase mutations (the latter are associated with the hereditary leiomyomatosis and renal cell carcinoma syndrome)	Pathogenesis unclear but probably arises *de novo* rather than from malignant transformation of leiomyoma although cases of the latter have been described; various chromosomal aberrations; subsets contain mutations of *TP53, ATRX,* and *MED12* (the frequency of *MED12* mutations is much lower than in leiomyomas)
Histology	1. Spindle cell neoplasm with fascicular architecture 2. The 2020 WHO Classification recommends the term leiomyoma with bizarre nuclei (symplastic leiomyoma); significant (moderate or severe) atypia evident at low- or intermediate-power magnification *(Fig. 4.1.1)*; may include symplastic/bizarre nuclei (enlarged with smudgy chromatin, +/− intranuclear inclusions) *(Figs. 4.1.2 and 4.1.3)*; fumarate hydratase-deficient leiomyomas show prominent nucleoli with perinucleolar halos, alveolar-type edema, staghorn vessels, and cytoplasmic eosinophilic inclusions 3. Variable mitotic index (<10 mitotic figures/10 high-power fields) 4. May have infarct-type/hyaline necrosis (intervening band of hyalinization or granulation tissue between necrosis and viable tumor; acute infarct may be indistinguishable from coagulative tumor cell necrosis, but the latter designation is generally reserved for leiomyosarcoma) *(Fig. 4.1.4)* 5. Criteria for atypical leiomyoma: lacks two of three criteria necessary for diagnosis of leiomyosarcoma	1. Spindle cell neoplasm with fascicular architecture 2. Significant (moderate or severe) atypia evident at low- or intermediate-power magnification; usually lacks symplastic/bizarre nuclei (enlarged with smudgy chromatin, +/− intranuclear inclusions) although occasionally can be present; some cases may have deceptively homogeneous (rather than pleomorphic) pattern of moderate atypia at low- or intermediate-power magnification (evaluation at high-power magnification can be helpful in such cases) *(Figs. 4.1.5 and 4.1.6)* 3. Elevated mitotic index (usually, ≥10 mitotic figures/10 high-power fields) *(Figs. 4.1.5 and 4.1.6)* 4. May have coagulative tumor cell necrosis (sharp interface between necrosis and viable tumor); infarct-type/hyaline necrosis can also be present, but the latter is not used as a diagnostic criterion for leiomyosarcoma *(Figs. 4.1.7-4.1.9)* 5. Criteria for leiomyosarcoma: ≥2 of 3 criteria present (significant atypia, mitotic index ≥10 mitotic figures/10 high-power fields, coagulative tumor cell necrosis)
Special studies	Immunohistochemistry of no help (exact role of p53, p16, and Ki-67 for this differential diagnosis unclear)	Immunohistochemistry of no help (exact role of p53, p16, and Ki-67 for this differential diagnosis unclear)

	Atypical Leiomyoma	**Leiomyosarcoma**
Treatment	Myomectomy or hysterectomy	Hysterectomy, +/− bilateral salpingo-oophorectomy; further management is stage dependent but can include observation or chemotherapy and/or radiation therapy
Prognosis	Risk of recurrence low (≤2%)	Stage dependent; 5-y survival: 15%-25%; tumors are not graded as they are conventionally considered high grade

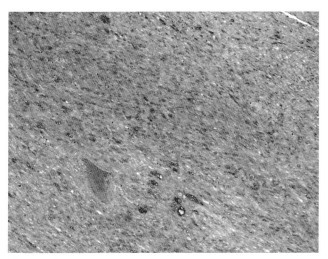

Figure 4.1.1 Atypical leiomyoma with significant nuclear atypia evident at intermediate-power magnification.

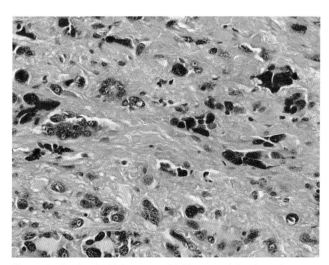

Figure 4.1.2 Atypical leiomyoma with bizarre nuclei and smudgy chromatin.

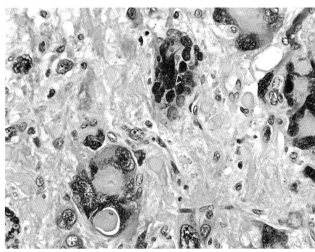

Figure 4.1.3 Atypical leiomyoma with bizarre nuclei and intranuclear inclusions.

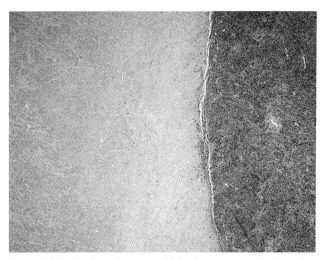

Figure 4.1.4 Atypical leiomyoma with hyaline-type necrosis. Necrotic tumor is at the **left** with viable tumor at the **right**. In the **middle**, a vertical intervening band of granulation tissue/hyalinization is present.

4 UTERINE CORPUS

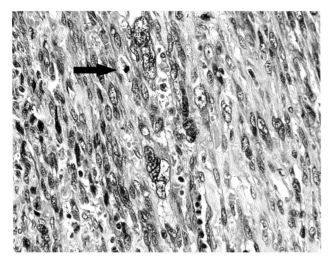

Figure 4.1.5   Leiomyosarcoma with significant nuclear atypia and mitotic activity (*arrow*).

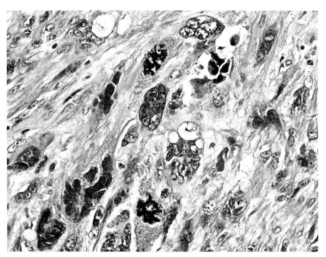

Figure 4.1.6   Leiomyosarcoma with significant nuclear atypia and atypical mitotic figures. The morphologic features of the atypical nuclei in this case overlap with those of bizarre/symplastic leiomyomas.

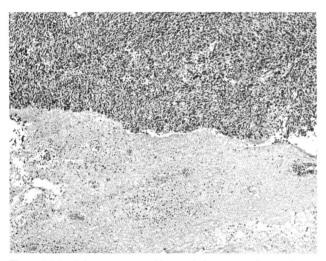

Figure 4.1.7   Leiomyosarcoma with coagulative tumor cell necrosis. Note the abrupt transition between viable tumor and necrosis.

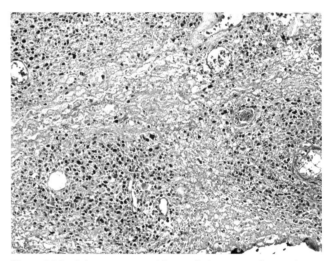

Figure 4.1.8   Leiomyosarcoma with coagulative tumor cell necrosis. Note the preserved atypical nuclei within zones of necrosis.

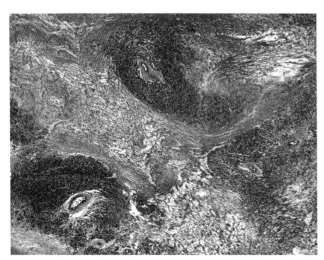

Figure 4.1.9   Leiomyosarcoma with coagulative tumor cell necrosis. Viable tumor cells are present around large thick-walled vessels ("peritheliomatous pattern").

	Infarcted Cellular Leiomyoma	**STUMP**
Age	Most common in pre- or perimenopausal women	Pre-, peri-, or postmenopausal
Location	Uterus	Uterus
Symptoms	Asymptomatic, menorrhagia, or pelvic pain/pressure	Asymptomatic, menorrhagia, or pelvic pain/pressure
Signs	May have enlarged uterus on clinical examination; gross mass within the myometrium	May have enlarged uterus on clinical examination; gross mass within the myometrium
Etiology	Acute infarction within a cellular leiomyoma, which can create histologic concern for leiomyosarcoma; may be related to progestin therapy; *MED12* mutations in majority; *HMGA2* or *HMGA1* fusions in a subset	STUMP has been variably defined; however, herein, it is considered a smooth muscle neoplasm with features concerning for leiomyosarcoma but that the ambiguous histologic findings preclude further classification (typically due to inability to determine the level of atypia, mitotic index, or type of necrosis); various genetic/molecular changes have been described, but heterogeneity in results likely reflects variability of diagnostic classification in the literature
Histology	1. Cellular tumor with spindle cell differentiation 2. Infarct-type/hyaline necrosis, often with hemorrhage (intervening band of hyalinization or granulation tissue between necrosis and viable tumor; acute infarct may be indistinguishable from coagulative tumor cell necrosis, but the latter designation is generally reserved for leiomyosarcoma) *(Figs. 4.2.1 and 4.2.2)* 3. No significant atypia *(Fig. 4.2.3)* 4. Mitotic index usually not elevated (mitotically active cellular leiomyomas may have mitotic index ≥5 mitotic figures/10 high-power fields); pyknotic nuclei can mimic mitotic figures *(Figs. 4.2.4 and 4.2.5)*	1. Spindle cell tumor with variable cellularity *(Fig. 4.2.6)* 2. Infarct-type/hyaline necrosis can be present; pattern of necrosis may be of indeterminate type, in which distinction between infarct-type/hyaline necrosis vs coagulative tumor cell necrosis (sharp interface between necrosis and viable tumor) may not be possible *(Fig. 4.2.7)* 3. No insignificant (mild), or significant (moderate or severe) atypia may be present; due to ambiguous morphologic features, determining insignificant vs significant atypia may not be possible *(Fig. 4.2.8)* 4. Variable mitotic index; in cases with significant atypia or coagulative tumor cell necrosis, the mitotic index may approach the level of 10 mitotic figures/10 high-power fields, but due to ambiguous morphologic features, determining the exact level of mitotic activity may not be possible *(Fig. 4.2.9)*

	Infarcted Cellular Leiomyoma	STUMP
	5. Does not fulfill criteria for leiomyosarcoma; caution should be exercised when diagnosing leiomyosarcoma based only on the mitotic index and necrosis in cases lacking atypia since mitotically active leiomyomas can have infarct-type necrosis indistinguishable from coagulative tumor cell necrosis	5. Does not fulfill criteria for leiomyosarcoma (lacks ≥2 of 3 criteria: significant atypia, mitotic index ≥10 mitotic figures/10 high-power fields, coagulative tumor cell necrosis)
Special studies	Immunohistochemistry of no help for this differential diagnosis	Immunohistochemistry of no help for this differential diagnosis
Treatment	Myomectomy or hysterectomy	Hysterectomy
Prognosis	Benign	Uncertain behavior (this is a heterogeneous category that likely includes morphologically problematic leiomyomas and leiomyosarcomas that cannot be distinguished from one another because of ambiguous histologic features)

Figure 4.2.1   Cellular leiomyoma with acute infarct simulating coagulative tumor cell necrosis of leiomyosarcoma.

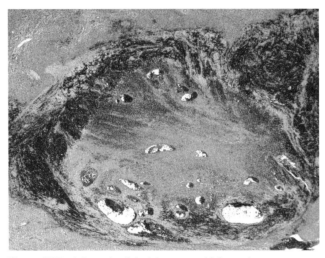

Figure 4.2.2   Infarcted cellular leiomyoma with hemorrhage.

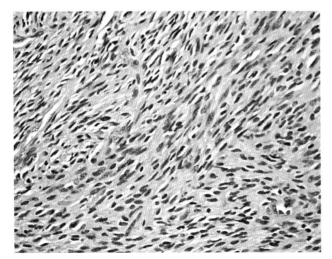

Figure 4.2.3   Region of viable tumor from infarcted cellular leiomyoma. Note the absence of atypia.

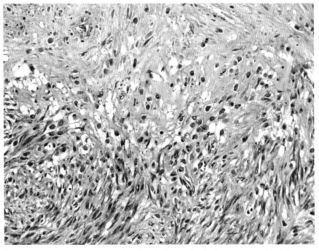

Figure 4.2.4   Pyknotic nuclei simulating mitotic figures at edge of infarct in cellular leiomyoma.

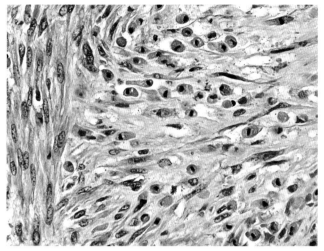

Figure 4.2.5   Pyknotic nuclei simulating mitotic figures at edge of infarct in cellular leiomyoma (same case as *Fig. 4.2.4*).

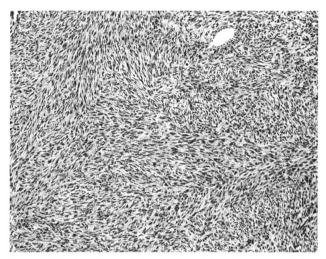

Figure 4.2.6   Smooth muscle tumor of uncertain malignant potential with increased cellularity and spindle cell differentiation.

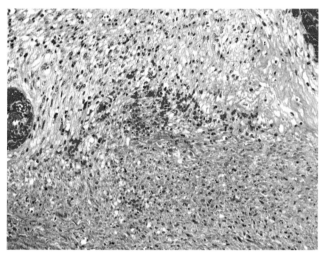

Figure 4.2.7   Smooth muscle tumor of uncertain malignant potential with necrosis of uncertain type.

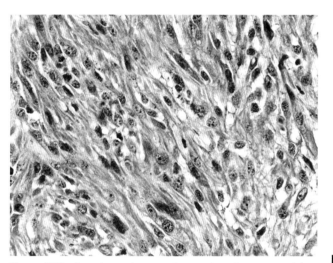

Figure 4.2.8   Smooth muscle tumor of uncertain malignant potential with level of atypia equivocal for mild (insignificant) vs moderate (significant).

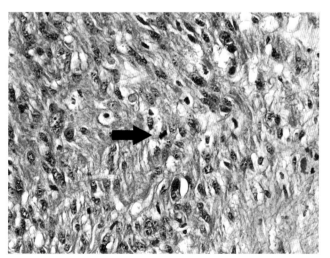

Figure 4.2.9   Smooth muscle tumor of uncertain malignant potential with mitotic activity (*arrow*).

4   UTERINE CORPUS

	Leiomyomas With Variant Growth Patterns (Dissecting Leiomyoma/Intravenous Leiomyomatosis)	Leiomyosarcoma
Age	Most common in pre- or perimenopausal women	Usually, >50 y
Location	Uterus	Uterus
Symptoms	Asymptomatic, menorrhagia, or pelvic pain/pressure	Abnormal vaginal bleeding and/or pelvic pain; clinical features can overlap with those of leiomyoma
Signs	May have enlarged uterus on clinical examination; gross mass within the myometrium, including nodular/worm-like growth within the myometrium or broad ligament; cotyledonoid dissecting leiomyoma (the "Sternberg tumor") may grossly resemble placental tissue within broad ligament	Pelvic mass; gross mass within the myometrium; clinical features can overlap with those of leiomyoma
Etiology	Variant growth patterns of leiomyomas that may create concern for leiomyosarcoma because of permeation into the myometrium or broad ligament; insufficient genetic/molecular data for dissecting leiomyoma; although data are also limited for intravenous leiomyomatosis, reported molecular/genetic aberrations include gains and losses of various chromosomal regions (*MED12* mutations appear to be uncommon)	Pathogenesis unclear but probably arises *de novo* rather than from malignant degeneration of leiomyoma although cases of the latter have been described; various chromosomal aberrations; subsets contain mutations of *TP53, ATRX,* and *MED12* (the frequency of *MED12* mutations is much lower than in leiomyomas)
Histology	1. Dissecting leiomyoma contains bundles of leiomyoma extending between preexisting myometrium; may extend into broad ligament *(Figs. 4.3.1 and 4.3.2)* 2. Intravenous leiomyomatosis contains extension of leiomyoma into vascular spaces beyond confines of leiomyoma; may extend into broad ligament; histologic variants have been described, including cellular, atypical, epithelioid, and lipoleiomyomatous types *(Figs. 4.3.3-4.3.5)* 3. Lacks histologic criteria for leiomyosarcoma *(Fig. 4.3.6)*	1. Frequently has pushing border, but infiltrative patterns may be seen *(Fig. 4.3.7)* 2. Lymphovascular space invasion may be seen *(Fig. 4.3.8)* 3. Criteria for leiomyosarcoma: ≥2 of 3 criteria present (significant atypia *[Figs. 4.3.9 and 4.3.10]*, mitotic index ≥10 mitotic figures/10 high-power fields, coagulative tumor cell necrosis) *(also see Figs. 4.1.7-4.1.9)*; significant (moderate or severe) atypia evident at low- or intermediate-power magnification *(Fig. 4.3.9)*; some cases may have deceptively homogeneous (rather than pleomorphic) pattern of moderate atypia at low- or intermediate-power magnification (evaluation at high-power magnification can be helpful in such cases); may have coagulative tumor cell necrosis (abrupt transition between necrosis and viable tumor); infarct-type/hyaline necrosis can also be present

	Leiomyomas With Variant Growth Patterns (Dissecting Leiomyoma/Intravenous Leiomyomatosis)	**Leiomyosarcoma**
Special studies	Immunohistochemistry of no help (exact role of p53, p16, and Ki-67 for this differential diagnosis unclear)	Immunohistochemistry of no help (exact role of p53, p16, and Ki-67 for this differential diagnosis unclear)
Treatment	Hysterectomy	Hysterectomy, +/− bilateral salpingo-oophorectomy; further management is stage dependent but can include observation or chemotherapy and/or radiation therapy
Prognosis	Benign; intravenous leiomyomatosis can recur (<5%), sometimes many years later, with sites of recurrence including the pelvis, vena cava, lung, and heart	Stage dependent; 5-y survival: 15%-25%; tumors are not graded as they are conventionally considered high grade

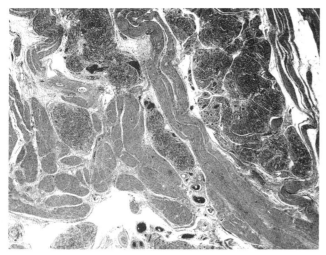

Figure 4.3.1 Dissecting leiomyoma with tumor present in between preexisting nonneoplastic myometrial bundles of smooth muscle.

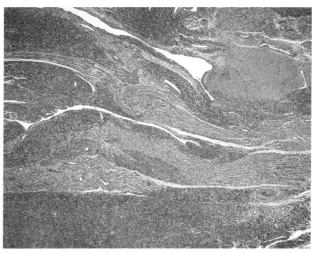

Figure 4.3.2 Dissecting leiomyoma.

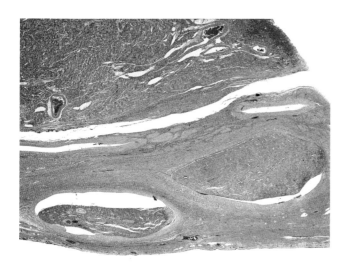

Figure 4.3.3 Intravenous leiomyomatosis. At low-power magnification, this appearance can create concern for either leiomyosarcoma with lymphovascular space invasion or low-grade endometrial stromal sarcoma.

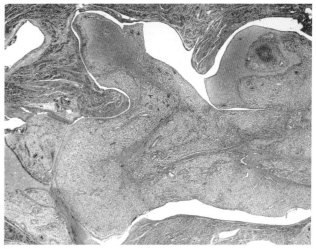

Figure 4.3.4 Intravenous leiomyomatosis.

4 UTERINE CORPUS

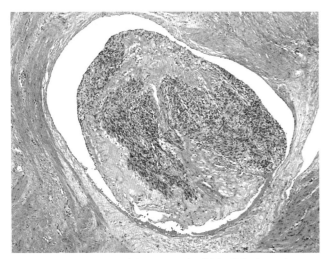

Figure 4.3.5 Intravenous leiomyomatosis with hyalinization and areas of increased cellularity.

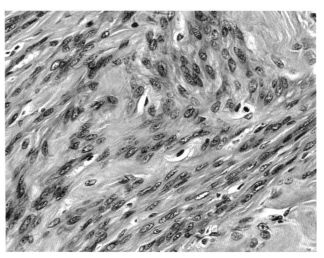

Figure 4.3.6 Intravenous leiomyomatosis. Note absence of atypia.

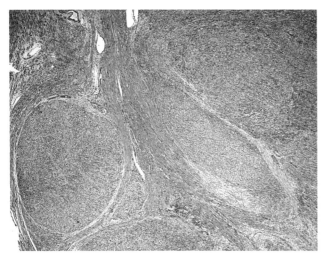

Figure 4.3.7 Leiomyosarcoma with infiltrating border.

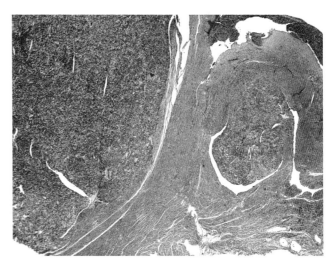

Figure 4.3.8 Leiomyosarcoma exhibiting lymphovascular space invasion. This appearance at low-power magnification can mimic cellular intravenous leiomyomatosis or low-grade endometrial stromal sarcoma.

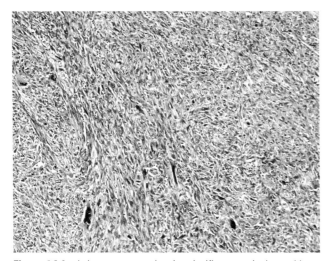

Figure 4.3.9 Leiomyosarcoma showing significant atypia detectable at intermediate-power magnification.

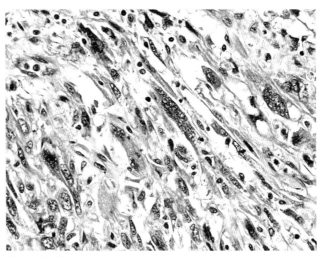

Figure 4.3.10 Leiomyosarcoma with significant nuclear atypia.

	Epithelioid Leiomyoma	Epithelioid Leiomyosarcoma
Age	Most common in pre- or perimenopausal women	Pre-, peri-, or postmenopausal
Location	Uterus	Uterus
Symptoms	Asymptomatic, menorrhagia, or pelvic pain/pressure	Abnormal vaginal bleeding and/or pelvic pain; clinical features can overlap with those of leiomyoma
Signs	May have enlarged uterus on clinical examination; gross mass within the myometrium	Pelvic mass; gross mass within the myometrium; clinical features can overlap with those of leiomyoma
Etiology	Pathogenesis unclear	Pathogenesis unclear; *PGR* rearrangements occur in a subset
Histology	1. Usually sheets of tumor cells with occasional corded, trabecular, and/or nested patterns *(Figs. 4.4.1 and 4.4.2)* 2. Polygonal to round cells with eosinophilic to pale cytoplasm 3. Necrosis is absent in most cases 4. Mild atypia can be present *(Fig. 4.4.3)* 5. Mitotic index typically low (<3 mitotic figures/10 high-power fields) 6. No lymphovascular space invasion 7. No infiltrating patterns 8. Criteria for malignancy: criteria are ill defined and based on limited data for uterine epithelioid smooth muscle neoplasms; however, most epithelioid leiomyomas lack significant atypia, mitotic activity, and/or necrosis; cases that have ambiguous features in between epithelioid leiomyoma and epithelioid leiomyosarcoma may be classified as smooth muscle tumor of uncertain malignant potential *(Fig. 4.4.4)*	1. Usually sheets of tumor cells with occasional corded, trabecular, and/or nested patterns *(Figs. 4.4.5-4.4.7)* 2. Polygonal to round cells with eosinophilic to pale cytoplasm 3. Coagulative tumor cell necrosis may be present *(Fig. 4.4.8)* 4. Atypia can be variable from mild–moderate to severe; in general, level of atypia is less than in conventional/spindle cell leiomyosarcomas *(Figs. 4.4.9 and 4.4.10)* 5. Mitotic index usually low but often >3 mitotic figures/10 high-power fields *(Fig. 4.4.7)*; in general, level of mitotic activity is less than in conventional/spindle cell leiomyosarcomas 6. Lymphovascular space invasion may be present 7. Borders are often pushing but may be infiltrative 8. Criteria for malignancy: 2020 WHO criteria for epithelioid leiomyosarcoma (1 or more of the following): moderate to severe atypia, tumor cell necrosis, or ≥4 mitotic figures/10 high-power fields; neoplasms that have ambiguous features in between epithelioid leiomyoma and epithelioid leiomyosarcoma may be classified as smooth muscle tumor of uncertain malignant potential
Special studies	Immunohistochemistry of no help for this differential diagnosis	Immunohistochemistry of no help for this differential diagnosis

	Epithelioid Leiomyoma	**Epithelioid Leiomyosarcoma**
Treatment	Myomectomy or hysterectomy; however, insufficient data for the level of risk associated with performing only myomectomy (see Prognosis below)	Hysterectomy, +/− bilateral salpingo-oophorectomy; further management is stage dependent but can include observation or chemotherapy and/or radiation therapy
Prognosis	Benign; however, rare cases without significant mitotic activity or atypia can recur	Stage dependent; limited survival data for epithelioid types (5-y survival of 35%); tumors are not graded as they are conventionally considered high grade

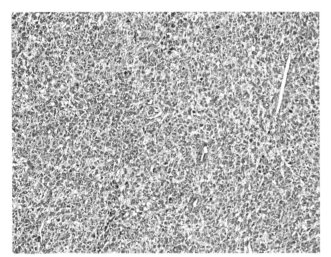

Figure 4.4.1   Epithelioid leiomyoma with diffuse sheets of tumor cells.

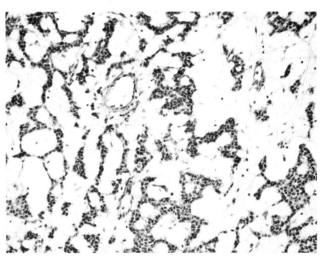

Figure 4.4.2   Epithelioid leiomyoma with corded pattern.

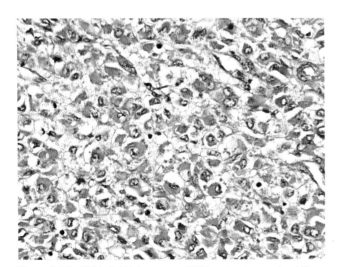

Figure 4.4.3   Epithelioid leiomyoma exhibiting abundant eosinophilic cytoplasm and lack of significant atypia.

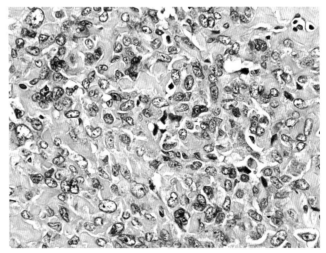

Figure 4.4.4   Atypical epithelioid smooth muscle tumor with other features too equivocal for definitive classification as leiomyoma or leiomyosarcoma (ie, best classified as smooth muscle tumor of uncertain malignant potential).

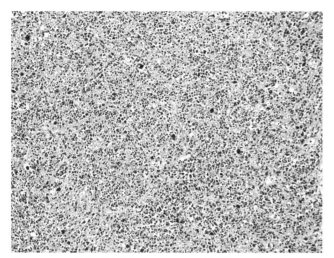

Figure 4.4.5 Epithelioid leiomyosarcoma with diffuse cellular pattern and significant atypia seen at intermediate-power magnification.

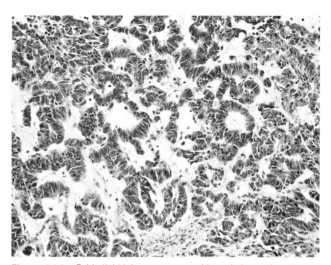

Figure 4.4.6 Epithelioid leiomyosarcoma with corded growth pattern.

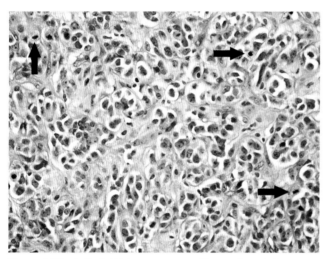

Figure 4.4.7 Epithelioid leiomyosarcoma with vaguely nested pattern and mitotic activity (*arrows*).

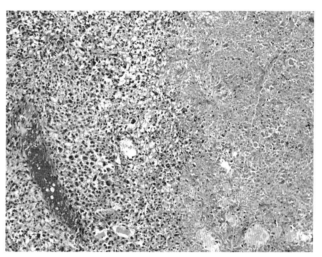

Figure 4.4.8 Epithelioid leiomyosarcoma with necrosis.

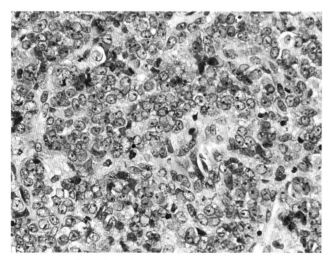

Figure 4.4.9 Epithelioid leiomyosarcoma showing uniform pattern of moderate (significant) atypia.

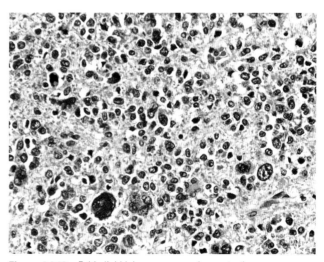

Figure 4.4.10 Epithelioid leiomyosarcoma demonstrating severe atypia.

	Cellular Leiomyoma	Endometrial Stromal Nodule
Age	Most common in pre- or perimenopausal women	53 y (mean)
Location	Uterus	Uterus
Symptoms	Asymptomatic, menorrhagia, or pelvic pain/pressure	Abnormal vaginal bleeding or abdominal pain
Signs	May have enlarged uterus on clinical examination; gross mass within the myometrium	Uterus may be enlarged, or a pelvic mass may be present; circumscribed gross mass within the myometrium; cut surface of tumor often yellow
Etiology	*MED12* mutations in majority; *HMGA2* or *HMGA1* fusions in a subset	Substantial proportion of cases has a translocation of chromosomes 7 and 17 with *JAZF1* rearrangement
Histology	1. Increased cellularity 2. Spindle cell differentiation with organization into fascicles *(Figs. 4.5.1 and 4.5.2)*; some spindle cells can have abundant eosinophilic cytoplasm, but many cells have scant cytoplasm with high nuclear-to-cytoplasmic ratios; nuclei are elongated; fascicles tangentially oriented may simulate the cytology of an endometrial stromal tumor *(Fig. 4.5.3)* 3. Large thick-walled vessels *(Fig. 4.5.4)* 4. Interface between tumor and myometrium may have cleft-like spaces *(Fig. 4.5.5)* 5. Usually lack hyaline bands/plaques 6. Foam cells often not present	1. Circumscribed nodule with increased cellularity *(Fig. 4.5.6)* 2. No spindle cell differentiation or fascicular architecture (occasional cases may have smooth muscle differentiation with some degree of spindle cell/fascicle formation *[Fig. 4.5.7]*); tumor cells are round to oval with scant cytoplasm, have high nuclear-to-cytoplasmic ratios, and resemble proliferative phase endometrial stroma; nuclei are round to oval *(Fig. 4.5.8)* 3. Large thick-walled vessels typically absent; spiral arteriolar or fine branching vasculature pattern usually present *(Fig. 4.5.8)*; cells may appear to circumferentially swirl around spiral arterioles 4. Cleft-like spaces at interface between tumor and myometrium typically absent 5. Hyaline bands/plaques may be present *(Fig. 4.5.9)* 6. Foam cells may be present *(Fig. 4.5.10)*
Special studies	• Smooth muscle actin/desmin: positive (usually diffuse pattern) • CD10: often negative; occasionally may have focal to patchy expression but not diffuse in most cases (a subset of cellular leiomyomas can have diffuse CD10 staining)	• Smooth muscle actin/desmin: typically negative; may occasionally have some smooth muscle actin expression but usually not diffuse; cases with smooth muscle differentiation can have smooth muscle actin/desmin expression in the latter component • CD10: usually diffuse expression

	Cellular Leiomyoma	**Endometrial Stromal Nodule**
Treatment	Myomectomy or hysterectomy	Hysterectomy (for an endometrial biopsy/curettage or a myomectomy specimen, distinction between a cellular leiomyoma and an endometrial stromal lesion is clinically important because distinguishing an endometrial stromal nodule from a low-grade endometrial stromal sarcoma in the aforementioned specimens usually requires a hysterectomy, which is not necessary for all leiomyomas)
Prognosis	Benign	Benign

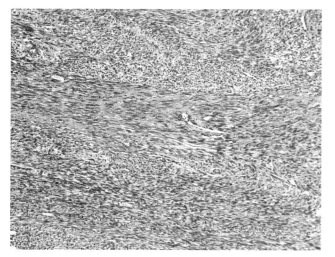

Figure 4.5.1   Cellular leiomyoma showing fascicular architecture.

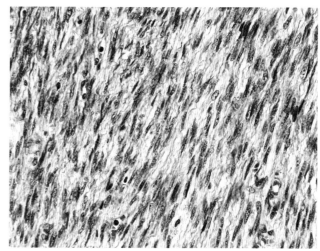

Figure 4.5.2   Cellular leiomyoma with spindle cell differentiation.

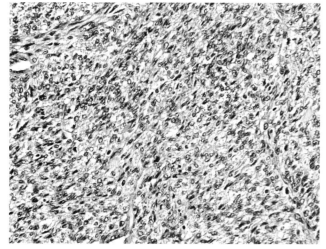

Figure 4.5.3   Cellular leiomyoma with fascicles oriented perpendicular to the plane of section simulating an endometrial stromal neoplasm.

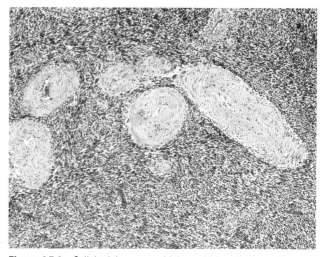

Figure 4.5.4   Cellular leiomyoma with large thick-walled vessels.

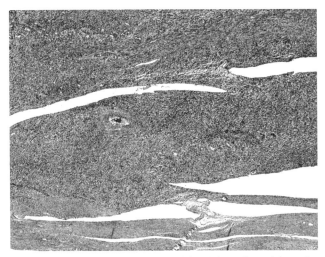

Figure 4.5.5 Cellular leiomyoma containing clefts at the periphery of the tumor.

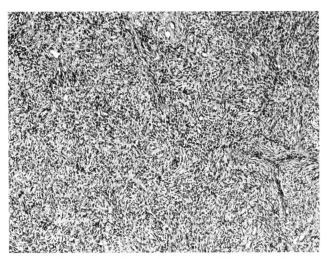

Figure 4.5.6 Endometrial stromal nodule with diffuse sheets of increased cellularity.

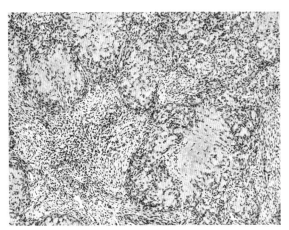

Figure 4.5.7 Endometrial stromal nodule with smooth muscle differentiation. The latter is identified by the nodular, corded, and hyalinized foci, while the area lacking these features in the lower-left quadrant exhibits endometrial stromal differentiation.

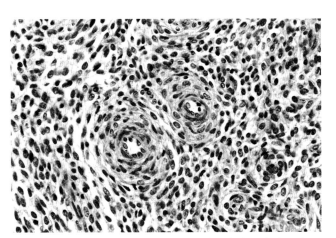

Figure 4.5.8 Endometrial stromal nodule with typical cytologic and vascular features.

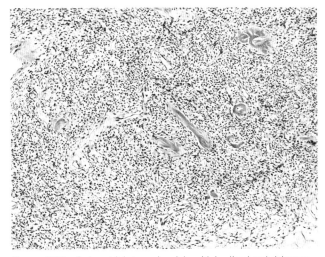

Figure 4.5.9 Endometrial stromal nodule with hyaline bands/plaques.

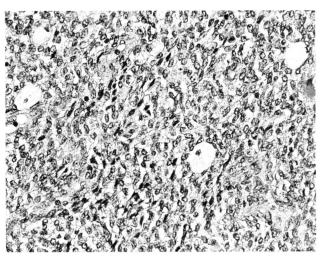

Figure 4.5.10 Endometrial stromal nodule with foam cells.

	Endometrial Stromal Nodule/Tumor With Irregular Margins	Low-Grade Endometrial Stromal Sarcoma
Age	53 y (mean)	52 y (mean)
Location	Uterus	Uterus
Symptoms	Abnormal vaginal bleeding or abdominal pain	Abnormal vaginal bleeding or abdominal pain
Signs	Uterus may be enlarged, or a pelvic mass may be present; gross circumscribed mass within the myometrium or endometrial cavity; cut surface of tumor often yellow	Uterus may be enlarged, or a pelvic mass may be present; gross mass within the myometrium or endometrial cavity (may exhibit tongue-like growth pattern); cut surface of tumor often yellow
Etiology	Substantial proportion of cases has a translocation of chromosomes 7 and 17 with *JAZF1* rearrangement	Substantial proportion of cases has a translocation of chromosomes 7 and 17 with *JAZF1* rearrangement; fusions of *PHF1*, *EPC1*, and *MEAF6* also may occur
Histology	1. Mostly circumscribed border *(Fig. 4.6.1)*, but focal projections extend <3 mm beyond tumor-myometrial interface *(Figs. 4.6.2 and 4.6.3)* (rare cases with extension >3 mm beyond tumor-myometrial interface but lacking the overt tongue-like growth pattern of low-grade endometrial stromal sarcoma have been designated "endometrial stromal tumor with limited infiltration"; however, the 2020 WHO Classification regards such cases as low-grade endometrial stromal sarcoma) 2. No lymph-vascular space invasion 3. Tumor cells are round to oval with scant cytoplasm, have high nuclear-to-cytoplasmic ratios, and resemble proliferative phase endometrial stroma; nuclei are round to oval 4. Spiral arteriolar or fine branching vasculature pattern usually present; cells may appear to circumferentially swirl around spiral arterioles 5. Hyaline bands/plaques may be present 6. Foam cells may be present 7. Smooth muscle, sex cord, glandular, fibromyxoid, and epithelioid differentiation can occur	1. Tongue-like pattern of growth: multiple round to oval nodules of varying size permeate throughout the myometrial wall *(Figs. 4.6.4 and 4.6.5)* 2. Lymph-vascular space invasion may be present 3. Same cytologic features as in endometrial stromal nodule *(Fig. 4.6.6)* 4. Same type of vasculature as in endometrial stromal nodule *(Fig. 4.6.7)* 5. Hyaline bands/plaques may be present 6. Foam cells may be present 7. Same histologic variants as in endometrial stromal nodule
Special studies	Immunohistochemistry of no help for this differential diagnosis	Immunohistochemistry of no help for this differential diagnosis
Treatment	Hysterectomy (for an endometrial biopsy/curettage or a myomectomy specimen, distinction of endometrial stromal nodule from low-grade endometrial stromal sarcoma usually requires a hysterectomy)	Dependent on stage; hysterectomy (+/− bilateral salpingo-oophorectomy); may include observation, hormonal therapy, and/or radiation therapy

	Endometrial Stromal Nodule/Tumor With Irregular Margins	**Low-Grade Endometrial Stromal Sarcoma**
Prognosis	Benign; in some studies, it has been suggested that endometrial stromal tumors with limited infiltration (*see above*) should be considered tumors of low malignant potential, whereas the 2020 WHO Classification considers such cases as low-grade endometrial stromal sarcoma	Stage dependent; 5-y survival: 90% for stages I-II vs 50% for stages III-IV

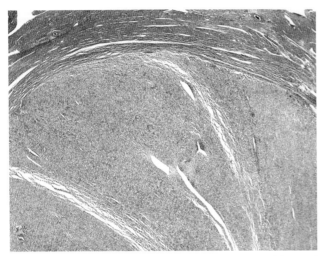

Figure 4.6.1 Typical tumor-myometrial interface of endometrial stromal nodule with smooth border.

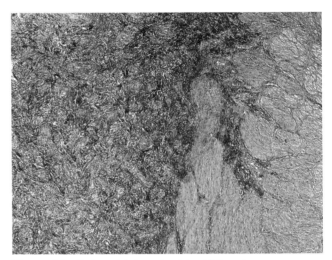

Figure 4.6.2 Endometrial stromal nodule with irregular tumor-myometrial interface.

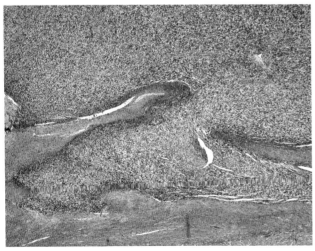

Figure 4.6.3 Endometrial stromal nodule with a more irregular tumor-myometrial interface than in *Figure 4.6.2*.

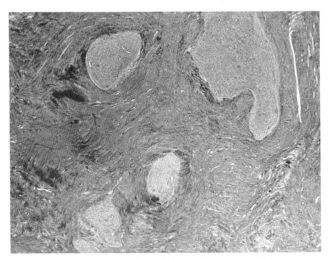

Figure 4.6.4 Low-grade endometrial stromal sarcoma with characteristic tongue-like pattern of invasion.

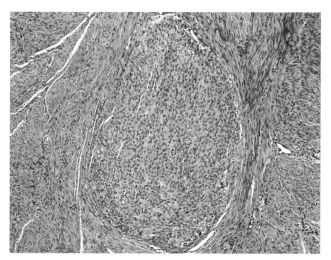

Figure 4.6.5 Invasive area from low-grade endometrial stromal sarcoma.

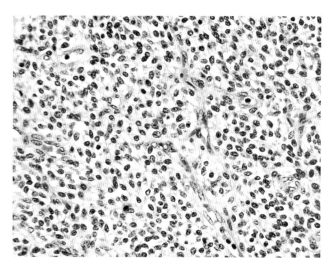

Figure 4.6.6 Low-grade endometrial stromal sarcoma showing cytologic features similar to those of endometrial stromal nodule.

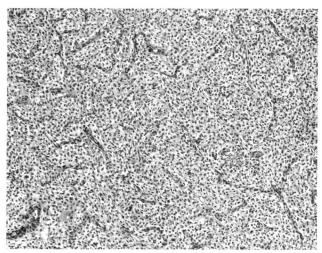

Figure 4.6.7 Low-grade endometrial stromal sarcoma with fine branching vascular pattern, which is also identical to that of endometrial stromal nodule.

4 UTERINE CORPUS

	Low-Grade Endometrial Stromal Sarcoma With Glandular Differentiation	Adenosarcoma
Age	52 y (mean)	Usually postmenopausal
Location	Uterus	Uterus
Symptoms	Abnormal vaginal bleeding or abdominal pain	Abnormal vaginal bleeding
Signs	Uterus may be enlarged, or a pelvic mass may be present; gross mass within the myometrium or endometrial cavity (may exhibit tongue-like growth pattern); cut surface of tumor often yellow	Pelvic mass may be present; gross mass within the endometrial cavity; cut surface may have a cystic component
Etiology	Substantial proportion of cases has a translocation of chromosomes 7 and 17 with *JAZF1* rearrangement; fusions of *PHF1, EPC1,* and *MEAF6* also may occur	Pathogenesis unclear; a subset have been associated with tamoxifen use
Histology	1. Mostly intramural myometrial mass; exophytic component is usually not prominent; tongue-like pattern of growth: multiple round to oval nodules of varying size permeate throughout myometrial wall *(Figs. 4.7.1 and 4.7.2)* 2. Small- to medium-sized, round, benign, and endometrial-type glands; however, areas of classic low-grade endometrial stromal sarcoma should be present elsewhere *(Fig. 4.7.3)* and could potentially mimic areas of sarcomatous overgrowth in adenosarcoma 3. No intraglandular polypoid projections with leaf-like or phyllodes-type architecture 4. No periglandular or subepithelial stromal condensation 5. Tumor cells are round to oval with scant cytoplasm, have high nuclear-to-cytoplasmic ratios, and resemble proliferative phase endometrial stroma; nuclei are low-grade and round to oval *(Fig. 4.7.4)* 6. Spiral arteriolar or fine branching vasculature pattern usually present; cells may appear to circumferentially swirl around spiral arterioles 7. Smooth muscle, sex cord, fibromyxoid, and epithelioid differentiation can occur	1. Polypoid/exophytic growth; no tongue-like growth pattern 2. Benign glandular component (variable in size and shape); may have metaplastic-type changes 3. Intraglandular polypoid projections with leaf-like or phyllodes-type architecture *(Figs. 4.7.5 and 4.7.6)* 4. Periglandular or subepithelial stromal condensation *(Figs. 4.7.6-4.7.8)* 5. Cells may resemble those of low-grade endometrial stromal sarcoma or have fibroblastic-type morphology *(Fig. 4.7.9)* 6. Vasculature as seen in low-grade endometrial stromal sarcoma can be seen but not characteristic 7. Variant patterns of stromal differentiation as seen in low-grade endometrial stromal sarcoma can occur; heterologous elements may be seen in some cases
Special studies	Immunohistochemistry of no help for this differential diagnosis	Immunohistochemistry of no help for this differential diagnosis

	Low-Grade Endometrial Stromal Sarcoma With Glandular Differentiation	Adenosarcoma
Treatment	Dependent on stage; hysterectomy (+/– bilateral salpingo-oophorectomy); may include observation, hormonal therapy, and/or radiation therapy	Hysterectomy and bilateral salpingo-oophorectomy
Prognosis	Stage dependent; 5-y survival: 90% for stages I-II vs 50% for stages III-IV	Dependent on stage and other risk factors; 5-y survival: ~80%

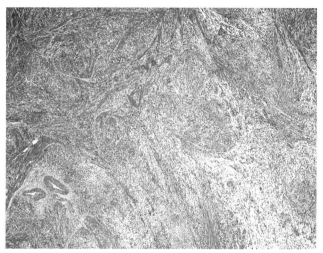

Figure 4.7.1 Typical tongue-like pattern of invasion in low-grade endometrial stromal sarcoma with glandular differentiation (glandular differentiation not present in this field).

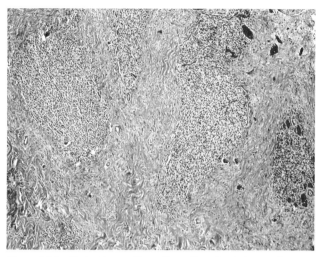

Figure 4.7.2 Typical tongue-like pattern of invasion in low-grade endometrial stromal sarcoma with glandular differentiation (glandular differentiation not present in this focus).

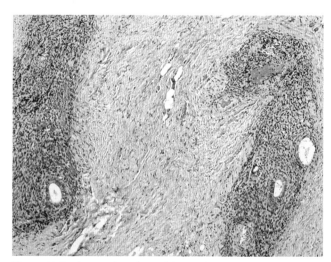

Figure 4.7.3 Low-grade endometrial stromal sarcoma with glandular differentiation. Areas such as the one shown in this case can be potentially confused with periglandular stromal condensation of adenosarcoma. This can also simulate adenomyosis (see Section 4.8).

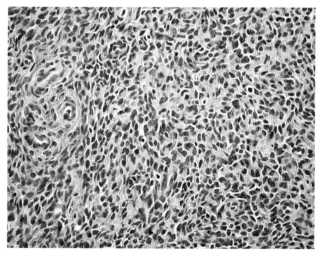

Figure 4.7.4 Low-grade endometrial stromal sarcoma with glandular differentiation showing typical cytologic features (glandular differentiation not present in this focus).

4   UTERINE CORPUS

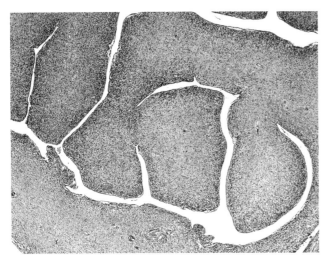

Figure 4.7.5   Adenosarcoma with phyllodes growth pattern.

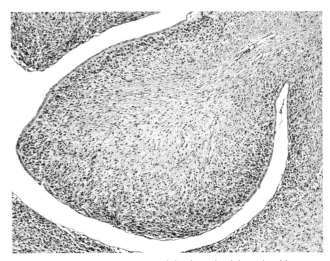

Figure 4.7.6   Adenosarcoma containing intraglandular polypoid projections and subepithelial condensation.

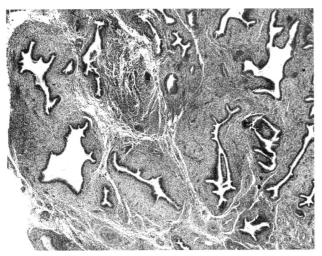

Figure 4.7.7   Adenosarcoma with periglandular stromal condensation. The vague multinodular pattern in this case has the potential to mimic the tongue-like pattern of invasion in low-grade endometrial stromal sarcoma with glandular differentiation.

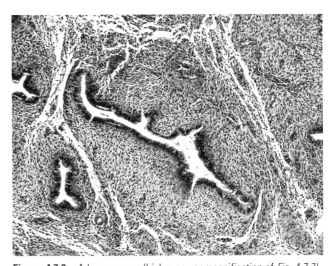

Figure 4.7.8   Adenosarcoma (higher-power magnification of *Fig. 4.7.7*).

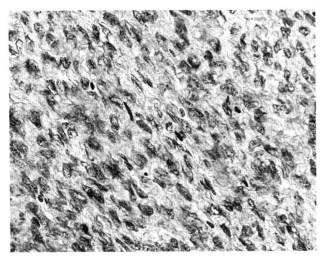

Figure 4.7.9   Adenosarcoma exhibiting fibromatous differentiation.

	Low-Grade Endometrial Stromal Sarcoma With Glandular Differentiation	Adenomyosis/Endometriosis
Age	52 y (mean)	Usually pre- or perimenopausal
Location	Uterus or extrauterine sites	Uterus (adenomyosis); extrauterine sites, including ovaries, uterine ligaments, rectovaginal septum, cul-de-sac, and peritoneum (endometriosis)
Symptoms	Abnormal vaginal bleeding or abdominal pain	Dysmenorrhea, abdominal/pelvic pain, dyspareunia, abnormal vaginal bleeding, and/or infertility
Signs	Uterus may be enlarged, or a pelvic mass may be present; gross mass within the myometrium or endometrial cavity (may exhibit tongue-like growth pattern on gross examination); cut surface of tumor often yellow	Uterus may be enlarged, and myometrium can be thickened with hemorrhagic foci (adenomyosis); although adenomyosis may be nodular, a mass should not be present; tender nodules in the cul-de-sac and uterosacral ligaments, and nonpigmented or pigmented lesions involving the peritoneum (endometriosis)
Etiology	Substantial proportion of cases has a translocation of chromosomes 7 and 17 with *JAZF1* rearrangement; fusions of *PHF1, EPC1,* and *MEAF6* also may occur	Endometrial diverticula containing glands and endometrial stroma extend into myometrium (adenomyosis); ectopic extrauterine endometrial tissue with glands and stroma (endometriosis); most cases of endometriosis believed to be a result of retrograde menstruation
Histology	1. Tongue-like pattern of growth: multiple round nodules of varying size permeate throughout the myometrial wall or extrauterine sites *(Figs. 4.8.1-4.8.3)*	1. No tongue-like pattern of growth; extent of proliferation, degree of crowding of foci, and size of foci in adenomyosis *(Figs. 4.8.7-4.8.9)*/ endometriosis *(Fig. 4.8.10)* not as great as in low-grade endometrial stromal sarcoma; foci are typically small; occasionally, endometriosis may produce a mass (polypoid endometriosis); foci of adenomyosis or endometriosis can be gland-poor mimicking low-grade endometrial stromal sarcoma (see Section 4.9); adenomyosis can be surrounded by smooth muscle hyperplasia
	2. Small- to medium-sized, round, benign, and endometrial-type glands; however, areas of classic low-grade endometrial stromal sarcoma should be present elsewhere; extent of glandular differentiation is variable *(Figs. 4.8.3-4.8.6)*	2. Appearance of glands similar to that in low-grade endometrial stromal sarcoma with glandular differentiation
	3. Stromal tumor cells are round to oval with scant cytoplasm, have high nuclear-to-cytoplasmic ratios, and resemble proliferative phase endometrial stroma; nuclei are low grade and round to oval	3. Cytologic features of endometrial stroma similar to that in low-grade endometrial stromal sarcoma with glandular differentiation
	4. Spiral arteriolar or fine branching vasculature pattern usually present; cells may appear to circumferentially swirl around spiral arterioles	4. Vascular pattern similar to that in low-grade endometrial stromal sarcoma with glandular differentiation
	5. Smooth muscle, sex cord, fibromyxoid, and epithelioid differentiation can occur	5. Histologic variants that occur in low-grade endometrial stromal sarcoma not seen

	Low-Grade Endometrial Stromal Sarcoma With Glandular Differentiation	Adenomyosis/Endometriosis
Special studies	Immunohistochemistry of no help for this differential diagnosis	Immunohistochemistry of no help for this differential diagnosis
Treatment	Dependent on stage; hysterectomy (+/− bilateral salpingo-oophorectomy); may include observation, hormonal therapy, and/ or radiation therapy	Surgical or hormonal/medical therapy
Prognosis	Stage dependent; 5-y survival: 90% for stages I-II vs 50% for stages III-IV	Benign

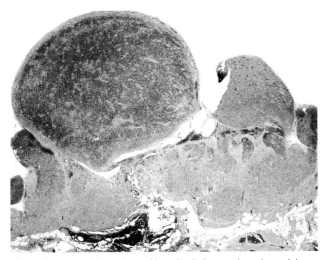

Figure 4.8.1 Nodular pattern of invasion in low-grade endometrial stromal sarcoma with glandular differentiation involving the peritoneum (glandular differentiation not present in this field).

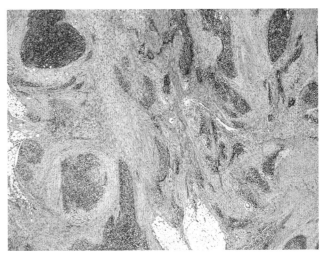

Figure 4.8.2 Typical pattern of invasion in low-grade endometrial stromal sarcoma with glandular differentiation involving the omentum (glandular differentiation not present in this focus).

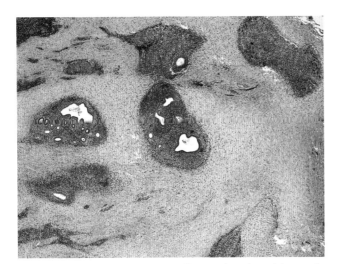

Figure 4.8.3 Typical growth pattern of low-grade endometrial stromal sarcoma. Note the presence of glandular differentiation.

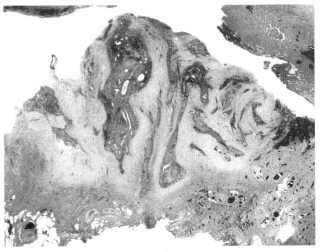

Figure 4.8.4 Low-grade endometrial stromal sarcoma with glandular differentiation involving serosa. The appearance in this case mimics that of endometriosis. At this magnification, a tongue-like growth pattern is evident.

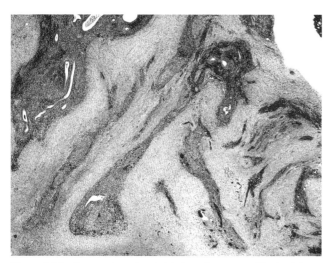

Figure 4.8.5 Low-grade endometrial stromal sarcoma with glandular differentiation involving serosa (higher-power magnification of *Fig. 4.8.4*). Note the associated smaller, crowded, and cellular foci without glands, which are haphazardly arranged and morphologically identical to typical low-grade endometrial stromal sarcoma.

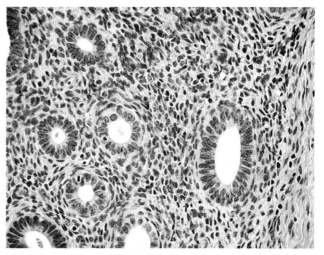

Figure 4.8.6 Low-grade endometrial stromal sarcoma with glandular differentiation. Out of context, the histologic appearance of the glands and stroma can be identical to endometriosis/adenomyosis.

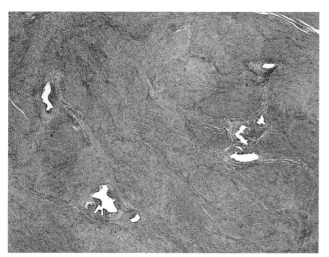

Figure 4.8.7 Adenomyosis with multiple foci in the myometrium. This appearance can overlap with that of low-grade endometrial stromal sarcoma with glandular differentiation; however, the tongue-like growth pattern, degree of crowding of foci, and size of foci are not as striking as seen in low-grade endometrial stromal sarcoma with glandular differentiation, and areas elsewhere lacking glands (as in low-grade endometrial stromal sarcoma) are absent.

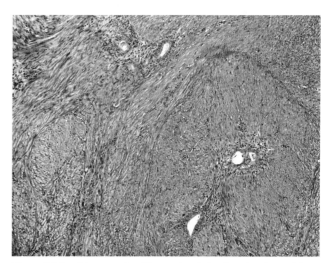

Figure 4.8.8 Adenomyosis with associated glands and endometrial stroma.

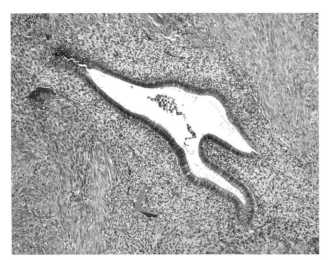

Figure 4.8.9 Adenomyosis with associated glands and endometrial stroma.

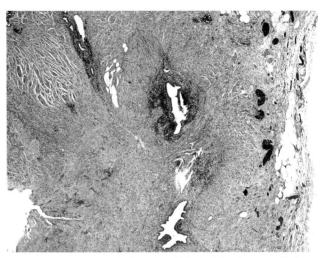

Figure 4.8.10 Endometriosis with multiple foci, but the constellation of features diagnostic of low-grade endometrial stromal sarcoma with glandular differentiation is not present.

	Gland-Poor Adenomyosis	Low-Grade Endometrial Stromal Sarcoma
Age	Pre-, peri-, or postmenopausal women	52 y (mean)
Location	Uterus	Uterus
Symptoms	Dysmenorrhea and abnormal vaginal bleeding	Abnormal vaginal bleeding or abdominal pain
Signs	Uterus may be enlarged, and myometrium can be thickened with hemorrhagic foci	Uterus may be enlarged, or a pelvic mass may be present; gross mass within the myometrium or endometrial cavity (may exhibit tongue-like growth pattern); cut surface of tumor often yellow
Etiology	Endometrial diverticula containing glands and endometrial stroma extending into the myometrium; may represent a form of adenomyosis with endometrial atrophy	Substantial proportion of cases has a translocation of chromosomes 7 and 17 with *JAZF1* rearrangement; fusions of *PHF1, EPC1,* and *MEAF6* also may occur
Histology	1. No tongue-like pattern of growth; extent of proliferation, degree of crowding of foci, and size of foci in adenomyosis not as great as in low-grade endometrial stromal sarcoma; foci are typically small 2. Foci lacking glands can occur simulating low-grade endometrial stromal sarcoma *(Figs. 4.9.1 and 4.9.2)*; other areas of typical adenomyosis should be seen elsewhere *(Fig. 4.9.3)* 3. Intravascular variants have been described *(Fig. 4.9.4)* 4. Circumferential smooth muscle hypertrophy around foci of question 5. Cytologic features similar to that in low-grade endometrial stromal sarcoma *(Fig. 4.9.5)* 6. Vascular pattern similar to that in low-grade endometrial stromal sarcoma 7. Other histologic variants that occur in low-grade endometrial stromal sarcoma not seen	1. Tongue-like pattern of growth: multiple round nodules of varying size permeate throughout myometrial wall *(Figs. 4.9.6 and 4.9.7)* 2. Adenomyosis typically not seen but can occur simultaneously given the relatively high frequency of adenomyosis in the general population (glandular variants of low-grade endometrial stromal sarcoma simulating extensive adenomyosis may occur) 3. Lymphovascular space invasion may be present *(Fig. 4.9.8)* 4. No circumferential smooth muscle hypertrophy around foci of question 5. Tumor cells are round to oval with scant cytoplasm, have high nuclear-to-cytoplasmic ratios, and resemble proliferative phase endometrial stroma; nuclei are round to oval *(Fig. 4.9.9)* 6. Spiral arteriolar or fine branching vasculature pattern usually present; cells may appear to circumferentially swirl around spiral arterioles *(Fig. 4.9.9)* 7. Smooth muscle, sex cord, fibromyxoid, and epithelioid differentiation can occur *(Figs. 4.9.8, 4.9.10, and 4.9.11)*
Special studies	Immunohistochemistry of no help for this differential diagnosis	Immunohistochemistry of no help for this differential diagnosis
Treatment	Hysterectomy or hormonal/medical therapy	Dependent on stage; hysterectomy (+/− bilateral salpingo-oophorectomy); may include observation, hormonal therapy, and/or radiation therapy
Prognosis	Benign	Stage dependent; 5-y survival: 90% for stages I-II vs 50% for stages III-IV

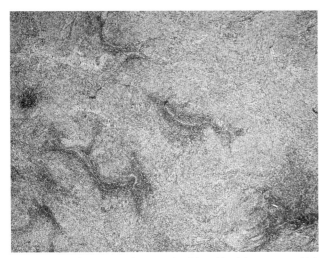

Figure 4.9.1 Gland-poor adenomyosis with multinodular pattern, which can simulate low-grade endometrial stromal sarcoma at low-power magnification.

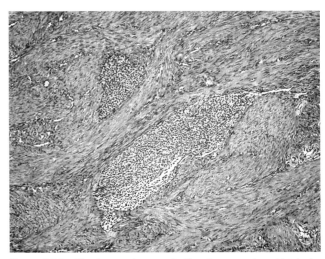

Figure 4.9.2 Gland-poor adenomyosis. Out of context, these histologic features can mimic low-grade endometrial sarcoma.

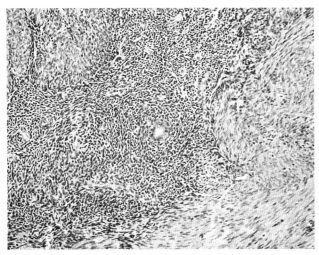

Figure 4.9.3 Gland-poor adenomyosis. The presence of focal glands **(center)** is a helpful diagnostic clue.

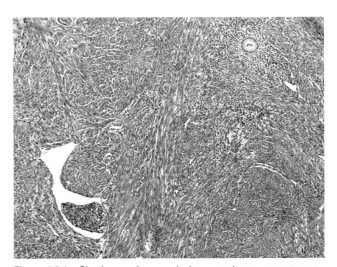

Figure 4.9.4 Gland-poor adenomyosis. Intravascular components may occur **(lower left)** causing concern for low-grade endometrial stromal sarcoma, but associated typical adenomyosis **(upper right)** helps facilitate the correct diagnosis.

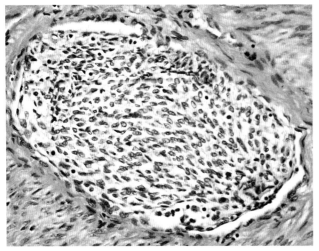

Figure 4.9.5 Gland-poor adenomyosis. The cytologic features are essentially identical to those of low-grade endometrial stromal sarcoma.

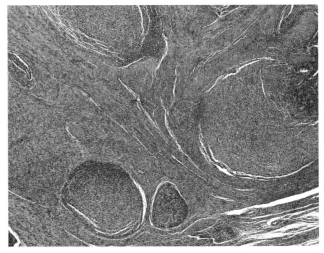

Figure 4.9.6 Low-grade endometrial stromal sarcoma with usual tongue-like pattern of invasion.

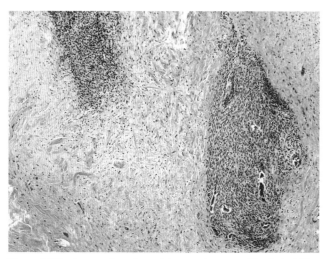

Figure 4.9.7 Low-grade endometrial stromal sarcoma. The foci within the myometrium tend to be larger than those of adenomyosis.

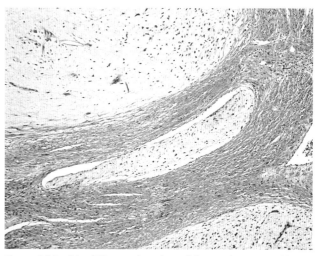

Figure 4.9.8 Myxoid low-grade endometrial stromal sarcoma with lymphovascular space invasion.

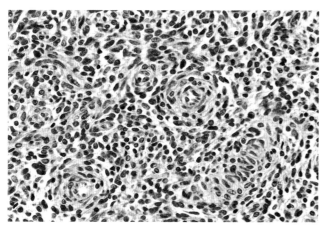

Figure 4.9.9 Low-grade endometrial stromal sarcoma showing characteristic cytologic and vascular features.

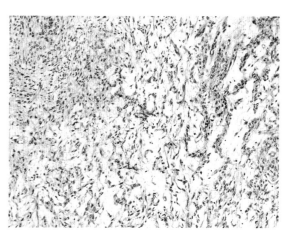

Figure 4.9.10 Low-grade endometrial stromal sarcoma exhibiting myxoid differentiation.

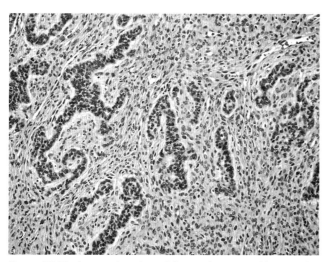

Figure 4.9.11 Low-grade endometrial stromal sarcoma with sex cord differentiation.

	High-Grade Endometrial Stromal Sarcoma	Low-Grade Endometrial Stromal Sarcoma
Age	Pre- and postmenopausal	52 y (mean)
Location	Uterus	Uterus
Symptoms	Abnormal vaginal bleeding	Abnormal vaginal bleeding or abdominal pain
Signs	Enlarged uterus or pelvic mass	Uterus may be enlarged, or a pelvic mass may be present; gross mass within the myometrium or endometrial cavity (may exhibit tongue-like growth pattern); cut surface of tumor often yellow
Etiology	A subset has translocations of chromosomes 10 and 17 with *YWHAE-NUTM2A/B* rearrangement (other cases have *BCOR/BCORL1* fusions or *BCOR* internal tandem duplications); a subset of other cases in some studies do not show the above alterations; believed to be unrelated to low-grade endometrial stromal sarcoma	Substantial proportion of cases has a translocation of chromosomes 7 and 17 with *JAZF1* rearrangement; fusions of *PHF1, EPC1,* and *MEAF6* also may occur
Histology	1. Biphasic pattern with low- and high-grade components may be present (more commonly seen in *YWHAE-NUTM2A/B* rearranged tumors); *BCOR/BCOL1* rearranged tumors show fascicular architecture with myxoid features reminiscent of myxoid leiomyosarcoma 2. Tongue-like pattern of growth can be present *(Figs. 4.10.1 and 4.10.2)* 3. Mitotic activity in higher-grade component 4. Necrosis often present 5. Cytology of lower-grade component resembles low-grade endometrial stromal sarcoma, often with fibromyxoid appearance (more commonly seen in *YWHAE-NUTM2A/B* rearranged tumors) *(Fig. 4.10.3)* 6. Higher-grade component (more commonly seen in *YWHAE-NUTM2A/B* rearranged tumors) has small round blue cell-like appearance with round nuclei; compared with low-grade endometrial stromal sarcoma, nuclei are larger with slightly irregular chromatin and nuclear membranes and more atypical although not pleomorphic; chromatin clearing may be seen *(Figs. 4.10.4-4.10.6)*; *BCOR/BCOL1* rearranged tumors show spindle cell morphology having oval to spindle cell nuclei with evenly distributed chromatin	1. No biphasic pattern 2. Tongue-like pattern of growth: multiple round nodules of varying size permeate throughout myometrial wall *(Fig. 4.10.8)* 3. Mitotic figures usually difficult to find, but occasionally may have mitotic activity 4. Necrosis occasionally present 5. Tumor cells are round to oval with scant cytoplasm, have high nuclear-to-cytoplasmic ratios, and resemble proliferative phase endometrial stroma; nuclei are bland and round to oval *(Figs. 4.10.9 and 4.10.10)* 6. No high-grade component present

	High-Grade Endometrial Stromal Sarcoma	Low-Grade Endometrial Stromal Sarcoma
	7. Lower-grade component has vasculature resembling low-grade endometrial stromal sarcoma; higher-grade component (more commonly seen in *YWHAE-NUTM2A/B* rearranged tumors) does not have spiral arteriolar pattern as well developed as in of low-grade endometrial stromal sarcoma, but vasculature is fine and branching with tumor cells segregated into small tightly packed nests *(Fig. 4.10.6)*	**7.** Spiral arteriolar or fine branching vasculature pattern usually present; cells may appear to circumferentially swirl around spiral arterioles *(Fig. 4.10.9)*
Special studies	• CD10: diffuse expression in lower-grade component (in *YWHAE-NUTM2A/B* rearranged tumors); limited to no expression in higher-grade component • ER/PR: diffuse expression in lower-grade component (in *YWHAE-NUTM2A/B* rearranged tumors); limited to no expression in higher-grade component • Cyclin D1: no diffuse pattern of expression in lower-grade component (in *YWHAE-NUTM2A/B* rearranged tumors); diffuse (>70% positive cells) expression in higher-grade component *(Fig. 4.10.7)* • BCOR: diffuse in high-grade component of *YWHAE-NUTM2A/B* rearranged tumors/limited expression in lower-grade component; variably expressed in *BCOR* rearranged/*BCOR* internal tandem duplication tumors (may be negative in *BCOR* rearranged tumors) • Ki-67 proliferation index: usually low in lower-grade component (in *YWHAE-NUTM2A/B* rearranged tumors); typically intermediate (occasionally low) in higher-grade component	• CD10: diffuse expression • ER/PR: diffuse expression • Cyclin D1: no diffuse pattern of expression • *BCOR*: usually negative • Ki-67 proliferation index: usually low, occasionally intermediate
Treatment	Hysterectomy, +/− bilateral salpingo-oophorectomy; further management is stage dependent but can include observation or chemotherapy and/or radiation therapy	Dependent on stage; hysterectomy (+/− bilateral salpingo-oophorectomy); may include observation, hormonal therapy, and/or radiation therapy
Prognosis	Behave more aggressively than low-grade endometrial stromal sarcoma	Stage dependent; 5-y survival: 90% for stages I-II vs 50% for stages III-IV

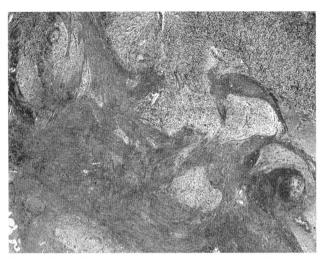

Figure 4.10.1 High-grade endometrial stromal sarcoma with tongue-like growth pattern.

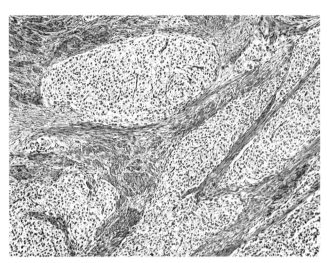

Figure 4.10.2 High-grade endometrial stromal sarcoma with tongue-like growth pattern.

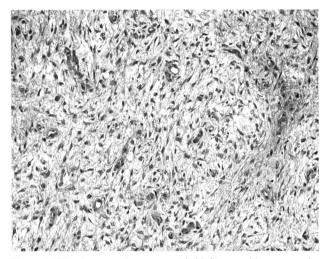

Figure 4.10.3 Lower-grade component (with fibromyxoid appearance) of high-grade endometrial stromal sarcoma.

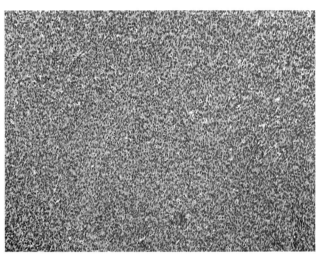

Figure 4.10.4 High-grade endometrial stromal sarcoma showing diffuse sheets of tumor cells.

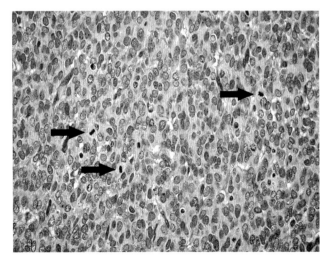

Figure 4.10.5 High-grade endometrial stromal sarcoma exhibiting uniform pattern of atypia with chromatin clearing. Mitotic activity (*arrows*) is present.

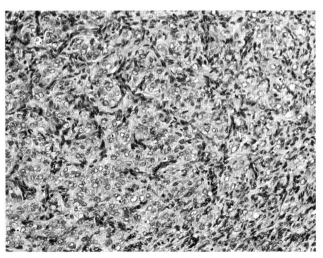

Figure 4.10.6 High-grade endometrial stromal sarcoma showing fine branching vasculature with tumor cells arranged in small solid nests.

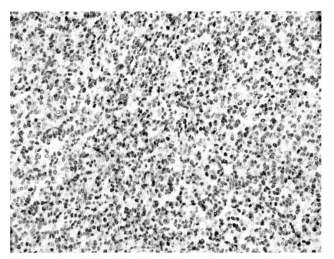

Figure 4.10.7 High-grade endometrial stromal sarcoma with diffuse expression of cyclin D1.

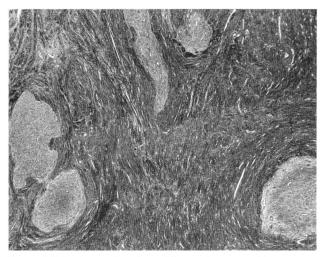

Figure 4.10.8 Low-grade endometrial stromal sarcoma with tongue-like growth pattern.

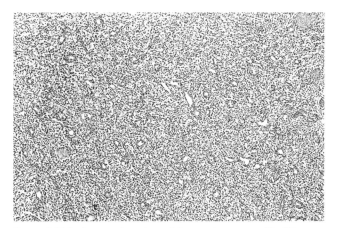

Figure 4.10.9 Low-grade endometrial stromal sarcoma with diffuse architecture and characteristic vasculature.

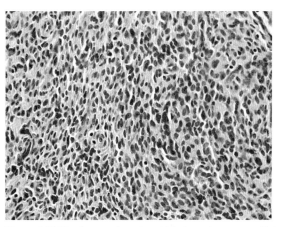

Figure 4.10.10 Low-grade endometrial stromal sarcoma with typical cytologic features (compare with *Figs. 4.10.5 and 4.10.6*).

	UTROSCT	Epithelioid Leiomyoma
Age	50 y (mean)	Most common in pre- or perimenopausal women
Location	Uterus	Uterus
Symptoms	Abnormal vaginal bleeding or pelvic pain	Asymptomatic, menorrhagia, or pelvic pain/pressure
Signs	Myometrial or endometrial mass	May have enlarged uterus on clinical examination; gross mass within myometrium
Etiology	Pathogenesis unclear, but thought to be unrelated to low-grade endometrial stromal tumors; *NCOA* fusions are common; rearrangements involving *ESR1* and *GREB1* have also been described	Pathogenesis unclear
Histology	1. Typically well-circumscribed border, but occasionally has infiltrative appearance *(Fig. 4.11.1)* 2. Tumor exhibits sheet-like, corded, nested, trabecular, tubular, and/or retiform/glomeruloid patterns; overall appearance resembles an ovarian sex cord-stromal tumor *(Figs. 4.11.1-4.11.7)* 3. Cells have epithelioid shapes; variable amount of cytoplasm, occasionally abundant eosinophilic or foamy cytoplasm with lipid-rich appearance *(Figs. 4.11.2-4.11.5, and 4.11.7)* 4. Typically lack atypia 5. Mitotic activity not usually present	1. Circumscribed borders 2. Usually sheets of tumor cells with occasional corded, trabecular, and/or nested patterns *(Figs. 4.11.8 and 4.11.9)* 3. Polygonal to round cells with eosinophilic to pale cytoplasm *(Fig. 4.11.10)* 4. Mild atypia can be present 5. Mitotic index typically low (<3 mitotic figures/10 high-power fields)
Special studies	• Inhibin/SF-1/calretinin/melan-A: +/− • Desmin: +/− • Cytokeratin: usually positive	• Inhibin/SF-1/calretinin/melan-A: (−) • Desmin: (+) • Cytokeratin: usually negative, occasionally positive
Treatment	Myomectomy or hysterectomy	Myomectomy or hysterectomy; however, insufficient data for the level of risk associated with performing only myomectomy (see Prognosis below)
Prognosis	Most are benign; however, malignant behavior has been reported in a subset (necrosis and significant mitotic activity have been associated with malignant behavior)	Benign; however, rare cases without significant mitotic activity or atypia can recur

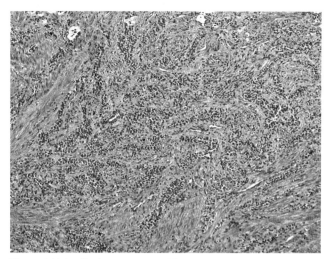

Figure 4.11.1 Uterine tumor resembling ovarian sex cord tumor (UTROSCT). Cords of tumor cells are present between smooth muscle.

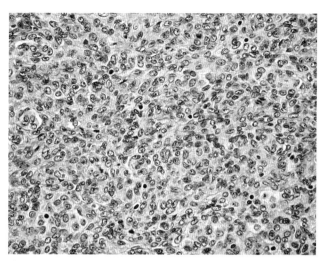

Figure 4.11.2 Uterine tumor resembling ovarian sex cord tumor (UTROSCT) with diffuse sheets of tumor cells. The cytologic features are similar to those of ovarian adult granulosa cell tumor.

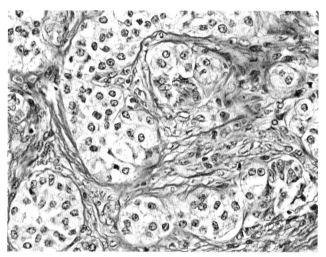

Figure 4.11.3 Uterine tumor resembling ovarian sex cord tumor (UTROSCT) with solid tubules similar to those of lipid-rich Sertoli cell tumor of the ovary.

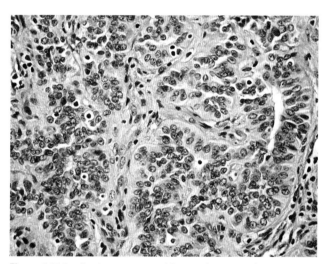

Figure 4.11.4 Uterine tumor resembling ovarian sex cord tumor (UTROSCT) with open tubules and low cuboidal cells.

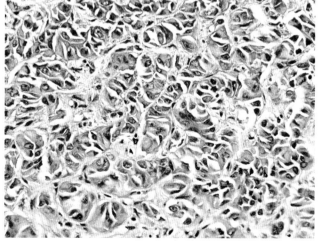

Figure 4.11.5 Uterine tumor resembling ovarian sex cord tumor (UTROSCT) demonstrating corded pattern and polygonal cells.

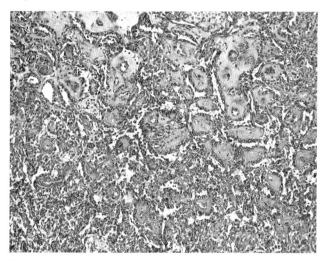

Figure 4.11.6 Uterine tumor resembling ovarian sex cord tumor (UTROSCT) showing retiform/pseudopapillary pattern.

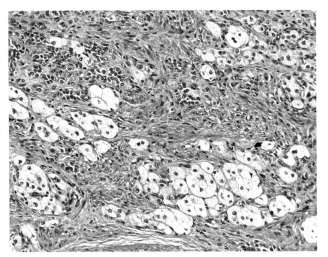

Figure 4.11.7 Uterine tumor resembling ovarian sex cord tumor (UTROSCT) with lipidized stromal cells.

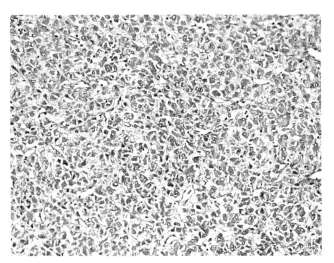

Figure 4.11.8 Epithelioid leiomyoma with diffuse architecture.

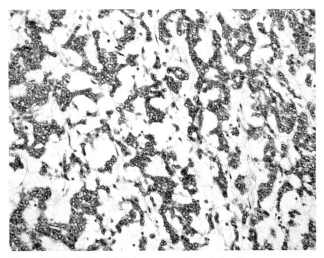

Figure 4.11.9 Epithelioid leiomyoma with corded pattern.

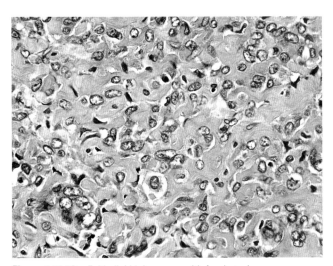

Figure 4.11.10 Epithelioid leiomyoma with focal atypia.

	Perivascular Epithelioid Cell Tumor (PEComa)	Epithelioid Smooth Muscle Tumor (Leiomyoma/Leiomyosarcoma)
Age	Most are perimenopausal	Pre-, peri-, or postmenopausal
Location	Uterus	Uterus
Symptoms	Abnormal vaginal bleeding and/or symptoms attributable to a pelvic mass; subset of cases associated with tuberous sclerosis complex	Asymptomatic, menorrhagia, or pelvic pain/pressure
Signs	Pelvis mass; gross mass within the myometrium	Enlarged uterus or pelvic mass; gross mass within the myometrium
Etiology	Part of the family of epithelioid clear cell tumors with HMB-45 expression and myomelanocytic differentiation; frequently have *TSC1/TSC2* mutations; subset of cases have *TFE3* gene rearrangements; believed to arise from the "perivascular epithelioid cell"	Pathogenesis unclear; *PGR* rearrangements occur in a subset of epithelioid leiomyosarcoma
Histology	1. Diffuse growth pattern; can have nested or fascicular architecture *(Figs. 4.12.1 and 4.12.2)* 2. Predominantly epithelioid cells; may have spindle cell component 3. Abundant clear to eosinophilic and pale or granular cytoplasm *(Figs. 4.12.3-4.12.5)* 4. Atypia can be variable from none to mild, moderate, or severe 5. Variable mitotic index 6. Necrosis may be present 7. Lymphovascular space invasion may be present 8. Borders can be well circumscribed or infiltrative 9. Stroma can be sclerotic/hyalinized *(Fig. 4.12.5)*	1. Usually sheets of tumor cells with occasional corded, trabecular, and/or nested patterns *(Figs. 4.12.6 and 4.12.7)* 2. Polygonal to round cells 3. Eosinophilic to pale cytoplasm *(Figs. 4.12.8 and 4.12.9)* 4. Atypia can be variable from none to mild, moderate, or severe *(Fig. 4.12.8)* 5. Variable mitotic index 6. Necrosis may be present *(Fig. 4.12.10)* 7. Lymphovascular space invasion may be present 8. Borders can be well circumscribed or infiltrative 9. Stroma can be sclerotic/hyalinized *(Fig. 4.12.8)*
Special studies	• HMB-45(+) (extent of staining can range from focal to diffuse) • Melan-A: +/− (extent of staining can range from focal to diffuse) • Cathepsin K: diffuse expression • Smooth muscle actin/desmin: +/− • FISH: *TFE3* gene rearrangement (subset of cases)	• HMB-45(−) • Melan-A(−) • Cathepsin K: variable expression • Smooth muscle actin/desmin(+) • *TFE3* rearrangement data lacking

	Perivascular Epithelioid Cell Tumor (PEComa)	**Epithelioid Smooth Muscle Tumor (Leiomyoma/Leiomyosarcoma)**
Treatment	Specific treatment guidelines unclear; potential for targeted therapy with mTOR inhibitors	Management dependent on diagnosis (leiomyoma, smooth muscle tumor of uncertain malignant potential, leiomyosarcoma), but options include myomectomy and hysterectomy, +/− bilateral salpingo-oophorectomy; further management for sarcoma is stage dependent but can include observation or chemotherapy and/or radiation therapy
Prognosis	Behavior is variable; 2020 WHO criteria for prognostic subclassification (based on the following features: >5 cm, high nuclear grade, >1 mitotic figure/50 high-power fields, necrosis, vascular invasion): a benign category is not recognized; uncertain malignant potential (<3 features); malignant (≥3 features)	• Leiomyoma: benign; however, rare cases without significant mitotic activity or atypia can recur • Leiomyosarcoma: stage dependent; limited survival data for epithelioid types (5-y survival of 35%)

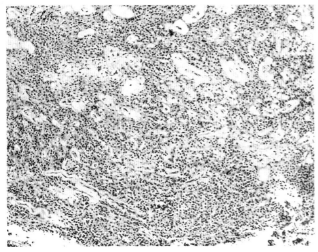

Figure 4.12.1 Perivascular epithelioid cell tumor (PEComa) with diffuse sheets of tumor cells.

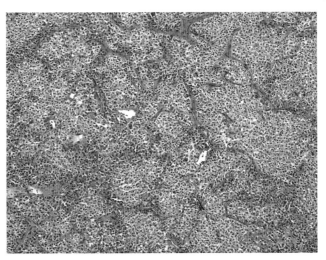

Figure 4.12.2 *TFE3*-translocated perivascular epithelioid cell tumor (PEComa) showing fine branching vasculature with tumor cells arranged in a nested pattern.

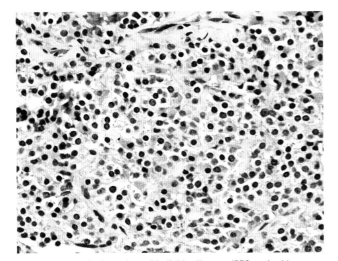

Figure 4.12.3 Perivascular epithelioid cell tumor (PEComa) with abundant clear cytoplasm.

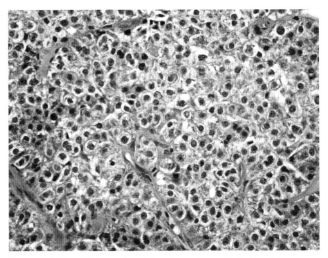

Figure 4.12.4 *TFE3*-translocated perivascular epithelioid cell tumor (PEComa) with pale eosinophilic and granular cytoplasm.

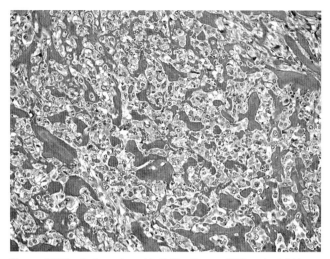

Figure 4.12.5 Perivascular epithelioid cell tumor (PEComa) exhibiting cells with abundant pale cytoplasm and sclerotic/hyalinized stroma.

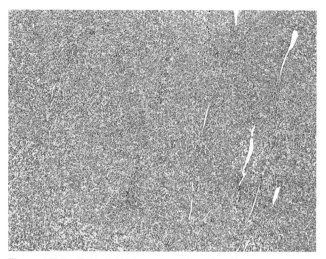

Figure 4.12.6 Epithelioid leiomyoma with solid architecture.

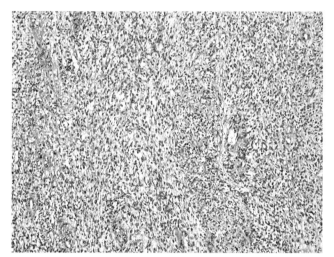

Figure 4.12.7 Epithelioid leiomyosarcoma exhibiting sheets of tumor cells.

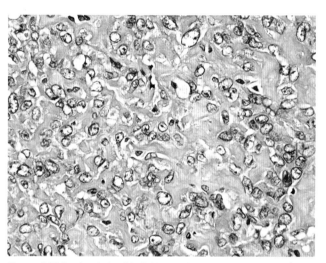

Figure 4.12.8 Atypical epithelioid smooth muscle tumor with scant cytoplasm and hyalinized stroma.

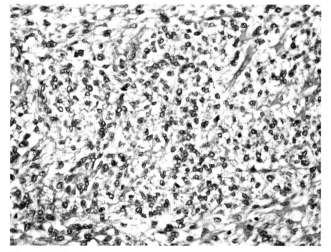

Figure 4.12.9 Epithelioid leiomyosarcoma with artifactual cytoplasmic clearing simulating abundant clear cytoplasm of perivascular epithelioid cell tumor (PEComa).

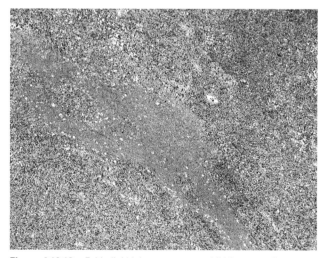

Figure 4.12.10 Epithelioid leiomyosarcoma exhibiting necrosis.

4 UTERINE CORPUS

	Lymphangiomyoma/Lymphangiomyomatosis	Leiomyoma
Age	Usually reproductive age	Most common in pre- or perimenopausal women
Location	Uterus; however, extrauterine sites (eg, lung) are more common	Uterus
Symptoms	May be associated with the tuberous sclerosis complex	Asymptomatic, menorrhagia, or pelvic pain/pressure
Signs	Typically a microscopic finding	May have enlarged uterus on clinical examination; gross mass within the myometrium
Etiology	Also referred to as lymphangioleiomyoma/lymphangioleiomyomatosis; rare in the uterus; part of the family of tumors related to the perivascular epithelioid cell with myomelanocytic differentiation	*MED12* mutations in majority; *HMGA2* or *HMGA1* fusions in a subset
Histology	1. May be solitary nodule (lymphangiomyoma) or exhibit multiple, small, and ill-defined nodules (lymphangiomyomatosis) *(Figs. 4.13.1 and 4.13.2)* 2. Predominantly spindle cell tumor with fascicular architecture *(Fig. 4.13.3)* 3. Fascicles are short and intimately associated with irregular, slit-like, and thin lymphovascular spaces *(Fig. 4.13.4)* 4. Cells are plump with abundant eosinophilic to pale cytoplasm with granular or vacuolated features *(Fig. 4.13.5)* 5. Nuclei are bland and round to oval 6. Usually no mitotic activity	1. Well-circumscribed nodule (leiomyoma); diffuse leiomyomatosis (rare) contains multiple circumscribed nodules 2. Spindle cell differentiation with organization into fascicles *(Fig. 4.13.6)* 3. Fascicles are elongated and interlacing; vascular leiomyomas have numerous thick-walled vessels; leiomyoma does not have the type of lymphovascular network seen in lymphangiomyomatosis *(Fig. 4.13.7)*; other architectural variants *(Fig. 4.13.8)* and stromal hyalinization *(Fig. 4.13.9)* can be seen 4. Cells have abundant and dense cytoplasm *(Fig. 4.13.10)* 5. Nuclei are elongated and bland 6. Variable mitotic activity
Special studies	• Smooth muscle actin (+) • Desmin: +/− • HMB-45/MART-1: usually positive	• Smooth muscle actin (+) • Desmin (+) • HMB-45/MART-1 (−)
Treatment	Myomectomy or hysterectomy	Myomectomy or hysterectomy
Prognosis	Benign; however, clinical correlation is advised to determine whether the lesion is part of a more generalized process	Benign

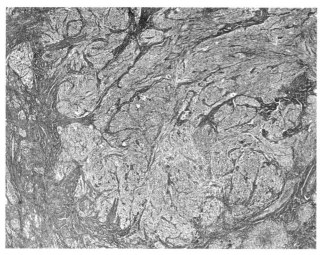

Figure 4.13.1   Lymphangiomyoma with fascicles in between preexisting myometrial bundles.

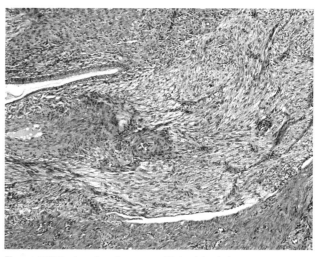

Figure 4.13.2   Lymphangiomyoma with fascicles in between preexisting myometrial bundles.

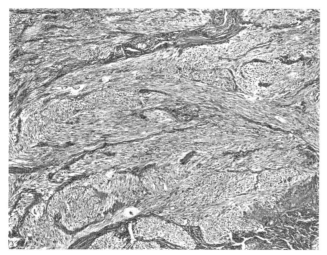

Figure 4.13.3   Lymphangiomyoma showing fascicular architecture, which can mimic leiomyoma.

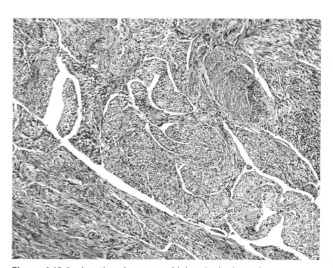

Figure 4.13.4   Lymphangiomyoma with lymphatic channels demonstrating irregular slit-like spaces.

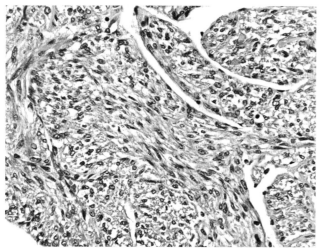

Figure 4.13.5   Lymphangiomyoma with typical cytologic features and lymphatic channels.

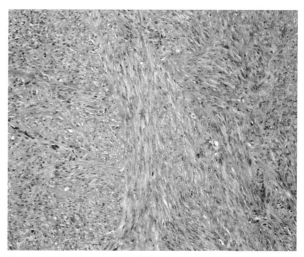

Figure 4.13.6   Leiomyoma with interlacing fascicles.

4   UTERINE CORPUS

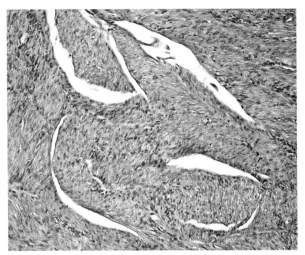

Figure 4.13.7 Leiomyoma with cleft-like spaces mimicking lymphangiomyoma.

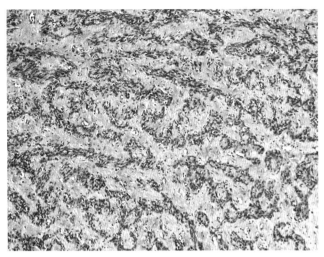

Figure 4.13.8 Leiomyoma demonstrating a sex cord–like pattern.

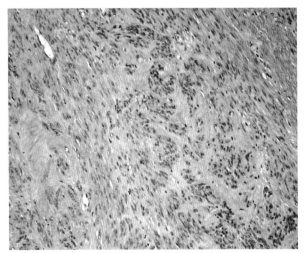

Figure 4.13.9 Leiomyoma with hyalinized stroma.

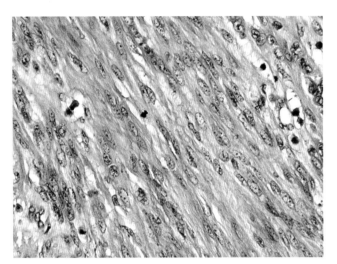

Figure 4.13.10 Leiomyoma showing spindle cells with eosinophilic cytoplasm.

	Inflammatory Myofibroblastic Tumor	Myxoid Leiomyosarcoma
Age	Usually premenopausal	Pre-, peri-, or postmenopausal
Location	Uterus	Uterus
Symptoms	Abnormal vaginal bleeding or pelvic pain/pressure	Abnormal vaginal bleeding and/or pelvic pain; clinical features can overlap with those of leiomyoma
Signs	Pelvic mass; gross mass within the myometrium	Pelvic mass; gross mass within the myometrium; clinical features can overlap with those of leiomyoma
Etiology	Similar to its nonuterine counterpart, inflammatory myofibroblastic tumor is associated with rearrangements of the *ALK* gene; other rearrangements, such as *ROS1* or *RET*, may be seen; rarely *NTRK3* rearrangements (described thus far in nongynecologic sites)	Pathogenesis unclear; a subset have *PLG1* rearrangements
Histology	1. Border may be smooth or infiltrative 2. Predominantly myxoid pattern (with fasciitis-like appearance) with minor fascicular component (with leiomyoma-like appearance); generally, myxoid areas are hypocelullar *(Figs. 4.14.1-4.14.3)* 3. Spindle- to stellate-shaped myofibroblastic cells with pale eosinophilic cytoplasm 4. Usually bland nuclei with evenly dispersed chromatin but may be vesicular with prominent nucleoli *(Fig. 4.14.4)* 5. Variable mitotic activity, but mitotic index is typically low 6. Edematous background with lymphocytes and plasma cells *(Fig. 4.14.5)* 7. No lymphovascular space invasion 8. Necrosis usually absent but has been described in a small subset of cases with aggressive behavior	1. Border may be smooth or infiltrative *(Fig. 4.14.6)* 2. Predominantly myxoid pattern; occasionally, may have component of conventional-type (spindle cell) or epithelioid leiomyosarcoma; cellularity of myxoid areas is variable but can be hypercellular *(Figs. 4.14.7 and 4.14.8)* 3. Spindle- to stellate-shaped cells often with scant cytoplasm 4. Hyperchromatic nuclei; nuclear atypia is variable *(Fig. 4.14.9)* 5. Variable mitotic index (may be low or high) 6. No significant inflammatory component 7. Lymphovascular space invasion can be present 8. Necrosis may be present *(Fig. 4.14.10)*
Special studies	• *ALK* (immunohistochemistry): positive in most cases • FISH: *ALK* rearrangement in most cases • Smooth muscle actin/desmin: variably positive • ER/PR: variably positive	• *ALK* (immunohistochemistry) (−) • FISH: no *ALK* rearrangement • Smooth muscle actin/desmin: variably positive • ER/PR: variably positive

	Inflammatory Myofibroblastic Tumor	**Myxoid Leiomyosarcoma**
Treatment	Myomectomy or hysterectomy	Hysterectomy, +/− bilateral salpingo-oophorectomy; further management is stage dependent but can include observation or chemotherapy and/or radiation therapy
Prognosis	Benign in most cases, but a small subset may exhibit aggressive behavior (histologic criteria for malignancy based on limited data); recurrences can occur, metastases are rare	Stage dependent; limited survival data for myxoid types (for conventional/spindle cell types, 5-y survival: 15%-25%); tumors are not graded as they are conventionally considered high grade

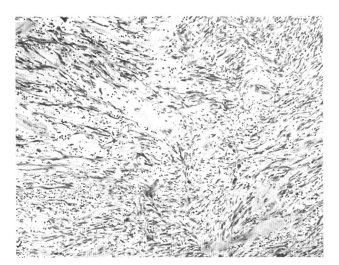

Figure 4.14.1 Inflammatory myofibroblastic tumor with myxoid stroma.

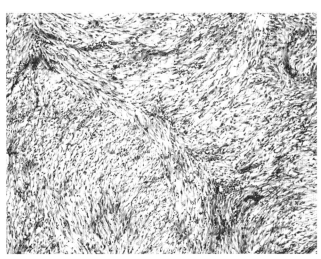

Figure 4.14.2 Inflammatory myofibroblastic tumor exhibiting fasciitis-like appearance.

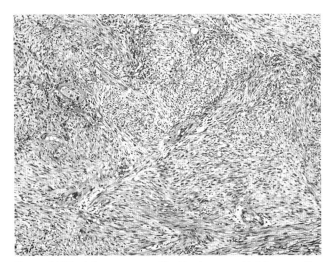

Figure 4.14.3 Inflammatory myofibroblastic tumor with leiomyoma-like morphology.

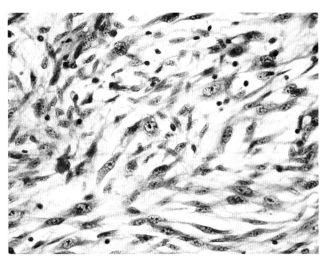

Figure 4.14.4 Inflammatory myofibroblastic tumor demonstrating atypical nuclei with ganglion cell–like features.

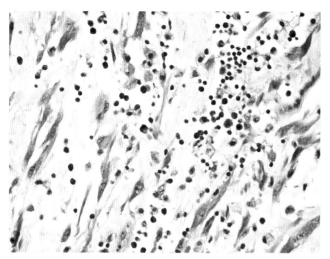

Figure 4.14.5 Inflammatory myofibroblastic tumor with inflammatory cells.

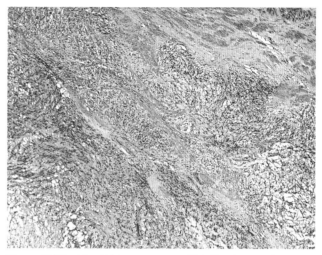

Figure 4.14.6 Myxoid leiomyosarcoma with infiltrating growth pattern.

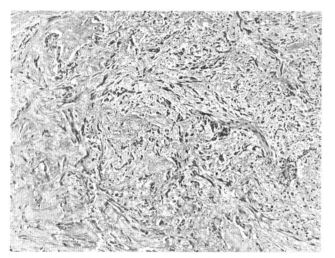

Figure 4.14.7 Myxoid leiomyosarcoma showing hypocellular appearance.

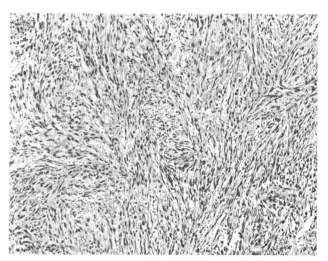

Figure 4.14.8 Myxoid leiomyosarcoma with cellular features.

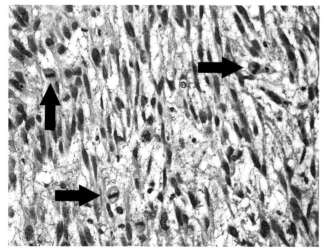

Figure 4.14.9 Myxoid leiomyosarcoma with atypia and mitotic figures (*arrows*).

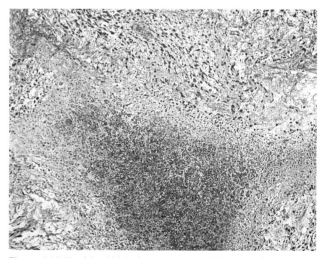

Figure 4.14.10 Myxoid leiomyosarcoma containing necrosis.

	Adenomatoid Tumor	Dilated Lymphatics/Veins
Age	Reproductive age	Variable
Location	Myometrium; also, broad ligament, adnexal soft tissue, and fallopian tube	Myometrium
Symptoms	No specific symptoms; usually incidental finding in hysterectomy specimen performed for other reasons	Dependent on reason for hysterectomy; dilated lymphatics/veins are an incidental finding
Signs	No specific signs; usually incidental finding in hysterectomy specimen performed for other reasons; typically small but can produce gross mass	Dependent on reason for hysterectomy; dilated lymphatics/veins are an incidental finding
Etiology	Mesothelial neoplasm; *TRAF7* mutations are common; an association with immunosuppression has been noted in some cases	Dilated lymphatics/veins within the myometrium, which can simulate adenomatoid tumor; incidental finding in hysterectomy specimens performed for variable indications
Histology	1. Circumscribed but can have irregular borders 2. Proliferation of cystically dilated tubules; tubules permeate between smooth muscle bundles *(Figs. 4.15.1-4.15.3)* 3. Tubules are empty 4. Tubules are lined by single layer of flat to low-cuboidal eosinophilic cells *(Fig. 4.15.4)* 5. Thin cytoplasmic strands may traverse the lumen of the tubule *(Fig. 4.15.4)* 6. Small cytoplasmic vacuoles can be present *(Fig. 4.15.5)* 7. Round to flat bland nuclei 8. Lymphoid aggregates may be present within stroma	1. Does not produce a mass or circumscribed lesion 2. Lymphatics/veins may be dilated and crowded *(Figs. 4.15.6 and 4.15.7)* 3. Lymphatics/veins may be empty or filled with serum or blood *(Figs. 4.15.8 and 4.15.9)* 4. Lymphatics/veins are lined by single layer of flat eosinophilic cells *(Fig. 4.15.10)* 5. No cytoplasmic strands traversing the lumen 6. No cytoplasmic vacuoles 7. Flat bland nuclei 8. No lymphoid aggregates
Special studies	• Cytokeratin: positive in tubules • Calretinin: diffuse expression in tubules • D2-40 (+)CD31 (−)	• Cytokeratin (−) • Calretinin: no diffuse expression • D2-40: +/−CD31: +/−
Treatment	Myomectomy or hysterectomy	None
Prognosis	Benign	Benign

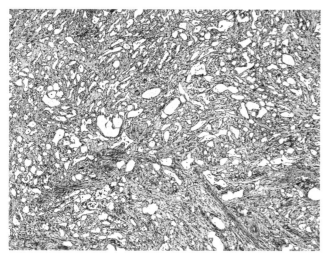

Figure 4.15.1 Adenomatoid tumor with markedly crowded tubules.

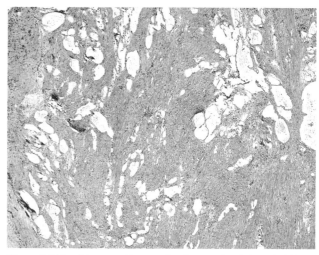

Figure 4.15.2 Adenomatoid tumor showing ectatic tubules mimicking dilated lymphatics/veins.

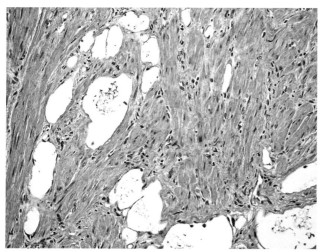

Figure 4.15.3 Adenomatoid tumor with tubules separated by smooth muscle.

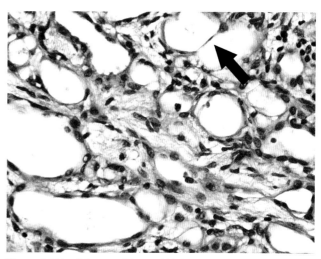

Figure 4.15.4 Adenomatoid tumor. Tubules are lined by flat eosinophilic cells containing oval to flat nuclei. Thin cytoplasmic strands bridging the diameter of the tubule are present (*arrow*).

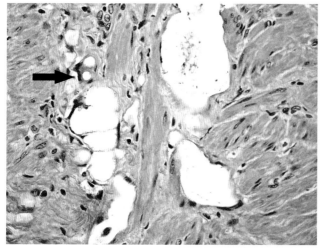

Figure 4.15.5 Adenomatoid tumor with cytoplasmic vacuoles (*arrow*).

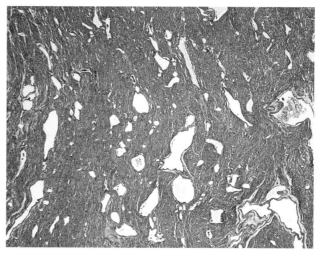

Figure 4.15.6 Abundant dilated lymphatics/veins, which may simulate adenomatoid tumor.

4 UTERINE CORPUS

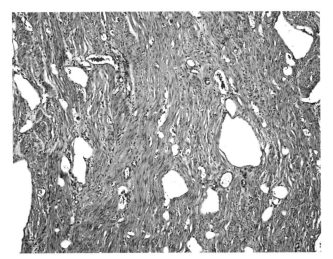

Figure 4.15.7   Dilated lymphatics/veins.

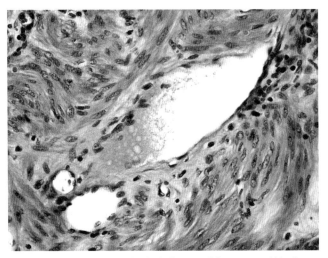

Figure 4.15.8   Dilated lymphatics/veins containing serum within the lumen.

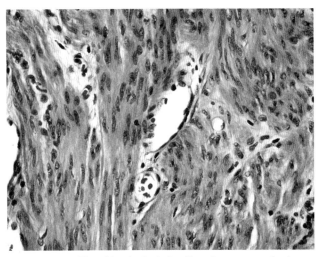

Figure 4.15.9   Dilated lymphatics/veins. Note the presence of red blood cells within the lumens.

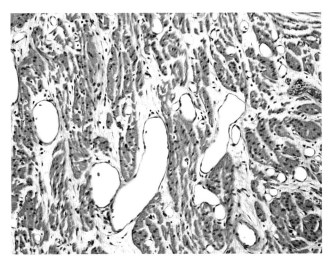

Figure 4.15.10   Dilated lymphatics/veins. The lining of the vessels does not contain the more prominent eosinophilic layer seen in adenomatoid tumor.

	Adenomatoid Tumor	**Lipoleiomyoma**
Age	Reproductive age	Most common in pre- or perimenopausal women
Location	Myometrium; also, broad ligament, adnexal soft tissue, and fallopian tube	Uterus
Symptoms	No specific symptoms; usually incidental finding in hysterectomy specimen performed for other reasons	Asymptomatic, menorrhagia, or pelvic pain/pressure
Signs	No specific signs; usually incidental finding in hysterectomy specimen performed for other reasons; typically small but can produce gross mass	May have enlarged uterus on clinical examination; gross mass (occasionally yellow) within myometrium
Etiology	Mesothelial neoplasm; *TRAF7* mutations are common; an association with immunosuppression has been noted in some cases	Leiomyoma with adipocytic differentiation
Histology	1. Circumscribed but can have irregular borders 2. Proliferation of cystically dilated tubules; tubules permeate between smooth muscle bundles *(Figs. 4.16.1-4.16.3)* 3. Tubules are lined by single layer of flat to low-cuboidal eosinophilic cells *(Fig. 4.16.4)* 4. Small cytoplasmic vacuoles can be present 5. Thin cytoplasmic strands may traverse the lumen of the tubule 6. Round to flat bland nuclei 7. Lymphoid aggregates may be present within stroma *(Fig. 4.16.5)*	1. Circumscribed border 2. Adipocytic component within background of conventional (spindle cell)-type leiomyoma with fascicular architecture; adipocytes may be separate or cluster together *(Figs. 4.16.6-4.16.8)* 3. No perceptible eosinophilic lining of adipocytic component *(Fig. 4.16.9)* 4. Cytoplasmic vacuoles occasionally can be seen 5. Thin cytoplasmic strands may be present between two back-to-back adipocytes *(Fig. 4.16.10)* 6. Nuclei lining adipocytic component imperceptible 7. No lymphoid aggregates, but occasional leiomyomas can have an inflammatory component
Special studies	• Cytokeratin: positive in tubules • Calretinin: diffuse expression in tubules • Smooth muscle actin/desmin: negative in tubules (positive in intervening myometrial smooth muscle bundles)	• Cytokeratin (−) • Calretinin: no diffuse expression • Smooth muscle actin/desmin: positive in smooth muscle component • S100 (+) in adipocytes
Treatment	Myomectomy or hysterectomy	Myomectomy or hysterectomy
Prognosis	Benign	Benign

303

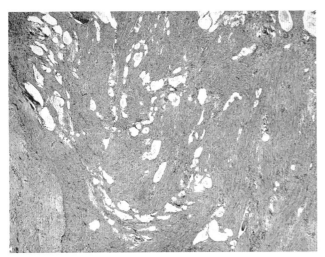

Figure 4.16.1 Adenomatoid tumor. This histologic appearance at low-power magnification can overlap with that of lipoleiomyoma.

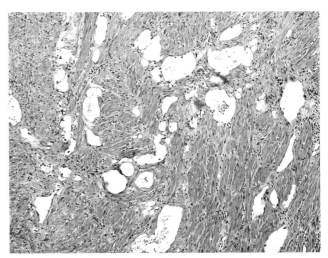

Figure 4.16.2 Adenomatoid tumor with proliferation of tubules.

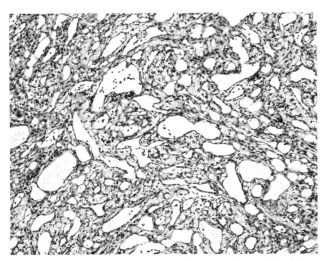

Figure 4.16.3 Adenomatoid tumor showing markedly crowded tubules.

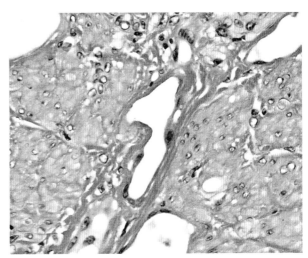

Figure 4.16.4 Adenomatoid tumor. The tubules are lined by a prominent eosinophilic flat layer.

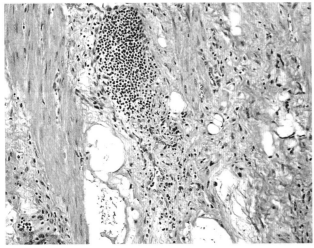

Figure 4.16.5 Adenomatoid tumor with lymphoid aggregates.

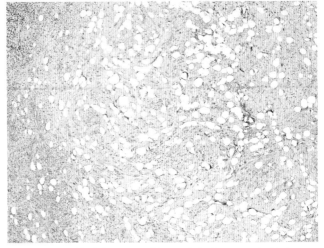

Figure 4.16.6 Lipoleiomyoma with crowded adipocytes. At this low-power magnification, the appearance can resemble an adenomatoid tumor.

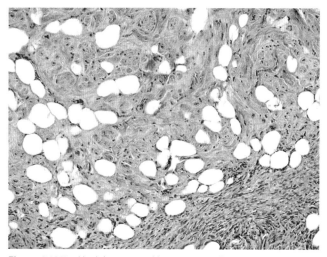

Figure 4.16.7 Lipoleiomyoma with numerous adipocytes.

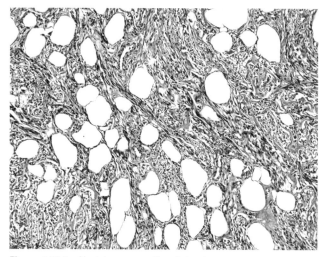

Figure 4.16.8 Lipoleiomyoma with cellular stroma.

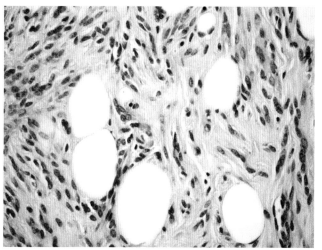

Figure 4.16.9 Lipoleiomyoma. The adipocytes lack the prominent eosinophilic flat layer seen in adenomatoid tumor.

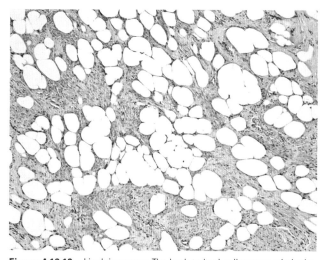

Figure 4.16.10 Lipoleiomyoma. The back-to-back adipocytes mimic the bridging cytoplasmic strands of adenomatoid tumor.

	Atypical Polypoid Adenomyoma (APA)	Invasive FIGO Grade 1 Endometrioid Carcinoma With Squamous Differentiation
Age	40 y (mean)	59–63 y (mean)
Location	Endometrium, commonly involving the lower uterine segment	Endometrium
Symptoms	Abnormal vaginal bleeding	Abnormal vaginal bleeding
Signs	Polypoid mass on hysteroscopy	Pelvic mass in some advanced stage cases; polypoid mass may be present at hysteroscopy or in gross specimen
Etiology	Biphasic lesion composed of benign (atypical) glands and benign mesenchymal component	Estrogen-driven pathogenesis with hyperplasia evolving to carcinoma
Histology	1. Glands within myomatous or myofibromatous stroma (Figs. 4.17.1-4.17.3) 2. Glands may demonstrate lobular architecture (Fig. 4.17.4) 3. Glandular crowding resembling hyperplasia, but myomatous/myofibromatous stroma present between glands; usually no confluent (cribriform or papillary) growth; however, focal FIGO grade 1 endometrioid carcinoma can arise within a small subset of APAs (Fig. 4.17.5) 4. Cytologic atypia may or may not be evident (Fig. 4.17.6) 5. Squamous morular metaplasia (characteristic feature) (Fig. 4.17.7)	1. Glands may be associated with desmoplastic stroma (Fig. 4.17.8) 2. No lobular architecture; glands can display haphazard arrangement within myometrium (Fig. 4.17.9) 3. Confluent (cribriform or papillary) growth typically present elsewhere (Fig. 4.17.10) 4. Cytologic atypia usually present, but glands can be deceptively bland 5. Squamous morules present in a subset of cases
Special studies	Immunohistochemistry usually of no help for this differential diagnosis although some studies suggest that p16 and SATB2 are more frequently expressed in the stroma of APA	Immunohistochemistry usually of no help for this differential diagnosis although some studies suggest that p16 and SATB2 are less frequently expressed in the stroma of myoinvasive carcinoma
Treatment	Hysterectomy or polypectomy; background (nonpolyp) endometrium should be evaluated for associated hyperplasia or endometrioid carcinoma	Dependent on stage and other risk factors; may include observation, hysterectomy with bilateral salpingo-oophorectomy, surgical staging, chemotherapy, and/or radiation therapy
Prognosis	Benign; however, patients have an associated increased (low) risk for endometrial carcinoma	Dependent on stage and other risk factors

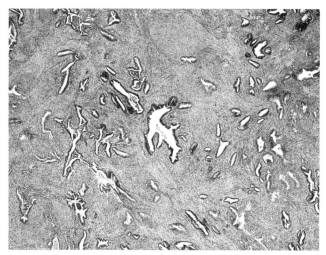

Figure 4.17.1 Atypical polypoid adenomyoma (APA). Crowded glands are present within myofibromatous stroma simulating invasive carcinoma.

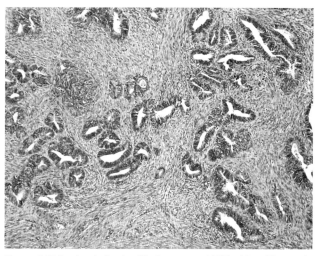

Figure 4.17.2 Atypical polypoid adenomyoma (APA) with architectural features mimicking FIGO grade 1 endometrioid carcinoma.

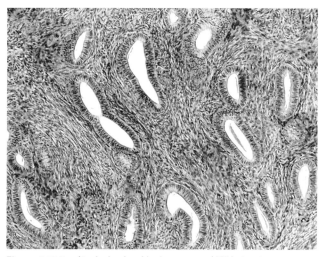

Figure 4.17.3 Atypical polypoid adenomyoma (APA) showing myofibromatous stroma.

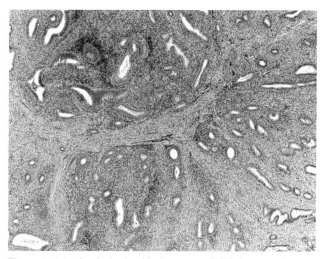

Figure 4.17.4 Atypical polypoid adenomyoma (APA) demonstrating lobular architecture.

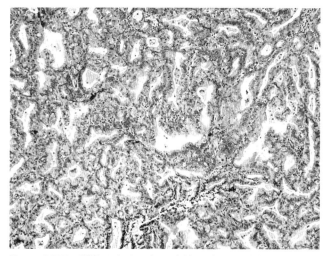

Figure 4.17.5 FIGO grade 1 endometrioid carcinoma arising within an atypical polypoid adenomyoma (APA). The APA is not illustrated in this field.

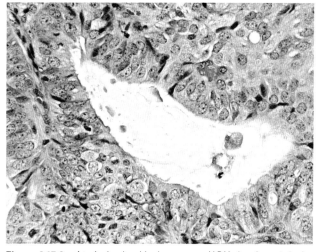

Figure 4.17.6 Atypical polypoid adenomyoma (APA) showing cytologic atypia similar to that seen in atypical hyperplasia.

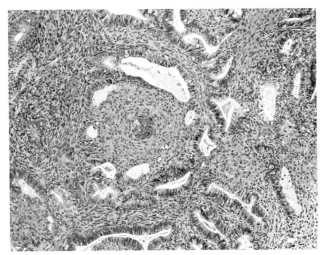

Figure 4.17.7 Atypical polypoid adenomyoma (APA) with squamous morular metaplasia (most evident in **center**).

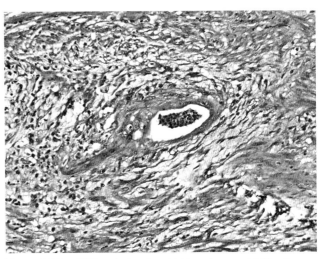

Figure 4.17.8 FIGO grade 1 endometrioid carcinoma exhibiting the MELF (microcystic, elongated, and fragmented) glandular pattern.

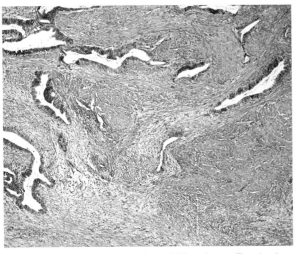

Figure 4.17.9 FIGO grade 1 endometrioid carcinoma. The glands are haphazardly arranged within altered stroma.

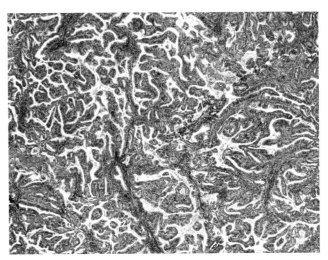

Figure 4.17.10 FIGO grade 1 endometrioid carcinoma with complex papillary growth pattern.

	Adenosarcoma	**Adenofibroma**
Age	Usually postmenopausal	Usually postmenopausal
Location	Uterus	Endometrium
Symptoms	Abnormal vaginal bleeding	Abnormal vaginal bleeding
Signs	Pelvic mass may be present; gross mass within endometrial cavity; cut surface may have a cystic component	Polypoid lesion within endometrial cavity
Etiology	Biphasic neoplasm with benign glands and malignant mesenchymal component; relatively much more common than adenofibroma	Biphasic neoplasm with benign glands and benign mesenchymal component; adenofibroma is not recognized in the 2020 WHO Classification, and some cases diagnosed as such may represent adenofibromatous polyps (or atypical adenofibromatous polyps with features falling short of a diagnosis of adenosarcoma; also see Section 4.19)
Histology	1. Polypoid configuration 2. Benign glandular component (variable in size and shape); may have metaplastic-type changes 3. Intraglandular polypoid projections with leaf-like or phyllodes-type architecture *(Fig. 4.18.1)* 4. Periglandular or subepithelial stromal condensation *(Figs. 4.18.2 and 4.18.3)* 5. Cellularity of mesenchymal component can vary but, in general, is hypercellular *(Figs. 4.18.3 and 4.18.4)* 6. Cells of mesenchymal component may resemble those of low-grade endometrial stromal sarcoma or have fibroblastic morphology 7. Atypia of mesenchymal component varies from none/minimal to low grade *(Fig. 4.18.5)* 8. Mitotic figures can be found (particularly in areas of periglandular or subepithelial stromal condensation), but mitotic index is usually low (2-4 mitotic figures per 10 high-power fields)	1. Polypoid configuration 2. Benign glandular component (variable in size and shape); may have metaplastic-type changes *(Fig. 4.18.6)* 3. Intraglandular polypoid projections with leaf-like or phyllodes-type architecture *(Figs. 4.18.7 and 4.18.8)* 4. No periglandular or subepithelial stromal condensation *(Fig. 4.18.9)* 5. Mesenchymal component not cellular 6. Cells of mesenchymal component have fibroblastic morphology 7. No atypia of mesenchymal component *(Fig. 4.18.10)* 8. No mitotic activity in adenofibroma
Special studies	Immunohistochemistry of no help for this differential diagnosis	Immunohistochemistry of no help for this differential diagnosis
Treatment	Hysterectomy and bilateral salpingo-oophorectomy	Hysterectomy or polypectomy
Prognosis	Dependent on stage and other risk factors; 5-y survival: ~80%	Benign

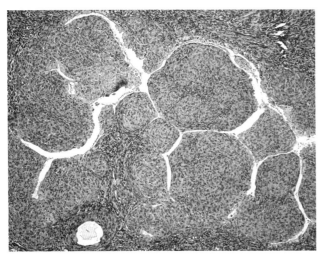

Figure 4.18.1   Adenosarcoma with leaf-like architecture.

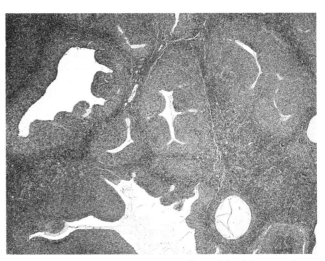

Figure 4.18.2   Adenosarcoma demonstrating periglandular stromal condensation.

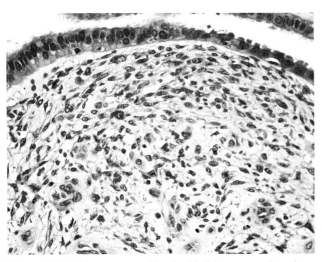

Figure 4.18.3   Adenosarcoma with subepithelial stroma condensation.

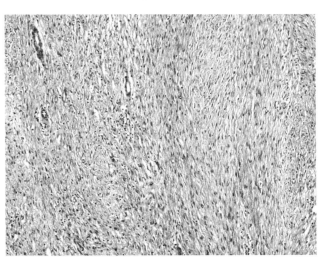

Figure 4.18.4   Adenosarcoma with hypocellular stroma resembling adenofibroma.

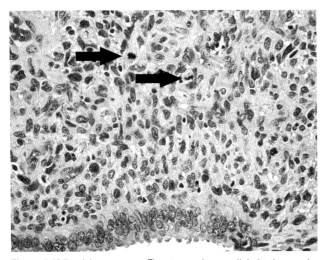

Figure 4.18.5   Adenosarcoma. The stroma shows cellularity, low-grade atypia, and mitotic activity (*arrows*).

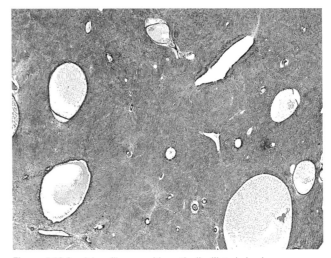

Figure 4.18.6   Adenofibroma with cystically dilated glands.

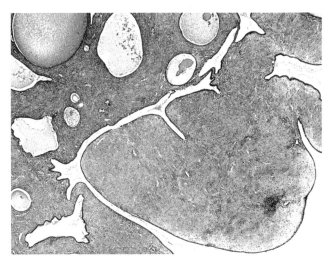

Figure 4.18.7   Adenofibroma with leaf-like architecture.

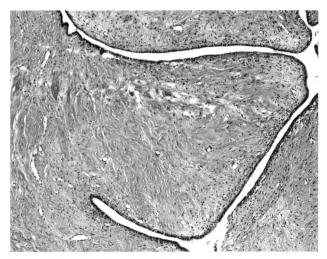

Figure 4.18.8   Adenofibroma with leaf-like architecture.

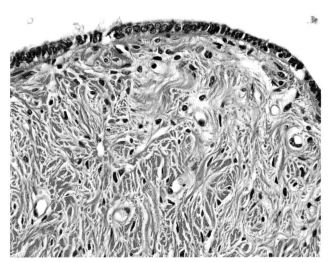

Figure 4.18.9   Adenofibroma without subepithelial stromal condensation.

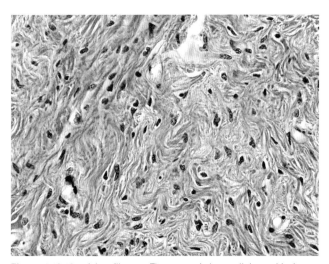

Figure 4.18.10   Adenofibroma. The stroma is hypocellular and lacks atypia and mitotic activity.

	Adenosarcoma	**Benign Endometrial Polyp**
Age	Usually postmenopausal	Pre- and postmenopausal
Location	Uterus	Endometrium
Symptoms	Abnormal vaginal bleeding	Abnormal vaginal bleeding
Signs	Pelvic mass may be present; gross mass within endometrial cavity; cut surface may have a cystic component; usually >3 cm	Polypoid lesion within endometrial cavity; usually <3 cm
Etiology	Biphasic neoplasm with benign glands and malignant mesenchymal component; pathogenesis unclear	Pathogenesis thought to be related to estrogen stimulation
Histology	1. Polypoid configuration 2. Benign glandular component (variable in size and shape); may have metaplastic-type changes *(Fig. 4.19.1)* 3. Intraglandular polypoid projections with leaf-like or phyllodes-type architecture *(Figs. 4.19.2 and 4.19.3)* 4. Periglandular or subepithelial stromal condensation *(Fig. 4.19.4)* 5. Cellularity of mesenchymal component can vary but, in general, is hypercellular 6. Cells of mesenchymal component may resemble those of low-grade endometrial stromal sarcoma or have fibroblastic morphology 7. Atypia of mesenchymal component varies from none/minimal to low grade *(Fig. 4.19.5)* 8. Mitotic figures can be found (particularly in areas of periglandular or subepithelial stromal condensation), but mitotic index is usually low (2-4 mitotic figures per 10 high-power fields)	1. Polypoid configuration *(Fig. 4.19.6)* 2. Benign glandular component (variable in size and shape); may have metaplastic-type changes 3. Small subset of benign endometrial polyps may have incompletely developed leaf-like architecture, which will be focal rather than diffuse *(Figs. 4.19.7 and 4.19.8)* 4. Small subset of benign endometrial polyps may have incompletely developed periglandular or subepithelial stromal condensation, which will be focal rather than diffuse *(Figs. 4.19.7 and 4.19.8)* 5. Cellularity of mesenchymal component varies but can be hypercellular 6. Cells of mesenchymal component may have fibroblastic or endometrial stroma-type morphology 7. Usually no atypia of mesenchymal component; however, a small subset of endometrial polyps can have atypical (bizarre) cells with enlarged nuclei and smudgy chromatin (without nucleoli or mitotic activity) *(Figs. 4.19.9 and 4.19.10)* 8. Usually no mitotic activity, but some benign endometrial polyps can have mitotically active stroma
Special studies	Immunohistochemistry of no help for this differential diagnosis	Immunohistochemistry of no help for this differential diagnosis

	Adenosarcoma	**Benign Endometrial Polyp**
Treatment	Hysterectomy and bilateral salpingo-oophorectomy	Polypectomy; in cases having some features that can raise concern for adenosarcoma (but in which the findings are insufficient for that diagnosis in the current specimen), clinical correlation is advised to assess whether the entire lesion has been removed
Prognosis	Dependent on stage and other risk factors; 5-y survival: ~80%	Benign

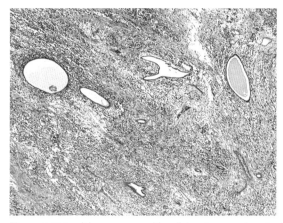

Figure 4.19.1   Adenosarcoma with cellular stroma and cystically dilated glands.

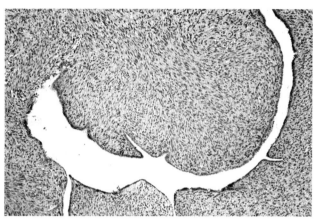

Figure 4.19.2   Adenosarcoma with well-developed leaf-like architecture.

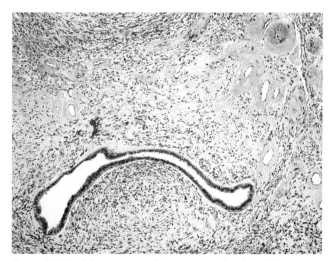

Figure 4.19.3   Adenosarcoma with suggestion of early leaf-like architecture.

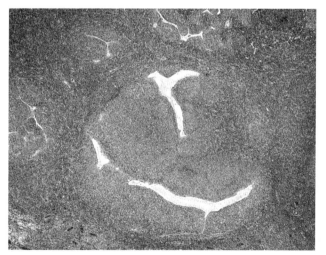

Figure 4.19.4   Adenosarcoma showing periglandular stromal condensation.

4   UTERINE CORPUS

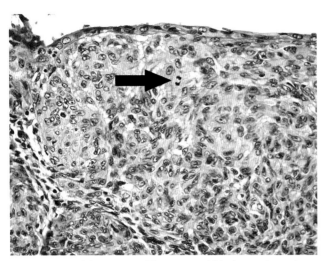

Figure 4.19.5 Adenosarcoma. The stroma exhibits low-grade atypia and mitotic activity (*arrow*).

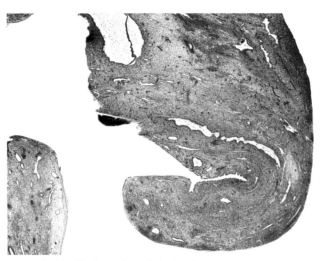

Figure 4.19.6 Benign endometrial polyp. Low-power appearance showing polypoid fragments of endometrial glands and stroma.

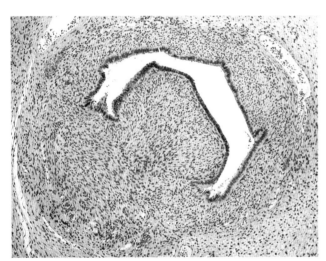

Figure 4.19.7 Benign endometrial polyp with periglandular stromal condensation and intraglandular polypoid projection simulating early changes of adenosarcoma.

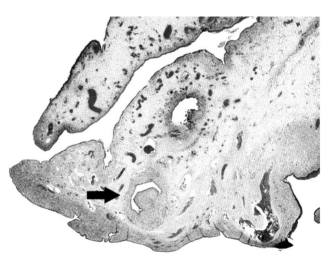

Figure 4.19.8 Benign endometrial polyp with periglandular stromal condensation and intraglandular polypoid projection simulating early changes of adenosarcoma. These combined findings were only focally present (*arrow*) in this endometrial polyp (same case as *Fig. 4.19.7*).

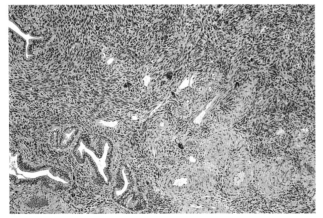

Figure 4.19.9 Benign endometrial polyp with cellular stroma and focally bizarre (symplastic) atypia **(center)**.

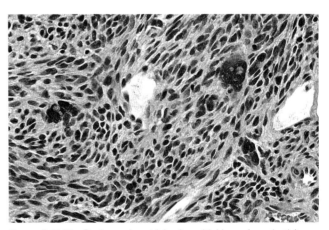

Figure 4.19.10 Benign endometrial polyp with bizarre (symplastic) atypia (same case as *Fig. 4.19.9*). Note the presence of intranuclear inclusions and smudgy chromatin in the enlarged atypical nuclei.

	Adenosarcoma With Sarcomatous Overgrowth	MMMT
Age	Postmenopausal	Postmenopausal
Location	Endometrium; can occur elsewhere in the gynecologic tract	Endometrium; can occur elsewhere in the gynecologic tract
Symptoms	Abnormal vaginal bleeding	Abnormal vaginal bleeding
Signs	Uterine enlargement or pelvic mass; polypoid mass in gross specimen	Uterine enlargement or pelvic mass; polypoid mass may be present at hysteroscopy or in gross specimen
Etiology	Biphasic epithelial-mesenchymal neoplasm, in which the sarcoma (low-grade) component of adenosarcoma undergoes high-grade transformation resulting in a high-grade sarcoma component in a background of conventional adenosarcoma	Biphasic epithelial-mesenchymal neoplasm, in which the sarcoma component is clonally related to the carcinoma component and believed to arise from the latter; *TP53* mutations common; a small subset of MMMTs is thought to evolve from adenosarcoma *(Fig. 4.20.6)*
Histology	1. Background of biphasic tumor composed of conventional adenosarcoma (benign epithelial component and malignant [low-grade] mesenchymal component) *(Figs. 4.20.1 and 4.20.2)* 2. No carcinoma component present 3. Additional pure poorly differentiated sarcoma component with high-grade nuclei and high mitotic index (proportion of sarcomatous overgrowth accounting for entire tumor is variable, but some authors reserve this diagnosis when the pure sarcoma component accounts for ≥25% of the tumor); heterologous types can occur *(Figs. 4.20.3-4.20.5)*	1. Biphasic appearance with intimate admixture of carcinoma and sarcoma components *(Figs. 4.20.7 and 4.20.8)* 2. High-grade carcinoma component is typically serous, endometrioid, or unclassified; other histologic types of carcinoma can occur *(Figs. 4.20.8 and 4.20.9)* 3. High-grade sarcoma component (with high-grade nuclei and high mitotic index) may be unclassified or of a specific type (eg, rhabdomyosarcoma, chondrosarcoma, etc.) *(Figs. 4.20.8 and 4.20.10)*
Special studies	• Immunohistochemistry of no help in assessment of sarcoma component • p53: no abnormal expression pattern (complete absence of expression or diffuse staining) in epithelial component • p16: no diffuse expression in epithelial component • Ki-67 index: low in epithelial component	• Immunohistochemistry of no help in assessment of sarcoma component • p53: often abnormal expression pattern (complete absence of expression or diffuse staining) in carcinoma component (if serous) • p16: often diffuse expression in carcinoma component (if serous) • Ki-67 index: high in carcinoma component

	Adenosarcoma With Sarcomatous Overgrowth	**MMMT**
Treatment	Specific treatment guidelines unclear; usually managed similar to other high-grade uterine sarcomas	Dependent on stage and other risk factors; may include hysterectomy with bilateral salpingo-oophorectomy and surgical staging, chemotherapy, and/or radiation therapy
Prognosis	Poor survival, similar to MMMT	5-y survival: 30%-40%; dependent on stage and other risk factors

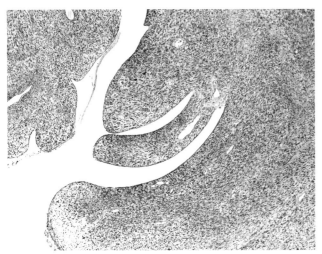

Figure 4.20.1 Adenosarcoma with leaf-like architecture from a case of adenosarcoma with sarcomatous overgrowth (*high-grade component not shown*).

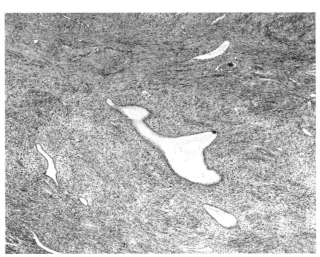

Figure 4.20.2 Adenosarcoma with benign glandular component from a case of adenosarcoma with sarcomatous overgrowth (*high-grade component not shown*).

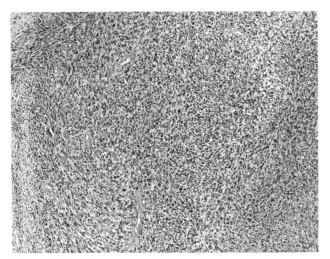

Figure 4.20.3 Adenosarcoma with sarcomatous overgrowth showing sheets of high-grade sarcoma without any glandular component.

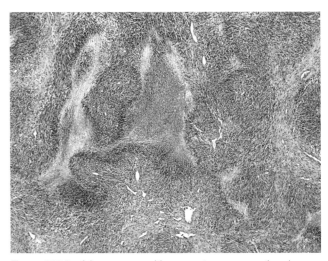

Figure 4.20.4 Adenosarcoma with sarcomatous overgrowth and geographic necrosis.

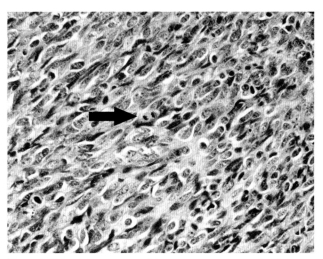

Figure 4.20.5 Adenosarcoma with sarcomatous overgrowth. High-grade nuclei and mitotic activity (*arrow*) are present.

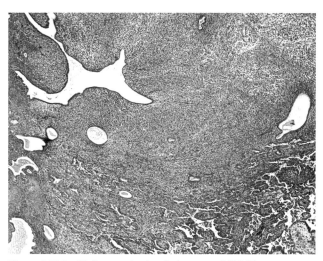

Figure 4.20.6 Malignant mixed müllerian tumor (MMMT; carcinosarcoma) **(lower right)** arising within an adenosarcoma **(upper left)**.

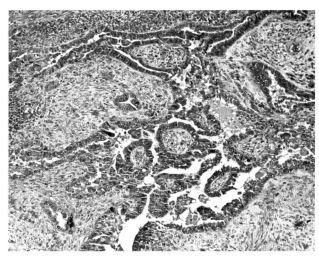

Figure 4.20.7 Malignant mixed müllerian tumor (MMMT; carcinosarcoma). Malignant glandular and stromal components are present.

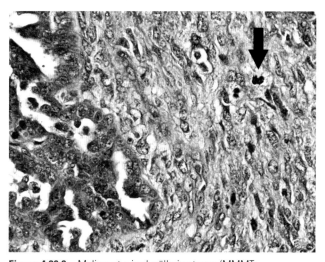

Figure 4.20.8 Malignant mixed müllerian tumor (MMMT; carcinosarcoma) showing high-grade glandular and stromal components with mitotic activity (*arrow*).

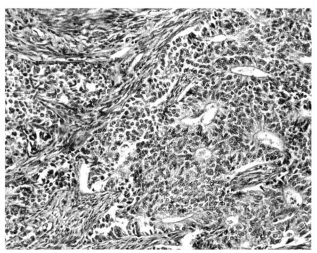

Figure 4.20.9 Malignant mixed müllerian tumor (MMMT; carcinosarcoma). The glandular component in this case consists of endometrioid carcinoma.

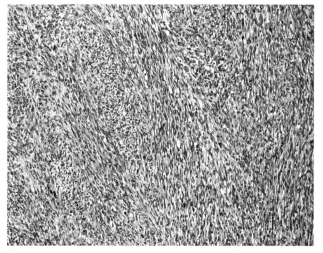

Figure 4.20.10 Malignant mixed müllerian tumor (MMMT; carcinosarcoma). The mesenchymal component in this case consists of a high-grade sarcoma with spindle cell differentiation.

4   UTERINE CORPUS

	Uterine Artery Embolization Gelatin Microspheres	Dilated Lymphatics/Veins
Age	Most patients premenopausal	Variable
Location	Intravascular spaces within infarcted leiomyomas or nonneoplastic myometrium; can be occasionally seen in broad ligament, ovarian hilar vessels, fallopian tube vessels, and endometrium	Myometrium
Symptoms	Typical symptoms related to uterine leiomyomas; no specific symptoms due to microspheres	Dependent on reason for hysterectomy; dilated lymphatics/veins are an incidental finding
Signs	Typical clinical and gross findings related to uterine leiomyomas; specific signs related to microspheres usually not present although, occasionally, small microspheres can been seen within the myometrial wall	Dependent on reason for hysterectomy; dilated lymphatics/veins are an incidental finding
Etiology	Intravascular foreign material used for embolization of uterine leiomyomas; when microspheres are not within the plane of section, the appearance can simulate dilated lymphatics/veins	Dilated lymphatics/veins within the myometrium; incidental finding in hysterectomy specimens performed for variable indications
Histology	1. Enlarged vascular spaces (thick-walled arteries as well as smaller-caliber vessels) are round and uniform; when microspheres are in extravascular locations, the resulting cystic spaces may cluster together *(Figs. 4.21.1 and 4.21.2)* 2. Inflammatory response, including multinucleated giant cells, may surround enlarged vascular spaces 3. Enlarged vascular spaces may contain microspheres (mean diameter: 0.43 mm); the former often rigid and conform to the shape of the microspheres *(Fig. 4.21.3)*; microspheres are round, homogeneous, and pale eosinophilic with appearance similar to colloid *(Fig. 4.21.4)*; microspheres may appear folded; sometimes, only fragments of microspheres remain within predominantly empty spaces *(Figs. 4.21.2 and 4.21.5)*	1. Lymphatics/veins may be dilated and crowded *(Figs. 4.21.6 and 4.21.7)*; they may be of variable size and shape (often not as round and uniform as spaces containing microspheres) 2. Usually no associated inflammatory response 3. Lymphatics/veins may be empty or filled with serum or blood *(Fig. 4.21.8)*
Special studies	PAS histochemical stains can highlight microspheres if present within vessels (positive staining at peripheral rim of microspheres)	Special stains of no use if microspheres are not present in vessels
Treatment	No specific treatment for microspheres	None
Prognosis	Benign	Benign

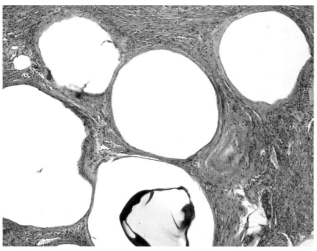

Figure 4.21.1 Uterine artery embolization gelatin microspheres. The myometrium contains rigid spaces, which are mostly empty. Focal residual embolization material is present **(lower center)**.

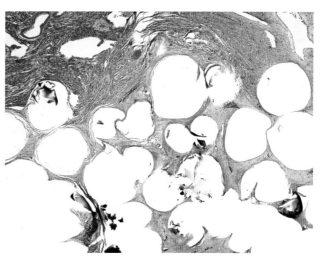

Figure 4.21.2 Uterine artery embolization gelatin microspheres. The myometrium contains rigid spaces that are clustered together. The spaces are predominantly empty but focally contain residual embolization material.

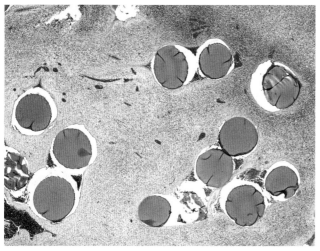

Figure 4.21.3 Numerous intact uterine artery embolization gelatin microspheres are present within a cellular leiomyoma.

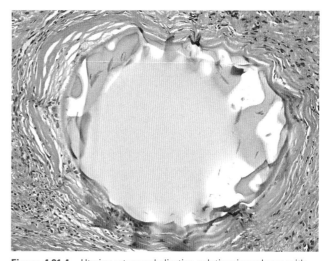

Figure 4.21.4 Uterine artery embolization gelatin microspheres with typical morphologic appearance and associated mild inflammation.

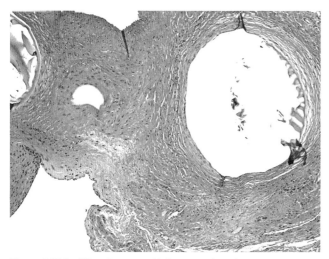

Figure 4.21.5 Dilated spaces with fragmented uterine artery embolization gelatin microspheres.

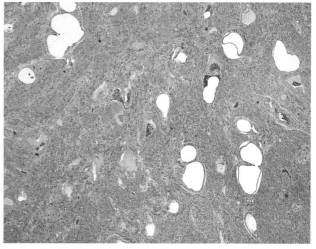

Figure 4.21.6 Dilated lymphatics/veins.

4 UTERINE CORPUS

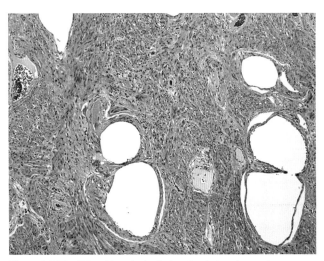

Figure 4.21.7   Dilated lymphatics/veins simulating clustered empty rigid spaces that may be seen in cases of uterine artery embolization gelatin microspheres.

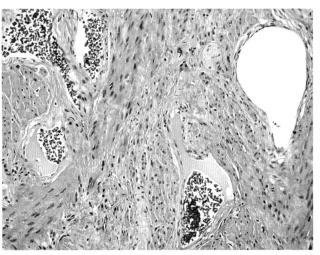

Figure 4.21.8   Dilated lymphatics/veins containing serum (morphologically similar to the material of uterine artery embolization gelatin microspheres) and red blood cells.

SUGGESTED READINGS

4.1 and 4.2

Bell SW, Kempson RL, Hendrickson MR. Problematic uterine smooth muscle neoplasms. A clinicopathologic study of 213 cases. *Am J Surg Pathol.* 1994;18:535-558.

Bennett JA, Lamb C, Young RH. Apoplectic leiomyomas: a morphologic analysis of 100 cases highlighting unusual features. *Am J Surg Pathol.* 2016;40:563-568.

Croce S, Young RH, Oliva E. Uterine leiomyomas with bizarre nuclei: a clinicopathologic study of 59 cases. *Am J Surg Pathol.* 2014;38:1330-1339.

Ip PPC, Bennett JA, Croce S, et al. Tumours of the uterine corpus: uterine leiomyoma. In: WHO Classification of Tumours Editorial Board, ed. *Female Genital Tumours. WHO Classification of Tumours.* 5th ed. International Agency for Research on Cancer; 2020:272-226.

Ip PPC, Croce S, Gupta M. Tumours of the uterine corpus: smooth muscle tumor of uncertain malignant potential of the uterine corpus. In: WHO Classification of Tumours Editorial Board, ed. *Female Genital Tumours. WHO Classification of Tumours.* 5th ed. International Agency for Research on Cancer; 2020:279-280.

Kempson RL, Hendrickson MR. Smooth muscle, endometrial stromal, and mixed Müllerian tumors of the uterus. *Mod Pathol.* 2000;13:328-342.

Ly A, Mills AM, McKenney JK, et al. Atypical leiomyomas of the uterus: a clinicopathologic study of 51 cases. *Am J Surg Pathol.* 2013;37:643-649.

Mittal KR, Chen F, Wei JJ, et al. Molecular and immunohistochemical evidence for the origin of uterine leiomyosarcomas from associated leiomyoma and symplastic leiomyoma-like areas. *Mod Pathol.* 2009;22:1303-1311.

Myles JL, Hart WR. Apoplectic leiomyomas of the uterus. A clinicopathologic study of five distinctive hemorrhagic leiomyomas associated with oral contraceptive usage. *Am J Surg Pathol.* 1985;9:798-805.

4.3

Carr RJ, Hui P, Buza N. Intravenous leiomyomatosis revisited: an experience of 14 cases at a single medical center. *Int J Gynecol Pathol.* 2015;34:169-176.

Clement PB, Young RH, Scully RE. Intravenous leiomyomatosis of the uterus. A clinicopathological analysis of 16 cases with unusual histologic features. *Am J Surg Pathol.* 1988;12:932-945.

Du J, Zhao X, Guo D, et al. Intravenous leiomyomatosis of the uterus: a clinicopathologic study of 18 cases, with emphasis on early diagnosis and appropriate treatment strategies. *Hum Pathol.* 2011;42:1240-1246.

Lu B, Liu Q, Tang L, et al. Intravenous leiomyomatosis: molecular analysis of 17 cases. *Pathology.* 2020;52:213-217.

Mittal KR, Chen F, Wei JJ, et al. Molecular and immunohistochemical evidence for the origin of uterine leiomyosarcomas from associated leiomyoma and symplastic leiomyoma-like areas. *Mod Pathol.* 2009;22:1303-1311.

Mulvany NJ, Slavin JL, Ostör AG, et al. Intravenous leiomyomatosis of the uterus: a clinicopathologic study of 22 cases. *Int J Gynecol Pathol.* 1994;13:1-9.

Norris HJ, Parmley T. Mesenchymal tumors of the uterus. V. Intravenous leiomyomatosis. A clinical and pathologic study of 14 cases. *Cancer.* 1975;36:2164-2178.

Ordulu Z, Chai H, Peng G, et al. Molecular and clinicopathologic characterization of intravenous leiomyomatosis. *Mod Pathol.* 2020;33:1844-1860.

Ordulu Z, Nucci MR, Dal Cin P, et al. Intravenous leiomyomatosis: an unusual intermediate between benign and malignant uterine smooth muscle tumors. *Mod Pathol.* 2016;29:500-510.

Roth LM, Reed RJ. Dissecting leiomyomas of the uterus other than cotyledonoid dissecting leiomyomas: a report of eight cases. *Am J Surg Pathol.* 1999;23:1032-1039.

Roth LM, Reed RJ, Sternberg WH. Cotyledonoid dissecting leiomyoma of the uterus. The Sternberg tumor. *Am J Surg Pathol.* 1996;20:1455-1461.

Wang L, Hu S, Xin F, et al. MED12 exon 2 mutation is uncommon in intravenous leiomyomatosis: clinicopathologic features and molecular study. *Hum Pathol.* 2020;99:36-42.

4.4

Chapel DB, Nucci MR, Quade BJ, et al. Epithelioid leiomyosarcoma of the uterus: modern outcome-based appraisal of diagnostic criteria in a large institutional series. *Am J Surg Pathol.* 2022;46:464-475.

Chiang S, Samore W, Zhang L, et al. PGR gene fusions identify a molecular subset of uterine epithelioid leiomyosarcoma with rhabdoid features. *Am J Surg Pathol.* 2019;43:810-818.

Kurman RJ, Norris HJ. Mesenchymal tumors of the uterus. VI. Epithelioid smooth muscle tumors including leiomyoblastoma and clear-cell leiomyoma: a clinical and pathologic analysis of 26 cases. *Cancer.* 1976;37:1853-1865.

Prayson RA, Goldblum JR, Hart WR. Epithelioid smooth-muscle tumors of the uterus: a clinicopathologic study of 18 patients. *Am J Surg Pathol.* 1997;21:383-391.

4.5

Dionigi A, Oliva E, Clement PB, et al. Endometrial stromal nodules and endometrial stromal tumors with limited infiltration: a clinicopathologic study of 50 cases. *Am J Surg Pathol.* 2002;26:567-581.

Oliva E, Clement PB, Young RH, et al. Mixed endometrial stromal and smooth muscle tumors of the uterus: a clinicopathologic study of 15 cases. *Am J Surg Pathol.* 1998;22:997-1005.

Oliva E, Young RH, Amin MB, et al. An immunohistochemical analysis of endometrial stromal and smooth muscle tumors of the uterus: a study of 54 cases emphasizing the importance of using a panel because of overlap in immunoreactivity for individual antibodies. *Am J Surg Pathol.* 2002;26:403-412.

Oliva E, Young RH, Clement PB, et al. Cellular benign mesenchymal tumors of the uterus. Comparative morphologic and immunohistochemical analysis of 33 highly cellular leiomyomas and six endometrial stromal nodules, two frequently confused tumors. *Am J Surg Pathol.* 1995;19:757-768.

Tavassoli FA, Norris HJ. Mesenchymal tumours of the uterus. VII. A clinicopathological study of 60 endometrial stromal nodules. *Histopathology.* 1981;5:1-10.

4.6

Chang KL, Crabtree GS, Lim-Tan SK, et al. Primary uterine endometrial stromal neoplasms. A clinicopathologic study of 117 cases. *Am J Surg Pathol.* 1990;14:415-438.

Conklin CM, Longacre TA. Endometrial stromal tumors: the new WHO classification. *Adv Anat Pathol.* 2014;21:383-393.

Dionigi A, Oliva E, Clement PB, et al. Endometrial stromal nodules and endometrial stromal tumors with limited infiltration: a clinicopathologic study of 50 cases. *Am J Surg Pathol.* 2002;26:567-581.

Lee CH, Nucci MR. Endometrial stromal sarcoma—the new genetic paradigm. *Histopathology.* 2015;67:1-19.

Moore M, McCluggage WG. Uterine endometrial stromal tumors with limited infiltration: first report of a case series indicating potential for malignant behavior. *Int J Gynecol Pathol.* 2020;39:221-226.

4.7-4.9

Clement PB. The pathology of endometriosis: a survey of the many faces of a common disease emphasizing diagnostic pitfalls and unusual and newly appreciated aspects. *Adv Anat Pathol.* 2007;14:241-260.

Clement PB, Scully RE. Endometrial stromal sarcomas of the uterus with extensive endometrioid glandular differentiation: a report of three cases that caused problems in differential diagnosis. *Int J Gynecol Pathol.* 1992;11:163-173.

Clement PB, Scully RE. Mullerian adenosarcoma of the uterus: a clinicopathologic analysis of 100 cases with a review of the literature. *Hum Pathol.* 1990;21:363-381.

Goldblum JR, Clement PB, Hart WR. Adenomyosis with sparse glands. A potential mimic of low-grade endometrial stromal sarcoma. *Am J Clin Pathol.* 1995;103:218-223.

McCluggage WG, Ganesan R, Herrington CS. Endometrial stromal sarcomas with extensive endometrioid glandular differentiation: report of a series with emphasis on the potential for misdiagnosis and discussion of the differential diagnosis. *Histopathology.* 2009;54:365-373.

4.10

Chiang S, Croce S, Lee CH, et al. Tumours of the uterine corpus: High-grade endometrial stromal sarcoma. In: WHO Classification of Tumours Editorial Board, ed. *Female Genital Tumours. WHO Classification of Tumours.* 5th ed. International Agency for Research on Cancer; 2020:289-291.

Chiang S, Lee CH, Stewart CJR, et al. BCOR is a robust diagnostic immunohistochemical marker of genetically diverse high-grade endometrial stromal sarcoma, including tumors exhibiting variant morphology. *Mod Pathol.* 2017;30:1251-1261.

Conklin CM, Longacre TA. Endometrial stromal tumors: the new WHO classification. *Adv Anat Pathol.* 2014;21:383-393.

Hoang LN, Aneja A, Conlon N, et al. Novel high-grade endometrial stromal sarcoma: a morphologic mimicker of myxoid leiomyosarcoma. *Am J Surg Pathol.* 2017;41:12-24.

Kommoss FKF, Chiang S, Köbel M, et al. Endometrial stromal sarcomas with BCOR internal tandem duplication and variant BCOR/BCORL1 rearrangements resemble high-grade endometrial stromal sarcomas with recurrent CDK4 pathway alterations and MDM2 amplifications. *Am J Surg Pathol.* 2022;46(8):1142-1152.

Kurihara S, Oda Y, Ohishi Y, et al. Endometrial stromal sarcomas and related high-grade sarcomas: immunohistochemical and molecular genetic study of 31 cases. *Am J Surg Pathol.* 2008;32:1228-1238.

Lee CH, Ali RH, Rouzbahman M, et al. Cyclin D1 as a diagnostic immunomarker for endometrial stromal sarcoma with YWHAE-FAM22 rearrangement. *Am J Surg Pathol.* 2012;36:1562-1570.

Lee CH, Mariño-Enriquez A, Ou W, et al. The clinicopathologic features of YWHAE-FAM22 endometrial stromal sarcomas: a histologically high-grade and clinically aggressive tumor. *Am J Surg Pathol.* 2012;36:641-653.

Lee CH, Nucci MR. Endometrial stromal sarcoma—the new genetic paradigm. *Histopathology.* 2015;67:1-19.

Lewis N, Soslow RA, Delair DF, et al. ZC3H7B-BCOR high-grade endometrial stromal sarcomas: a report of 17 cases of a newly defined entity. *Mod Pathol.* 2018;31:674-684.

Lin DI, Huang RSP, Mata DA, et al. Clinicopathological and genomic characterization of BCORL1-driven high-grade endometrial stromal sarcomas. *Mod Pathol.* 2021;34:2200-2210.

Mariño-Enriquez A, Lauria A, Przybyl J, et al. BCOR internal tandem duplication in high-grade uterine sarcomas. *Am J Surg Pathol.* 2018;42:335-341.

Sciallis AP, Bedroske PP, Schoolmeester JK, et al. High-grade endometrial stromal sarcomas: a clinicopathologic study of a group of tumors with heterogenous morphologic and genetic features. *Am J Surg Pathol.* 2014;38:1161-1172.

Zou Y, Turashvili G, Soslow RA, et al. High-grade transformation of low-grade endometrial stromal sarcomas lacking YWHAE and BCOR genetic abnormalities. *Mod Pathol.* 2020;33:1861-1870.

4.11

Bennett JA, Lastra RR, Barroeta JE, et al. Uterine tumor resembling ovarian sex cord stromal tumor (UTROSCT): a series of 3 cases with extensive rhabdoid differentiation, malignant behavior, and ESR1-NCOA2 fusions. *Am J Surg Pathol.* 2020;44:1563-1572.

Clement PB, Scully RE. Uterine tumors resembling ovarian sex-cord tumors. A clinicopathologic analysis of fourteen cases. *Am J Clin Pathol.* 1976;66:512-525.

Croce S, Lesluyes T, Delespaul L, et al. GREB1-CTNNB1 fusion transcript detected by RNA-sequencing in a uterine tumor resembling ovarian sex cord tumor (UTROSCT): a novel CTNNB1 rearrangement. *Genes Chromosomes Cancer.* 2019;58:155-163.

Czernobilsky B. Uterine tumors resembling ovarian sex cord tumors: an update. *Int J Gynecol Pathol.* 2008;27:229-235.

de Leval L, Lim GS, Waltregny D, et al. Diverse phenotypic profile of uterine tumors resembling ovarian sex cord tumors: an immunohistochemical study of 12 cases. *Am J Surg Pathol.* 2010;34:1749-1761.

Dickson BC, Childs TJ, Colgan TJ, *et al.* Uterine tumor resembling ovarian sex cord tumor: a distinct entity characterized by recurrent NCOA2/3 gene fusions. *Am J Surg Pathol.* 2019;43:178–86.

Irving JA, Carinelli S, Prat J. Uterine tumors resembling ovarian sex cord tumors are polyphenotypic neoplasms with true sex cord differentiation. *Mod Pathol.* 2006;19:17-24.

Goebel EA, Hernandez Bonilla S, et al. Uterine tumor resembling ovarian sex cord tumor (UTROSCT): a morphologic and molecular study of 26 cases confirms recurrent NCOA1-3 rearrangement. *Am J Surg Pathol.* 2020;44:30-42.

Lee CH, Kao YC, Lee WR, et al. Clinicopathologic characterization of GREB1-rearranged uterine sarcomas with variable sex-cord differentiation. *Am J Surg Pathol.* 2019;43:928-942.

Moore M, McCluggage WG. Uterine tumour resembling ovarian sex cord tumour: first report of a large series with follow-up. *Histopathology.* 2017;71:751-759.

4.12

Bennett JA, Braga AC, Pinto A, et al. Uterine PEComas: a morphologic, immunohistochemical, and molecular analysis of 32 tumors. *Am J Surg Pathol.* 2018;42:1370-1383.

Bennett JA, Ordulu Z, Pinto A, et al. Uterine PEComas: correlation between melanocytic marker expression and TSC alterations/TFE3 fusions. *Mod Pathol.* 2022;35:515-523.

Bennett JA, Schoolmeester JK. Tumours of the uterine corpus: perivascular epithelioid cell tumor (PEComa). In: WHO Classification of Tumours Editorial Board, ed. *Female Genital Tumours. WHO Classification of Tumours.* 5th ed. International Agency for Research on Cancer; 2020:296-297.

Folpe AL, Mentzel T, Lehr HA, et al. Perivascular epithelioid cell neoplasms of soft tissue and gynecologic origin: a clinicopathologic study of 26 cases and review of the literature. *Am J Surg Pathol.* 2005;29:1558-1575.

Schoolmeester JK, Dao LN, Sukov WR, et al. TFE3 translocation-associated perivascular epithelioid cell neoplasm (PEComa) of the gynecologic tract: morphology, immunophenotype, differential diagnosis. *Am J Surg Pathol.* 2015;39:394-404.

Schoolmeester JK, Howitt BE, Hirsch MS, et al. Perivascular epithelioid cell neoplasm (PEComa) of the gynecologic tract: clinicopathologic and immunohistochemical characterization of 16 cases. *Am J Surg Pathol.* 2014;38:176-188.

Selenica P, Conlon N, Gonzalez C, et al. Genomic profiling aids classification of diagnostically challenging uterine mesenchymal tumors with myomelanocytic differentiation. *Am J Surg Pathol.* 2021;45:77-92.

Vang R, Kempson RL. Perivascular epithelioid cell tumor ('PEComa') of the uterus: a subset of HMB-45-positive epithelioid mesenchymal neoplasms with an uncertain relationship to pure smooth muscle tumors. *Am J Surg Pathol.* 2002;26:1-13.

4.13

Ando H, Ogawa M, Watanabe Y, et al. Lymphangioleiomyoma of the uterus and pelvic lymph nodes: a report of 3 cases, including the potentially earliest manifestation of extrapulmonary lymphangioleiomyomatosis. *Int J Gynecol Pathol.* 2020;39:227-232.

Gyure KA, Hart WR, Kennedy AW. Lymphangiomyomatosis of the uterus associated with tuberous sclerosis and malignant neoplasia of the female genital tract: a report of two cases. *Int J Gynecol Pathol.* 1995;14:344-351.

Lim GS, Oliva E. The morphologic spectrum of uterine PEC-cell associated tumors in a patient with tuberous sclerosis. *Int J Gynecol Pathol.* 2011;30:121-128.

Longacre TA, Hendrickson MR, Kapp DS, et al. Lymphangioleiomyomatosis of the uterus simulating high-stage endometrial stromal sarcoma. *Gynecol Oncol.* 1996;63:404-410.

4.14

Arias-Stella JA, Benayed R, Oliva E, et al. Novel PLAG1 gene rearrangement distinguishes a subset of uterine myxoid leiomyosarcoma from other uterine myxoid mesenchymal tumors. *Am J Surg Pathol.* 2019;43:382-388.

Bennett JA, Croce S, Pesci A, et al. Inflammatory myofibroblastic tumor of the uterus: an immunohistochemical study of 23 cases. *Am J Surg Pathol.* 2020;44:1441-1449.

Bennett JA, Nardi V, Rouzbahman M, et al. Inflammatory myofibroblastic tumor of the uterus: a clinicopathological, immunohistochemical, and molecular analysis of 13 cases highlighting their broad morphologic spectrum. *Mod Pathol.* 2017;30:1489-1503.

Burch DM, Tavassoli FA. Myxoid leiomyosarcoma of the uterus. *Histopathology.* 2011;59:1144-1155.

Cheek EH, Fadra N, Jackson RA, et al. Uterine inflammatory myofibroblastic tumors in pregnant women with and without involvement of the placenta: a study of 6 cases with identification of a novel TIMP3-RET fusion. *Hum Pathol.* 2020;97:29-39.

Fuehrer NE, Keeney GL, Ketterling RP, et al. ALK-1 protein expression and ALK gene rearrangements aid in the diagnosis of inflammatory myofibroblastic tumors of the female genital tract. *Arch Pathol Lab Med.* 2012;136:623-626.

Haimes JD, Stewart CJR, Kudlow BA, et al. Uterine inflammatory myofibroblastic tumors frequently harbor ALK fusions with IGFBP5 and THBS1. *Am J Surg Pathol.* 2017;41:773-780.

King ME, Dickersin GR, Scully RE. Myxoid leiomyosarcoma of the uterus. A report of six cases. *Am J Surg Pathol.* 1982;6:589-598.

Kuisma H, Jokinen V, Pasanen A, et al. Histopathologic and molecular characterization of uterine leiomyoma-like inflammatory myofibroblastic tumor: comparison to molecular subtypes of uterine leiomyoma. *Am J Surg Pathol.* 2022;46(8):1126-1136.

Mohammad N, Haimes JD, Mishkin S, et al. ALK is a specific diagnostic marker for inflammatory myofibroblastic tumor of the uterus. *Am J Surg Pathol.* 2018;42:1353-1359.

Parra-Herran C. ALK immunohistochemistry and molecular analysis in uterine inflammatory myofibroblastic tumor: proceedings of the ISGyP Companion Society Session at the 2020 USCAP Annual Meeting. *Int J Gynecol Pathol.* 2021;40:28-31.

Parra-Herran C, Quick CM, Howitt BE, et al. Inflammatory myofibroblastic tumor of the uterus: clinical and pathologic review of 10 cases including a subset with aggressive clinical course. *Am J Surg Pathol.* 2015;39:157-168.

Parra-Herran C, Schoolmeester JK, Yuan L, et al. Myxoid leiomyosarcoma of the uterus: a clinicopathologic analysis of 30 cases and review of the literature with reappraisal of its distinction from other uterine myxoid mesenchymal neoplasms. *Am J Surg Pathol.* 2016;40:285-301.

Rabban JT, Zaloudek CJ, Shekitka KM, et al. Inflammatory myofibroblastic tumor of the uterus: a clinicopathologic study of 6 cases emphasizing distinction from aggressive mesenchymal tumors. *Am J Surg Pathol.* 2005;29:1348-1355.

4.15 and 4.16

Chen HF, Liu XL, Liu AZ, et al. Uterine adenomatoid tumor: a clinicopathologic study of 102 cases. *Int J Clin Exp Pathol.* 2017;10:9627-9632.

Goode B, Joseph NM, Stevers M, et al. Adenomatoid tumors of the male and female genital tract are defined by TRAF7 mutations that drive aberrant NF-kB pathway activation. *Mod Pathol.* 2018;31:660-673.

Itami H, Fujii T, Nakai T, et al. TRAF7 mutations and immunohistochemical study of uterine adenomatoid tumor compared with malignant mesothelioma. *Hum Pathol.* 2021;111:59-66.

Karpathiou G, Hiroshima K, Peoc'h M. Adenomatoid tumor: a review of pathology with focus on unusual presentations and sites, histogenesis, differential diagnosis, and molecular and clinical aspects with a historic overview of its description. *Adv Anat Pathol.* 2020;27:394-407.

Lerias S, Ariyasriwatana C, Agaimy A, et al. Adenomatoid tumor of the uterus: a report of 6 unusual cases with prominent cysts including 4 with diffuse myometrial involvement, 4 with uterine serosal involvement, and 2 presenting in curettage specimens. *Int J Gynecol Pathol.* 2021;40:248-256.

Nogales FF, Isaac MA, Hardisson D, et al. Adenomatoid tumors of the uterus: an analysis of 60 cases. *Int J Gynecol Pathol.* 2002;21:34-40.

Tamura D, Maeda D, Halimi SA, et al. Adenomatoid tumour of the uterus is frequently associated with iatrogenic immunosuppression. *Histopathology.* 2018;73:1013-1022.

Wang X, Kumar D, Seidman JD. Uterine lipoleiomyomas: a clinicopathologic study of 50 cases. *Int J Gynecol Pathol.* 2006;25:239-242.

4.17

Kihara A, Amano Y, Yoshimoto T, et al. Stromal p16 expression helps distinguish atypical polypoid adenomyoma from myoinvasive endometrioid carcinoma of the uterus. *Am J Surg Pathol.* 2019;43:1526-1535.

Longacre TA, Chung MH, Rouse RV, et al. Atypical polypoid adenomyofibromas (atypical polypoid adenomyomas) of the uterus. A clinicopathologic study of 55 cases. *Am J Surg Pathol.* 1996;20:1-20.

McCluggage WG, Van de Vijver K. SATB2 is consistently expressed in squamous morules associated with endometrioid proliferative lesions and in the stroma of atypical polypoid adenomyoma. *Int J Gynecol Pathol.* 2019;38:397-403.

Worrell HI, Sciallis AP, Skala SL. Patterns of SATB2 and p16 reactivity aid in the distinction of atypical polypoid adenomyoma from myoinvasive endometrioid carcinoma and benign adenomyomatous polyp on endometrial sampling. *Histopathology.* 2021;79:96-105.

Young RH, Treger T, Scully RE. Atypical polypoid adenomyoma of the uterus. A report of 27 cases. *Am J Clin Pathol.* 1986;86:139-145.

4.18 and 4.19

Chapel DB, Howitt BE, Sholl LM, et al. Atypical uterine polyps show morphologic and molecular overlap with mullerian adenosarcoma but follow a benign clinical course. *Mod Pathol.* 2022;35:106-116.

Clement PB, Scully RE. Mullerian adenosarcoma of the uterus: a clinicopathologic analysis of 100 cases with a review of the literature. *Hum Pathol.* 1990;21:363-381.

Gallardo A, Prat J. Mullerian adenosarcoma: a clinicopathologic and immunohistochemical study of 55 cases challenging the existence of adenofibroma. *Am J Surg Pathol.* 2009;33:278-288.

Howitt BE, Quade BJ, Nucci MR. Uterine polyps with features overlapping with those of Müllerian adenosarcoma: a clinicopathologic analysis of 29 cases emphasizing their likely benign nature. *Am J Surg Pathol.* 2015;39:116-126.

Soslow RA, Ali A, Oliva E. Mullerian adenosarcomas: an immunophenotypic analysis of 35 cases. *Am J Surg Pathol.* 2008;32:1013-1021.

Tai LH, Tavassoli FA. Endometrial polyps with atypical (bizarre) stromal cells. *Am J Surg Pathol.* 2002;26:505-509.

Zaloudek CJ, Norris HJ. Adenofibroma and adenosarcoma of the uterus: a clinicopathologic study of 35 cases. *Cancer.* 1981;48:354-366.

4.20

Clement PB. Müllerian adenosarcomas of the uterus with sarcomatous overgrowth. A clinicopathological analysis of 10 cases. *Am J Surg Pathol.* 1989;13:28-38.

Hodgson A, Amemiya Y, Seth A, et al. High-grade müllerian adenosarcoma: genomic and clinicopathologic characterization of a distinct neoplasm with prevalent TP53 pathway alterations and aggressive behavior. *Am J Surg Pathol.* 2017;41:1513-1522.

Krivak TC, Seidman JD, McBroom JW, et al. Uterine adenosarcoma with sarcomatous overgrowth versus uterine carcinosarcoma: comparison of treatment and survival. *Gynecol Oncol.* 2001;83:89-94.

Seidman JD, Chauhan S. Evaluation of the relationship between adenosarcoma and carcinosarcoma and a hypothesis of the histogenesis of uterine sarcomas. *Int J Gynecol Pathol.* 2003;22:75-82.

4.21

Dundr P, Mára M, Masková J, et al. Pathological findings of uterine leiomyomas and adenomyosis following uterine artery embolization. *Pathol Res Pract.* 2006;202:721-729.

Maleki Z, Kim HS, Thonse VR, et al. Uterine artery embolization with trisacryl gelatin microspheres in women treated for leiomyomas: a clinicopathologic analysis of alterations in gynecologic surgical specimens. *Int J Gynecol Pathol.* 2010;29:260-268.

Weichert W, Denkert C, Gauruder-Burmester A, et al. Uterine arterial embolization with tris-acryl gelatin microspheres: a histopathologic evaluation. *Am J Surg Pathol.* 2005;29:955-961.

5

Ovary

Preface (A note on terminology)

The category of ovarian epithelial tumors which display epithelial proliferation and are accordingly not clearly benign, but lack unequivocal evidence of invasive carcinoma, has been referred to by several different names over the past few decades. The terms "atypical proliferative tumor," "borderline tumor," and "tumor of low malignant potential" have been considered equivalent but have been variously preferred, or argued against, by different investigators/experts. Although an NIH-sponsored Borderline Ovarian Tumor Workshop in 2003, and the 2003 and 2014 World Health Organization Classification of Tumours (WHO), did not arrive at a single consensus term, "borderline tumor" has been favored by a majority of pathologists and has been the most widely used.

The serous borderline tumor category has been divided into typical and micropapillary variants. The micropapillary variant has also been referred to as noninvasive low grade/micropapillary serous carcinoma, but these latter terms are not recommended in the 2020 WHO.

In the first edition of this book, we used "borderline tumor" and "atypical proliferative tumor," as well as "noninvasive low-grade/micropapillary serous carcinoma." In this new edition, we are following the 2020 World Health Organization Classification of Tumours recommendations in which "borderline tumor" is the preferred term and the other terms are not recommended. In addition, we use (typical) "serous borderline tumor" and "micropapillary serous borderline tumor."

	Typical Serous Borderline Tumor (SBT)	Micropapillary Serous Borderline Tumor (MP-SBT)
Age	Median 49 y	Median 54 y
Location	Within ovary with or without exophytic surface component; may be confined to surface	Within ovary with or without exophytic surface component; may be confined to ovarian surface
Symptoms	Commonly asymptomatic; may have nonspecific pelvic pain or urinary symptoms	Commonly asymptomatic; may have nonspecific pelvic pain, increasing abdominal girth, bloating, early satiety
Signs	Pelvic/adnexal mass	Pelvic/adnexal mass
Etiology	Unknown; originates from serous-type inclusions, possibly originating from tubal epithelial implantation; *KRAS* or *BRAF* mutations	Evolves in a stepwise manner from SBT. Often harbor *BRAF* or *KRAS* mutations
Gross and histology	1. Intracystic and exophytic components 2. Hierarchical branching, tufting, and apparent detachment of cell clusters; some micropapillae may be present but not as numerous as in MP-SBT; no invasion *(Figs. 5.1.1-5.1.4)* 3. Tubal-type epithelium, often ciliated, focally with hobnail or dense eosinophilic cytoplasm *(Figs. 5.1.4 and 5.1.5)*; mild cytologic atypia; may have psammoma bodies; extracellular mucin may be present 4. 12% have noninvasive peritoneal implants; 1% have invasive implants; those with exophytic component/surface involvement are more often associated with implants (see Chapter 6)	1. Intracystic and exophytic components 2. Nonhierarchical branching with abundant micropapillae (at least 5 times as long as they are wide); Medusa head-like appearance *(Figs. 5.1.6 and 5.1.7)*; papillary fusion with cribriform pattern *(Figs. 5.1.8 and 5.1.9)*; SBT component usually present (quantitative criteria for distinction from SBT: pure MP-SBT areas without intervening foci of typical SBT must measure at least 5 mm in greatest extent); no invasion 3. Tubal-type epithelium may be ciliated; mild to occasionally moderate cytologic atypia with small prominent nucleoli *(Figs. 5.1.9 and 5.1.10)*; psammoma bodies common; extracellular mucin may be present *(Fig. 5.1.10)* 4. Peritoneal implants usually present and often are invasive (see Chapter 6)
Special studies	Not useful in this differential	Not useful in this differential
Treatment	Salpingo-oophorectomy +/− staging	Hysterectomy with bilateral salpingo-oophorectomy, comprehensive staging +/− debulking; if invasive implants present (ie, invasive low-grade serous carcinoma), options include chemotherapy and hormonal therapy

	Typical Serous Borderline Tumor (SBT)	**Micropapillary Serous Borderline Tumor (MP-SBT)**
Prognosis	Increased risk of invasive serous carcinoma (vast majority low grade) (HR = 9.2; 95% CI: 6.8-12.2); if confined to ovaries (ie, without associated peritoneal implants), 1.7% develop carcinoma; noninvasive implants confer risk of invasive low-grade serous carcinoma of ~16% (HR = 7.7; 95% CI: 3.9-15.0)	If confined to ovaries, 7.3% develop carcinoma; if invasive peritoneal implants (ie, peritoneal low-grade serous carcinoma) present, advanced stage is indolent with 5-/10-y survival ~75%/45%, respectively

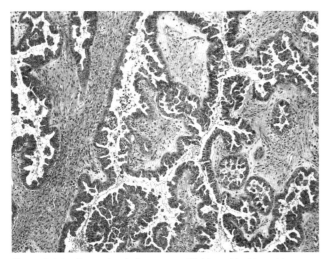

Figure 5.1.1 Serous borderline tumor with hierarchical branching pattern, tufting, and detachment of cell clusters.

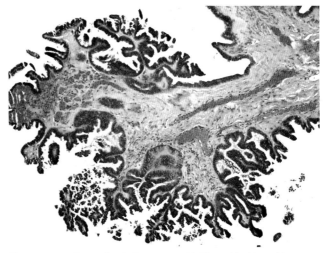

Figure 5.1.2 Serous borderline tumor with hierarchical branching, detachment of cell clusters, and apparent detachment of larger papillary processes.

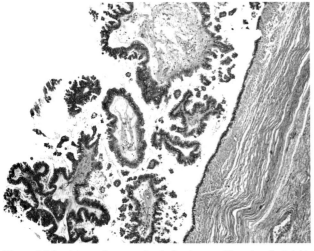

Figure 5.1.3 Intracystic serous borderline tumor with cyst wall at right lined by single layer of benign-appearing serous epithelium.

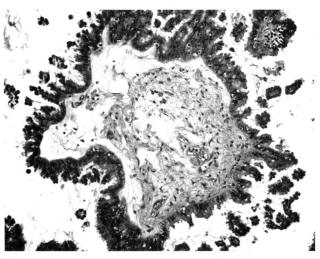

Figure 5.1.4 Serous borderline tumor showing ciliated epithelium and apparent detachment of individual cells and cell clusters.

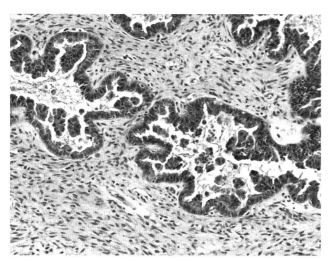

Figure 5.1.5 Serous borderline tumor with detachment of atypical cell clusters.

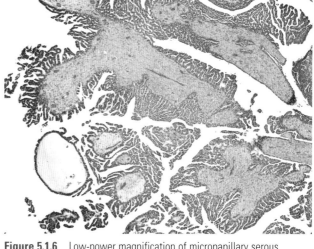

Figure 5.1.6 Low-power magnification of micropapillary serous borderline tumor displaying diffuse micropapillary architecture with "Medusa head" configuration.

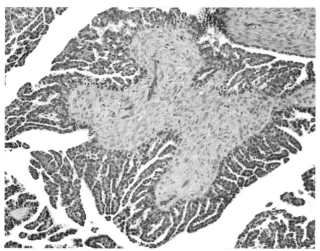

Figure 5.1.7 Micropapillary serous borderline tumor with large papilla containing elongated micropapillary projections ("Medusa head" appearance). Same case as in *Figure 5.1.6*, higher magnification.

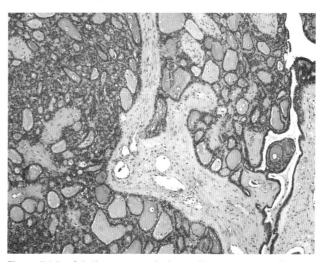

Figure 5.1.8 Cribriform pattern of micropapillary serous borderline tumor.

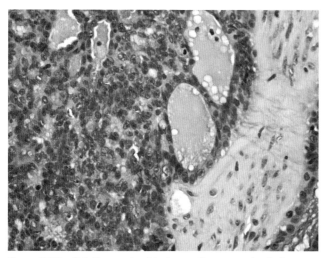

Figure 5.1.9 Cribriform and solid micropapillary serous borderline tumor displaying mild nuclear atypia with small prominent nucleoli. Same case as in *Figure 5.1.8*, higher magnification.

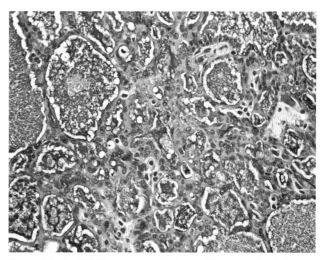

Figure 5.1.10 Cribriform pattern of micropapillary serous borderline tumor. Extracellular mucin is noted.

	Seromucinous Borderline Tumor (SMBT)	Low-Grade Seromucinous Carcinoma
Age	Mean 38-40 y	Mean 47 y
Location	Intracystic within ovarian stroma	Within ovarian stroma
Symptoms	Commonly asymptomatic; may have pelvic or abdominal pain or other endometriosis-associated symptoms	Very limited data suggest pelvic pain or other endometriosis-associated symptoms
Signs	Pelvic/adnexal mass	Pelvic/adnexal mass
Etiology	Endometriosis; limited data suggest *KRAS* and *ARID1A* mutations present	Likely arise through progression of SMBT, which is derived from endometriosis
Gross and histology	1. Usually unilocular and associated with endometriosis; about one-third bilateral; mean 8 cm 2. Hierarchical branching pattern; invasion absent *(Figs. 5.2.1-5.2.3)* 3. Endocervical-like mucinous epithelium admixed with serous and other cell types (including indifferent-type cells); neutrophils and extracellular mucin usually present; mild atypia, rare mitotic figures *(Figs. 5.2.3-5.2.5)* 4. Rarely associated with peritoneal implants	1. Usually confined to ovaries; 16% bilateral; mean 10.5 cm; solid or mixed solid/cystic 2. Considered a variant of low-grade endometrioid carcinoma with metaplastic features; complex papillary, glandular, microglandular, and solid patterns *(Figs. 5.2.6-5.2.8)*; occasional stromal hyalinization; invasion is based on confluent growth; occasional destructive invasion *(Fig. 5.2.9)*; SMBT component usually present 3. Endocervical-like mucinous cells and eosinophilic indifferent cells; may also contain hobnail, squamous, clear, endometrioid-like, and focal signet ring–like cells; neutrophils and extracellular mucin usually present; mild to focally moderate cytologic atypia with low mitotic activity *(Figs. 5.2.9 and 5.2.10)* 4. Rarely associated with peritoneal metastases
Special studies	Not useful in this differential	Not useful in this differential
Treatment	Salpingo-oophorectomy +/− staging	Insufficient data to justify difference from other low-grade ovarian carcinomas
Prognosis	Generally benign behavior; cases with implants may be at increased risk for recurrence/progression	Limited data suggest very good prognosis given predominance of stage I

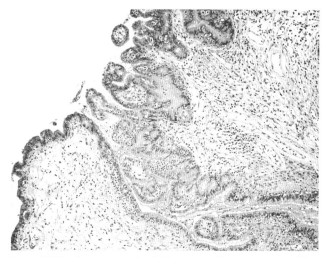

Figure 5.2.1　Seromucinous borderline tumor with hierarchical papillary branching.

Figure 5.2.2　Seromucinous borderline tumor with marked neutrophilic infiltration and edema.

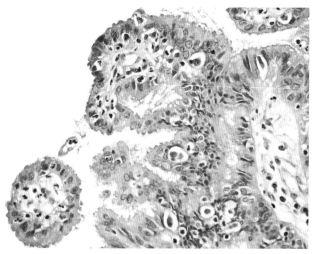

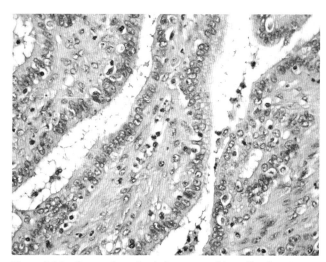

Figure 5.2.3　Seromucinous borderline tumor with pseudostratified epithelium with tufting and occasional neutrophils.

Figure 5.2.4　Seromucinous borderline tumor with papillae lined by single layer of mildly atypical indifferent-type and tubal-type cells with small nucleoli. Some cells display cilia.

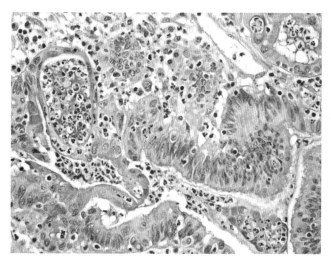

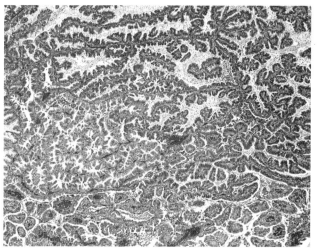

Figure 5.2.5　Seromucinous borderline tumor with pseudostratified epithelium with some ciliated cells, mild atypia, prominent neutrophilic infiltrate, and both intracellular and extracellular mucin.

Figure 5.2.6　Low-grade seromucinous carcinoma with confluent papillary pattern.

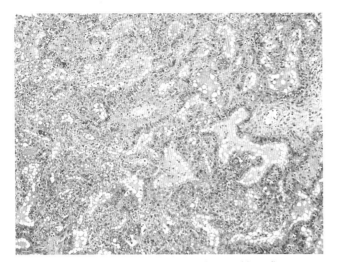

Figure 5.2.7 Low-grade seromucinous carcinoma with confluent glandular pattern.

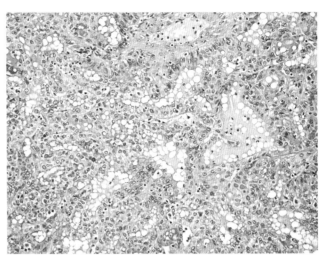

Figure 5.2.8 Low-grade seromucinous carcinoma with confluence of glands with cribriforming, in many areas lacking fibrovascular support.

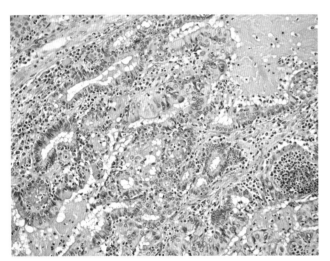

Figure 5.2.9 Low-grade seromucinous carcinoma displaying marked gland crowding, infiltrative pattern of stromal invasion, abundant neutrophils, and extracellular mucin.

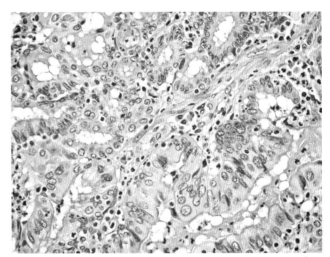

Figure 5.2.10 Low-grade seromucinous carcinoma with pseudostratification of mucinous epithelium and mild to focally moderate nuclear atypia. Note presence of neutrophils **(upper right)**.

	Autoimplants of Serous Borderline Tumor (SBT)	Serous Borderline Tumor With Microinvasion/ Microinvasive Carcinoma
Age	Mean 36 y	Mean 42 y
Location	Exophytic portion of primary ovarian tumor, often between papillae; rarely in intracystic component	Primary ovarian tumor
Symptoms	Commonly asymptomatic; may have nonspecific pelvic pain or urinary symptoms	Commonly asymptomatic; may have nonspecific pelvic pain or urinary symptoms
Signs	Pelvic or adnexal mass	Pelvic or adnexal mass
Etiology	Unknown; possibly arise from detachment of exophytic papillae from SBT, perhaps due to infarction, and subsequent reattachment/ adhesion	Unknown; possibly SBT epithelium may undergo mutation (ie, *BRAF*), infarction, terminal differentiation, or senescence Size criteria vary for distinction of microinvasion from invasive low-grade serous carcinoma (LGSC): 5 mm is most commonly used upper limit for microinvasion
Gross and histology	1. Two-thirds are multifocal; range in size up to 2.5 cm; 93% have been associated with and resemble desmoplastic peritoneal implants (see Chapter 6); 10% have invasive LGSC (invasive implants) involving the peritoneum. Lesional cells present on ovarian surface or within fibrous tissue between large papillae *(Fig. 5.3.1)*. Fibroblastic stroma, often with chronic inflammation, overshadows the epithelial component with which it merges *(Figs. 5.3.2-5.3.5)* and has circumscribed border with underlying tissue. Fibrinous inflammatory exudate *(Figs. 5.3.3 and 5.3.5)* and calcification often present 2. Single cells, cell clusters, small, smoothly contoured glands and papillae with mild or moderate atypia without invasive features *(Figs. 5.3.2-5.3.5)*; 37% associated with infarcted papillae 3. 20% of SBTs with autoimplants have micropapillary features (MP-SBT)	1. No gross correlates of microinvasion; stroma of SBT may be dense and hyalinized or edematous; rarely cellular and fibroblastic when inflammation or infarction present. Lesional cells located within stroma of tumor 2. Eosinophilic type *(Figs. 5.3.6 and 5.3.7)*: epithelial cells with central, bland nuclei and abundant eosinophilic cytoplasm bud into the stromal cores of the papillae singly and in small clusters, occasionally forming glands, often surrounded by a space, which may be lined by flattened cells 3. Micropapillary type *(Figs. 5.3.8 and 5.3.9)*: solid nests and micropapillae usually surrounded by a space display an infiltrative pattern ("small focus of low-grade carcinoma" or "microinvasive carcinoma" terminology may be used); frequent psammomatous calcification *(Figs. 5.3.8 and 5.3.9)*; larger papillae occasionally present and are referred to as "macropapillary" *(Figs. 5.3.10 and 5.3.11)*. In both eosinophilic and micropapillary types, the cytologic features are similar to the noninvasive epithelium lining the papillae
Special studies	Autoimplants presumed to have similar immunoprofile as desmoplastic implants; remainder of tumor same as SBT	Microinvasive cells often lose ER, PR, and WT1 expression, and Ki67 proliferation index low, compared to background tumor; otherwise same as SBT
Treatment	Same as SBT	Same as SBT
Prognosis	Limited data; same as SBT stratified by implant type	Same as SBT when stratified by stage and implant type

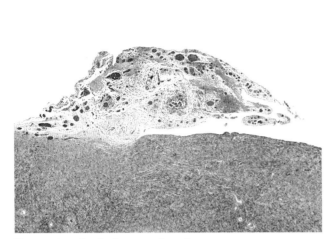

Figure 5.3.1 Autoimplant on surface of ovary.

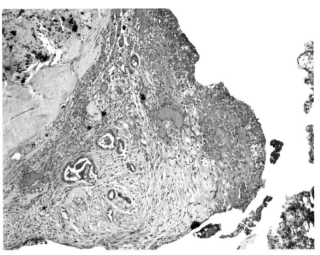

Figure 5.3.2 Autoimplant with a few glands overshadowed by an inflamed fibroblastic stroma resembling a desmoplastic implant (see Chapter 6). Note fibrosis and calcification at **upper left**.

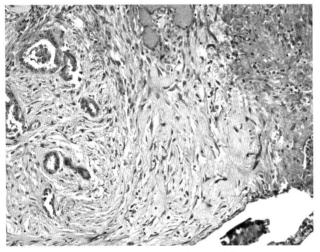

Figure 5.3.3 Autoimplant. Higher magnification of *Figure 5.3.2* showing a few glands embedded in fibroblastic stroma with focal hemorrhage and fibrinous exudate at **right**.

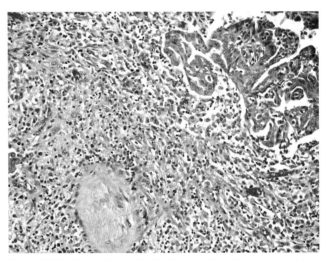

Figure 5.3.4 Autoimplant with fibroblastic inflamed stroma containing small glands and papillae at **upper right**.

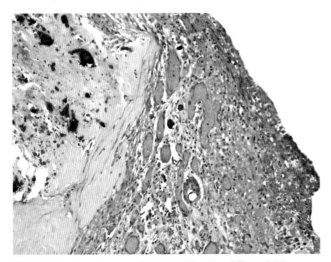

Figure 5.3.5 Autoimplant. Higher magnification of *Figure 5.3.2* showing inflamed fibroblastic stroma covered by fibrinous exudate, with both psammomatous and nonpsammomatous calcifications at **left**.

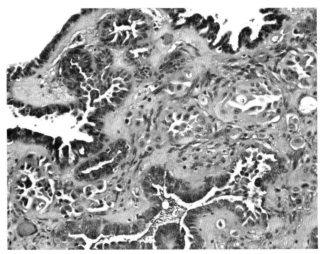

Figure 5.3.6 Eosinophilic type of microinvasion displaying glands lined by eosinophilic cells with a hobnail pattern, and single epithelial cells, most of which are surrounded by a space. The nuclei of these eosinophilic cells resemble those of some cells in the overlying noninvasive epithelium.

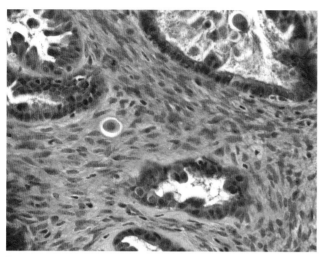

Figure 5.3.7 Eosinophilic type of microinvasion displaying a single ovoid epithelial cell with eosinophilic cytoplasm in the stroma, surrounded by a space.

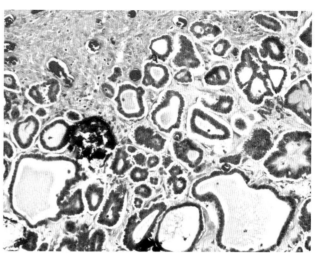

Figure 5.3.8 Microinvasive carcinoma displaying micropapillae surrounded by spaces and psammomatous calcification. Note that the qualitative appearance is similar to frankly invasive low-grade serous carcinoma.

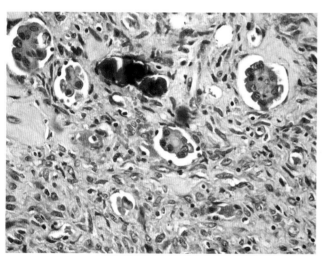

Figure 5.3.9 Microinvasive carcinoma displaying micropapillae surrounded by spaces and psammomatous calcification.

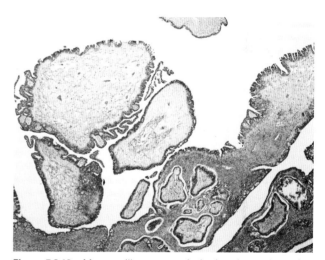

Figure 5.3.10 Macropapillary pattern of microinvasive carcinoma (see Section 5.5).

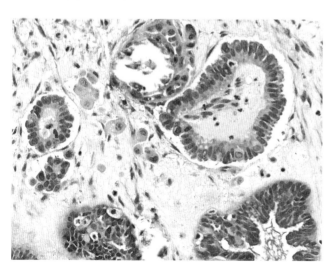

Figure 5.3.11 Microinvasive carcinoma and eosinophilic type of microinvasion. Eosinophilic cells **(center)**, micropapillae **(left)**, and a macropapilla **(right)**. Higher magnification of *Figure 5.3.10*.

	Lymph Node "Involvement" by Serous Borderline Tumor (SBT)	Lymph Node With Endosalpingiosis
Age	Mean 40 y	Wide age range of adults
Location	Nodal sinuses including subcapsular sinus; pelvic and paraaortic groups; rarely seen in other lymph node groups	Intracapsular and within fibrous trabeculae; pelvic and paraaortic lymph node groups
Symptoms	No symptoms referable to the lymph nodes	Asymptomatic
Signs	None	None
Etiology	Likely due to lymphatic filtration of peritoneal fluid containing exfoliated cells from ovarian tumor surface; alternative possibilities include origin from nodal endosalpingiosis	Associated with salpingitis, SBT, and low-grade serous carcinoma; endosalpingiosis is more common in women with low-grade serous tumors compared to women without such tumors
Gross and histology	1. Eosinophilic cells resembling those seen in microinvasion, singly and in clusters and small papillae, in sinuses and, in florid cases, in parenchyma *(Figs. 5.4.1 and 5.4.2)* 2. Endosalpingiosis usually present, often closely associated with the eosinophilic cells; endosalpingiotic glands may display intraglandular tufting with detachment of cell clusters *(Figs. 5.4.3-5.4.5)*; *psammomatous calcification often present (Figs. 5.4.1 and 5.4.3)*	1. Simple glands lined by flattened cuboidal to columnar ciliated tubal-type epithelium, usually within node capsule *(Figs. 5.4.6 and 5.4.7)* 2. Occasionally with minimal and blunt papillae; isolated eosinophilic cells not present; psammomatous calcification may be present
Special studies	Serous cells in lymph node often lose ER, PR, and WT1 expression and have decreased Ki 67 proliferation index in comparison to similar cells in primary SBT; other markers same as SBT	ER+, PR+, WT1+, PAX8+, CK7+, calretinin−
Treatment	Same as SBT	None
Prognosis	Same as SBT after correction for implant type	Benign

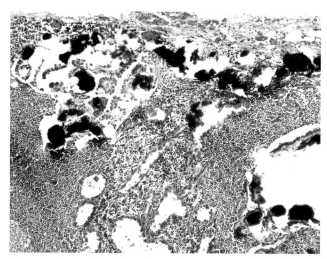

Figure 5.4.1　Lymph node involvement by serous borderline tumor showing detached papillary clusters with abundant psammomatous calcification.

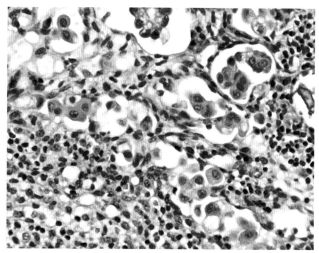

Figure 5.4.2　Lymph node involvement by ovarian serous borderline tumor showing detached small clusters and individual cells with abundant eosinophilic cytoplasm.

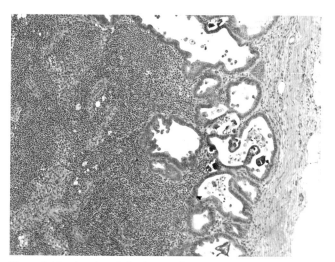

Figure 5.4.3　Lymph node involvement by serous borderline tumor (SBT). The lymph node capsule and nodal parenchyma contain endosalpingiotic-type glands showing prominent tufting and cell clusters within glands. Alternatively, this could also represent SBT arising within nodal endosalpingiosis.

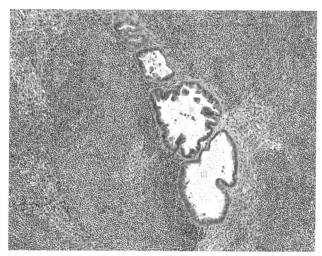

Figure 5.4.4　Lymph node involvement by serous borderline tumor. The epithelial stratification, including detached cell clusters, exceeds that of endosalpingiosis.

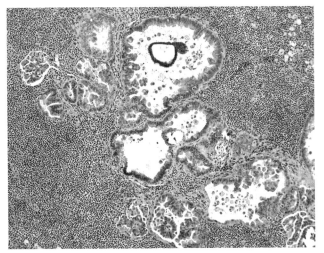

Figure 5.4.5 Lymph node involvement by serous borderline tumor (SBT). The nodal parenchyma contains endosalpingiotic-type glands showing prominent tufting and cell clusters within glands, as well as clusters of epithelial cells outside of glands. Alternatively, this could also represent SBT arising within nodal endosalpingiosis.

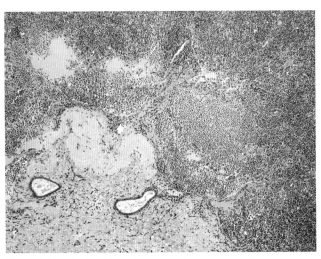

Figure 5.4.6 Endosalpingiosis characterized by two benign glands within the lymph node capsule.

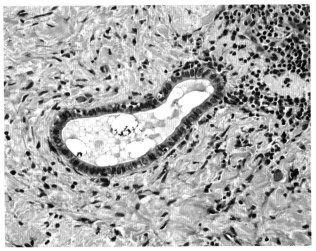

Figure 5.4.7 Higher magnification of *Figure 5.4.6* displays benign tubal-type epithelium lacking atypia or mitotic figures.

	Macropapillary Pattern of Invasive Low-Grade Serous Carcinoma (LGSC)	Serous Adenofibroma/Cystadenofibroma
Age	Mean 50 y	Mean 61 y; wide age range of adults
Location	Within ovary	Within ovary
Symptoms	Commonly asymptomatic; may have nonspecific pelvic pain, increasing abdominal girth, bloating, and early satiety	Commonly asymptomatic; may have pelvic pain or discomfort
Signs	Pelvic/adnexal mass	Pelvic/adnexal mass
Etiology	Limited data suggest *KRAS* or *BRAF* mutations present in macropapillary component	May arise from surface epithelial inclusions and surrounding stroma; epithelium is polyclonal and nonneoplastic in most cases; copy number aberrations (often gain of chromosome 12) may be found in stromal fibroblasts in the majority of cases
Gross and histology	1. Mean size 12 cm; often bilateral; otherwise grossly same as micropapillary serous borderline tumor (MP-SBT) 2. Invasive papillae characteristic of LGSC with papillary structures ≥0.3 cm in diameter, surrounded by a space, usually involving >50% of the tumor *(Figs. 5.5.1-5.5.4)*; often seen in combination with MP-SBT and typical LGSC *(Fig. 5.5.5)* 3. Epithelium bland, cuboidal to columnar, mild atypia, often ciliated, similar to typical LGSC *(Figs. 5.5.3 and 5.5.4)*; serous borderline tumor component usually present	1. One-third of benign ovarian serous tumors are adenofibromas/cystadenofibromas (remainder are unilocular or multilocular serous cystadenomas without significant fibromatous components); usually solid, often with cystic component 2. Broad fibrous papillary processes may be exophytic or endophytic within cysts; rarely, endophytic appearance in noncystic fibrous areas resembles macropapillary pattern of LGSC *(Figs. 5.5.6-5.5.8)* 3. Papillae are lined by benign tubal-type epithelium lacking atypia *(Figs. 5.5.8 and 5.5.9)*; focal small papillary proliferations with minimal stroma may be present
Special studies	Not useful in this differential	Not useful in this differential
Treatment	Same as LGSC	Unilateral salpingo-oophorectomy or cystectomy
Prognosis	Limited data; likely same as LGSC	Benign

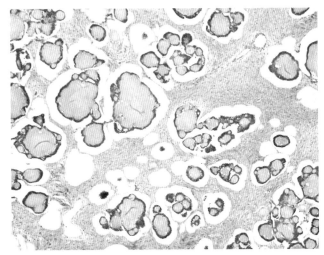

Figure 5.5.1 Invasive low-grade serous carcinoma, macropapillary pattern, displays an infiltrative pattern of papillae of varying sizes, some >3 mm in diameter

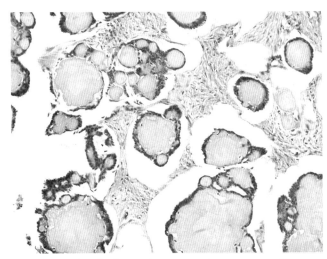

Figure 5.5.2 Invasive low-grade serous carcinoma, macropapillary pattern (same case as *Fig. 5.5.1*), displays prominent spaces surrounding the papillae.

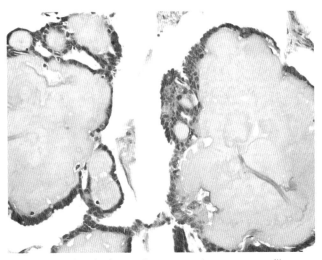

Figure 5.5.3 Invasive low-grade serous carcinoma, macropapillary pattern, displays minimal atypia and cilia in the serous epithelium lining the papillae.

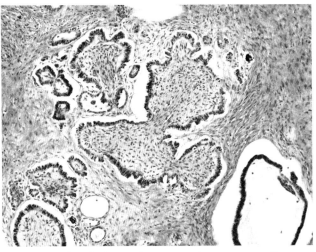

Figure 5.5.4 Invasive low-grade serous carcinoma, macropapillary pattern, with large papillae lined by serous epithelium with minimal atypia and focal areas with ciliated cells.

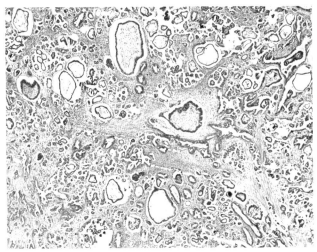

Figure 5.5.5 Invasive low-grade serous carcinoma with macropapillae and micropapillae.

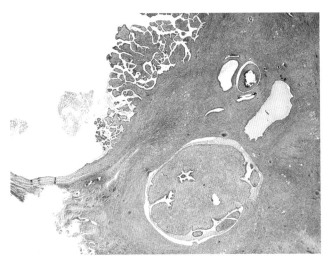

Figure 5.5.6 Serous cystadenofibroma with intracystic papillae at **top left**, and endophytic papillae within the fibrous stroma toward **bottom right**.

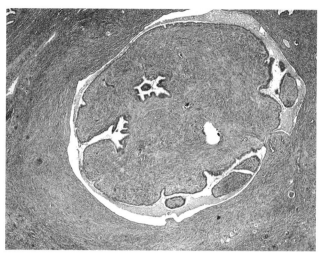

Figure 5.5.7 Serous cystadenofibroma, higher magnification of *Figure 5.5.6,* showing endophytic papilla.

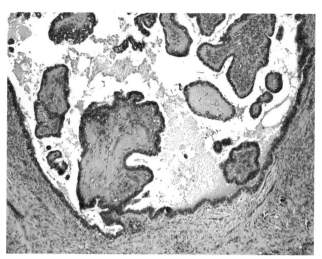

Figure 5.5.8 Serous cystadenofibroma with papillae in small cyst, lined by benign serous epithelium.

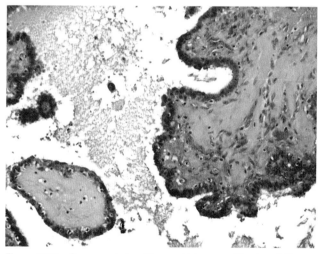

Figure 5.5.9 Serous cystadenofibroma, higher magnification of *Figure 5.5.8,* with papillae lined by benign serous epithelium.

	High-Grade Serous Carcinoma	Low-Grade Serous Carcinoma
Age	Mean 60-63 y	Mean 47-57 y
Location	Ovarian surface, within ovarian stroma, tubal fimbriae, commonly invades nonfimbrial tube	Ovarian surface, within ovarian stroma, can invade fallopian tube
Symptoms	Pelvic pain, increasing abdominal girth, bloating, early satiety, urinary symptoms	Pelvic pain, increasing abdominal girth, bloating, early satiety, urinary symptoms
Signs	Pelvic/abdominal mass, ascites	Pelvic/abdominal mass, ascites
Etiology	Majority derive from serous tubal intraepithelial carcinoma (STIC), usually of fimbrial origin; nearly all have *TP53* mutations; a substantial proportion have either germline or somatic mutation in *BRCA1*, *BRCA2* or other homologous recombination repair gene or epigenetic silencing of these genes; high levels of genomic instability	Derive from progression of serous borderline tumor (SBT) through micropapillary SBT; *KRAS* and *BRAF* mutations
Gross and histology	1. Ovaries normal sized or slightly enlarged in one-third to one-half of cases with subcentimeter surface nodules; remaining show enlarged solid and/or cystic ovaries, 8-10 cm; fallopian tube fimbriae may be prominent and tumorous and may be splayed across ovarian surface; usually bilateral adnexal involvement with extensive tubal invasion and nearly always with peritoneal carcinomatosis or extensive bowel invasion; bilateral adnexa may be obliterated by tumor 2. Papillary, glandular, slit-like, and solid patterns, commonly intermixed *(Figs. 5.6.1-5.6.3)*; infiltrative small nests and micropapillae *(Figs. 5.6.4-5.6.7)*; less commonly thick urothelial-like papillae (see Section 5.30) 3. Large epithelial cells with marked atypia, often with bizarre nuclear forms *(Figs. 5.6.3-5.6.5, and 5.6.7)*; large prominent nucleoli, abundant mitotic activity with abnormal forms; psammoma bodies are usually present but may sometimes be seen only focally 4. STIC is the only morphologically noninvasive component	1. Intracystic and exophytic components; peritoneal involvement or carcinomatosis usually present 2. Haphazard infiltrative pattern of nests and micropapillae, often surrounded by a space *(Figs. 5.6.8-5.6.12)* 3. Serous (tubal)-type epithelium, occasionally ciliated; mild to occasionally moderate cytologic atypia with small prominent nucleoli *(Figs. 5.6.9, 5.6.10, 5.6.12)*; psammoma bodies common *(Fig. 5.6.8)*; mitotic figures are absent or infrequent 4. Noninvasive component with nonhierarchical branching, Medusa appearance, papillary fusion (see Section 5.1); SBT component often present; ciliated cells more commonly seen in SBT component
Special studies	Aberrant p53 expression; p16+ (extensive, often diffuse); Ki 67 index high	p53 wild-type staining pattern; no diffuse p16 expression; Ki 67 index low (mildly elevated)

	High-Grade Serous Carcinoma	**Low-Grade Serous Carcinoma**
Treatment	Hysterectomy with bilateral salpingo-oophorectomy, staging (with debulking when indicated); chemotherapy (in neoadjuvant, adjuvant +/− maintenance setting)	Hysterectomy with bilateral salpingo-oophorectomy, comprehensive staging +/− debulking; adjuvant therapeutic options include chemotherapy and hormonal therapy
Prognosis	Stage III patients have 5-y survival of 45%-50% if optimally debulked; suboptimal debulking has 20%-30% 5-y survival	Indolent with 5-/10-y survival ~75%/45%, respectively, for stage III

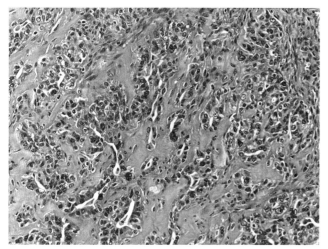

Figure 5.6.1 High-grade serous carcinoma displays interanastomosing slit-like spaces and high-grade nuclear atypia.

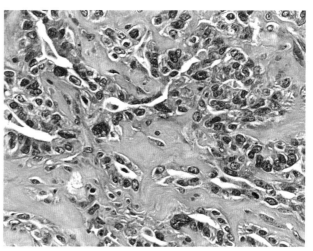

Figure 5.6.2 High-grade serous carcinoma, same case as *Figure 5.6.1*, with glands and slit-like spaces lined by markedly atypical epithelium.

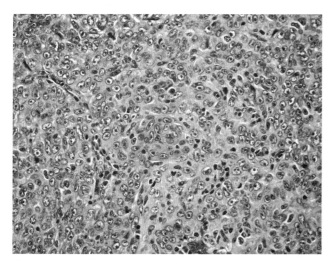

Figure 5.6.3 Solid pattern of high-grade serous carcinoma with relatively uniform but high-grade nuclei with large prominent nucleoli and chromatin clumping.

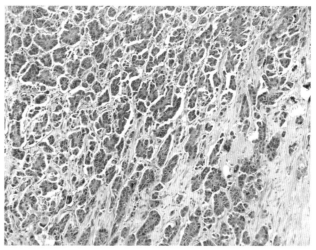

Figure 5.6.4 High-grade serous carcinoma with infiltrative small nests and clustered cells, high-grade nuclear features and fibrotic stroma.

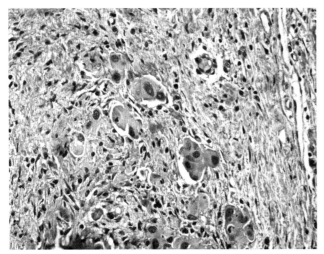

Figure 5.6.5 High-grade serous carcinoma (HGSC) with isolated and clustered large cells with abundant eosinophilic cytoplasm and marked nuclear atypia. Isolated cells in the stroma, as seen here, are more commonly seen in treated HGSCs and rare in chemotherapy-naive tumors.

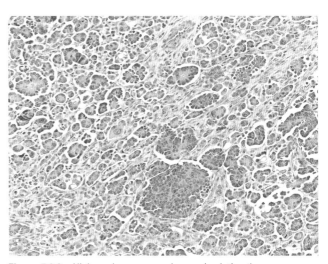

Figure 5.6.6 High-grade serous carcinoma simulating the micropapillary pattern of low-grade serous carcinoma.

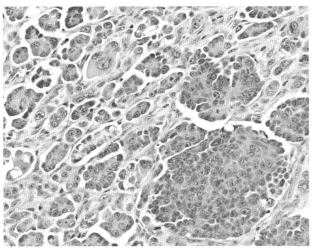

Figure 5.6.7 High-grade serous carcinoma simulating low-grade serous carcinoma (same case as *Fig. 5.6.6*).

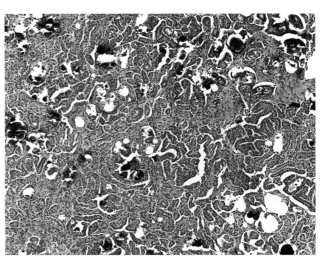

Figure 5.6.8 Low-grade serous carcinoma showing infiltrative pattern of small papillae and numerous psammoma bodies.

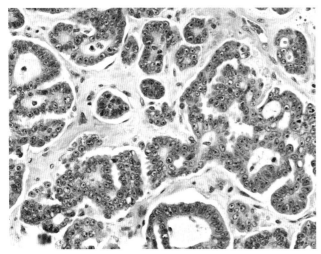

Figure 5.6.9 Low-grade serous carcinoma with invasive micropapillae displaying uniform and round nuclei, evenly dispersed chromatin, and small nucleoli. Mitotic figures are not seen.

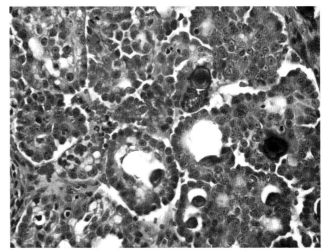

Figure 5.6.10 Low-grade serous carcinoma with psammomatous calcification within the cores of several papillae; note mild atypia with small prominent nucleoli.

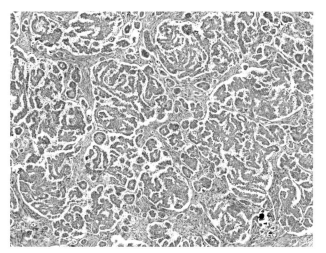

Figure 5.6.11 Low-grade serous carcinoma showing infiltrative pattern of small papillae.

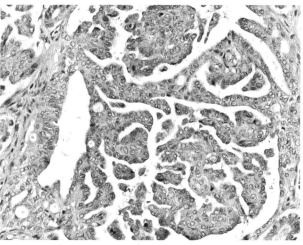

Figure 5.6.12 Low-grade serous carcinoma with micropapillae displaying uniform and round nuclei, evenly dispersed chromatin, and small nucleoli. Mitotic figures are not seen. Same case as *Figure 5.6.11*.

	High-Grade Serous Carcinoma With Serous Borderline Tumor (SBT)–Like Pattern	Typical Serous Borderline Tumor (SBT)
Age	Mean 60-63 y	Median 49 y
Location	Ovarian surface and within ovarian stroma, tubal fimbriae, commonly invade nonfimbrial tube	Within ovary with or without exophytic surface component; may be confined to surface
Symptoms	Pelvic pain, increasing abdominal girth, bloating, early satiety, urinary symptoms	Commonly asymptomatic; may have nonspecific pelvic pain or urinary symptoms
Signs	Pelvic/abdominal mass, ascites	Pelvic/adnexal mass
Etiology	Majority derive from serous tubal intraepithelial carcinoma (STIC), usually of fimbrial origin; nearly all have *TP53* mutations; a substantial proportion have either germline or somatic mutation in *BRCA1*, *BRCA2*, or other homologous recombination repair gene or epigenetic silencing of these genes; high genomic instability	Unknown; originates from serous-type inclusions, possibly originating from tubal epithelial implantation; *KRAS* and *BRAF* mutations
Gross and histology	1. Bilateral, intracystic tumors 2. Hierarchical papillary branching resembling SBT architecture *(Figs. 5.7.1-5.7.4)* 3. Typical high-grade cytology of serous carcinoma *(Figs. 5.7.5 and 5.7.6)* with high mitotic index 4. This high-grade "noninvasive" pattern is occasionally seen focally in otherwise typical HGSC but may be pure in <0.5% of HGSC	1. Intracystic and exophytic components 2. Hierarchical branching, tufting, and apparent detachment of cell clusters; no invasion *(Figs. 5.7.7-5.7.10)* 3. Tubal-type epithelium, ciliated, focally with hobnail or dense eosinophilic cytoplasm; mild cytologic atypia *(Figs. 5.7.9 and 5.7.10)*; may have psammoma bodies; low mitotic index 4. 12% have noninvasive peritoneal implants; those with exophytic component more often with implants
Special studies	Aberrant p53 staining pattern; p16+ (extensive, often diffuse); Ki 67 index high	p53 wild-type staining pattern; no diffuse p16 expression; Ki 67 index low
Treatment	Staging (with debulking when indicated), chemotherapy (in adjuvant, neoadjuvant +/− maintenance setting)	Salpingo-oophorectomy +/− staging
Prognosis	Patient described was alive and well after 6 y; expected outcome should be similar to classic high-grade serous carcinoma (stage III patients have 5-y survival of 45%-50% if optimally debulked; suboptimal debulking has 20%-30% 5-y survival) (limited data on the significance of this histological appearance)	Increased risk of serous carcinoma (vast majority low grade) (HR = 9.2; 95% CI: 6.8-12.2); if confined to ovaries (ie, without associated peritoneal implants) 1.7% develop carcinoma; noninvasive implants confer risk of invasive low-grade serous carcinoma of ~16% (HR = 7.7; 95% CI: 3.9-15.0)

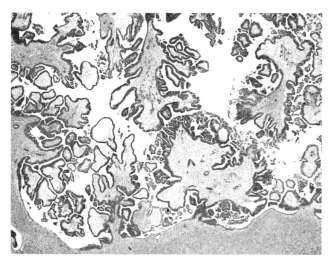

Figure 5.7.1 High-grade serous carcinoma with serous borderline tumor–like pattern characterized by hierarchical branching without obvious stromal invasion.

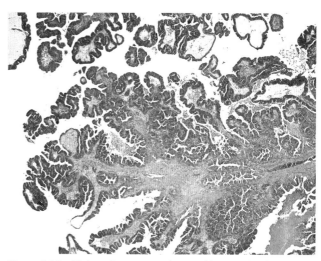

Figure 5.7.2 High-grade serous carcinoma with serous borderline tumor–like pattern with hierarchical branching, tufting, and detachment of cell clusters. There is no obvious stromal invasion.

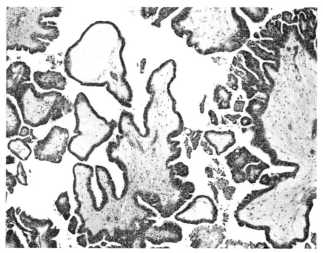

Figure 5.7.3 High-grade serous carcinoma with serous borderline tumor–like pattern, same case as *Figure 5.7.1*, showing epithelial proliferation, detachment of cell clusters, focal bridging of surface papillae, and no invasion of the stromal cores of the papillae.

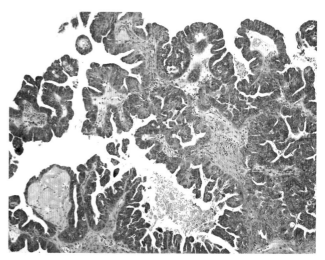

Figure 5.7.4 High-grade serous carcinoma with serous borderline tumor–like pattern, same case as *Figure 5.7.2*. Epithelial proliferation with stratification and detachment of cell clusters.

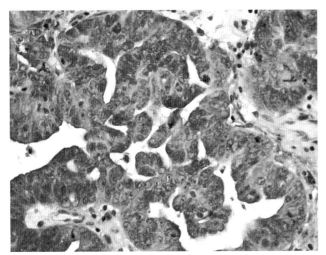

Figure 5.7.5 High-grade serous carcinoma with serous borderline tumor–like pattern, same case as *Figure 5.7.2*. The cytologic features of high-grade serous carcinoma are more evident at high magnification; nuclear enlargement, hyperchromasia, prominent nucleoli, and a few mitotic figures are seen.

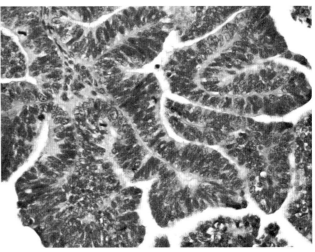

Figure 5.7.6 High-grade serous carcinoma with serous borderline tumor–like pattern (same case as *Figs. 5.7.1 and 5.7.3)*; high-grade cytologic features with epithelial stratification, nuclear enlargement, hyperchromasia, and occasional mitotic figures.

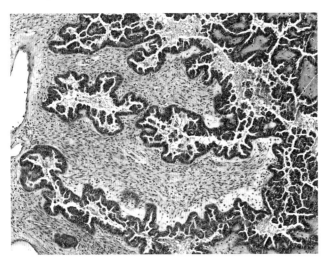

Figure 5.7.7 Serous borderline tumor with hierarchical branching pattern. Stromal invasion is absent.

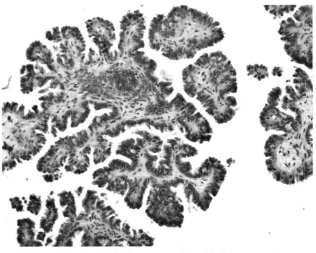

Figure 5.7.8 Serous borderline tumor with epithelial stratification, tufting, and focal detachment of cell clusters.

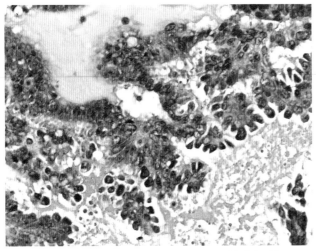

Figure 5.7.9 Serous borderline tumor displaying epithelial tufting, a hobnail-like pattern, and mild cytologic atypia. Cilia are present.

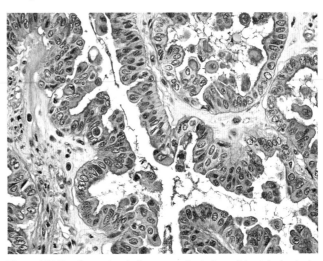

Figure 5.7.10 Serous borderline tumor displaying mild cytologic atypia, prominent eosinophilic cytoplasm, and detached individual cells and cell clusters. Mitotic figures are not seen.

	High-Grade Serous Carcinoma	Carcinosarcoma (Malignant Müllerian Mixed Tumor; MMMT)
Age	Mean 60-63 y	Mean 65-66 y
Location	Ovarian surface, and within ovarian stroma, tubal fimbriae, commonly invade nonfimbrial tube	Ovarian surface, and within ovarian stroma, tubal fimbriae, commonly invade nonfimbrial tube
Symptoms	Pelvic pain, increasing abdominal girth, bloating, early satiety, urinary symptoms	Pelvic pain, increasing abdominal girth, bloating, early satiety, urinary symptoms
Signs	Pelvic/abdominal mass, ascites	Pelvic/abdominal mass, ascites
Etiology	Majority derive from serous tubal intraepithelial carcinoma (STIC), usually of fimbrial origin; nearly all have *TP53* mutations; a substantial proportion have either germline or somatic mutation in *BRCA1*, *BRCA2* or other homologous recombination repair gene or epigenetic silencing of these genes; high genomic instability	Majority evolve from HGSCs that derive from STIC, usually of fimbrial origin; nearly all have *TP53* mutations
Gross and histology	1. Ovaries normal sized or slightly enlarged in one-third to one-half of cases with subcentimeter surface nodules; remaining show enlarged solid and/or cystic ovaries, 8-10 cm; fallopian tube fimbriae may be prominent and tumorous and may be splayed across ovarian surface; usually bilateral adnexal involvement with extensive tubal invasion and nearly always with peritoneal carcinomatosis or extensive bowel invasion 2. Papillary, glandular, slit-like, and solid patterns, commonly intermixed *(Figs. 5.8.1-5.8.5)*; less commonly thick urothelial-like papillae (see Section 5.30) 3. Large epithelial cells with marked atypia, often with bizarre nuclear forms *(Figs. 5.8.3-5.8.5)*; large prominent nucleoli and abundant mitotic activity with abnormal forms; psammomatous calcification usually present 4. Sarcomatous component absent; carcinomatous component may on occasion have spindle cell features (see Section 5.17)	1. Ovaries normal sized or slightly enlarged in one-third to one-half of cases with subcentimeter surface nodules; remaining show markedly enlarged solid and/or cystic ovaries, mean 14 cm, can be up to 15-20 cm; fallopian tube fimbriae may be prominent and tumorous and may be splayed across ovarian surface; usually bilateral adnexal involvement with extensive tubal invasion and nearly always with peritoneal carcinomatosis or extensive bowel invasion 2. Epithelial component usually displays high-grade serous patterns with papillary, glandular, and solid patterns, commonly intermixed *(Figs. 5.8.6-5.8.8)*; endometrioid patterns may be present 3. Large epithelial cells with marked atypia *(Fig. 5.8.7)*, often with bizarre nuclear forms; large prominent nucleoli and abundant mitotic activity with abnormal forms; psammomatous calcification usually present 4. Sarcomatous component with high-grade spindle cell differentiation with high mitotic activity and marked cytologic atypia *(Figs. 5.8.6-5.8.8)*; myxoid or small cell areas may be present; heterologous elements commonly present (>50%), most often cytologically malignant cartilage, rhabdomyoblasts, occasionally osteoid, and liposarcoma *(Fig. 5.8.9)*

	High-Grade Serous Carcinoma	**Carcinosarcoma (Malignant Müllerian Mixed Tumor; MMMT)**
Special studies	Aberrant p53 expression, CK7+, p16+ (diffuse), WT1+, CAM5.2+, PAX8+; stromal cells, including reactive desmoplastic areas, will be negative; no aberrant p53 expression in the stroma	**Epithelial component**: aberrant p53 expression, CK7+, p16+ (diffuse), WT1+, CAM5.2+; **sarcomatous component** generally has similar profile but may stain more weakly or focally for epithelial markers or completely lack their expression; PAX8 often negative in sarcomatous component
Treatment	Staging (with debulking when indicated), chemotherapy (in neoadjuvant/adjuvant +/− maintenance setting)	Staging (with debulking when indicated), chemotherapy (in neoadjuvant/adjuvant +/− maintenance setting)
Prognosis	Stage III patients have 5-y survival of 45%-50% if optimally debulked; suboptimal debulking has 20%-30% 5-y survival	Stage III patients have 5-y survival of 20%-25%

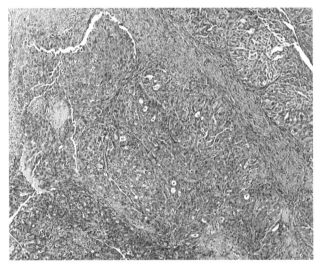

Figure 5.8.1 High-grade serous carcinoma with poorly differentiated solid and glandular patterns with slit-like spaces.

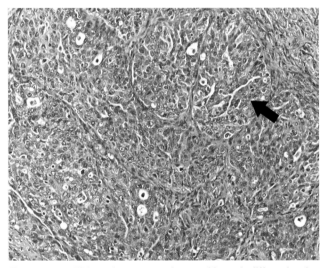

Figure 5.8.2 High-grade serous carcinoma with poorly differentiated glandular pattern. Note slit-like spaces (*arrow*).

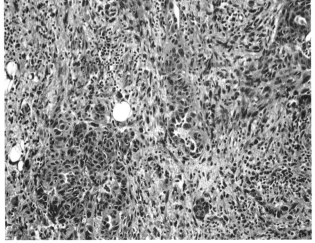

Figure 5.8.3 High-grade serous carcinoma with glands lined by high-grade epithelium infiltrating a spindle cell stroma lacking significant atypia in the spindle cells.

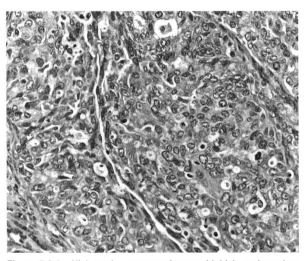

Figure 5.8.4 High-grade serous carcinoma with high-grade nuclear atypia.

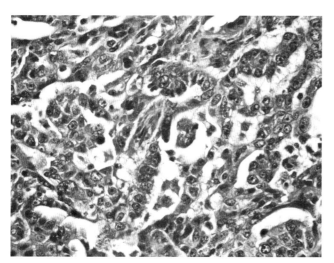

Figure 5.8.5   High-grade serous carcinoma with marked nuclear atypia, glands, and slit-like spaces.

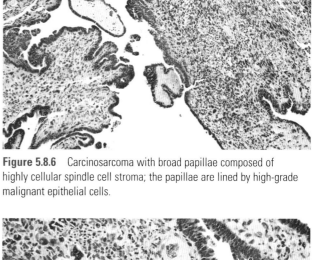

Figure 5.8.6   Carcinosarcoma with broad papillae composed of highly cellular spindle cell stroma; the papillae are lined by high-grade malignant epithelial cells.

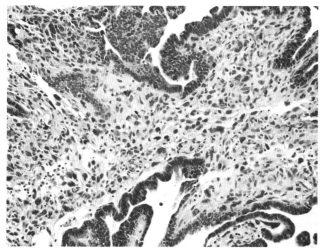

Figure 5.8.7   Carcinosarcoma, same case as *Figure 5.8.6*, with marked atypia of spindle cell stroma with markedly enlarged hyperchromatic nuclei.

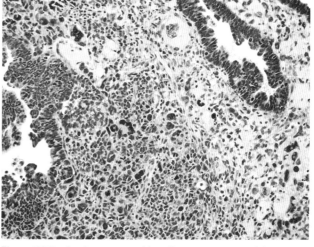

Figure 5.8.8   Carcinosarcoma with malignant stroma-containing tumor giant cells with bizarre hyperchromatic nuclei, and high-grade malignant glands resembling high-grade serous carcinoma.

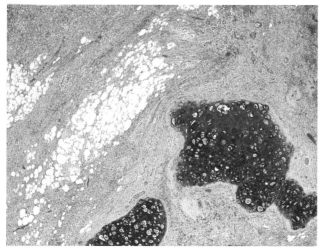

Figure 5.8.9   Carcinosarcoma with heterologous chondrosarcomatous and liposarcomatous components.

	High-Grade Serous Carcinoma	High-Grade Endometrioid Carcinoma
Age	Mean 60-63 y	Mean 55-58 y
Location	Ovarian surface, and within ovarian stroma, tubal fimbriae, commonly invade nonfimbrial tube	Within ovary
Symptoms	Pelvic pain, increasing abdominal girth, bloating, early satiety, urinary symptoms	Pelvic pain, increasing abdominal girth, bloating, early satiety, vaginal bleeding, urinary symptoms
Signs	Pelvic/abdominal mass, ascites	Pelvic/abdominal mass, ascites
Etiology	Majority derive from serous tubal intraepithelial carcinoma (STIC), usually of fimbrial origin; nearly all have *TP53* mutations; a substantial proportion have either germline or somatic mutation in *BRCA1, BRCA2* or other homologous recombination repair gene or epigenetic silencing of these genes; high genomic instability	Endometriosis; germline *MLH1, MSH2, PMS2,* or *MSH6* mutation (Lynch syndrome) in a small subset; *PTEN,* β-*catenin* (*CTNNB1*), *KRAS, ARID1A,* and *PIK3CA* mutations; a subset of cases may have *TP53* mutations
Gross and histology	1. Ovaries normal sized or slightly enlarged in one-third to one-half of cases with subcentimeter surface nodules; remaining show enlarged solid and/or cystic ovaries, 8-10 cm; fallopian tube fimbriae may be prominent and tumorous and may be splayed across ovarian surface; usually bilateral adnexal involvement with extensive tubal invasion and nearly always with peritoneal carcinomatosis or extensive bowel invasion 2. Papillary, glandular, slit-like, and solid patterns, commonly intermixed *(Figs. 5.9.1-5.9.5)*; SET (solid, pseudoendometrioid, transitional) patterns often present *(Figs. 5.9.6 and 5.9.7)*; pseudoendometrioid pattern may have solid areas containing spaces mimicking endometrioid glands *(Fig. 5.9.7)*, or well-formed glands but with classic high-grade serous nuclear features; thick urothelial (transitional)-like papillae may be present 3. Large epithelial cells with marked atypia, often with bizarre nuclear forms *(Figs. 5.9.4 and 5.9.5)*; large prominent nucleoli, abundant mitotic activity with abnormal forms; psammomatous calcification usually present	1. Usually unilateral, stage I in almost half; mean size 15 cm; cystic or cystic and solid; cysts contain dark brown viscous fluid (old blood +/− mucus); papillary or nodular growths arise from cyst lining 2. Poorly differentiated areas may have solid growth with infiltrative pattern of glands, cribriform growth, nests, and solid masses with jagged edges *(Figs. 5.9.8-5.9.10)*; architecturally well-differentiated areas with confluent glandular epithelial proliferation and/or cribriform growth resembling endometrial endometrioid carcinoma are often present *(Fig. 5.9.9)* 3. Columnar epithelium with sharp luminal gland margins in architecturally well-differentiated areas *(Fig. 5.9.11)*; may display variable range of nuclear atypia/mitotic activity, including enlarged, round to ovoid nuclei with hyperchromasia, prominent nucleoli, and high mitotic index in both glandular and solid areas; psammomatous calcification usually absent

	High-Grade Serous Carcinoma	**High-Grade Endometrioid Carcinoma**
	4. STIC is the only noninvasive component present	4. Squamous differentiation in half *(Fig. 5.9.12)*; adenofibromatous component often present; associated endometriosis is present in majority and often shows atypia, hyperplasia, and other features reflecting origin within endometriotic cyst or associated endometrioid borderline tumor; sex cord–like differentiation may be present *(Fig. 5.9.10)*
Special studies	• Aberrant p53 expression; p16+ (extensive, often diffuse), WT1+ • No loss of staining for DNA mismatch repair proteins (MLH1, PMS2, MSH2, and/or MSH6)	• p53 may show aberrant staining pattern in a subset; no diffuse p16 expression; WT1 usually (−) • Loss of staining for DNA mismatch repair proteins (MLH1, PMS2, MSH2, and/or MSH6) in a subset
Treatment	Staging (with debulking when indicated), chemotherapy (in adjuvant/neoadjuvant +/− maintenance setting)	Staging (with debulking when indicated), chemotherapy (in adjuvant or neoadjuvant setting) except for low-grade stage IA/B; hormonal suppression may be used for recurrence
Prognosis	Stage III patients have 5-y survival of 45%-50% if optimally debulked; suboptimal debulking has 20%-30% 5-y survival	Stage I >90% survival; stage-stratified analyses show somewhat better prognosis compared to high-grade serous carcinoma in advanced stage

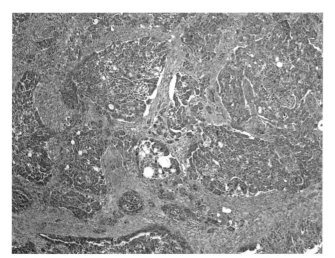

Figure 5.9.1   High-grade serous carcinoma with solid, papillary, and glandular patterns.

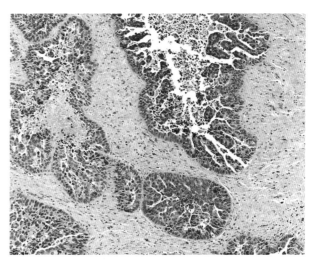

Figure 5.9.2   High-grade serous carcinoma with intraglandular papillary pattern with necrosis.

5 OVARY

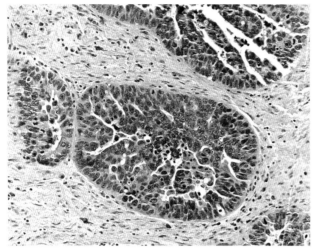

Figure 5.9.3 High-grade serous carcinoma with high-grade nuclear atypia (higher magnification of *Fig. 5.9.2*). The gland at the **left** resembles an endometrioid-type gland but displays the same high-grade atypia seen in the papillary areas.

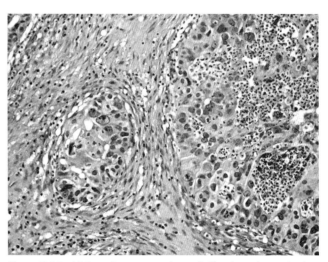

Figure 5.9.4 High-grade serous carcinoma infiltrating a desmoplastic stroma with bizarre nuclear features and necrosis.

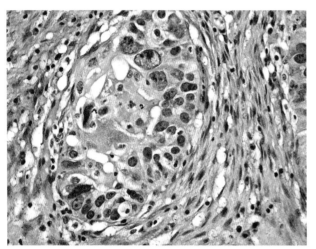

Figure 5.9.5 High-grade serous carcinoma. Higher magnification of *Figure 5.9.4* with marked nuclear atypia and large prominent nucleoli.

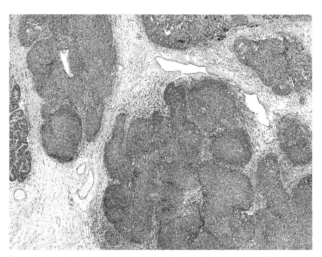

Figure 5.9.6 High-grade serous carcinoma showing solid SET pattern.

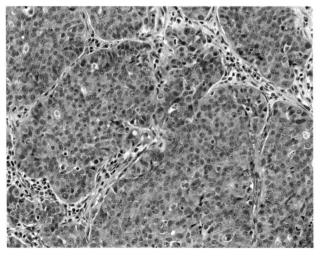

Figure 5.9.7 SET pattern of high-grade serous carcinoma with lumen-like spaces mimicking endometrioid differentiation **(top left)**. Same case as *Figure 5.9.6*.

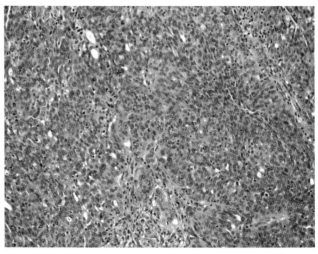

Figure 5.9.8 High-grade endometrioid carcinoma showing solid pattern.

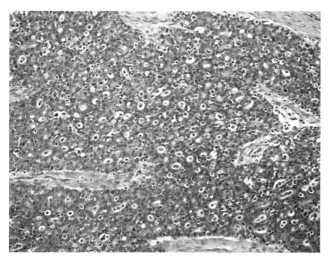

Figure 5.9.9   Cribriform pattern of high-grade endometrioid carcinoma.

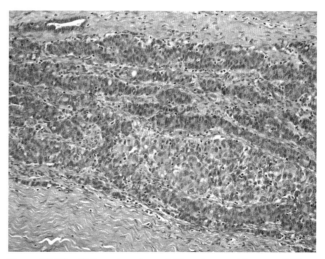

Figure 5.9.10   High-grade endometrioid carcinoma with sex cord–like pattern (see Section 5.16).

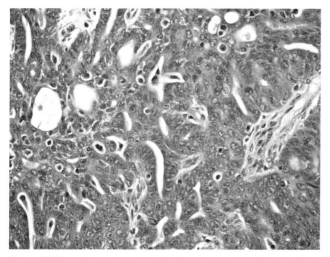

Figure 5.9.11   High-grade endometrioid carcinoma. Note the cuboidal to columnar cells with flat luminal edges. The degree of atypia is not as severe as in high-grade serous carcinoma.

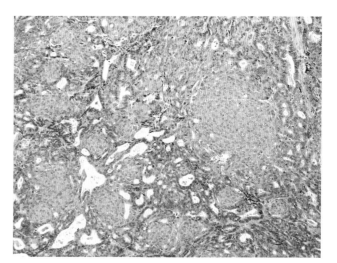

Figure 5.9.12   High-grade endometrioid carcinoma with squamous differentiation. This area of the tumor is better differentiated than in other areas.

	Mucinous Borderline Tumor (MBT)	MBT With Intraepithelial Carcinoma
Age	Mean 50 y	Mean 50 y
Location	Within ovary	Within ovary
Symptoms	Pelvic/abdominal pain and increasing abdominal girth	Pelvic/abdominal pain and increasing abdominal girth
Signs	Large pelvic/abdominal mass	Large pelvic/abdominal mass
Etiology	Arise in mucinous cystadenomas; *KRAS* mutations; low frequency of *TP53* mutations; rarely *BRAF* mutations	Arise in mucinous cystadenomas; *KRAS* mutations; low frequency of *TP53* mutations; rarely *BRAF* mutations
Gross and histology	1. Nearly always unilateral, mean size 22 cm; grossly similar to mucinous cystadenomas, with large, mucin-filled cysts; papillary growths sometimes arise in cyst walls 2. Architectural complexity with glandular crowding and cystic areas with epithelial stratification, intraglandular papillary growth, and detached epithelial clusters *(Figs. 5.10.1 and 5.10.2)*; mucinous epithelial lining displays abundant basophilic or eosinophilic cytoplasm with grade 1-2 atypia; areas of cystadenoma with small basal nuclei may be present; proliferative areas with atypical architecture and cytology constitute >10% of the tumor, displaying nuclear enlargement, mild hyperchromasia, prominent nucleoli, and pseudostratification, often with mitotic figures *(Figs. 5.10.2 and 5.10.3)* 3. Tumors should be well sampled to exclude invasion	1. Nearly always unilateral, mean size 22 cm; grossly similar to mucinous cystadenomas, with large, mucin-filled cysts; papillary growths sometimes arise in cyst walls 2. Architectural complexity with glandular crowding and cystic areas with epithelial stratification, intraglandular papillary growth, and detached epithelial clusters *(Figs. 5.10.4 and 5.10.5)*; mucinous epithelial lining displays abundant basophilic or eosinophilic cytoplasm; areas of cystadenoma with small basal nuclei; areas of grade 3 atypia are present, displaying unequivocal cytologic features of malignancy with nuclear enlargement, hyperchromasia, prominent nucleoli, pseudostratification, and often with mitotic figures *(Figs. 5.10.5 and 5.10.6)* 3. Tumors should be well sampled to exclude invasion
Special studies	Of no use for this differential diagnosis	Of no use for this differential diagnosis
Treatment	Unilateral salpingo-oophorectomy +/− staging +/− appendectomy	Unilateral salpingo-oophorectomy +/− staging +/− appendectomy
Prognosis	Benign	Rare cases recur or metastasize; virtually 100% survival if well sampled (two blocks/centimeter maximum diameter) and metastatic carcinoma to the ovary is rigorously excluded

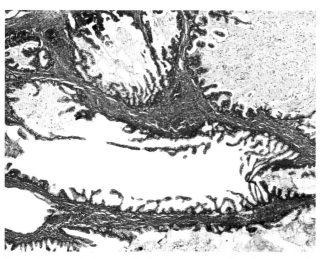

Figure 5.10.1 Mucinous borderline tumor with cystic architecture and epithelial stratification/intraglandular papillary growth.

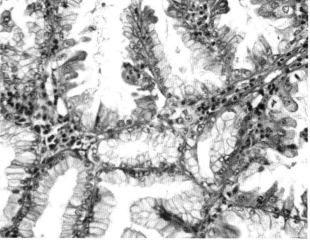

Figure 5.10.2 Mucinous borderline tumor with mild nuclear pseudostratification and cytologic atypia with small prominent nucleoli.

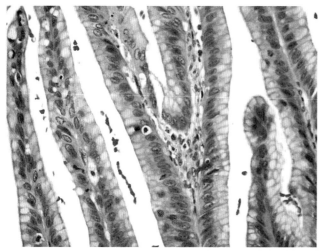

Figure 5.10.3 Mucinous borderline tumor. The nuclear features are insufficient for intraepithelial carcinoma.

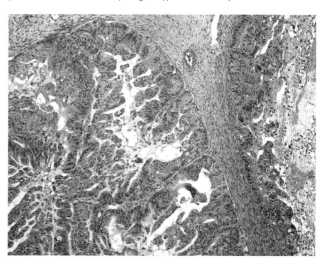

Figure 5.10.4 Mucinous borderline tumor with intraepithelial carcinoma. The architecture is similar to mucinous borderline tumor without intraepithelial carcinoma.

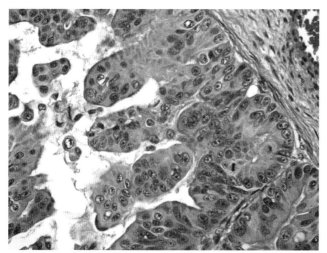

Figure 5.10.5 Mucinous borderline tumor with intraepithelial carcinoma. The epithelium is stratified with cells showing high-grade atypia, enlarged and prominent nucleoli, and occasional mitotic figures. Note the loss of mucin compared with *Figure 5.10.3*.

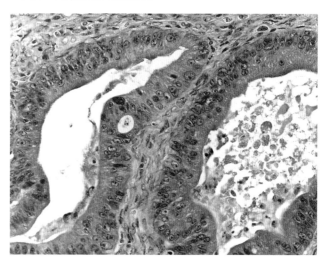

Figure 5.10.6 Mucinous borderline tumor with intraepithelial carcinoma. The cells show round and large vesicular nuclei with prominent nucleoli.

	Mucinous Borderline Tumor (MBT) With Microinvasion/Microinvasive Carcinoma	MBT With Gland Rupture
Age	Mean 50 y	Mean 50 y
Location	Within ovary	Within ovary
Symptoms	Pelvic/abdominal pain, increasing abdominal girth	Pelvic/abdominal pain, increasing abdominal girth
Signs	Large pelvic/abdominal mass	Large pelvic/abdominal mass
Etiology	MBT arises in mucinous cystadenomas; *KRAS* mutations; rarely *BRAF* mutations; low frequency of TP53 mutations; pathogenesis of microinvasion unclear	MBT arises in mucinous cystadenomas; *KRAS* mutations; low frequency of TP53 mutations; rarely *BRAF* mutations; gland rupture may be due to infarction or possibly due to intraoperative manipulation
Gross and histology	1. Nearly always unilateral, mean size 22 cm; grossly similar to mucinous cystadenomas, with large, mucin-filled cysts; papillary growths sometimes arise in cyst walls 2. Architectural complexity with glandular crowding and cystic areas with epithelial stratification, intraglandular papillary growth, and detached epithelial clusters; mucinous epithelial lining displays abundant basophilic or eosinophilic cytoplasm with grade 1-2 atypia (grade 3 atypia warrants a designation of MBT with intraepithelial carcinoma, with marked nuclear enlargement, hyperchromasia, and prominent nucleoli, often with mitotic figures); proliferative areas with atypical architecture and cytology constitute >10% of the tumor; areas of cystadenoma with small basal nuclei may be present 3. Microinvasion is characterized by budding of single and small nests of atypical mucinous epithelium haphazardly into the stroma, showing the same degree of cytologic atypia as the main tumor; each focus <5 mm in diameter; multiple foci of microinvasion permissible; stromal reaction may be myxoid or fibrous, sometimes with mucin dissection in stroma; mucin granulomas often present *(Figs. 5.11.1-5.11.5)*; per the 2020 WHO Classification, tumors satisfying the above definition but with marked cytologic atypia should be classified as "microinvasive carcinoma." 4. Tumors should be well sampled to exclude more extensive areas of invasion	1. Nearly always unilateral, mean size 22 cm; grossly similar to mucinous cystadenomas, with large, mucin-filled cysts; papillary growths sometimes arise in cyst walls 2. Architectural complexity with glandular crowding and cystic areas with epithelial stratification, intraglandular papillary growth, and detached epithelial clusters; mucinous epithelial lining displays abundant basophilic or eosinophilic cytoplasm with grade 1-2 atypia (grade 3 atypia warrants a designation of MBT with intraepithelial carcinoma, with marked nuclear enlargement, hyperchromasia, and prominent nucleoli, often with mitotic figures); proliferative areas with atypical architecture and cytology constitute >10% of the tumor; areas of cystadenoma with small basal nuclei may be present 3. Areas of gland rupture display mucin dissection through the stroma (pseudomyxoma ovarii) *(Figs. 5.11.6-5.11.8)* and inflammation *(Figs. 5.11.0 and 5.11.9)*, mucin granulomas characterized by clustered foamy macrophages are often present and may also contain lymphocytes and multinucleated giant cells; isolated or clustered mucinous epithelial cells or disrupted glands may be present within the stroma *(Fig. 5.11.7)*; features of infarction may be present; stromal reaction may be fibrous 4. Tumors should be well sampled to exclude invasion

	Mucinous Borderline Tumor (MBT) With Microinvasion/Microinvasive Carcinoma	**MBT With Gland Rupture**
Special studies	Not useful in this differential	Not useful in this differential
Treatment	Unilateral salpingo-oophorectomy +/− staging +/− appendectomy	Unilateral salpingo-oophorectomy +/− staging +/− appendectomy
Prognosis	Rare cases recur or metastasize; virtually 100% survival if well sampled (two blocks/centimeter maximum diameter) and metastatic carcinoma to the ovary is rigorously excluded	Benign

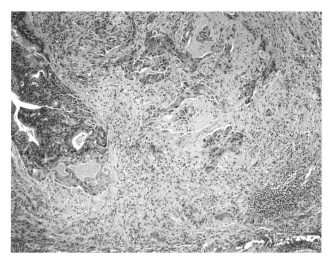

Figure 5.11.1   Mucinous borderline tumor with microinvasion/microinvasive carcinoma displays a haphazard infiltrative pattern of angulated glands in a reactive desmoplastic stroma. Noninvasive component is at **left**.

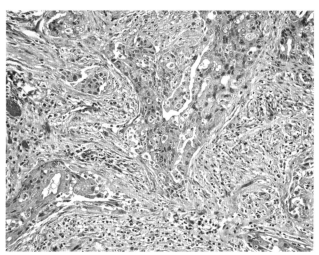

Figure 5.11.2   Same case as *Figure 5.11.1* with microinvasion/microinvasive carcinoma displaying infiltrative glands with moderate cytologic atypia.

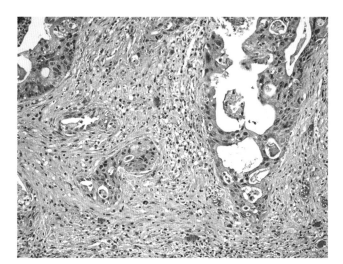

Figure 5.11.3   Mucinous borderline tumor with microinvasion with several irregularly shaped glands in a reactive stroma.

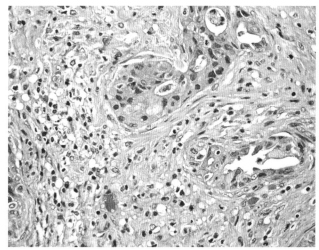

Figure 5.11.4   Mucinous borderline tumor with microinvasion, same case as *Figure 5.11.3*, displaying moderate cytologic atypia.

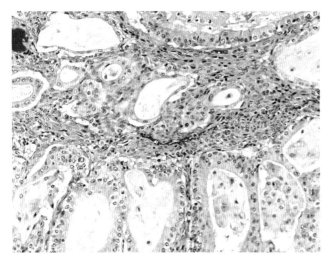

Figure 5.11.5 Mucinous borderline tumor with microinvasion shows a cluster of small glands with an infiltrative pattern in the **center**; noninvasive component is seen at **top** and **bottom**.

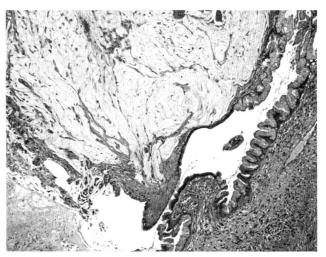

Figure 5.11.6 Mucinous borderline tumor with gland rupture at low magnification shows large pools of mucin dissecting the stroma (pseudomyxoma ovarii).

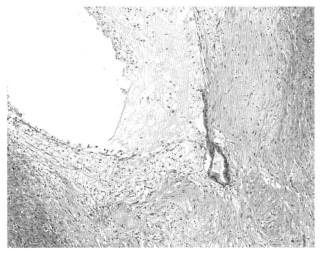

Figure 5.11.7 Mucinous borderline tumor with a solitary disrupted gland accompanied by mucin dissection. Note chronic inflammation and numerous foamy macrophages surrounding space at **top left**.

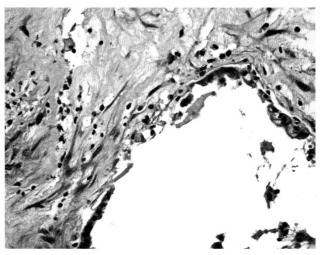

Figure 5.11.8 High magnification of stromal reaction to gland rupture with mucin dissection showing edema and chronic inflammation; disrupted glandular epithelium partially lines space.

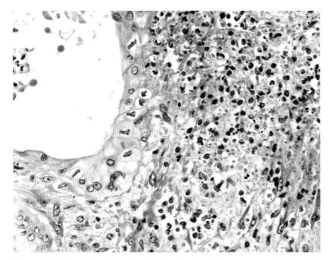

Figure 5.11.9 Round glands within site of rupture are associated with marked acute and chronic inflammation.

	Mucinous Borderline Tumor (MBT), Intestinal Type	Invasive Mucinous Carcinoma, Primary Ovarian
Age	Mean 50 y	Mean 50 y
Location	Within ovary	Within ovary
Symptoms	Pelvic/abdominal pain, increasing abdominal girth	Pelvic/abdominal pain, increasing abdominal girth
Signs	Large pelvic/abdominal mass	Large pelvic/abdominal mass
Etiology	Arise in mucinous cystadenomas; *KRAS* mutations; rarely *BRAF* mutations; low frequency of *TP53* mutations	Arise from mucinous cystadenomas through MBT; majority have *KRAS* and *TP53* mutations; rarely *BRAF* mutations; majority have copy number loss of *CDKN2A*
Gross and histology	1. Nearly always unilateral, mean size 22 cm; grossly similar to mucinous cystadenomas, with large, mucin-filled cysts; papillary growths sometimes arise in cyst walls 2. Architectural complexity with glandular crowding and cystic areas with epithelial stratification, intraglandular papillary growth, and detached epithelial clusters. Mucinous epithelial lining displays abundant basophilic or eosinophilic cytoplasm with grade 1-2 atypia (grade 3 atypia warrants a designation of MBT with intraepithelial carcinoma [see Section 5.10], with marked nuclear enlargement, hyperchromasia, and prominent nucleoli, often with mitotic figures); proliferative areas with atypical architecture and cytology constitute >10% of the tumor. Areas of cystadenoma with small basal nuclei may be present *(Figs. 5.12.1-5.12.5)*; tumors should be well sampled to exclude invasion	1. Nearly always unilateral, mean size 21 cm; 90% stage I; grossly similar to mucinous cystadenomas and MBT, with large, mucin-filled cysts; papillary growths sometimes arise in cyst walls 2. Complex papillary and/or glandular growth (including back-to-back glands without intervening stroma and/or presence of anastomosing epithelium) exceeding that seen in MBT reflects invasion in the confluent/expansile pattern *(Figs. 5.12.6-5.12.8)*; less commonly, a haphazard infiltrative pattern of small and moderately sized mucinous glands, nests, and single cells reflect destructive stromal invasion *(Figs. 5.12.9 and 5.12.10)*; a background of cystadenoma/MBT may be present (≥5 mm of confluent/invasive growth is required for distinguishing carcinoma from MBT); mucinous epithelial lining displays abundant basophilic or eosinophilic cytoplasm; invasive areas may display range of atypia (grades 1-3)
Special studies	Not useful in this differential	Not useful in this differential
Treatment	Unilateral salpingo-oophorectomy +/− staging, +/− appendectomy	Staging (with debulking when indicated) (omission of lymph nodes acceptable); +/− appendectomy; chemotherapy (in neoadjuvant or adjuvant setting) except for stage IA/B low-grade tumors
Prognosis	Benign	95% survival for stage I; advanced stage, which is rare, has dismal prognosis

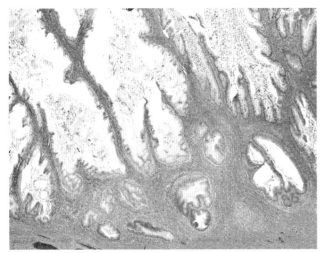

Figure 5.12.1   Mucinous borderline tumor showing multicystic appearance and epithelial stratification. Glands in stroma at the **bottom of the photograph** represent tangential sectioning of the base of the mucinous tumor rather than invasive carcinoma.

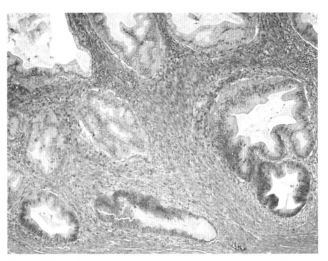

Figure 5.12.2   Mucinous borderline tumor (same case as *Fig. 5.12.1*) with glands separated by unaltered fibromatous stroma.

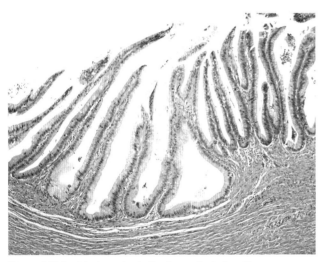

Figure 5.12.3   Mucinous borderline tumor displaying villous architecture.

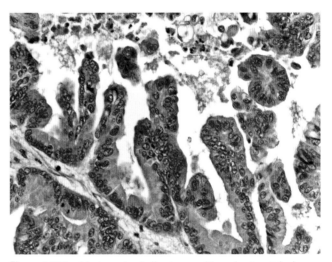

Figure 5.12.4   Mucinous borderline tumor with moderate cytologic atypia and focal detachment of cell clusters.

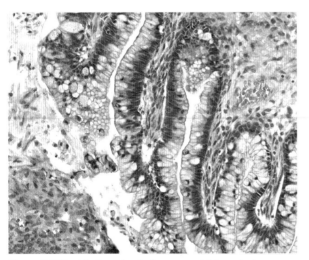

Figure 5.12.5   Mucinous borderline tumor with intestinal-type mucinous epithelium with goblet cells and mild cytologic atypia.

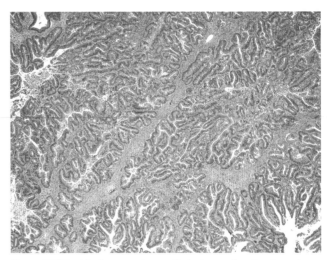

Figure 5.12.6   Mucinous carcinoma displaying confluent pattern of invasion, which is best appreciated at low magnification.

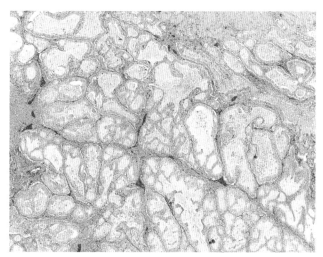

Figure 5.12.7 Mucinous carcinoma with confluent/expansile pattern of invasion appreciated at low magnification.

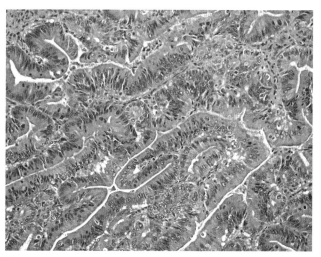

Figure 5.12.8 Mucinous carcinoma (confluent pattern) displaying intestinal-type mucinous epithelium with complex glandular and papillary pattern.

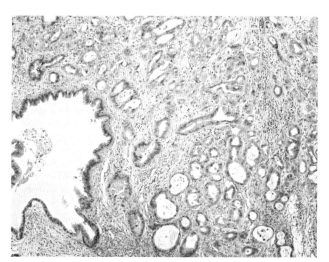

Figure 5.12.9 Mucinous carcinoma with haphazard infiltrative pattern of rounded and angulated glands of varying sizes. When this pattern is encountered in an ovarian mucinous tumor, a metastasis with secondary ovarian involvement must be excluded.

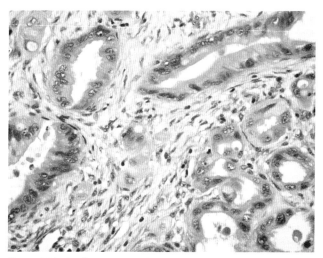

Figure 5.12.10 Same case as *Figure 5.12.9* showing moderate cytologic atypia in the infiltrative mucinous glands.

	Endometrioid Borderline Tumor (EBT)	**Endometrioid Carcinoma, FIGO Grade 1**
Age	Mean 53 y	Mean 55-58 y
Location	Within ovary	Within ovary
Symptoms	Pelvic/abdominal pain, vaginal bleeding	Pelvic pain, increasing abdominal girth, bloating, early satiety, vaginal bleeding, urinary symptoms
Signs	Pelvic mass; over a third have endometrial hyperplasia or carcinoma	Pelvic/abdominal mass, ascites
Etiology	Endometriosis; *CTNNB1* mutation in cases associated with carcinoma	Endometriosis; germline *MLH1*, *MSH2*, *PMS2*, or *MSH6* mutation (Lynch syndrome); *PTEN*, β-catenin (*CTNNB1*), *KRAS*, *ARID1A*, and *PIK3CA* mutation
Gross and histology	1. Mean 9 cm; 95% unilateral, 2% with peritoneal implants; solid or cystic, often with old blood reflecting endometriosis 2. Two major growth patterns: adenofibromatous pattern displays crowded, often back-to-back endometrioid glands *(Figs. 5.13.1-5.13.3)*; intracystic papillary/glandular pattern resembles endometrial hyperplasia or grade 1 carcinoma 3. Glands and papillae are lined by tall columnar cells with sharp luminal margins, mild to moderate cytologic atypia, round to ovoid nuclei, and sparse mitotic activity *(Fig. 5.13.3)* 4. Endometriosis is commonly present, and features often suggest an origin in the endometriosis. Squamous (morular) metaplasia is commonly seen 5. There may be glandular confluence or microinvasion, which does not exceed 5 mm	1. Usually unilateral, stage I in almost half; mean 15 cm; cystic or cystic and solid; cysts contain dark brown viscous fluid (old blood +/− mucus); papillary or nodular growths arise from cyst lining 2. Architecturally well differentiated with confluent glandular epithelial proliferation resembling endometrial endometrioid carcinoma; cribriform *(Figs. 5.13.4-5.13.7)*, papillary, glandular, and occasionally solid patterns; less commonly with infiltrative pattern of glands and nests. Confluence or invasion exceeds 5 mm 3. Tall columnar epithelium with sharp luminal gland margins, round to ovoid nuclei with hyperchromasia, and prominent nucleoli *(Figs. 5.13.6 and 5.13.7)*; mitotic activity variable, often high 4. Squamous differentiation in half; adenofibromatous component often present; associated endometriosis is present in majority and often shows atypia, hyperplasia, and other features reflecting origin within endometriotic cyst or associated EBT 5. Secretory, ciliated, and sertoliform variants may occur
Special studies	Not useful in this differential	Not useful in this differential
Treatment	Salpingo-oophorectomy +/− hysterectomy +/− staging	Staging (with debulking when indicated), chemotherapy (except for low-grade stage IA/B); hormonal suppression often used for recurrence
Prognosis	<1% recur; no deaths reported	Stage I >90% survival; stage-stratified analyses show somewhat better prognosis compared to high-grade serous carcinoma in advanced stage

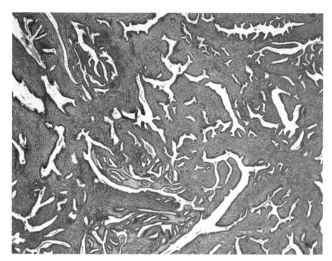

Figure 5.13.1   Endometrioid borderline tumor displays an adenofibromatous appearance with gland crowding but lacking confluence.

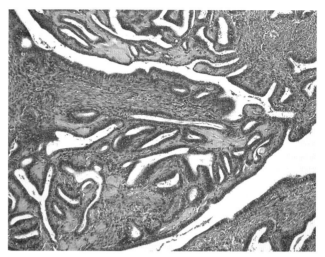

Figure 5.13.2   Endometrioid borderline tumor, same case as *Figure 5.13.1*, with crowded endometrioid glands.

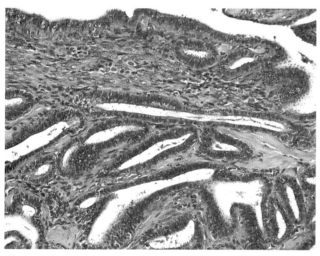

Figure 5.13.3   Endometrioid borderline tumor, same case as *Figure 5.13.1*, with mild cytologic atypia of endometrioid epithelium.

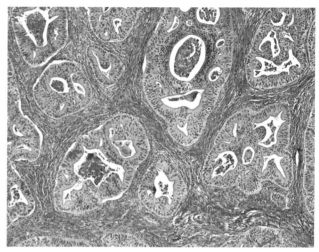

Figure 5.13.4   Low-grade endometrioid carcinoma with infiltrative pattern of cribriform glands.

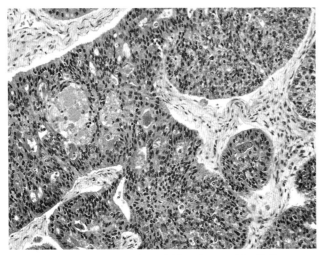

Figure 5.13.5 Low-grade endometrioid carcinoma with cribriform pattern showing sharp luminal margins and moderate cytologic atypia.

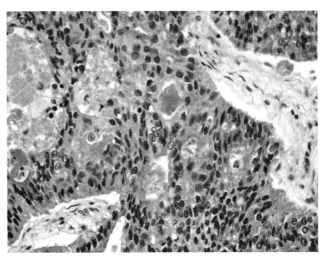

Figure 5.13.6 Same case as *Figure 5.13.5* displaying moderate cytologic atypia.

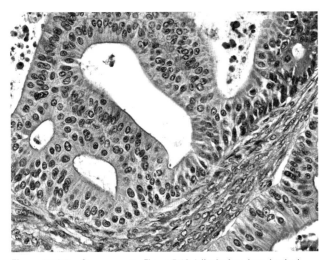

Figure 5.13.7 Same case as *Figure 5.13.4* displaying sharp luminal margins and mild to moderate cytologic atypia.

	Endometrioid Carcinoma	Metastatic Colonic Carcinoma
Age	Mean 55-58 y	Mean 48 y from undiagnosed colon cancers; mean 61 y from known colon cancers
Location	Within ovary	Within ovary and on ovarian surface
Symptoms	Pelvic pain, increasing abdominal girth, bloating, early satiety, vaginal bleeding, urinary symptoms	Pelvic/abdominal pain; a few patients have blood in stool
Signs	Pelvic/abdominal mass, ascites	Pelvic/abdominal mass; serum CA125 or CEA may be elevated; primary colonic tumor may be undiagnosed
Etiology	Endometriosis; germline *MLH1, MSH2, PMS2,* or *MSH6* mutation (Lynch syndrome); *PTEN,* β-*catenin* (*CTNNB1*), *KRAS, ARID1A,* and *PIK3CA* mutations	Metastasis from primary colorectal carcinoma with secondary involvement of ovary A subset can be associated with Lynch syndrome
Gross and histology	1. Usually unilateral, stage I in almost half; mean 15 cm; cystic or cystic and solid; cysts contain dark brown viscous fluid (old blood with mucus); papillary or nodular growths arise from cyst lining 2. Most are architecturally well differentiated with confluent glandular epithelial proliferation resembling endometrial endometrioid carcinoma; cribriform, papillary, glandular, and occasionally solid patterns; less commonly with infiltrative pattern of glands, nests, and solid masses with jagged edges *(Figs. 5.14.1-5.14.4)* 3. Tall columnar epithelium with sharp luminal gland margins, round to ovoid nuclei with hyperchromasia, prominent nucleoli *(Figs. 5.14.3-5.14.5)*; mitotic activity variable, often high; necrosis may occasionally be present *(Figs. 5.14.1-5.14.4)*; mucinous differentiation can be present 4. Squamous differentiation in half; adenofibromatous component often present; associated endometriosis is present in majority and often shows atypia, hyperplasia, and other features reflecting origin within endometriotic cyst or associated endometrioid borderline tumor 5. Secretory, ciliated, and sertoliform variants may occur	1. Mean 13-14 cm, 40% bilateral; typically cystic; not infrequently unilateral and >10 cm 2. Confluent invasive well-differentiated glandular architecture with garland pattern of dirty necrosis; may have infiltrating pattern of invasion with desmoplasia; tumor on ovarian surface and/or nodular growth within parenchyma *(Figs. 5.14.6-5.14.9)* 3. May be typical or mucinous type of colon carcinoma; typical type most often mimics endometrioid carcinoma *(Figs. 5.14.8-5.14.10)* 4. No squamous differentiation 5. No secretory, ciliated, or sertoliform differentiation
Special studies	CK7 patchy or diffuse; CK20 negative, focal, or patchy (extent of CK7 > CK20); CDX-2 negative (may be [+] in a component with mucinous differentiation); SATB2−; ER/PR+; usually PAX8+	CK20 usually diffuse; CDX-2 usually diffuse; minority are CK7+ (ascending colon and poorly differentiated tumors); in general, extent of CK20 > CK7; SATB2+, ER/PR−, PAX8−

	Endometrioid Carcinoma	**Metastatic Colonic Carcinoma**
Treatment	Staging (with debulking when indicated); chemotherapy (in neoadjuvant or adjuvant setting) except for low-grade stage IA/B; hormonal suppression often used for recurrence	As per advanced-stage colon carcinoma
Prognosis	Stage I >90% survival	The median survival for stage IV colon carcinoma can be over 2 y, particularly when isolated metastases (usually liver) can be completely resected

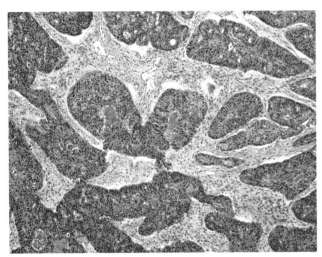

Figure 5.14.1   Endometrioid carcinoma displaying a haphazard infiltrative pattern of rounded, ovoid, and focally angulated islands of cribriform glands.

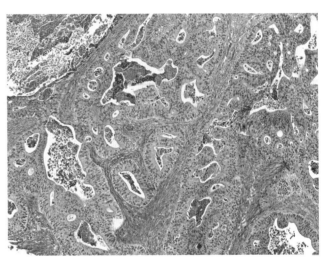

Figure 5.14.2   Low-grade endometrioid carcinoma with infiltrative pattern of smoothly contoured islands of cribriform glands. Necrosis is present within the larger glands toward **top left**.

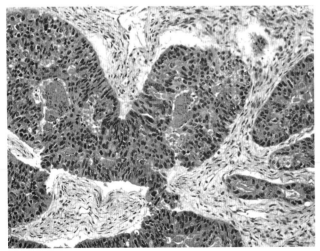

Figure 5.14.3   Endometrioid carcinoma. Same case as *Figure 5.14.1* showing tall columnar stratified epithelium closely resembling endometrial endometrioid carcinoma. Necrosis is present within glands.

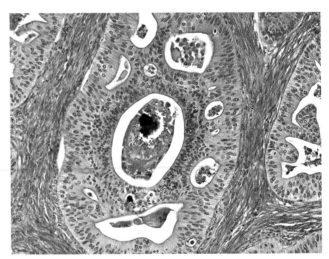

Figure 5.14.4   Low-grade endometrioid carcinoma. Same case as *Figure 5.14.2* with cribriform glands lined by tall columnar epithelium with sharp luminal margins. Necrosis is present in the **center**.

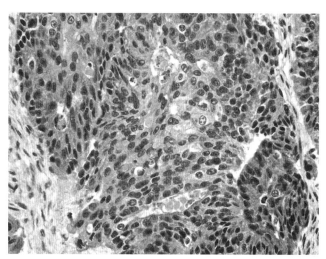

Figure 5.14.5 Endometrioid carcinoma with round to ovoid nuclei with moderate atypia.

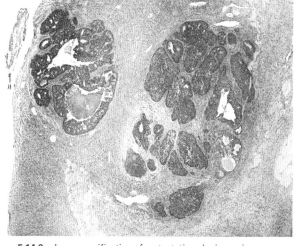

Figure 5.14.6 Low magnification of metastatic colonic carcinoma showing discrete nodules of carcinoma with focal garland pattern of necrosis **left of center**.

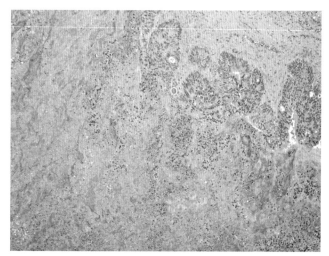

Figure 5.14.7 Metastatic colonic adenocarcinoma with **lower left** field displaying abundant dirty necrosis and irregular gland aggregates at **top right**.

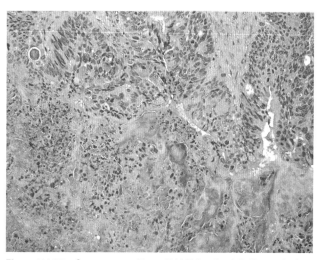

Figure 5.14.8 Same case as *Figure 5.14.7* showing cribriform colonic-type glands associated with extracellular mucin and necrosis.

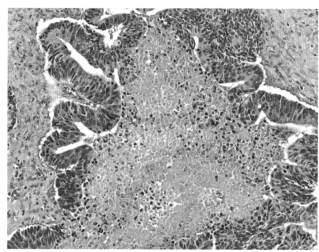

Figure 5.14.9 Same case as *Figure 5.14.6* showing garland pattern with central dirty necrosis, surrounded by undulating malignant colonic-type epithelium.

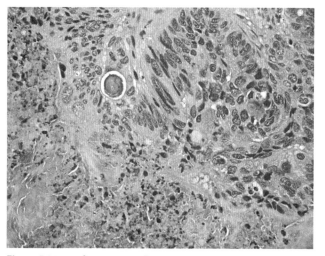

Figure 5.14.10 Same case as *Figure 5.14.7* showing goblet cells typical of colonic adenocarcinoma, moderate to severe atypia, and necrosis.

	Endometrioid Carcinoma	Mucinous Carcinoma, Primary Ovarian
Age	Mean 55-58 y	Mean 50 y
Location	Within ovary	Within ovary
Symptoms	Pelvic pain, increasing abdominal girth, bloating, early satiety, vaginal bleeding, urinary symptoms	Pelvic/abdominal pain, increasing abdominal girth
Signs	Pelvic/abdominal mass, ascites	Large pelvic/abdominal mass
Etiology	Endometriosis; germline *MLH1*, *MSH2*, *PMS2*, or *MSH6* mutation (Lynch syndrome); *PTEN*, β-*catenin* (*CTNNB1*), *KRAS*, *ARID1A*, and *PIK3CA* mutations	Arise from mucinous cystadenomas through mucinous borderline tumors (MBT); majority have *KRAS* and *TP53* mutations; rarely *BRAF* mutations; majority have copy number loss of *CDKN2A*
Gross and histology	1. Usually unilateral, stage I in almost half; mean 15 cm; cystic or cystic and solid; cysts contain dark brown viscous fluid (old blood +/− mucus); papillary or nodular growths arise from cyst lining 2. Most are architecturally well differentiated with confluent glandular epithelial proliferation resembling endometrial endometrioid carcinoma; cribriform, papillary, glandular, and occasionally solid patterns *(Figs. 5.15.1-5.15.3)*; less commonly with infiltrative pattern of glands, nests, and solid masses with jagged edges 3. Tall columnar epithelium with sharp luminal gland margins, round to ovoid nuclei with hyperchromasia, and prominent nucleoli *(Fig. 5.15.3)*; mitotic activity variable, often high; foci of intracellular and extracellular mucin may occasionally be present 4. Squamous differentiation in half *(Fig. 5.15.2)*; adenofibromatous component may be present; associated endometriosis is present in majority and often shows atypia, hyperplasia, and other features reflecting origin within endometriotic cyst or associated endometrioid borderline tumor 5. Secretory, ciliated, and sertoliform variants may occur	1. Nearly always unilateral, mean size 21 cm; 90% stage I; grossly similar to mucinous cystadenomas and MBT, with large, mucin-filled cysts; papillary growths sometimes arise in cyst walls 2. Most are architecturally well differentiated with complex papillary and glandular growth; the extent and complexity reflect invasion in the confluent/expansile pattern *(Figs. 5.15.4-5.15.6)*; less commonly, a haphazard infiltrative pattern of small- and moderately sized mucinous glands, nests, and single cells reflects destructive stromal invasion; ≥5 mm of confluent or invasive growth is required for a diagnosis of carcinoma 3. Mucinous epithelial lining displays abundant basophilic or eosinophilic cytoplasm *(Figs. 5.15.6 and 5.15.7)*; areas of cystadenoma display small basal nuclei; in other areas, there is a spectrum of atypia present from mild to severe, with nuclear enlargement, hyperchromasia, prominent nucleoli, and pseudostratification, often with numerous mitotic figures; extracellular mucin is often seen within glands 4. Endometriosis may occasionally be present; adenofibromatous background and squamous differentiation absent 5. No secretory, ciliated, or sertoliform differentiation

	Endometrioid Carcinoma	**Mucinous Carcinoma, Primary Ovarian**
Special Studies	• ER/PR+; PAX8 usually (+) • Loss of staining for DNA mismatch repair (MMR) proteins (MLH1, MSH2, PMS2, MSH6) in a subset	• ER/PR− (very focal weak staining is seen occasionally); PAX8 usually (−) but can be (+) in a subset of cases • No loss of staining for MMR proteins
Treatment	Staging (with debulking when indicated); chemotherapy (in neoadjuvant or adjuvant setting) except for low-grade stage IA/B; hormonal suppression may be used for recurrence	Staging (with debulking when indicated) (omission of lymph nodes acceptable); chemotherapy (in neoadjuvant or adjuvant setting) except for low-grade stage IA/B tumors; +/− appendectomy
Prognosis	Stage I >90% survival	95% survival for stage I; advanced stage, which is rare, has dismal prognosis

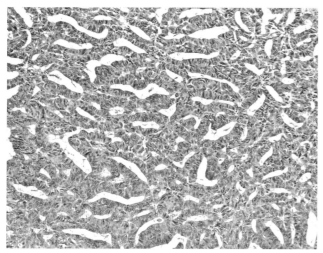

Figure 5.15.1   Endometrioid carcinoma with confluent pattern displaying cribriform and glandular architecture.

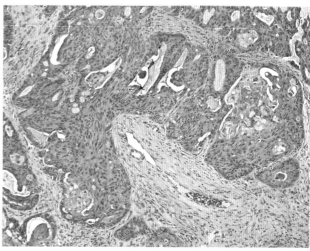

Figure 5.15.2   Endometrioid carcinoma showing infiltrating glandular pattern, squamous differentiation, and desmoplastic stroma.

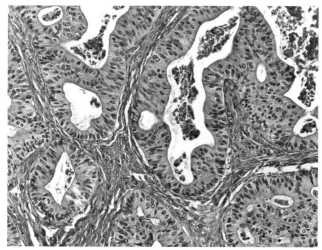

Figure 5.15.3   Endometrioid carcinoma displaying invasive cribriform glands with tall columnar epithelium and sharp luminal margins resembling endometrial endometrioid adenocarcinoma.

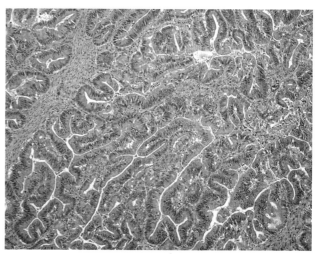

Figure 5.15.4   Confluent or expansile pattern of invasive mucinous carcinoma with complex and interconnecting glands and exclusion of stroma.

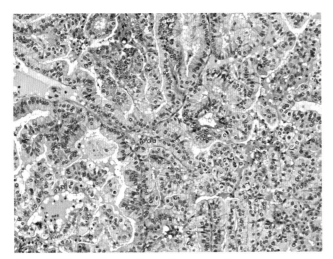

Figure 5.15.5 Confluent pattern of invasive mucinous carcinoma with very minimal intervening stroma and abundant intracytoplasmic mucin.

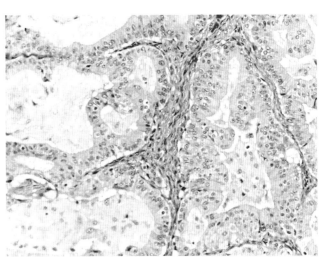

Figure 5.15.6 Mucinous carcinoma displaying abundant amphophilic to eosinophilic cytoplasm in cribriform glands.

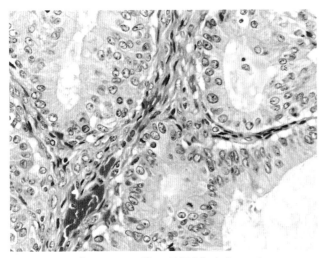

Figure 5.15.7 Same case as *Figure 5.15.6* displaying moderate cytologic atypia and both intracellular and extracellular mucin.

	Endometrioid Carcinoma, Sertoliform Variant	Sertoli Cell Tumor
Age	60-70 y	Mean 30 y
Location	Within ovary	Within ovary
Symptoms	Pelvic pain, increasing abdominal girth, bloating, early satiety, vaginal bleeding, urinary symptoms	Pelvic/abdominal pain, swelling, vaginal bleeding
Signs	Pelvic/abdominal mass; postmenopausal bleeding; may have virilization	40% have estrogenic manifestations
Etiology	Endometriosis; *PTEN*, β-*catenin* (*CTNNB1*), *KRAS*, *ARID1A*, and *PIK3CA* mutations	Rarely seen in patients with Peutz-Jeghers syndrome; *DICER1* mutations
Gross and histology	1. Predominantly solid, focally cystic; 10% bilateral; mean 13.6 cm; most commonly stage I 2. Solid or hollow slender anastomosing cords with stratified appearance, merge with tubules; low-grade nuclear features (in general, the level of nuclear atypia is greater than that seen in Sertoli cell tumor) *(Figs. 5.16.1-5.16.4)*; occasionally, secretions may be present within gland lumens; abundant fibromatous stroma, occasionally with calcification; stroma often luteinized 3. Areas of usual low-grade endometrioid carcinoma typically merge with sertoliform areas; mucin may be present at apical cell borders; occasional cilia may be seen *(Figs. 5.16.5-5.16.7)* 4. Background endometriosis, squamous differentiation, or adenofibromatous component may be present *(Fig. 5.16.5)*	1. Unilateral, stage I, mean 8-9 cm 2. Uniform tubular pattern; hollow tubules lined by tall cuboidal or columnar cells; solid tubules may be elongated, round, or ovoid; closely packed solid tubules may mimic diffuse sheets; less commonly cords, trabecular, and spindled patterns *(Figs. 5.16.8-5.16.11)*; no secretions within tubule lumens 3. Bland round to ovoid uniform nuclei, pale to eosinophilic cytoplasm, mitotically inactive *(Fig. 5.16.12)*; rare lipid-rich and oxyphilic variants 4. No endometriosis in the background; squamous differentiation is not seen
Special studies	• CK7+, EMA+, ER/PR+, usually PAX8+ • WT1, inhibin, and calretinin are usually (−) but may be focally (+) or strong (+) in small minority; SF-1 negative • Loss of staining for DNA mismatch repair (MMR) proteins (MLH1, MSH2, PMS2, and/or MSH6) in a subset of cases	• CK7−, EMA−, ER/PR+, PAX8− (other cytokeratin stains are nonspecific as they can be positive in Sertoli cell tumor) • WT1+, SF-1+, inhibin+, calretinin+ • No loss of MMR protein staining expected
Treatment	Limited data; presumed same as usual endometrioid carcinoma (staging [with debulking when indicated], chemotherapy [in adjuvant or neoadjuvant setting] except for stage IA/IB low-grade tumors; hormonal suppression may be used for recurrence)	Unilateral salpingo-oophorectomy
Prognosis	Based on limited data, same as stage-stratified usual endometrioid carcinoma	Usually benign; rare abdominopelvic recurrences

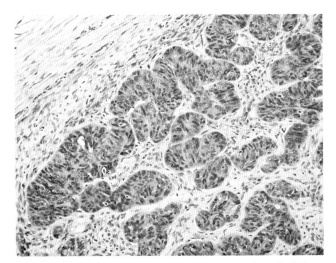

Figure 5.16.1   Endometrioid carcinoma, sertoliform variant, displaying solid nests and cords resembling Sertoli cell tumor.

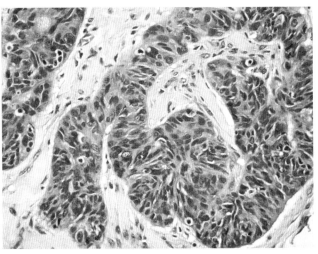

Figure 5.16.2   Endometrioid carcinoma, sertoliform variant (same case as *Fig. 5.16.1*), displaying cords of columnar cells with elongated, ovoid nuclei.

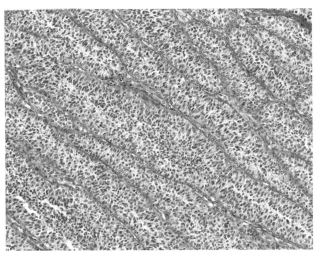

Figure 5.16.3   Endometrioid carcinoma, sertoliform variant, with cords and glands of columnar cells.

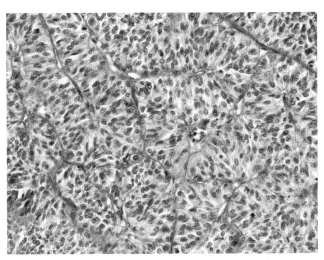

Figure 5.16.4   Endometrioid carcinoma, sertoliform variant (same case as *Fig. 5.16.3*), with cords of columnar cells mimicking the paired cell arrangement of Sertoli differentiation.

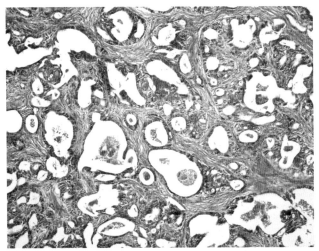

Figure 5.16.5   Endometrioid carcinoma, usual type, showing a haphazard infiltrative pattern of variably sized glands, which focally show squamous differentiation.

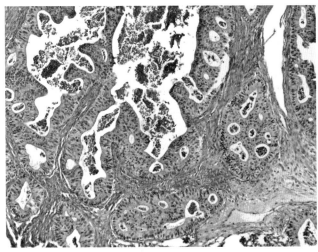

Figure 5.16.6   Endometrioid carcinoma, usual type, showing cribriform features and tall columnar epithelium lining glands with sharp luminal margins.

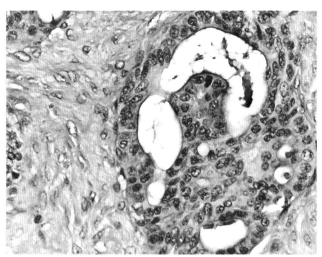

Figure 5.16.7   Endometrioid carcinoma, usual type, with columnar epithelium lining glands with sharp luminal margins.

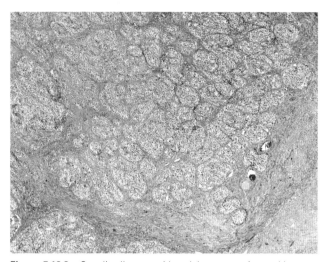

Figure 5.16.8   Sertoli cell tumor with nodular groups of smoothly contoured nests and islands.

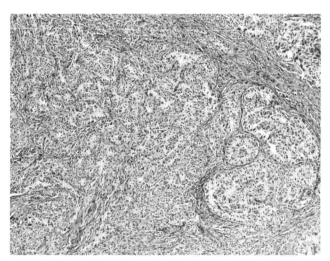

Figure 5.16.9   Sertoli cell tumor displaying crowded small tubules and cords with well-oriented basal nuclei.

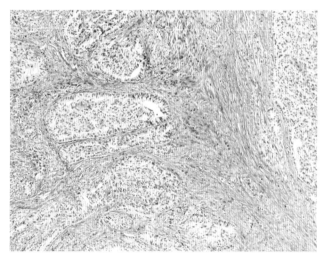

Figure 5.16.10   Sertoli cell tumor with crowded tubules and some degree of architectural complexity.

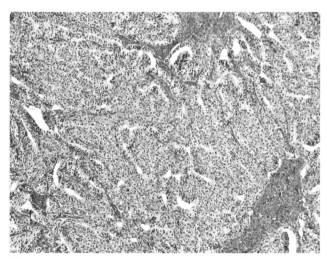

Figure 5.16.11   Sertoli cell tumor with back-to-back tubules mimicking a confluent pattern of endometrioid carcinoma.

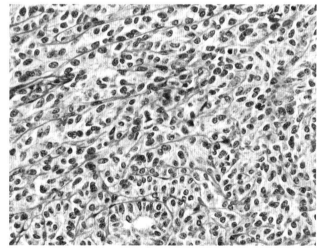

Figure 5.16.12   Sertoli cell tumor with open and solid tubules lined by columnar cells with round to ovoid nuclei and pale cytoplasm (same case as *Fig. 5.16.11*).

	Endometrioid Carcinoma With Spindled Squamous Component	Carcinosarcoma (MMMT)
Age	Mean 61 y	Mean 65-66 y
Location	Within ovary	Ovarian surface, and within ovarian stroma, tubal fimbriae, commonly invade nonfimbrial tube
Symptoms	Pelvic pain/dysmenorrhea	Pelvic pain, increasing abdominal girth, bloating, early satiety, urinary symptoms
Signs	Pelvic mass	Pelvic/abdominal mass, ascites
Etiology	Endometriosis; *PTEN*, β-*catenin* (*CTNNB1*), *KRAS*, *ARID1A*, and *PIK3CA* mutations expected	Majority derive from serous tubal intraepithelial carcinoma, usually of fimbrial origin; nearly all have *TP53* mutations
Gross and histology	1. Mean 13 cm, solid and cystic, about one-third stage I 2. Extensive spindle cell component, usually >50% of tumor, in nests, creating a lobulated appearance; less commonly, diffuse spindle cell pattern; may display whorls and focal palisading *(Figs. 5.17.1-5.17.3)*; squamous component may incite a foreign body–type giant cell reaction 3. Typical endometrioid glands present in all cases; in half, discrete component of typical low-grade endometrioid carcinoma *(Figs. 5.17.3-5.17.5)*; half have sertoliform areas 4. Nuclear features of the spindle cells similar to those of the endometrioid glands, generally low grade *(Fig. 5.17.4)*; usually low mitotic index	1. Ovaries normal sized or slightly enlarged in one-third to one-half of cases with subcentimeter surface nodules; remaining show enlarged solid and/or cystic ovaries, mean 14 cm, can be up to 15-20 cm; fallopian tube fimbriae may be prominent and tumorous and may be splayed across ovarian surface; usually bilateral adnexal involvement and nearly always with peritoneal carcinomatosis or extensive bowel invasion 2. Epithelial component usually displays high grade serous patterns with papillary, glandular, and solid patterns, commonly intermixed; less commonly thick urothelial-like papillae; endometrioid patterns may be present *(Figs. 5.17.6-5.17.9)* 3. Large epithelial cells with marked atypia *(Figs. 5.17.8 and 5.17.9)*, often with bizarre nuclear forms; large prominent nucleoli and abundant mitotic activity with abnormal forms 4. Sarcomatous component with high-grade spindle cell differentiation with high mitotic activity, marked cytologic atypia *(Figs. 5.17.8-5.17.10)*; myxoid or small cell areas may be present; heterologous elements commonly present (>50%), most often cytologically malignant cartilage, rhabdomyoblasts, occasionally osteoid, and liposarcoma
Special studies	• CK7+, ER/PR+, EMA+; WT1, and p16 are usually (−) but may be focally (+) or strongly (+) in small minority; usually nonaberrant pattern of p53 expression • Loss of staining for DNA mismatch repair proteins (MLH1, MSH2, PMS2, and/or MSH6) in a subset of cases	• Epithelial component: aberrant p53 expression; CK7+, p16+ (diffuse), WT1+, CAM5.2+, and ER+ in majority; sarcomatous component generally has similar profile but may stain more weakly or focally for epithelial markers

	Endometrioid Carcinoma With Spindled Squamous Component	**Carcinosarcoma (MMMT)**
Treatment	Staging (with debulking when indicated); chemotherapy (in neoadjuvant or adjuvant setting) except for low-grade stages IA/IB; hormonal therapy may be used for recurrences	Staging (with debulking when indicated); chemotherapy (in neoadjuvant or adjuvant +/− maintenance setting)
Prognosis	Presumed similar to usual endometrioid carcinoma: stage I >90% survival; stage-stratified analyses show somewhat better prognosis compared to high-grade serous carcinoma in advanced stage	Stage III patients have 5-y survival of 20%-25%

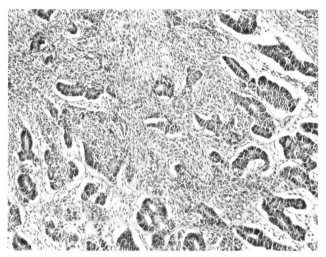

Figure 5.17.1 Spindle cell variant of endometrioid carcinoma with intimate admixture of glandular and spindle cell components.

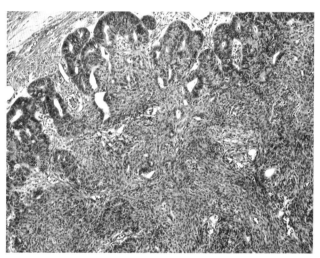

Figure 5.17.2 Spindle cell variant of endometrioid carcinoma displaying low-grade glandular pattern at periphery **(top portion of photograph)**, gradually merging with spindled squamous component toward **center** and **bottom**.

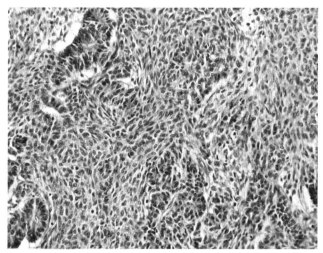

Figure 5.17.3 Spindle cell variant of endometrioid carcinoma with prominent spindle cell component. Although an intimate admixture of glandular and spindle components is seen as in carcinosarcoma, the spindle cell component is bland rather than high grade.

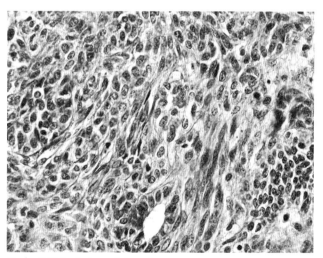

Figure 5.17.4 Endometrioid carcinoma with glands and cords surrounded by a low-grade spindled squamous component.

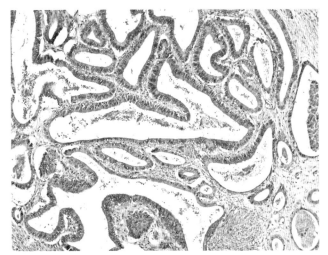

Figure 5.17.5 Conventional glandular component from a case of a spindle cell variant of endometrioid carcinoma (spindle cell component not shown in this field); this pattern can also be seen in endometrioid borderline tumor.

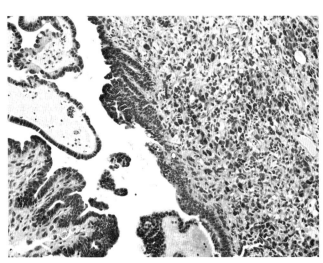

Figure 5.17.6 Carcinosarcoma with large papillae containing diffusely growing high-grade sarcoma, lined by single layer of malignant epithelial component.

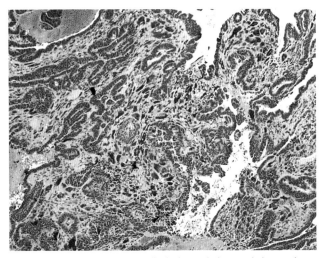

Figure 5.17.7 Carcinosarcoma displaying an intimate admixture of high-grade glands and high-grade spindle cell stroma.

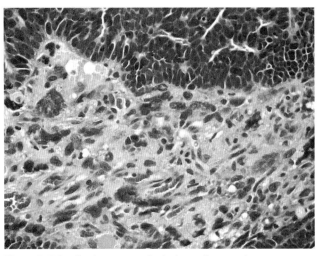

Figure 5.17.8 Carcinosarcoma displaying malignant columnar epithelium with stratification at **top** overlying malignant spindle cell stroma.

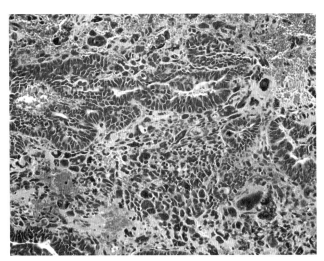

Figure 5.17.9 Carcinosarcoma displaying rounded and elongated malignant glands intermixed with a high-grade sarcomatous stromal component containing numerous bizarre nuclei.

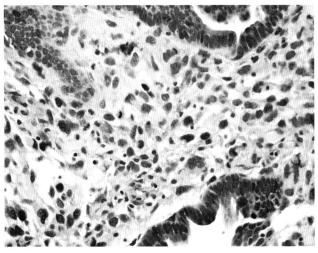

Figure 5.17.10 Carcinosarcoma with sarcomatous stroma and malignant columnar epithelial component.

	Endometrioid Carcinoma	Granulosa Cell Tumor, Adult Type
Age	Mean 55-58 y	Mean 50-55 y
Location	Within ovary	Within ovary
Symptoms	Pelvic pain, increasing abdominal girth, bloating, early satiety, vaginal bleeding, urinary symptoms	Pelvic/lower abdominal pain; postmenopausal bleeding; 10% have acute abdomen with hemoperitoneum
Signs	Pelvic/abdominal mass, ascites	Pelvic/lower abdominal mass; may have estrogenic manifestations
Etiology	Endometriosis; germline *MLH1*, *MSH2*, *PMS2*, or *MSH6* mutation (Lynch syndrome) in a subset of cases; *PTEN*, β-*catenin* (*CTNNB1*), *KRAS*, *ARID1A*, and *PIK3CA* mutations	*FOXL2* mutations
Gross and histology	1. Usually unilateral, stage I in almost half; mean size 15 cm; cystic or cystic and solid; cysts contain dark brown viscous fluid (old blood +/− mucus); papillary or nodular growths arise from cyst lining 2. Most are architecturally well differentiated with confluent glandular epithelial proliferation resembling endometrial endometrioid carcinoma; cribriform, papillary, glandular, and occasionally solid patterns; less commonly with infiltrative pattern of glands, nests, and solid masses with jagged edges *(Figs. 5.18.1 and 5.18.2)* 3. Tall columnar epithelium with sharp luminal gland margins, round to ovoid nuclei with hyperchromasia, and prominent nucleoli *(Fig. 5.18.3)*; peripheral palisading of nuclei may be seen at edge of nests and islands; mitotic activity variable, often high 4. Squamous differentiation in half; adenofibromatous component often present; associated endometriosis is present in majority and often shows atypia, hyperplasia, and other features reflecting origin within endometriotic cyst or associated endometrioid borderline tumor 5. Secretory, ciliated, and sertoliform variants may occur *(Figs. 5.18.4 and 5.18.5)*	1. Solid and cystic, hemorrhagic; mean size 10-12 cm; <5% bilateral; >90% stage I; solid and cystic with tan or yellow cut surfaces, hemorrhage with clotted blood within cysts common 2. Insular pattern is characterized by islands and nests of granulosa cells divided into lobules by fibrothecomatous stroma, but cords of tumor cells may be admixed; solid tubular pattern mimics Sertoli tumor; wide variety of other architectural patterns: diffuse, microfollicular, macrofollicular, trabecular, tubular, and combinations; microfollicular pattern may have Call-Exner bodies *(Figs. 5.18.6-5.18.8)*; rarely pseudopapillary 3. Small cells with ovoid or angulated/folded uniform nuclei, often with grooves *(Figs. 5.18.9 and 5.18.10)*; peripheral palisading of nuclei may be seen at edge of nests and islands; mitoses rare or absent; 2% contain bizarre nuclei 4. No squamous component; not associated with endometriosis except incidentally 5. No secretory or ciliated differentiation; sertoliform patterns can be seen

	Endometrioid Carcinoma	**Granulosa Cell Tumor, Adult Type**
Special studies	• CK7+, EMA+, ER/PR+, PAX8+ • WT1, inhibin, and calretinin are usually (−) but may be focally (+) or strongly (+) in small minority; SF-1 negative • Loss of staining for DNA mismatch repair (MMR) proteins (MLH1, MSH2, PMS2, or MSH6) in a subset of cases	• Calretinin+, inhibin+, SF-1+, WT-1+, and ER/PR+ • Usually PAX8−, CK7−, and EMA− • Other types of cytokeratins are nonspecific as they can be positive in adult granulosa cell tumor • No loss of MMR protein staining expected
Treatment	Staging (with debulking when indicated); chemotherapy (in neoadjuvant or adjuvant setting) except for low-grade stage IA/B; hormonal suppression may be used for recurrence	Hysterectomy-bilateral salpingo-oophorectomy; unilateral salpingo-oophorectomy if fertility desired
Prognosis	Stage I >90% survival	Those with recurrent disease or tumors of advanced stage may be indolent, some with late recurrences after 5-10 y or more, stage I has about 90% survival at 10 y

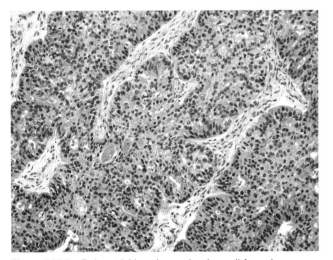

Figure 5.18.1   Endometrioid carcinoma showing well-formed interanastomosing and cribriform glands lined by tall columnar epithelium resembling endometrial endometrioid carcinoma.

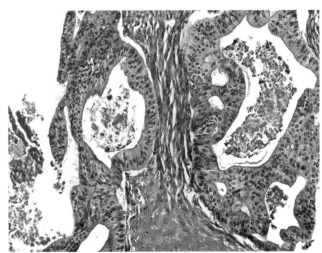

Figure 5.18.2   Endometrioid carcinoma with intraglandular cribriform pattern and sharp luminal margins.

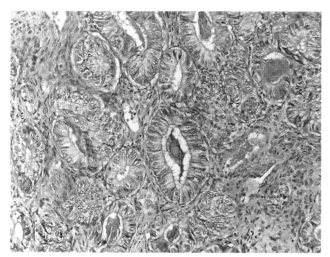

Figure 5.18.3 Endometrioid carcinoma displaying rounded glands lined by tall columnar epithelium with sharp luminal margins, round to ovoid nuclei, and pale cytoplasm.

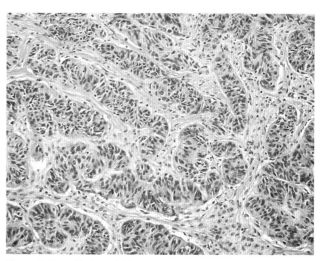

Figure 5.18.4 Endometrioid carcinoma, sertoliform variant, which can resemble patterns of granulosa cell tumor as well as Sertoli cell tumor (see Section 5.16).

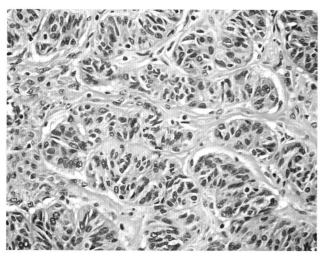

Figure 5.18.5 Endometrioid carcinoma, sertoliform variant, with columns and cords of columnar epithelium (same case as *Fig. 5.18.4*).

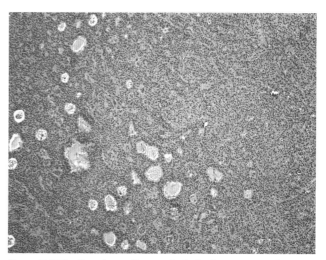

Figure 5.18.6 Granulosa cell tumor displaying interanastomosing columns and cords with occasional gland-like spaces.

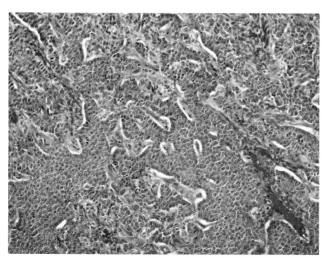

Figure 5.18.7 Granulosa cell tumor displaying interanastomosing cords and trabeculae containing uniform, evenly spaced nuclei.

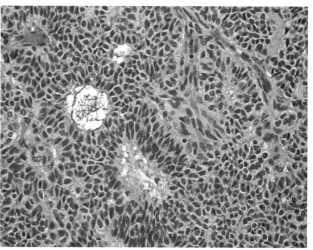

Figure 5.18.8 Same case as *Figure 5.18.6* displaying ovoid to elongated nuclei, which line up in columns and cords.

5 OVARY

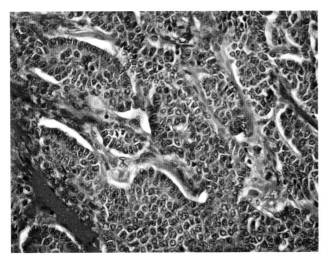

Figure 5.18.9   Granulosa cell tumor displays pale, ovoid nuclei with prominent longitudinal grooves.

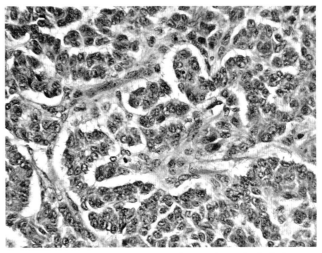

Figure 5.18.10   Granulosa cell tumor with slender cords displaying finely clumped chromatin with occasional nuclear grooves.

	Endometrioid Carcinoma With Secretory Features	Yolk Sac Tumor
Age	Mean 55-58 y	Under 30 y (occasional cases may occur in older adults and postmenopausal women)
Location	Within ovary	Within ovarian stroma; rarely in other midline sites (ie, retroperitoneum)
Symptoms	Pelvic pain, increasing abdominal girth, bloating, early satiety, vaginal bleeding, urinary symptoms	Abdominal enlargement, pain
Signs	Pelvic/abdominal mass, ascites	Lower abdominal/pelvic mass; elevated serum AFP
Etiology	Endometriosis; germline *MLH1, MSH2, PMS2,* or *MSH6* mutation (Lynch syndrome) in a subset of cases; *PTEN,* β-*catenin* (*CTNNB1*), *KRAS, ARID1A,* and *PIK3CA* mutations	Germ cell origin (rare cases are of somatic origin in older women when associated with a component of carcinoma); isochromosome 12p [i(12p)] often present; rarely arise from gonadoblastoma in gonadal dysgenesis
Gross and histology	1. Usually unilateral, stage I in almost half; mean 15 cm; cystic or cystic and solid; cysts contain dark brown viscous fluid (old blood +/− mucus); papillary or nodular growths arise from cyst lining 2. Most are architecturally well differentiated with confluent glandular epithelial proliferation resembling endometrial endometrioid carcinoma; cribriform, papillary, glandular, and occasionally solid patterns; less commonly with infiltrative pattern of glands, nests, and solid masses with jagged edges (*Figs. 5.19.1 and 5.19.2*) 3. Tall columnar epithelium with sharp luminal gland margins, round to ovoid nuclei with hyperchromasia and prominent nucleoli; secretory features are reflected by uniform subnuclear or supranuclear vacuoles resembling secretory endometrium (*Figs. 5.19.3-5.19.5*); mitotic activity variable, often high 4. Squamous differentiation in half; adenofibromatous component often present; associated endometriosis is present in majority and often shows atypia, hyperplasia, and other features reflecting origin within endometriotic cyst or associated endometrioid borderline tumor	1. Unilateral, >10 cm, frequently with hemorrhage and necrosis 2. Common patterns feature loose edematous microcystic/reticular network, myxomatous tissue, perivascular formations (Schiller-Duvall bodies), alveolar/gland-like architecture, larger cysts lined by flattened epithelium (polyvesicular vitelline), papillae, and solid growth (*Figs. 5.19.6 and 5.19.7*). Less commonly, hepatoid pattern with granular eosinophilic cytoplasm; primitive endodermal pattern resembling mucinous intestinal glands 3. Clear cytoplasm and primitive large nuclei with prominent nucleoli commonly seen in most of the above architectural patterns (*Fig. 5.19.8*); endometrioid-like cytologic features can resemble secretory endometrium and secretory variant of endometrioid carcinoma (*Figs. 5.19.9-5.19.12*) 4. Not associated with endometriosis; often combined with other germ cell component, particularly embryonal carcinoma

	Endometrioid Carcinoma With Secretory Features	Yolk Sac Tumor
Special studies	• CK7+, EMA+, ER/PR+, usually PAX8+ • AFP, glypican-3, and SALL4 usually (−) • Loss of staining for DNA mismatch repair (MMR) proteins (MLH1, MSH2, PMS2, and/or MSH6) in a subset of cases	• CK7−, EMA−, ER/PR− • AFP+, glypican-3+, SALL4+, frequently PAX8− but may be +; villin and CDX2+ (if glandular intestinal differentiation present) • No loss of MMR protein staining expected
Treatment	Staging (with debulking when indicated); chemotherapy (in adjuvant or neoadjuvant setting) except for low-grade stage IA/B; hormonal suppression may be used for recurrence	Combination chemotherapy with germ cell regimen
Prognosis	Stage I >90% survival	80% cure rate; pure hepatoid and primitive intestinal types have poor prognosis

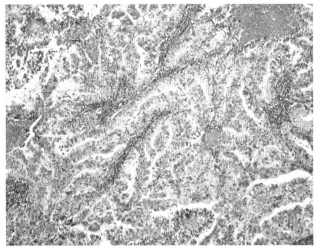

Figure 5.19.1 Endometrioid carcinoma with secretory features with architecturally well-formed glands displaying vacuolated clear cytoplasm.

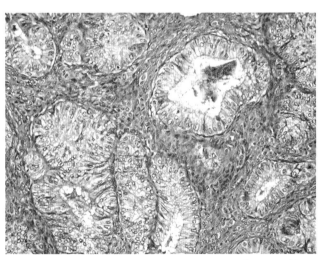

Figure 5.19.2 Endometrioid carcinoma with secretory features with well-formed rounded glands displaying sharp luminal margins.

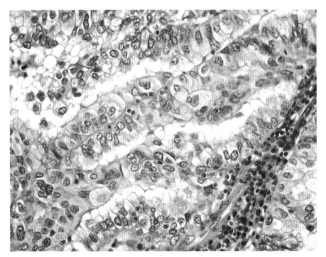

Figure 5.19.3 Endometrioid carcinoma with secretory features, same case as *Figure 5.19.1*, resembling secretory phase endometrium.

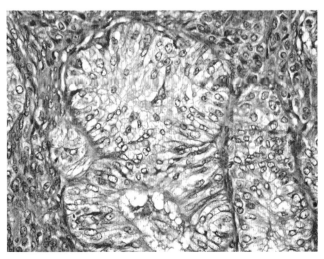

Figure 5.19.4 Endometrioid carcinoma with secretory features resembling secretory phase endometrium.

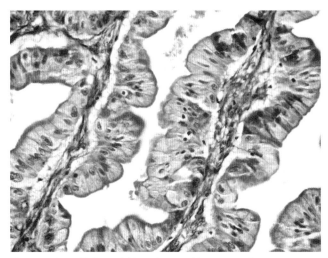

Figure 5.19.5   Endometrioid carcinoma with secretory features displaying supranuclear vacuoles and bland predominantly basally oriented round and ovoid nuclei.

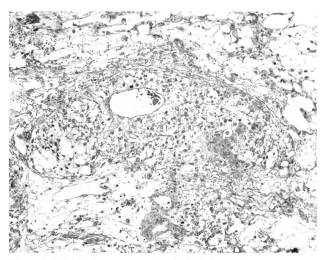

Figure 5.19.6   Yolk sac tumor with reticular/microcystic pattern.

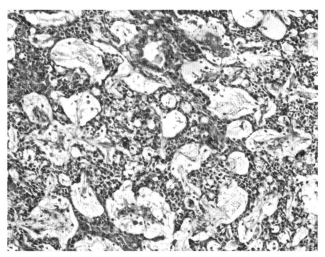

Figure 5.19.7   Yolk sac tumor with reticular/microcystic pattern.

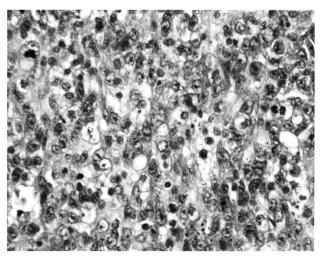

Figure 5.19.8   Yolk sac tumor with primitive, high-grade nuclei.

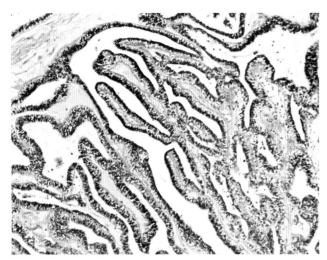

Figure 5.19.9   Endometrioid-like variant of yolk sac tumor mimicking the secretory variant of endometrioid carcinoma.

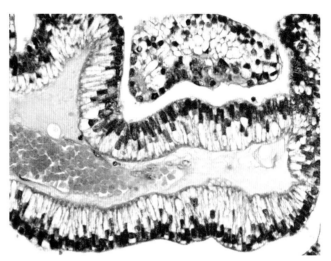

Figure 5.19.10   Endometrioid-like variant of yolk sac tumor mimicking the secretory variant of endometrioid carcinoma.

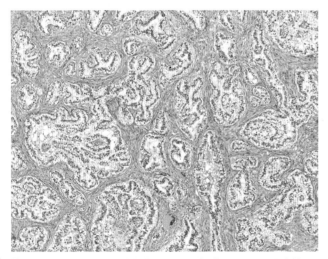

Figure 5.19.11   Endometrioid-like variant of yolk sac tumor mimicking the secretory variant of endometrioid carcinoma. The glands mimic early secretory endometrium with subnuclear vacuoles.

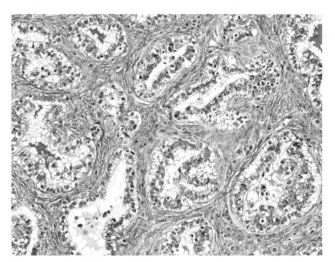

Figure 5.19.12   Endometrioid-like variant of yolk sac tumor mimicking the secretory variant of endometrioid carcinoma. The glands mimic early secretory endometrium with subnuclear vacuoles. Same case as *Figure 5.19.11*.

	Clear Cell Carcinoma	Yolk Sac Tumor
Age	Mean 50-53 y	Under 30 y (occasional cases may occur in older adults and postmenopausal women)
Location	Within ovary; rarely arises in extraovarian sites from endometriosis	Within ovarian stroma; rarely in other midline sites (ie, retroperitoneum)
Symptoms	Pelvic pain, increasing abdominal girth, bloating, early satiety, vaginal bleeding, urinary symptoms	Abdominal enlargement, pain
Signs	Pelvic/adnexal mass; rarely thromboembolic events or paraneoplastic hypercalcemia	Lower abdominal/pelvic mass; elevated serum AFP
Etiology	Vast majority arise in endometriosis; *ARID1A, PIK3CA, PTEN, KRAS, TGF-βII* mutations, *TERT* promoter mutations; germline *MLH1, MSH2, PMS2,* or *MSH6* mutations (Lynch syndrome) in a small subset of cases	Germ cell origin (rare cases are of somatic origin in older women when associated with a component of carcinoma); isochromosome 12p [i(12p)] often present; rarely arise from gonadoblastoma in gonadal dysgenesis
Gross and histology	1. One-third to one-half are stage I; endometriosis and adhesions often present; high incidence of tumor rupture; <10% bilateral; mean 13-15 cm 2. Two-thirds arise in endometriotic cysts as a nodular or polypoid growth of the cyst wall; one-third have adenofibromatous architecture, often with yellow-white honeycomb cut surface 3. Characteristic architectural patterns are papillary, tubulocystic, tubulopapillary (including ring-like structures) and hobnail. Infiltrative small glands and solid growth may also occur *(Figs. 5.20.1-5.20.4)*; adenofibromatous background in one-third; stroma often dense, eosinophilic, and hyalinized *(Fig. 5.20.4)* (particularly evident in some papillary patterns) 4. Range of nuclear atypia from mild to severe (generally, not as marked as in high-grade serous carcinoma) *(Figs. 5.20.4 and 5.20.5)*; nucleoli often prominent and enlarged; cytoplasm is often but not always clear; abundant eosinophilic cytoplasm also commonly seen; hyaline globules may be present; mitotic figures very scant in most cases but occasionally over 10/10 hpf 5. Rare cases may represent mixed clear cell carcinoma-yolk sac tumor	1. Unilateral, >10 cm, frequently with hemorrhage and necrosis 2. Not associated with endometriosis or adenofibromatous architecture 3. Common patterns feature loose edematous microcystic/reticular network, myxomatous tissue, perivascular formations (Schiller-Duvall bodies), alveolar/gland-like architecture, larger cysts lined by flattened epithelium (polyvesicular vitelline), papillae, and solid growth *(Figs. 5.20.6-5.20.9)*; less commonly, hepatoid pattern with granular eosinophilic cytoplasm; primitive endodermal pattern resembling mucinous intestinal glands; can occasionally have some degree of stromal hyalinization 4. Clear cytoplasm and primitive large nuclei with prominent nucleoli commonly seen in most of the above architectural patterns *(Figs. 5.20.9 and 5.20.10)*; the cells can show some degree of hobnail shapes; hyaline globules may be present 5. Often combined with other germ cell component, particularly embryonal carcinoma

	Clear Cell Carcinoma	**Yolk Sac Tumor**
Special studies	• HNF1β+, CK7+, EMA+, Napsin A+, PAX8+, racemase+; AFP–, glypican-3–, ER/PR– in about 90%; SALL4– (may be focal/weak+)	• CK7–, EMA–, ER/PR–, HNF1β–, racemase–; napsin A usually – (may occasionally be focally +); frequently PAX8– but may be + • AFP+, glypican-3+, SALL4+; villin and CDX2+ (if glandular intestinal differentiation present)
Treatment	Staging (with debulking when indicated); chemotherapy (in neoadjuvant or adjuvant setting)	Combination chemotherapy with germ cell regimen
Prognosis	Stage I has 90% survival	80% cure rate; pure hepatoid and primitive intestinal types have poor prognosis

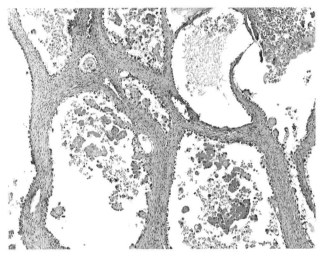

Figure 5.20.1 Clear cell carcinoma with tubulocystic pattern. The cysts contain both attached and detached papillary fragments of tumor. The papillae have hyalinized stromal cores.

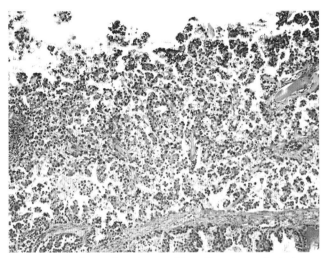

Figure 5.20.2 Clear cell carcinoma with papillary pattern displaying thin, delicate, and branching papillae lined by cells with clear cytoplasm.

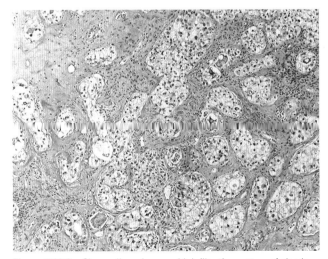

Figure 5.20.3 Clear cell carcinoma with infiltrative pattern of glands lined by epithelial cells with abundant clear cytoplasm.

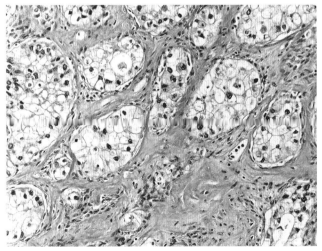

Figure 5.20.4 Same case as *Figure 5.20.3* displaying clear to eosinophilic cytoplasm and variable nuclear atypia, which is focally notable; eosinophilic hyalinized stroma can be seen in lower half of photograph.

Figure 5.20.5   Clear cell carcinoma with hobnail cell pattern showing protrusion of the nuclei and apical cytoplasm. Note that the cytoplasm is eosinophilic rather than clear.

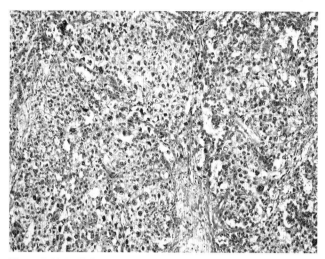

Figure 5.20.6   Yolk sac tumor with solid pattern displaying sheets of primitive cells with prominent clear cytoplasm.

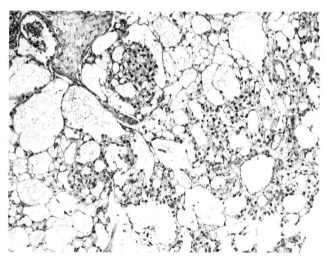

Figure 5.20.7   Yolk sac tumor with reticular/microcystic pattern.

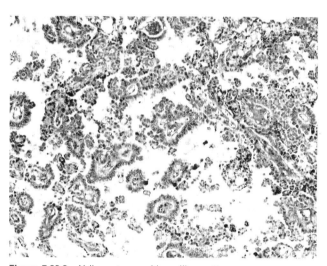

Figure 5.20.8   Yolk sac tumor with papillary pattern.

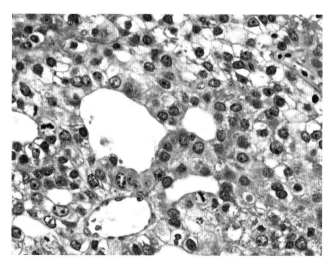

Figure 5.20.9   Yolk sac tumor with glandular differentiation. Note that the cells can resemble clear cell carcinoma.

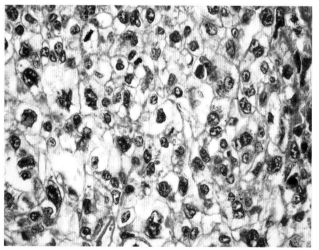

Figure 5.20.10   Solid pattern of yolk sac tumor with clear cytoplasm, marked nuclear atypia, coarsely clumped chromatin, and a mitotic figure.

	Serous Borderline Tumor (SBT)	Clear Cell Carcinoma With Papillary Pattern
Age	Median of 49 y	Mean 50-53 y
Location	Within ovary with or without exophytic surface component; may be confined to surface	Within ovary; rarely arises in extraovarian sites from endometriosis
Symptoms	Commonly asymptomatic; may have nonspecific pelvic pain or urinary symptoms	Pelvic pain, increasing abdominal girth, bloating, early satiety, vaginal bleeding, urinary symptoms
Signs	Pelvic/adnexal mass	Pelvic/adnexal mass; rarely thromboembolic events or paraneoplastic hypercalcemia
Etiology	Unknown; originates from serous-type inclusions, possibly originating from tubal epithelial implantation; *KRAS* and *BRAF* mutations	Vast majority arise in endometriosis; *ARID1A, PIK3CA, PTEN, KRAS, TGF-βRII* mutations; *TERT* promoter mutations; germline *MLH1, MSH2, PMS2,* or *MSH6* mutations (Lynch syndrome) in a small subset of cases
Gross and histology	1. Intracystic and exophytic components 2. Not associated with endometriosis except occasionally or incidentally 3. Hierarchical branching, tufting, and apparent detachment of cell clusters; no invasion *(Figs. 5.21.1-5.21.3)* 4. Tubal-type epithelium, often ciliated *(Figs. 5.21.2 and 5.21.3)*, focally with hobnail or dense eosinophilic cytoplasm; no hyaline globules; mild cytologic atypia; may have psammoma bodies 5. 12% have noninvasive peritoneal implants; those with exophytic component more often with implants	1. One-third to one-half are stage I; endometriosis and adhesions often present; high incidence of tumor rupture; <10% bilateral; mean 13-15 cm 2. Two-thirds arise in endometriotic cysts as a nodular or polypoid growth of the cyst wall; one-third have adenofibromatous architecture 3. Papillary pattern displays delicate, elongated, slender papillae with thin fibrovascular support and hobnail lining cells *(Figs. 5.21.4 and 5.21.5)*; cells lining papillae usually a monolayer without degree of stratification seen in SBT; other characteristic architectural patterns are tubulocystic, tubulopapillary (including ring-like structures), and hobnail; infiltrative small glands and solid growth may also occur; adenofibromatous background in one-third; stroma (especially within cores of small papillae) often dense, eosinophilic, and hyalinized *(Figs. 5.21.6-5.21.8)* 4. Range of nuclear atypia from mild to severe *(Figs. 5.21.5, 5.21.7, and 5.21.8)*; nucleoli often prominent and enlarged; cytoplasm is often but not always clear; abundant eosinophilic cytoplasm also commonly seen; hyaline globules may be present; mitotic figures very scant in most cases but occasionally over 10/10 hpf 5. Extraovarian disease may be present
Special studies	• WT1+, ER/PR+ • HNF1β−; Napsin A−, racemase (AMACR) − (limited data)	• WT1−, ER/PR− • HNF1β+, racemase (AMACR)+, Napsin A+

	Serous Borderline Tumor (SBT)	**Clear Cell Carcinoma With Papillary Pattern**
Treatment	Salpingo-oophorectomy with staging	Staging (with debulking when indicated); chemotherapy (in neoadjuvant or adjuvant setting)
Prognosis	Increased risk of serous carcinoma (vast majority low grade) (HR = 9.2; 95% CI: 6.8-12.2); if confined to ovaries (ie, without associated peritoneal implants) 1.7% develop carcinoma; noninvasive implants confer risk of invasive low-grade serous carcinoma of ~16% (HR = 7.7; 95% CI: 3.9-15.0)	Stage I has 90% survival; advanced stage appears to have worse prognosis than high-grade serous carcinoma

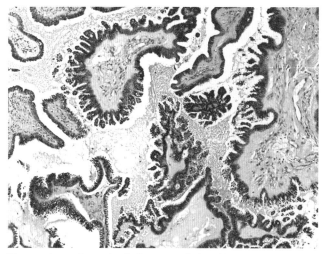

Figure 5.21.1 Serous borderline tumor displays hierarchical branching pattern with proliferation and tufting of epithelium at the surfaces of the papillae.

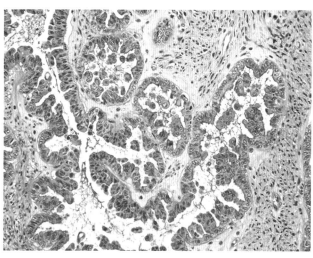

Figure 5.21.2 Serous borderline tumor with tufting and detachment of atypical cells and cell clusters.

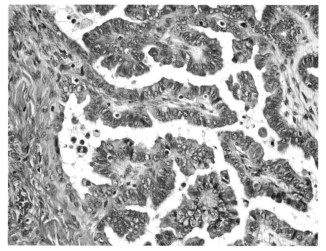

Figure 5.21.3 Serous borderline tumor with complex papillae, exfoliated tufts of cells, and only mild atypia.

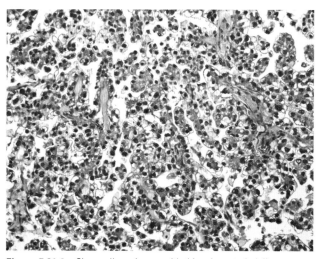

Figure 5.21.4 Clear cell carcinoma with thin, elongated, delicate papillae lined by cells with abundant clear cytoplasm.

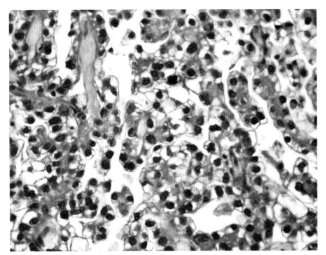

Figure 5.21.5 Clear cell carcinoma. Same case as *Figure 5.21.4* showing moderate cytologic atypia and abundant clear cytoplasm with prominent cell borders.

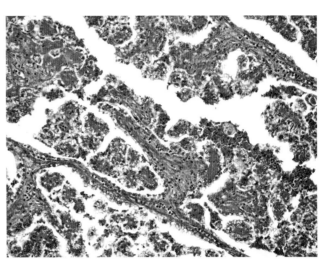

Figure 5.21.6 Clear cell carcinoma with papillae thickened by characteristic hyalinized eosinophilic stroma.

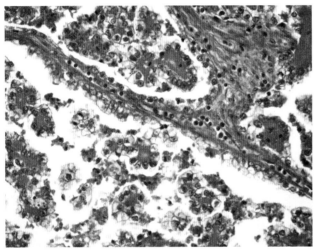

Figure 5.21.7 Clear cell carcinoma. Same case as *Figure 5.21.6* showing a range of nuclear atypia from mild to moderate.

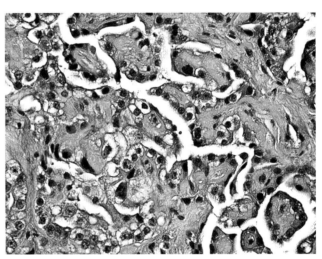

Figure 5.21.8 Clear cell carcinoma with papillae displaying hyalinized stroma and lined by markedly atypical cells.

	High-Grade Serous Carcinoma (HGSC) With Clear Cells	Clear Cell Carcinoma (CCC)
Age	Mean 60-63 y	Mean 50-53 y
Location	Ovarian surface and within ovarian stroma, tubal fimbriae, commonly invade nonfimbrial tube	Within ovary; rarely arises in extraovarian sites from endometriosis
Symptoms	Pelvic pain, increasing abdominal girth, bloating, early satiety, urinary symptoms	Pelvic pain, increasing abdominal girth, bloating, early satiety, vaginal bleeding, urinary symptoms
Signs	Pelvic/abdominal mass, ascites	Pelvic/adnexal mass; rarely thromboembolic events or paraneoplastic hypercalcemia
Etiology	Majority derive from serous tubal intraepithelial carcinoma, usually of fimbrial origin; nearly all have *TP53* mutations; a substantial proportion have germline or somatic mutation in *BRCA1*, *BRCA2*, or other homologous recombination repair genes, or epigenetic silencing of these genes; high genomic instability	Vast majority arise in endometriosis; *ARID1A*, *PIK3CA*, *PTEN*, *KRAS*, *TGF-βII* mutations; *TERT* promoter mutations; germline *MLH1*, *MSH2*, *PMS2*, or *MSH6* mutations (Lynch syndrome) in a small subset of cases
Gross and histology	1. Ovaries normal sized or slightly enlarged in one-third to one-half of cases with subcentimeter surface nodules; remaining show enlarged solid and/or cystic ovaries, 8-10 cm; fallopian tube fimbriae may be prominent and tumorous and may be splayed across ovarian surface; usually bilateral adnexal involvement with extensive tubal invasion and nearly always with peritoneal carcinomatosis or extensive bowel invasion 2. Endometriosis may be incidentally present in about 20% of cases 3. Papillary, glandular, and solid patterns, commonly intermixed *(Figs. 5.22.1-5.22.3)*; less commonly display thick urothelial (transitional)-like papillae 4. Large epithelial cells with marked atypia, often with bizarre nuclear forms; large prominent nucleoli and abundant mitotic activity with abnormal forms; cytoplasm may be clear or brightly eosinophilic *(Figs. 5.22.2-5.22.6)*; no hyaline globules; classic tubulopapillary and tubulocystic patterns of clear cell carcinoma are absent; psammomatous calcification usually present	1. One-third to one-half are stage I; endometriosis and adhesions often present; high incidence of tumor rupture; <10% bilateral; mean 13-15 cm 2. Two-thirds arise in endometriotic cyst as a nodular or polypoid growth of the cyst wall; one-third have adenofibromatous architecture 3. Characteristic architectural patterns are papillary, tubulocystic, tubulopapillary (including ring-like structures) and hobnail *(Figs. 5.22.7-5.22.10)*. Infiltrative small glands and solid growth may also occur; adenofibromatous background in one-third; stroma often dense, eosinophilic, and hyalinized but may also be edematous 4. Range of nuclear atypia from mild to severe (generally, not as marked as in HGSC; CCC tends to have nuclei more uniform than HGSC); nucleoli often prominent and enlarged; cytoplasm is often but not always clear; abundant eosinophilic cytoplasm also commonly seen; hyaline globules may be present; mitotic figures very scant in most cases but occasionally over 10/10 hpf *(Fig. 5.22.11)*; psammomatous calcification usually absent

	High-Grade Serous Carcinoma (HGSC) With Clear Cells	Clear Cell Carcinoma (CCC)
Special studies	WT1+, HNF1β−, napsin A−, racemase (AMACR) expected to be −; aberrant p53 expression; ER+/PR+ in majority	WT1−, HNF1β+, Napsin A+, racemase (AMACR)+, p53 wild type in most cases, ER/PR− in about 90%
Treatment	Staging (with debulking when indicated); chemotherapy (in neoadjuvant or adjuvant +/− maintenance setting)	Staging (with debulking when indicated); chemotherapy (in neoadjuvant or adjuvant setting)
Prognosis	Stage III patients have 5-y survival of 45%-50% if optimally debulked; suboptimal debulking has 20%-30% 5-y survival	Stage I has 90% survival; advanced stage appears to have worse prognosis as compared to HGSC

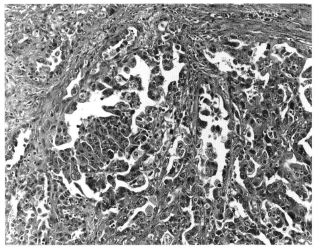

Figure 5.22.1 Papillary, glandular, and slit-like pattern of high-grade serous carcinoma with focal hobnail shapes but lacking classic clear cell carcinoma features.

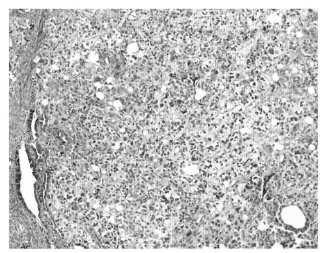

Figure 5.22.2 High-grade serous carcinoma with solid pattern, gland-like spaces, high-grade nuclear atypia, and numerous cells containing clear cytoplasm.

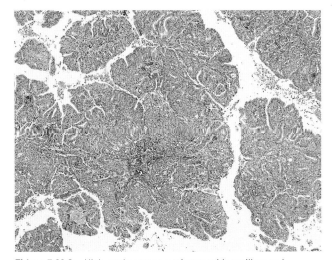

Figure 5.22.3 High-grade serous carcinoma with papillary and glandular pattern.

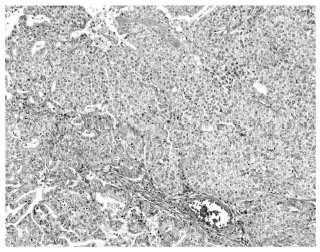

Figure 5.22.4 High-grade serous carcinoma with papillary and glandular pattern displaying pale eosinophilic to clear cytoplasm (same case as *Fig. 5.22.3*).

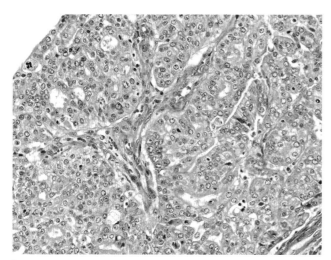

Figure 5.22.5 High-grade serous carcinoma with papillary and glandular pattern displaying pale eosinophilic to clear cytoplasm (same case as *Fig. 5.22.3*).

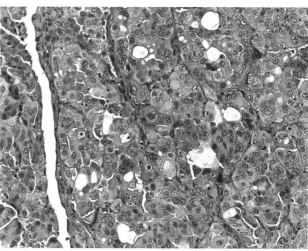

Figure 5.22.6 High-grade serous carcinoma with a solid pattern displaying predominantly brightly eosinophilic cytoplasm. This area shows more of a conventional appearance of high-grade serous carcinoma (areas with clear cells not shown). This example may resemble the oxyphilic variant of clear cell carcinoma. Nuclear grade is high with prominent nucleoli.

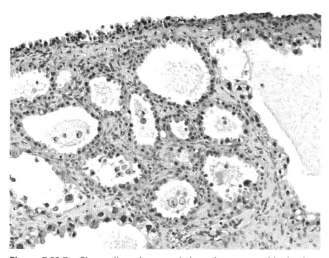

Figure 5.22.7 Clear cell carcinoma, tubulocystic pattern, with glands and cysts lined by hobnail cells with clear and eosinophilic cytoplasm.

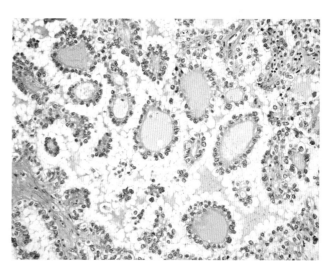

Figure 5.22.8 Clear cell carcinoma with ring-like structures (medium-sized papillae with empty stromal cores cut tangentially).

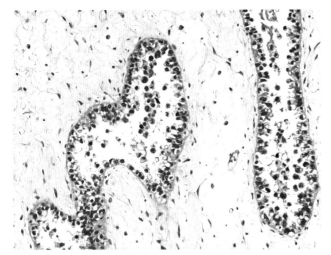

Figure 5.22.9 Clear cell carcinoma with glands lined by hobnail cells with clear cytoplasm.

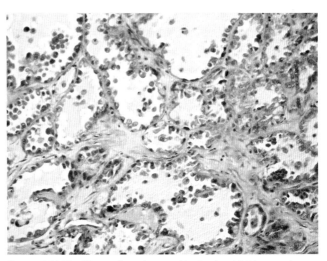

Figure 5.22.10 Clear cell carcinoma with glands exhibiting prominent hobnail cells.

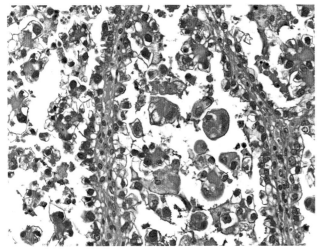

Figure 5.22.11 Clear cell carcinoma, papillary pattern, with moderate nuclear atypia, hobnail cells, and clear cytoplasm.

	Adenofibromatous Clear Cell Carcinoma	Sertoli Cell Tumor
Age	Mean 50-53 y	Mean 30 y
Location	Within ovary; rarely arises in extraovarian sites from endometriosis	Within ovary
Symptoms	Pelvic pain, increasing abdominal girth, bloating, early satiety, vaginal bleeding, urinary symptoms	Pelvic/abdominal pain, swelling, vaginal bleeding
Signs	Pelvic/adnexal mass; rarely thromboembolic events or paraneoplastic hypercalcemia	40% have estrogenic manifestations
Etiology	Majority arise in endometriosis; *ARID1A, PIK3CA, PTEN, KRAS, TGF-βII* mutations; *TERT* promoter mutations; germline *MLH1, MSH2, PMS2,* or *MSH6* mutations (Lynch syndrome) in a small subset of cases	Rarely seen in patients with Peutz-Jeghers syndrome; *DICER1* mutations
Gross and histology	1. One-third to one-half are stage I; endometriosis and adhesions often present; high incidence of tumor rupture; <10% bilateral; mean 13-15 cm; fibromatous gross appearance with yellow-white cut surface with honeycomb appearance; cystic component in small minority 2. Tumor predominantly shows adenofibromatous background often containing tubulocystic pattern of growth; infiltrative small glands and solid growth may also occur; other admixed patterns may be present (papillary, tubulopapillary [including ring-like structures], and hobnail); stroma predominantly fibromatous but can be dense, eosinophilic, and hyalinized; stroma may also be pale and edematous in some areas *(Figs. 5.23.1-5.23.4)* 3. Range of nuclear atypia from mild to severe *(Figs. 5.23.4 and 5.23.5)*; nucleoli often prominent and enlarged; cytoplasm is often but not always clear; abundant eosinophilic cytoplasm also commonly seen; hyaline globules may be present; mitotic figures very scant in most cases but occasionally over 10/10 hpf	1. Unilateral, stage I, mean 8-9 cm 2. Uniform tubular pattern; hollow tubules lined by tall cuboidal or columnar cells; solid tubules may be elongated, round, or ovoid; closely packed solid tubules may mimic sheets; less commonly cords, trabecular, and spindled patterns *(Figs. 5.23.6-5.23.8)* 3. Bland round to ovoid uniform nuclei, pale to eosinophilic cytoplasm, and mitotically inactive *(Figs. 5.23.8 and 5.23.9)*; rare lipid-rich and oxyphilic variants; no hyaline globules
Special studies	• HNF1β+, CK7+, EMA+, PAX8+; WT1−, ER/PR− in about 90% • Inhibin−, calretinin−, SF-1−	• WT1+, SF-1+, inhibin+, calretinin+; ER/PR may be (+) • EMA−, CK7−, HNF1β−, PAX8−; other cytokeratins are nonspecific as they may be (+) in Sertoli cell tumor

	Adenofibromatous Clear Cell Carcinoma	**Sertoli Cell Tumor**
Treatment	Staging (with debulking when indicated); chemotherapy (in neoadjuvant or adjuvant setting)	Unilateral salpingo-oophorectomy
Prognosis	Stage I has 90% survival; advanced stage appears to have worse prognosis as compared to high-grade serous carcinoma	Usually benign; rare abdominopelvic recurrences

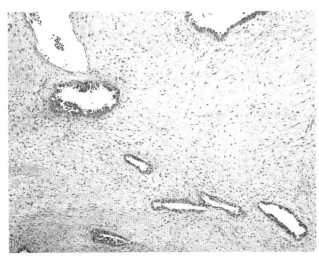

Figure 5.23.1   Adenofibromatous clear cell carcinoma displays abundant fibromatous stroma, which may be edematous as seen here, with a sparse glandular component.

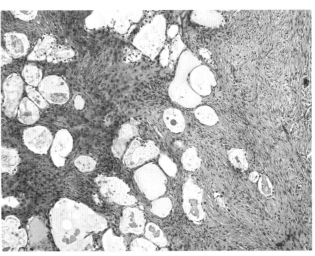

Figure 5.23.2   Tubulocystic pattern of clear cell carcinoma with abundant fibromatous stroma.

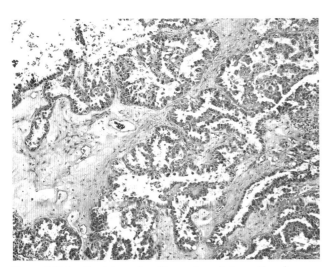

Figure 5.23.3   Glandular and papillary pattern of clear cell carcinoma with abundant fibromatous stroma and patchy edema.

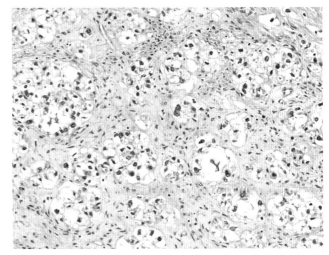

Figure 5.23.4   Adenofibromatous clear cell carcinoma displaying nests and glands of clear cells with severe cytologic atypia with focally bizarre nuclear features.

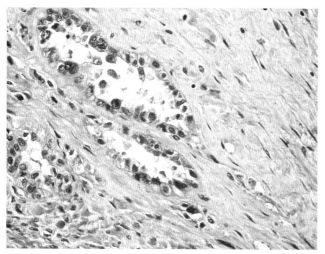

Figure 5.23.5   Adenofibromatous clear cell carcinoma with dense, eosinophilic fibrous stroma. Note hobnail pattern of clear cells lining glands and high-grade nuclear atypia.

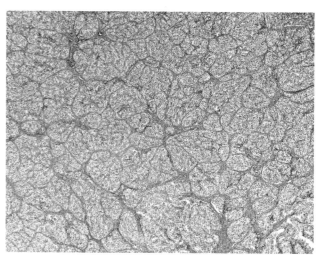

Figure 5.23.6   Sertoli cell tumor with evenly distributed, smoothly contoured islands and nests surrounded by thin bands of ovarian-type stroma.

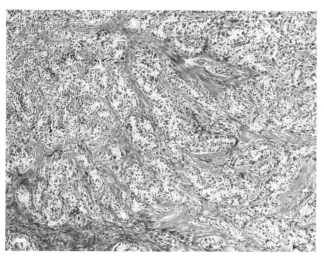

Figure 5.23.7   Sertoli cell tumor with well-formed cords and tubules.

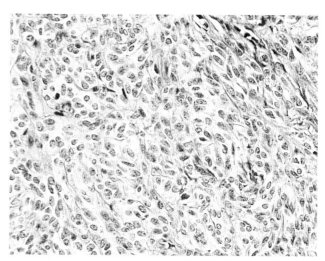

Figure 5.23.8   Sertoli cell tumor with solid tubules displaying bland ovoid nuclei and pale to clear cytoplasm.

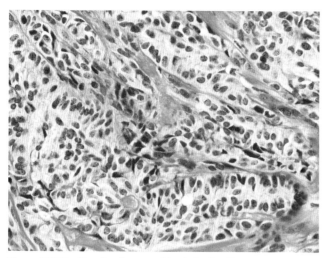

Figure 5.23.9   Sertoli cell tumor with tubules lined by cuboidal to columnar cells with bland ovoid nuclei and clear cytoplasm.

	Benign Brenner Tumor	Borderline Brenner Tumor
Age	Mean 53 y	Mean 59-61 y
Location	Within ovary; small tumors located close to junction of hilus with ovarian surface epithelium	Within ovary
Symptoms	Majority are incidentally found small or microscopic tumors	Pelvic/abdominal pain
Signs	Asymptomatic; large tumors may have pelvic/adnexal mass	Pelvic mass
Etiology	Likely arises from Walthard nests, which in turn probably arise from the tubal-peritoneal junction; *KRAS* mutations at codon 12 and *CTNNB1* mutations reported	Arise in benign Brenner tumor; *CDKN2A*, *PIK3CA*, *KRAS* mutations reported
Gross and histology	1. Mean 1.7 cm; 6% bilateral; solid, yellowish cut surface; confined to ovary 2. Transitional-type nests are ovoid or rounded and dispersed within a fibrotic ovarian stroma *(Figs. 5.24.1-5.24.4)*; half have spiculated calcification *(Fig. 5.24.3)*; nests may develop cystic spaces, which may be lined by mucinous epithelium 3. Neoplastic cells resemble normal urothelium, with ovoid nuclei, often with grooves parallel to the long axis; prominent cell borders and pale eosinophilic cytoplasm; no atypia, mitotically inactive *(Figs. 5.24.2-5.24.4)* 4. 30% contain benign mucinous epithelium originating within the transitional nests	1. Large, unilateral, cystic tumors, mean 17 cm; cyst walls display papillary masses; solid nodule may reflect benign Brenner component; occasionally completely solid 2. Tumor has solid markedly crowded transitional cell nests (+/− cystic change), some angulated and irregular; tumor nests larger than in benign Brenner tumor and show more complexity of epithelium *(Fig. 5.24.5)*; intracystic papillary component resembles noninvasive low-grade urothelial (transitional cell) neoplasm *(Figs. 5.24.6 and 5.24.7)*; mucinous epithelium may develop and line cystic spaces *(Fig. 5.24.8)*; infiltrative growth (stromal invasion) is absent 3. Cytologic atypia and mitotic activity may be present in papillae or nests *(Fig. 5.24.9)* 4. Benign mucinous epithelium may be present, rarely with atypia
Special studies	Not useful in this differential	Not useful in this differential
Treatment	Unilateral salpingo-oophorectomy	Unilateral salpingo-oophorectomy
Prognosis	Benign	Benign, rarely recurs

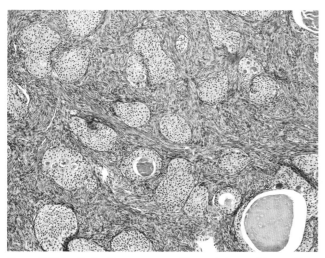

Figure 5.24.1 Benign Brenner tumor with rounded to ovoid smoothly contoured nests dispersed in a fibrotic ovarian-type stroma.

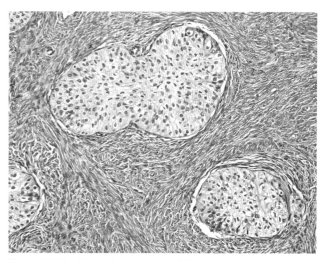

Figure 5.24.2 Benign Brenner tumor with nests composed of transitional-type cells resembling urothelium.

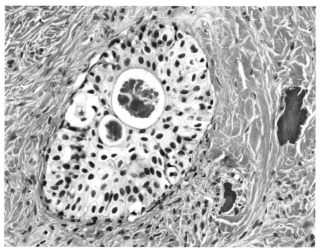

Figure 5.24.3 Benign Brenner tumor nest with cavities containing eosinophilic material. Spiculated calcification is noted.

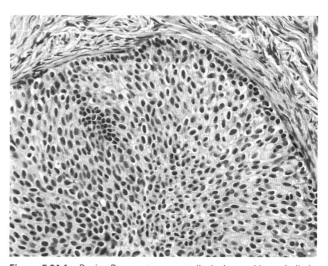

Figure 5.24.4 Benign Brenner tumor nest displaying ovoid to spindled uniform bland nuclei lacking mitotic activity. Nuclear grooves are inconspicuous.

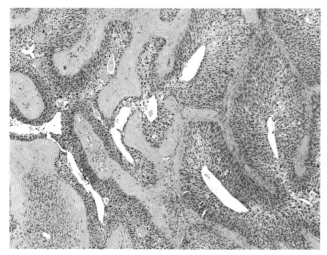

Figure 5.24.5 Borderline Brenner tumor with enlarged, interconnected nests lined by proliferating transitional-type epithelium resembling urothelium.

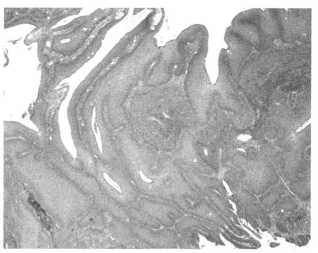

Figure 5.24.6 Borderline Brenner tumor resembling low-grade papillary urothelial (transitional cell) neoplasm.

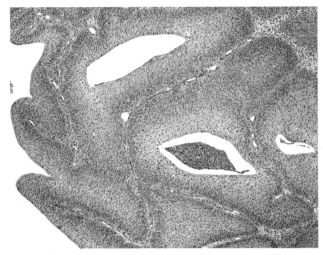

Figure 5.24.7   Borderline Brenner tumor with endophytic papillary growth resembling inverted urothelial (transitional cell) papilloma.

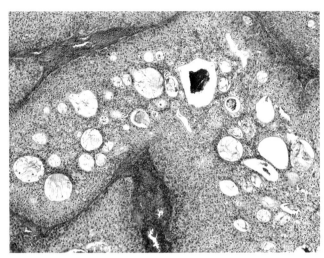

Figure 5.24.8   Borderline Brenner tumor with cystic spaces containing eosinophilic material. Spaces may be lined by mucinous epithelium.

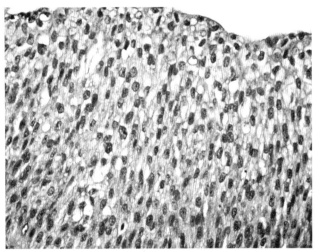

Figure 5.24.9   Borderline Brenner tumor with highly stratified transitional-type epithelium with mild to moderate atypia and longitudinal nuclear grooves.

	Borderline Brenner Tumor	Malignant Brenner Tumor
Age	Mean 59-61 y	Mean 63 y
Location	Within ovary	Within ovary
Symptoms	Pelvic pain	Pelvic/abdominal pain
Signs	Pelvic mass	Pelvic/abdominal mass
Etiology	Arise in benign Brenner tumor; *CDKN2A*, *PIK3CA*, *KRAS* mutations reported	Arise from benign Brenner tumor through borderline Brenner tumor; *PIK3CA* mutation, *CDKN2A/2B* deletion, *MDM2* amplification and *FGFR3* alterations reported
Gross and histology	1. Large, unilateral, cystic tumors, mean 18 cm; cyst walls display papillary masses; solid nodule may reflect benign Brenner component; occasionally completely solid 2. Intracystic papillary component resembles noninvasive low-grade urothelial (transitional cell) neoplasm *(Figs. 5.25.1-5.25.4)*; cavities containing eosinophilic material may develop within the proliferation and are often lined by mucinous epithelium; infiltrative growth (stromal invasion) is absent 3. Tumor may also be solid with markedly crowded transitional nests, some angulated and irregular 4. Cytologic atypia and mitotic activity may be present in papillae or nests *(Figs. 5.25.3 and 5.25.4)*	1. Mean 14-16 cm; 12% bilateral; 80% confined to the ovary; large, solid, or solid and cystic 2. Invasive multilayered urothelial-type epithelium (usually resembling transitional cell carcinoma, sometimes squamous cell carcinoma) *(Figs. 5.25.5-5.25.7)*; papillary component, which may be intracystic, may display invasion at the base or into the fibrovascular stroma; a benign or borderline Brenner component must be present to establish the diagnosis *(Fig. 5.25.5)*; if absent, consider diagnosis of high-grade serous carcinoma with transitional-like pattern (see Section 5.30) 3. A purely solid tumor may display irregularly dispersed and angulated transitional cell nests, clusters, and single cells with a haphazard infiltrative pattern 4. Usually high-grade malignant nuclear features and mitotic activity *(Figs. 5.25.6 and 5.25.8)*
Special studies	Not useful in this differential	Not useful in this differential
Treatment	Unilateral salpingo-oophorectomy	Limited data; presumed as per other ovarian carcinomas (staging [with debulking when indicated]; chemotherapy [in adjuvant or neoadjuvant setting])
Prognosis	Benign, rarely recurs	>90% survival for stage I; insufficient data for advanced stage

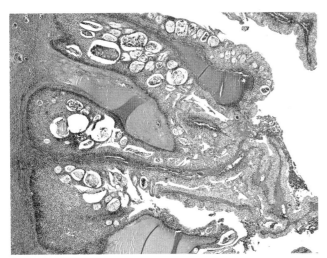

Figure 5.25.1 Borderline Brenner tumor with proliferating transitional-type epithelium resembling low-grade urothelial neoplasm. Cystic spaces are noted within the proliferating epithelium.

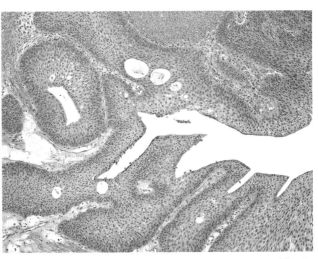

Figure 5.25.2 Borderline Brenner tumor with proliferating transitional-type epithelium resembling low-grade papillary urothelial neoplasm.

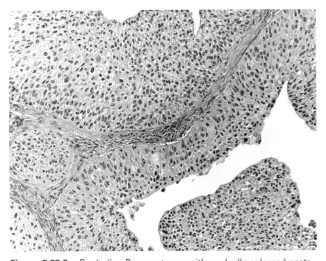

Figure 5.25.3 Borderline Brenner tumor with markedly enlarged nests lined by undulating transitional-type epithelium with prominent spaces within the enlarged nests; moderate cytologic atypia is present.

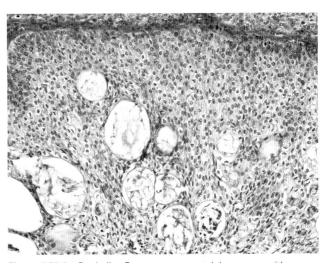

Figure 5.25.4 Borderline Brenner tumor containing spaces with eosinophilic material within the proliferating epithelium, which displays mild cytologic atypia; such spaces may be lined by mucinous epithelium (not obvious in this photograph).

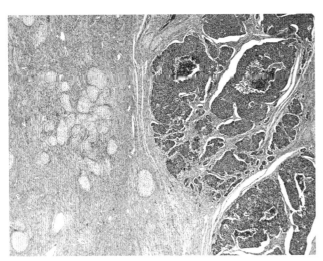

Figure 5.25.5 Malignant Brenner tumor. Invasive transitional cell (urothelial) carcinoma component on **right** and benign Brenner tumor component on **left**.

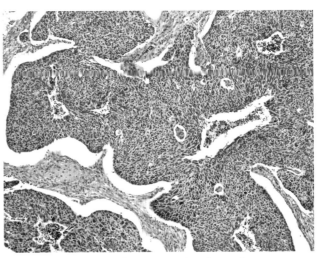

Figure 5.25.6 Malignant Brenner tumor. Invasive carcinoma component resembles transitional cell (urothelial) carcinoma.

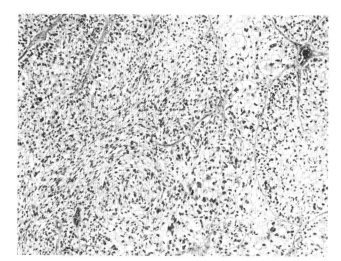

Figure 5.25.7 Malignant Brenner tumor. Invasive carcinoma component consists of sheets with some degree of spindle cell differentiation and clear cytoplasm resembling squamous cell carcinoma with glycogenation.

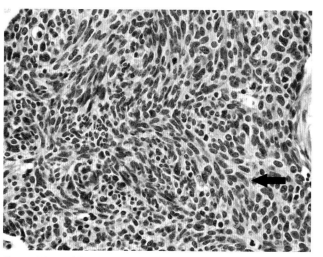

Figure 5.25.8 Malignant Brenner tumor. Transitional cell carcinoma component exhibits hyperchromasia, high nuclear-to-cytoplasmic ratios, and some degree of oval to elongated nuclei. Rare longitudinal nuclear grooves are present (*arrow*).

	Immature Teratoma, Low Grade	Mature Cystic Teratoma With Nonimmature Neuroepithelial Tubules
Age	<20 y	Most commonly 20-29 y
Location	Within ovary	Within ovary
Symptoms	Abdominal/pelvic pain	Abdominal/pelvic pain, swelling
Signs	Pelvic/lower abdominal mass	Pelvic/lower abdominal mass
Etiology	Premeiotic germ cell origin; associated with contralateral mature cystic teratoma in 10%-15%; chromosome 12 alterations only when part of mixed germ cell tumor	Arise from primordial germ cells after the first and before the second meiotic divisions; diploid with normal 46XX karyotype
Gross and histology	1. 9-28 cm, soft, lobulated, may be cystic, often hemorrhagic, and necrotic; 25% have associated mature cystic teratoma (hair or fat may be seen); one-third associated with peritoneal mature glial nodules (gliomatosis peritonei) 2. Immature neuroepithelium, in tubules, rosettes, or solid growth; lined by stratified hyperchromatic columnar cells with elongated nuclei, inconspicuous cell borders, high nuclear-to-cytoplasmic ratios, abundant apoptotic bodies, and high mitotic activity; sharp luminal margins and cilia often present (Figs. 5.26.1-5.26.4); immature neuroepithelium should constitute a limited area to qualify for low grade (no greater than one 4× low-power field, in aggregate) 3. Glial and neuronal tissue common; glia sometimes very cellular and mitotically active; admixed with wide variety of other teratomatous elements in varying stages of maturity 4. May be mixed with other germ cell elements, for example, dysgerminoma	1. Typically unilocular cyst; 10%-15% bilateral; mean 6-8 cm; hair and sebaceous material often present; rarely solid 2. Wide variety of differentiation, most commonly skin, respiratory mucosa, cartilage, adipose tissue, smooth muscle, thyroid, and gastrointestinal mucosa; cyst wall may display lipogranulomas; dense lymphocytic infiltrate may be present (Fig. 5.26.5); no true immature neuroectodermal tissue; neuroectodermal tubules with some degree of maturation may be present but lack the primitive cytologic features of the neuroepithelium in immature teratoma (ie, nuclear enlargement, high nuclear-to-cytoplasmic ratios, hyperchromasia, apoptotic bodies, and/or mitotic activity) ("nonimmature neuroepithelial tubules"); these can resemble the central canal of the spinal cord in children, and fetal-type ependymal differentiation may be present (Figs. 5.26.6-5.26.8) 3. Glial tissue commonly present; neuronal and other CNS elements may accompany glia; cerebellar tissue, particularly the granular cell layer, may be present and resemble primitive neuroepithelium of immature teratoma (Figs. 5.26.9 and 5.26.10) 4. Mature cystic teratoma can arise with other malignant germ cell tumors
Special studies	Neuroepithelium: SOX2+, glypican-3+, SALL4+, CD99+, and bcl-2+; may be NSE+; GFAP−; SALL4 is also (+) in intestinal elements; Ki 67 proliferation index for immature neuroectodermal tubules should be high	Variety of elements generally stain similarly to their normal tissue counterparts; insufficient data on profile of mature vs immature neuroepithelium; however, the expected Ki 67 proliferation index for nonimmature neuroectodermal tubules would be low

	Immature Teratoma, Low Grade	**Mature Cystic Teratoma With Nonimmature Neuroepithelial Tubules**
Treatment	Unilateral salpingo-oophorectomy or unilateral oophorectomy; combination chemotherapy for high-grade tumors	Cystectomy or unilateral salpingo-oophorectomy
Prognosis	Low-grade tumors (grade 1) have favorable outcome	Benign

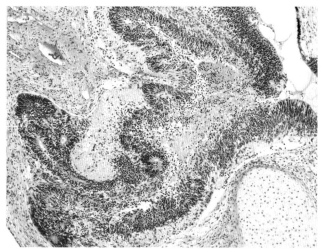

Figure 5.26.1   Immature teratoma with prominent immature neuroepithelium. Other teratomatous elements (cartilage) are present **(lower right)**.

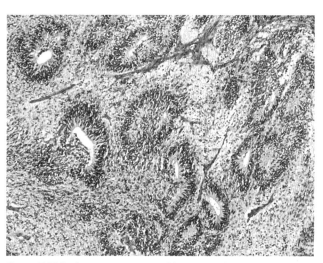

Figure 5.26.2   Immature teratoma with numerous immature neuroepithelial tubules.

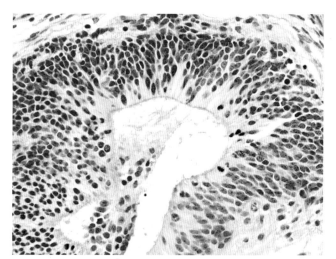

Figure 5.26.3   Immature teratoma with immature neuroepithelial tubule showing enlarged hyperchromatic nuclei, high nuclear-to-cytoplasmic ratios, and mitotic activity.

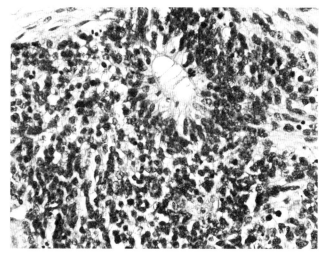

Figure 5.26.4   Immature teratoma with immature neuroepithelial tubule and solid sheets containing primitive cells with hyperchromasia, high nuclear-to-cytoplasmic ratios, and mitotic activity.

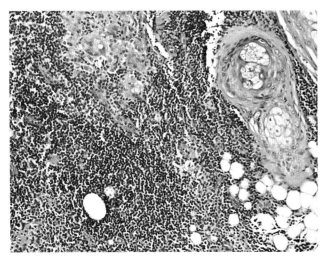

Figure 5.26.5 Mature teratoma with skin appendages and intense lymphocytic infiltrate.

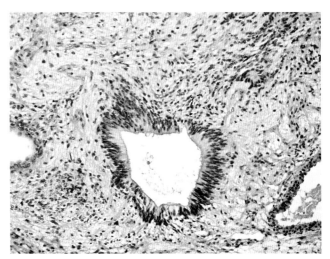

Figure 5.26.6 Mature teratoma with fetal-type ependymal epithelium resembling the central canal of the spinal cord in children. Note the elongated bland nuclei, in a background of glial tissue. The high nuclear-to-cytoplasmic ratios, hyperchromasia, mitotic activity, and apoptotic debris as seen in primitive neuroepithelium of immature teratoma are absent (contrast with *Figs. 5.26.1-5.26.3*).

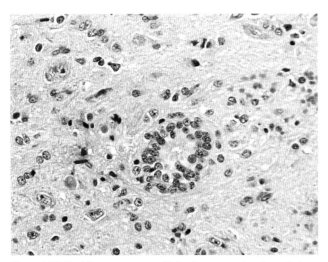

Figure 5.26.7 Mature teratoma with fetal-type ependymal rosette in a glial background. The high nuclear-to-cytoplasmic ratios, hyperchromasia, mitotic activity, and apoptotic debris as seen in primitive neuroepithelium of immature teratoma are absent (contrast with *Fig. 5.26.4*).

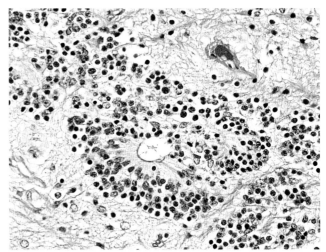

Figure 5.26.8 Mature teratoma with fetal-type ependymal rosette in a glial background. The high nuclear-to-cytoplasmic ratios, hyperchromasia, mitotic activity, and apoptotic debris as seen in primitive neuroepithelium of immature teratoma are absent (contrast with *Fig. 5.26.4*).

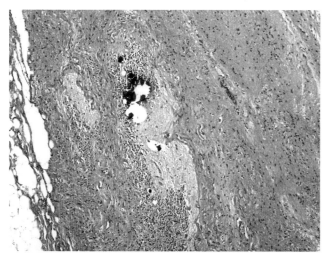

Figure 5.26.9 Mature teratoma with glial tissue associated with a hypercellular area of small round cells reflecting mature cerebellar differentiation.

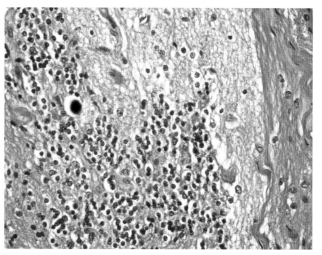

Figure 5.26.10 Mature teratoma. Same case as *Figure 5.26.9* with mature cerebellar tissue.

	Malignant Sex Cord-Stromal Tumor (Adult Granulosa Cell Tumor/Poorly Differentiated Sertoli-Leydig Cell Tumor/Unclassified Sex Cord-Stromal Tumor)	Cellular Fibroma
Age	Mean 50-55 y (adult granulosa cell tumor); mean, 25 y (poorly differentiated Sertoli-Leydig cell tumor)	Mean 41-51 y
Location	Within ovary	Within ovary
Symptoms	Pelvic/low abdominal pain; dysmenorrhea; increased abdominal girth	Pelvic/low abdominal pain; urinary symptoms; increased abdominal girth
Signs	Pelvic/adnexal mass; ascites; occasional virilization; occasionally diagnosed during pregnancy	Adnexal mass; ascites in >10 cm tumors in 10%-15%; Meigs syndrome; Gorlin (hereditary basal cell nevus) syndrome
Etiology	*FOXL2* mutations in adult granulosa cell tumor; *DICER1* mutations in Sertoli-Leydig cell tumor	Cellular variant of fibroma; LOH at 9q22.3 (*PTCH1*) and 19p13.3 (*STK11*) frequent; trisomy and/or tetrasomy 12; rarely *IDH1* mutation; *FOXL2* mutations absent
Gross and histology	1. Unilateral, usually stage I; mean size 9-12 cm 2. May have classic patterns of adult granulosa cell tumor or poorly differentiated Sertoli-Leydig cell tumor or show cords, trabeculae, follicle-like structures, and tubules with ambiguous features overlapping Sertoli-Leydig cell and adult granulosa cell groups; unclassified tumors may have diffuse cellular spindle cell proliferation lacking hyaline/fibrous plaques; oval or angulated/folded nuclei with longitudinal nuclear grooves in adult granulosa cell tumor; Leydig cells in Sertoli-Leydig cell tumor *(Figs. 5.27.1-5.27.6)* 3. Variable mitotic index with poorly differentiated Sertoli-Leydig cell tumor having increased mitotic activity; bizarre nuclei present in 10% of cases	1. <10% bilateral; wide size range from microscopic to >10 cm; hard, chalky white cut surface; larger cellular ones may be soft; 10% have adhesions and extraovarian involvement 2. Intersecting bundles of plump spindle cells with intercellular collagen *(Figs. 5.27.7-5.27.12)*; tumors are cellular, but there may be alternating highly cellular and hypocellular regions; storiform pattern may be present *(Figs. 5.27.7 and 5.27.11)*; calcification in <10%; rarely contains minor sex cord elements, but prominent sex cord patterns argue against a diagnosis of cellular fibroma; some undergo cystic degeneration (pseudocysts); spindle cell nuclei without longitudinal nuclear grooves 3. Mild to moderate atypia can be present *(Fig. 5.27.12)*; cellular fibromas frequently have >4 mitoses per 10 hpf
Special studies	Immunohistochemistry of no use for this differential diagnosis	Immunohistochemistry of no use for this differential diagnosis
Treatment	Hysterectomy and bilateral salpingo-oophorectomy with exploration and staging if indicated	Unilateral salpingo-oophorectomy

	Malignant Sex Cord-Stromal Tumor (Adult Granulosa Cell Tumor/Poorly Differentiated Sertoli-Leydig Cell Tumor/Unclassified Sex Cord-Stromal Tumor)	Cellular Fibroma
Prognosis	• Adult granulosa cell tumor: Those with malignant behavior may be indolent, some with late recurrences after 5-10 y or more; stage I has about 90% survival at 10 y • Poorly differentiated Sertoli-Leydig cell tumor: clinically malignant behavior has been observed in up to 50% of cases	Benign; may occasionally recur, but virtually never fatal; some authors regard these as "tumors of low malignant potential"

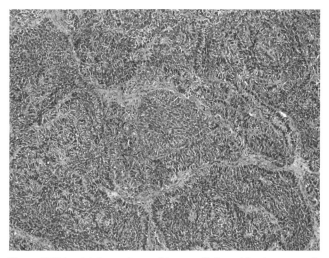

Figure 5.27.1 Adult granulosa cell tumor with large islands composed of interanastomosing cords and tubules. Peripheral palisading of nuclei is present.

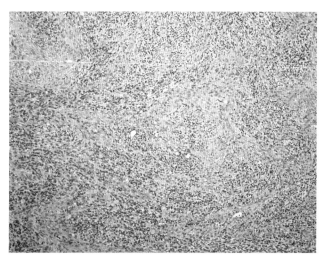

Figure 5.27.2 Adult granulosa cell tumor simulating cellular fibroma.

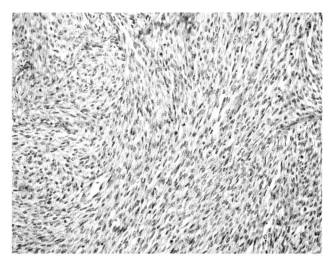

Figure 5.27.3 Poorly differentiated Sertoli-Leydig cell tumor with predominantly spindle cell architecture and mitotic activity mimicking cellular fibroma (other areas of more obvious sertoliform differentiation and Leydig cells not shown in this photograph).

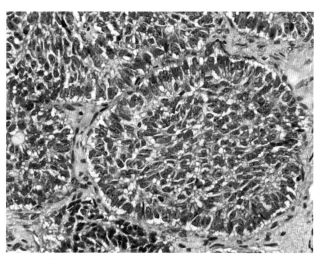

Figure 5.27.4 Adult granulosa cell tumor. Small island with peripheral palisading; the nuclei are round to ovoid and some display grooves.

5   OVARY

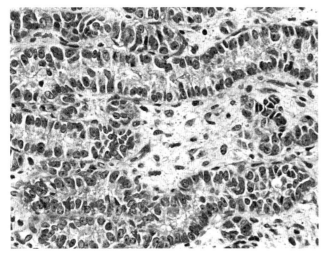

Figure 5.27.5   Malignant sex cord tumor with sertoliform differentiation.

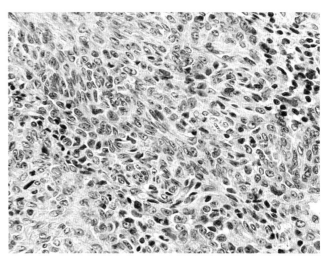

Figure 5.27.6   Adult granulosa cell tumor with spindle cells showing angulated/folded nuclei and occasional nuclear grooves.

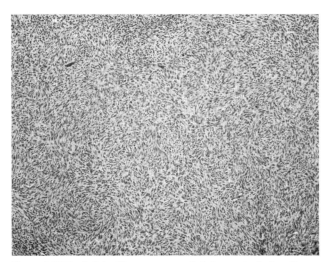

Figure 5.27.7   Cellular fibroma composed of sheets of spindle cells with storiform areas.

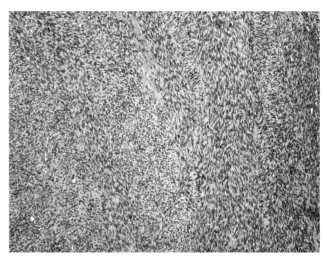

Figure 5.27.8   Cellular fibroma with spindle cells forming fascicles.

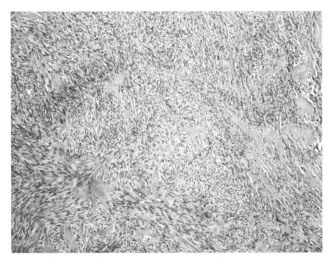

Figure 5.27.9 Cellular fibroma with hyalinized bands between patches of spindle cells.

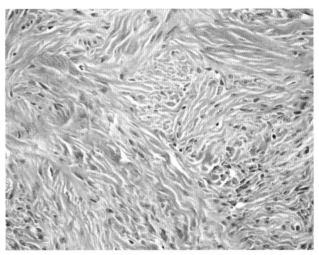

Figure 5.27.10 Area of hypocellularity from a case of cellular fibroma (cellular areas not shown in this photograph). Areas such as this with bland spindle cells and intercellular collagen are typical of fibroma and support a diagnosis of cellular fibroma for a difficult-to-classify cellular sex cord-stromal tumor.

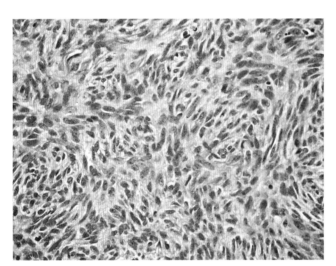

Figure 5.27.11 Cellular fibroma with storiform pattern. Tumor cells lack cytologic features of adult granulosa cell tumor.

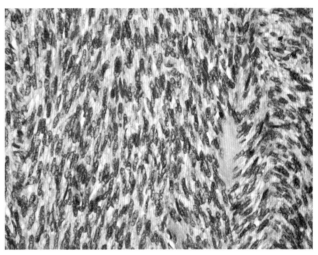

Figure 5.27.12 Cellular fibroma with mild cytologic atypia of spindle cells.

	Adult Granulosa Cell Tumor	Sertoli-Leydig Cell Tumor
Age	Mean 50-55 y	Mean 25 y (35 y for well differentiated; 16 y for retiform variant)
Location	Within ovary	Within ovary
Symptoms	Pelvic/lower abdominal pain; postmenopausal bleeding; 10% have acute abdomen with hemoperitoneum	Abdominal swelling and pelvic/low abdominal pain
Signs	Pelvic/lower abdominal mass; may have estrogenic manifestations	Pelvic/lower abdominal mass; virilization in one-third; occasionally estrogenic clinical features
Etiology	*FOXL2* mutations	3 molecular subtypes: *DICER1* mutations in moderately/poorly differentiated, retiform, and heterologous types; *FOXL2* reported in postmenopausal moderately/poorly differentiated without retiform pattern or heterologous elements; *DICER1/FOXL2* wild type in well differentiated without retiform pattern or heterologous elements
Gross and histology	1. Solid and cystic, hemorrhagic; mean 10-12 cm; <5% bilateral; >90% stage I; solid and cystic with tan or yellow cut surfaces, hemorrhage with clotted blood within cysts common 2. Wide variety of architectural patterns: diffuse, microfollicular, macrofollicular, insular, trabecular, tubular, and combinations *(Figs. 5.28.1-5.28.4)*; microfollicular pattern may have Call-Exner bodies 3. Small cells with ovoid or angulated/folded uniform nuclei, often with grooves *(Figs. 5.28.4 and 5.28.5)*; high mitotic activity rare or absent; 2% contain bizarre nuclei; luteinized stromal cells resembling Leydig cells may be present; Leydig cells generally absent, but rare adult granulosa cell tumors containing Leydig cells have been described	1. Nearly always unilateral and stage I, mean 13.5 cm; solid and cystic; heterologous variant may contain mucinous cysts; poorly differentiated tumors larger and more often with hemorrhage and necrosis 2. Sertoli cell pattern with hollow or solid tubules/cords; intermediate/poorly differentiated have poorly defined lobulated masses of immature Sertoli cells *(Figs. 5.28.6-5.28.10)* 3. Cuboidal to columnar Sertoli cells, round–ovoid nuclei, minimal atypia, and low mitotic activity in well-differentiated tumors; immature Sertoli cells usually have bland nuclear features *(Figs. 5.28.9 and 5.28.10)*, occasionally more atypia, and rarely scattered bizarre nuclei; nuclear grooves may be present infrequently but not as characteristic as in adult granulosa cell tumor; poorly differentiated tumors have increased atypia, mitotic activity, and spindle cell differentiation resembling sarcoma; variable numbers of intermixed Leydig cells with small round nuclei and abundant eosinophilic cytoplasm are present but may be inconspicuous *(Figs. 5.28.10 and 5.28.11)*

	Adult Granulosa Cell Tumor	Sertoli-Leydig Cell Tumor
	4. No heterologous elements	**4.** Heterologous elements, present in 20%; most commonly GI-type mucinous epithelium *(Figs. 5.28.12-5.28.14)*; rarely cartilage or skeletal muscle with sarcomatous features
	5. No retiform features	**5.** Retiform variant in 15%, tubules resemble rete ovarii; highly branched, sometimes with papillae or edematous polypoid growth *(Fig. 5.28.15)*
Special studies	Immunohistochemistry of no use for this differential diagnosis	Immunohistochemistry of no use for this differential diagnosis
Treatment	Hysterectomy and bilateral salpingo-oophorectomy; unilateral salpingo-oophorectomy if fertility desired	Unilateral salpingo-oophorectomy
Prognosis	Those with malignant behavior may be indolent, some with late recurrences after 5-10 y or more; stage I has about 90% survival at 10 y	Most stage I tumors are cured by oophorectomy; grade (well, intermediate, and poorly differentiated) correlates with outcome; poorly differentiated (up to 50% clinically malignant), heterologous, and retiform tumors more likely to recur

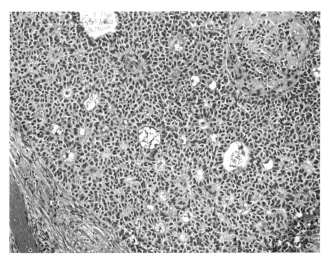

Figure 5.28.1 Granulosa cell tumor with microfollicular pattern.

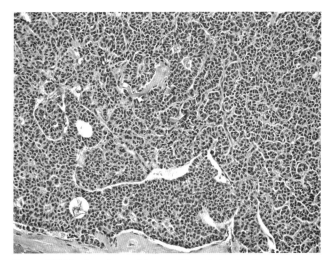

Figure 5.28.2 Granulosa cell tumor with corded and trabecular pattern, with focal areas of microfollicular pattern.

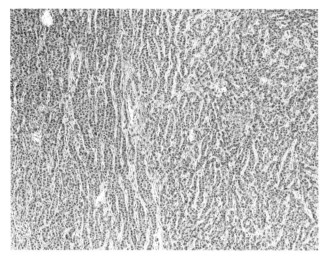

Figure 5.28.3 Granulosa cell tumor with watered-silk **(left)** and gyriform **(right)** patterns.

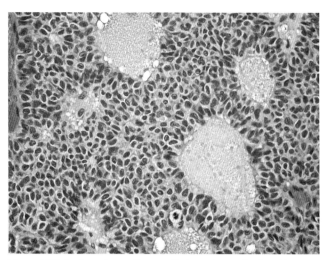

Figure 5.28.4 Granulosa cell tumor displays sheets of cells with ovoid grooved nuclei and microfollicular spaces containing eosinophilic material.

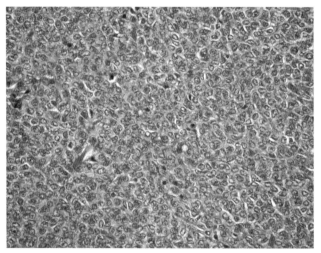

Figure 5.28.5 Granulosa cell tumor with solid pattern displaying nuclear grooves.

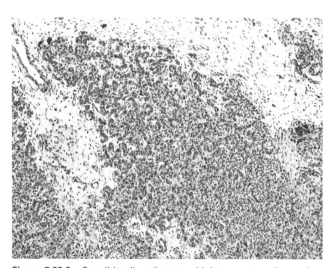

Figure 5.28.6 Sertoli-Leydig cell tumor with interanastomosing cords and tubules.

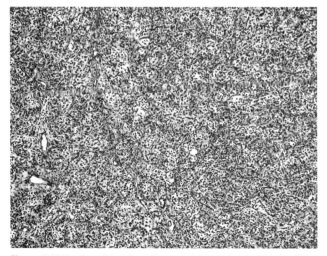

Figure 5.28.7 Sertoli-Leydig cell tumor with rounded, back-to-back solid tubules.

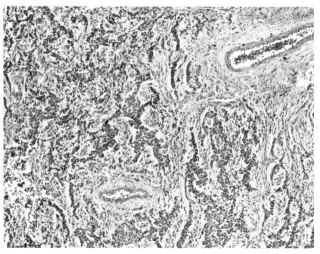

Figure 5.28.8 Sertoli-Leydig cell tumor with interanastomosing cords and ribbons of immature Sertoli cells.

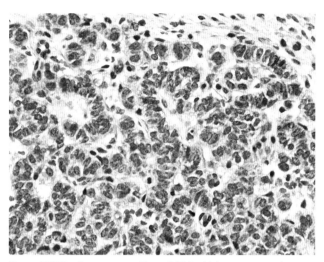

Figure 5.28.9   Same case as *Figure 5.28.8* with interanastomosing cords and ribbons of immature Sertoli cells with tall ovoid nuclei.

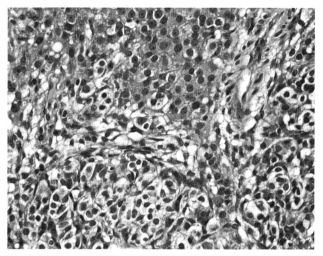

Figure 5.28.10   Sertoli-Leydig cell tumor with rounded solid tubules at **bottom** and Leydig cells with round nuclei and bright eosinophilic cytoplasm at **top**.

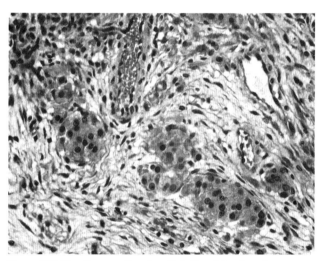

Figure 5.28.11   Clusters of Leydig cells in Sertoli-Leydig cell tumor. Leydig cells are more easily seen within edematous stroma just outside the periphery of the main tumor, as in this case.

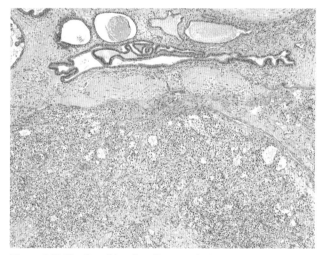

Figure 5.28.12   Sertoli-Leydig cell tumor with heterologous elements. Benign mucinous glands at the **top**, adjacent to the Sertoli-Leydig component with solid and glandular growth. Note well-circumscribed border between the two components.

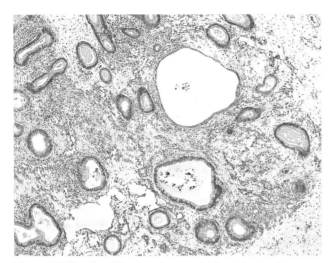

Figure 5.28.13   Sertoli-Leydig cell tumor with heterologous elements. Benign mucinous glands are intermixed throughout the Sertoli-Leydig component.

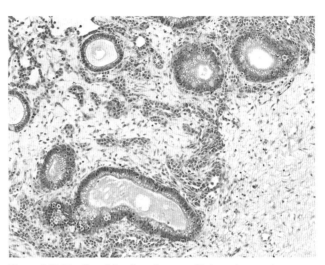

Figure 5.28.14   Sertoli-Leydig cell tumor with heterologous elements. Benign mucinous glands are intermixed throughout the Sertoli-Leydig component (same case as *Fig. 5.28.13*).

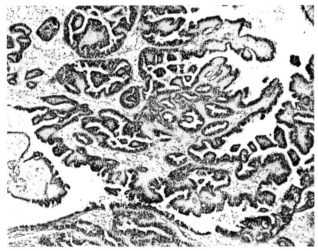

Figure 5.28.15   Sertoli-Leydig cell tumor with retiform pattern. Slit-like and papillary growth resembling the rete ovarii or rete testis.

	Luteinized Adult Granulosa Cell Tumor	Thecoma
Age	Mean 53 y	Mean 50-59 y
Location	Within ovary	Within ovary
Symptoms	Postmenopausal or dysfunctional uterine bleeding, amenorrhea	Pelvic/low abdominal pain; postmenopausal bleeding
Signs	Adnexal mass; hyperestrinism (association with endometrial hyperplasia and low-grade carcinoma)	Pelvic mass; estrogenic manifestations
Etiology	Insufficient data for the luteinized variant; adult granulosa cell tumors in general are associated with *FOXL2* mutations	Insufficient data; *FOXL2* mutations have been reported in a small subset of cases
Gross and histology	1. Solid, lobulated, and yellow or red-brown; mean 5 cm; unilateral, stage IA 2. Usually diffuse pattern, with large nodules separated by thin fibrous septa *(Figs. 5.29.1 and 5.29.2)*; also trabecular, with cords, ribbons, and nests 3. In luteinized variant, cells are large with abundant eosinophilic, often vacuolated, cytoplasm; ovoid uniform nuclei and nucleoli may be prominent; occasional nuclear grooves; no atypia; mitoses rare or absent *(Figs. 5.29.3-5.29.5)* 4. Minor nonluteinized component may be present	1. 5-10 cm, unilateral, solid, yellow-white cut surface, occasionally focally cystic, hemorrhage, or necrosis 2. Ovoid to spindled cells, intersected by fibrous/hyaline plaques, moderate to abundant pale, vacuolated, or eosinophilic cytoplasm, ovoid bland nuclei *(Figs. 5.29.7-5.29.11)*; occasional myxoid change and rarely calcified; often have luteinized cytoplasm *(Fig. 5.29.11)* 3. Low mitotic index (rare mitotically active examples); rare cases contain bizarre nuclei; nuclear grooves are not a typical feature although occasional cases have limited numbers of grooved nuclei 4. Sex cord differentiation (cords, trabeculae, tubules, well-defined islands/nests with peripheral palisading) generally absent although rare gonadal stromal tumors with minor sex cord elements have been described
Special studies	Reticulin surrounds nests of tumor cells; Relative loss of reticulin framework *(Fig. 5.29.6)*. Immunohistochemistry of no use for this differential diagnosis	Reticulin surrounds individual tumor cells *(Fig. 5.29.12)*; immunohistochemistry of no use for this differential diagnosis
Treatment	Bilateral or unilateral salpingo-oophorectomy	Unilateral salpingo-oophorectomy
Prognosis	No data; presumed similar to usual granulosa cell tumor	Benign

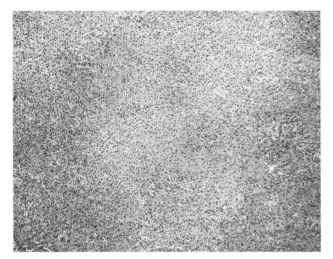

Figure 5.29.1   Luteinized adult granulosa cell tumor with solid pattern.

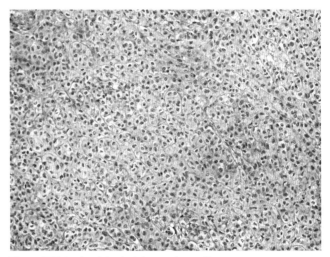

Figure 5.29.2   Luteinized adult granulosa cell tumor, same case as *Figure 5.29.1*, with rounded to polygonal cells with abundant eosinophilic cytoplasm.

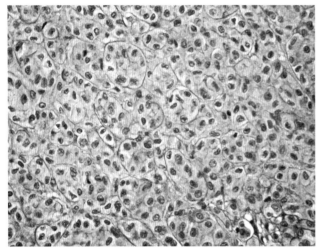

Figure 5.29.3   Luteinized adult granulosa cell tumor, same case as *Figure 5.29.1*, with round to ovoid nuclei, some with grooves, and abundant eosinophilic cytoplasm.

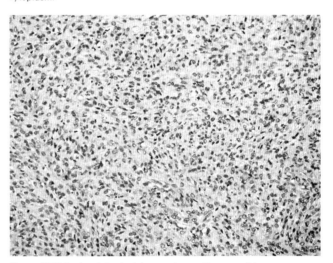

Figure 5.29.4   Luteinized adult granulosa cell tumor with vague suggestion of spindle cell differentiation.

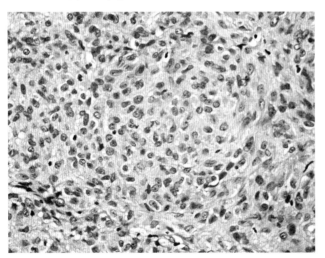

Figure 5.29.5   Luteinized adult granulosa cell tumor, same case as *Figure 5.29.4*, with folded/angulated nuclei, nuclear grooves, and moderate to abundant eosinophilic cytoplasm.

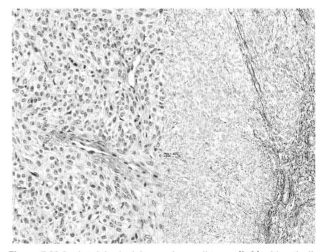

Figure 5.29.6   Luteinized adult granulosa cell tumor **(left)** with reticulin stain **(right)** showing sparse reticulin framework surrounding groups of neoplastic cells.

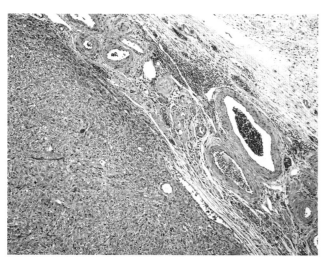

Figure 5.29.7 Thecoma displaying well-circumscribed margin with surrounding ovary.

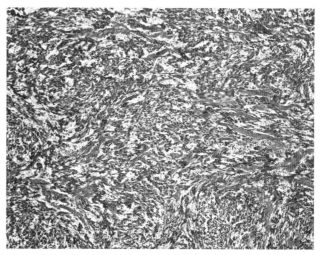

Figure 5.29.8 Thecoma/fibrothecoma with cellular spindle cell proliferation interrupted by thin collagenous plaques.

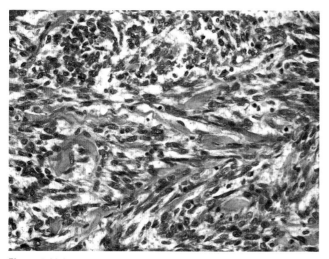

Figure 5.29.9 Thecoma/fibrothecoma. Same case as *Figure 5.29.8* with ovoid nuclei without atypia, and collagen deposition.

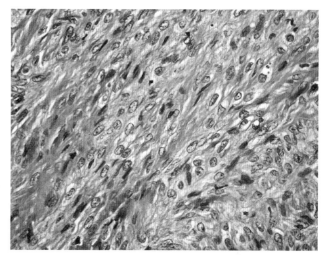

Figure 5.29.10 Thecoma with elongated spindle cells with ovoid nuclei without significant atypia. In this case, a few cells have nuclear grooves, which occurs occasionally in thecomas. That finding is allowed for thecomas as long as grooved nuclei are in limited numbers and that other diagnostic features of adult granulosa cell tumor are lacking.

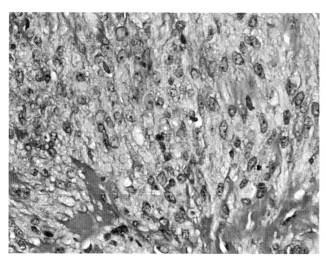

Figure 5.29.11 Thecoma with abundant eosinophilic cytoplasm reflecting luteinization, and collagen plaques at the **bottom**.

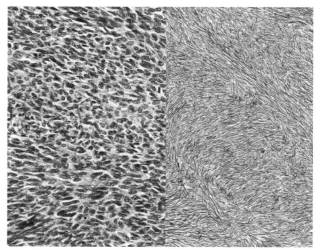

Figure 5.29.12 Thecoma **(left)** with reticulin stain **(right)** showing prominent reticulin framework surrounding individual neoplastic cells.

	Adult Granulosa Cell Tumor With Pseudopapillary Pattern	High-Grade Serous Carcinoma (HGSC)
Age	Mean 50-55 y	Mean 60-63 y
Location	Within ovary	Ovarian surface and within ovarian stroma, tubal fimbriae, commonly invade nonfimbrial tube
Symptoms	Pelvic/lower abdominal pain; postmenopausal bleeding; 10% have acute abdomen with hemoperitoneum	Pelvic pain, increasing abdominal girth, bloating, early satiety, urinary symptoms
Signs	Pelvic/lower abdominal mass; may have estrogenic manifestations	Pelvic/abdominal mass, ascites
Etiology	*FOXL2* mutations	Majority derive from serous tubal intraepithelial carcinoma, usually of fimbrial origin; virtually all have *TP53* mutations; a substantial proportion have germline or somatic mutation in *BRCA1*, *BRCA2*, or other homologous recombination repair gene or epigenetic silencing of these genes; high genomic instability
Gross and histology	1. Solid and cystic, hemorrhagic; mean 10-12 cm; <5% bilateral; >90% stage I; solid and cystic with tan or yellow cut surfaces, hemorrhage with clotted blood within cysts common	1. Ovaries normal sized or slightly enlarged in one-third to one-half of cases with subcentimeter surface nodules; remaining show enlarged solid and/or cystic ovaries, 8-10 cm; fallopian tube fimbriae may be prominent and tumorous and may be splayed across ovarian surface; usually bilateral adnexal involvement and nearly always with peritoneal carcinomatosis or extensive bowel invasion
	2. Small cells with ovoid to angulated/folded uniform nuclei, often with grooves; mitoses rare or absent; 2% contain bizarre nuclei	2. Papillary, micropapillary *(Figs. 5.30.5-5.30.9)*, glandular, slit-like, and solid patterns, commonly intermixed; infiltrative small nests and micropapillae; less commonly thick urothelial-like papillae lined by stratified epithelium mimicking urothelial dysplasia or malignant urothelial (transitional cell) carcinoma
	3. Pseudopapillary pattern, most notable at low magnification, is characterized by apparently papillary-like processes *(Figs. 5.30.1-5.30.4)*; this appearance may in some cases be artifactually created by fixation and sectioning problems; pseudopapillae are composed of typical small, granulosa cells with nuclear grooves, minimal cytologic atypia, and low mitotic index *(Fig. 5.30.4)*; fibrovascular support may be present further mimicking vasculature of true papillae *(Figs. 5.30.2-5.30.4)*	3. Large epithelial cells with marked atypia *(Figs. 5.30.6 and 5.30.9)*, often with bizarre nuclear forms; large prominent nucleoli and abundant mitotic activity with abnormal forms

	Adult Granulosa Cell Tumor With Pseudopapillary Pattern	**High-Grade Serous Carcinoma (HGSC)**
	4. Wide variety of architectural patterns, which may be disrupted by the same process creating the pseudopapillary pattern: diffuse, microfollicular, macrofollicular, insular, trabecular, tubular, and combinations; microfollicular pattern may have Call-Exner bodies	**4.** Other architectural patterns seen in adult granulosa cell tumor absent
Special studies	• Calretinin+, inhibin+, SF-1+, WT-1+, ER/PR+ • CK7−, EMA−; other cytokeratin stains are nonspecific as they can be positive in adult granulosa cell tumor; PAX8−	• CK7+, EMA+, WT1+, PAX8+, ER+ in majority • Inhibin may be focally (+) but is usually negative; calretinin often (−) but can be (+); SF-1−
Treatment	Hysterectomy and bilateral salpingo-oophorectomy; unilateral salpingo-oophorectomy if fertility desired	Staging (with debulking if indicated); chemotherapy (in neoadjuvant or adjuvant setting)
Prognosis	Those with malignant behavior may be indolent, some with late recurrences after 5-10 y or more; stage I has about 90% survival at 10 y	Stage III patients have 5-y survival of 45%-50% if optimally debulked; suboptimal debulking has 20%-30% 5-y survival

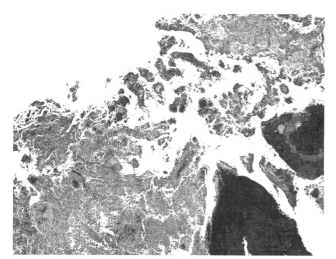

Figure 5.30.1 Pseudopapillary adult granulosa cell tumor showing fragmentation of solid tumor into narrow elongated fragments resembling papillae.

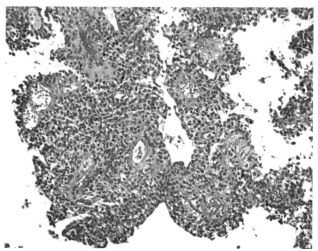

Figure 5.30.2 Pseudopapillary adult granulosa cell tumor, same case as *Figure 5.30.1*, with papillary-like structures having central vascular support.

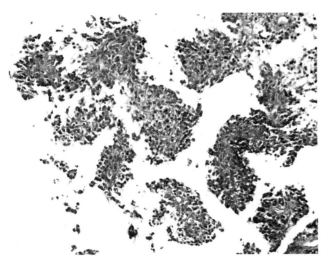

Figure 5.30.3　Pseudopapillary adult granulosa cell tumor displaying irregular, jagged, and sawtooth appearance of the surfaces of the pseudopapillae.

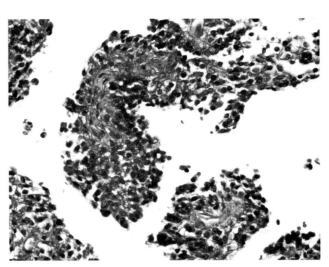

Figure 5.30.4　Pseudopapillary adult granulosa cell tumor with bland granulosa cells with ovoid nuclei. Note irregular surfaces where the cells are falling apart.

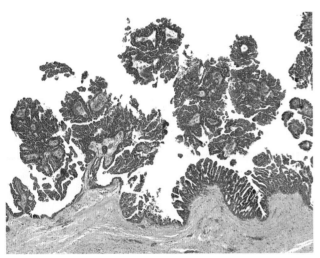

Figure 5.30.5　High-grade serous carcinoma. Micropapillary features are present.

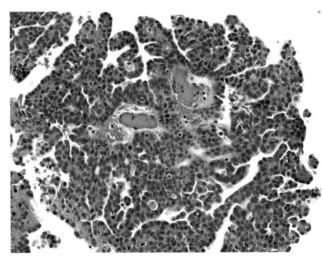

Figure 5.30.6　High-grade serous carcinoma. Micropapillary growth with moderate to severe nuclear atypia and scattered mitotic figures (same case as *Fig. 5.30.5*).

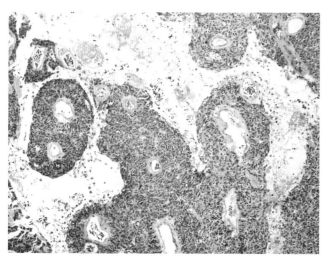

Figure 5.30.7   High-grade serous carcinoma, transitional cell carcinoma–like variant, with true papillae with fibrovascular cores.

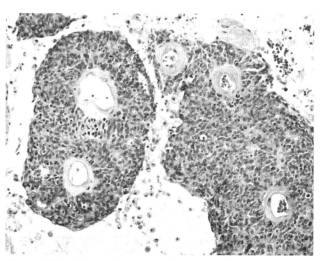

Figure 5.30.8   High-grade serous carcinoma, transitional cell carcinoma–like variant. Same case as *Figure 5.30.5*, displaying a cohesive epithelial proliferation with smooth papillary surfaces.

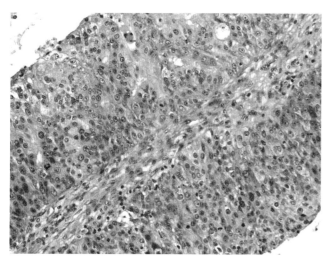

Figure 5.30.9   High-grade serous carcinoma, transitional cell carcinoma–like variant, with high-grade nuclear atypia, mitotic activity, cohesive epithelial growth, and smooth papillary surfaces. Note focal glandular differentiation at the **top of the photograph**.

	Cystic Adult Granulosa Cell Tumor	Follicle Cyst
Age	Mean 46 y	Premenopausal
Location	Within ovary	Within ovary
Symptoms	Pelvic/lower abdominal pain; abdominal distension, urinary frequency, dyspareunia, amenorrhea	Asymptomatic (normal variant); rarely may rupture causing pelvic pain
Signs	Pelvic/lower abdominal mass; may have estrogenic manifestations; reports are inconsistent on whether cystic variant is more likely to have androgenic manifestations	Typically none; rarely acute abdomen and hemoperitoneum with rupture
Etiology	*FOXL2* mutations in majority	Cystic dilatation of normal developing follicle
Gross and histology	1. Unilocular cystic *(Fig. 5.31.1)*, containing hemorrhagic fluid; mean 10 cm; unilateral; stage I 2. Granulosa cell proliferations often compressed and elongated within the cyst wall *(Fig. 5.31.2)*; most common architectural patterns: diffuse, macrofollicular, microfollicular, trabecular *(Figs. 5.31.2-5.31.4)*; Call-Exner bodies occasionally present; in general, a theca interna layer is absent in adult granulosa cell tumor, but a theca interna layer has been reported in some androgenic cystic variants 3. Small cells with ovoid to angulated/folded uniform nuclei, often with grooves *(Fig. 5.31.4)*; mitoses 2-7/10 hpf	1. Grossly smooth outer surface, thin-walled unilocular cyst with smooth lining, >3 cm but usually <7 cm 2. Follicle lined by one to three layers of normal granulosa cells with small round nuclei and basophilic cytoplasm *(Figs. 5.31.5 and 5.31.6)*; underlying theca interna layer is always present but may be inconspicuous *(Fig. 5.31.7)* 3. Lacks solid growth or other patterns of granulosa cell tumor; mitoses absent in granulosa cells; theca interna may display mitotic activity
Special studies	Not useful in this differential	Not useful in this differential
Treatment	Hysterectomy and bilateral salpingo-oophorectomy; unilateral salpingo-oophorectomy if fertility desired	No treatment needed
Prognosis	Limited data, but malignant behavior can occur	Benign

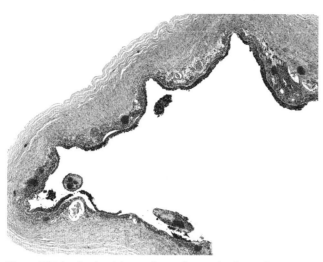

Figure 5.31.1 Cystic adult granulosa cell tumor is often unilocular with a narrow layer of granulosa cell proliferation surrounded by ovarian-type stroma.

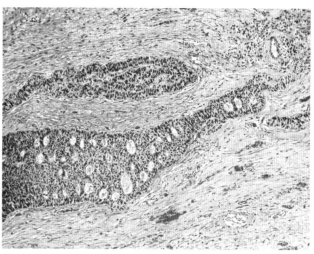

Figure 5.31.2 Cystic adult granulosa cell tumor may display any of the granulosa patterns including microfollicular and trabecular architecture, which are compressed and elongated within the cyst wall as seen in this example.

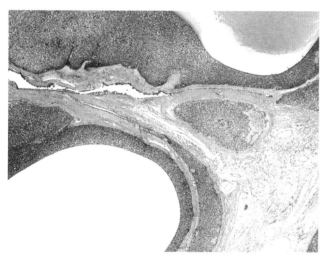

Figure 5.31.3 Cystic adult granulosa cell tumor may be multilocular and display the macrofollicular pattern of typical granulosa cell tumors.

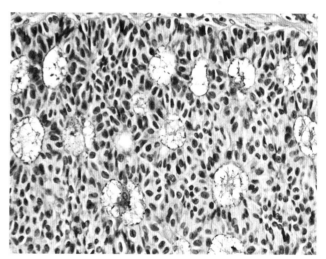

Figure 5.31.4 Cystic adult granulosa cell tumor with microfollicular pattern displaying bland ovoid nuclei with grooves. Same case as in *Figure 5.31.2.*

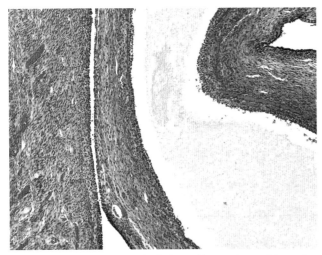

Figure 5.31.5   Follicle cyst typically has a thin granulosa cell layer of about two cells in thickness.

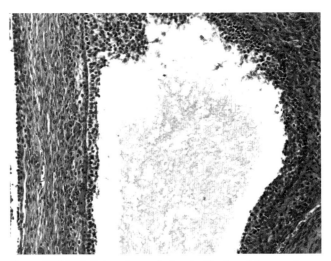

Figure 5.31.6   Follicle cyst may display stratification of the granulosa cell layer up to four to five cells or may appear thicker with tangential sectioning.

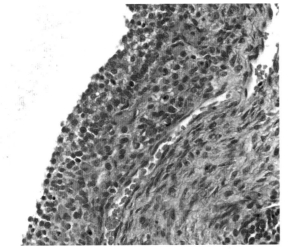

Figure 5.31.7   Follicle cyst shows theca interna layer with prominent congested capillaries subjacent to the granulosa cell layer.

	Juvenile Granulosa Cell Tumor	Small Cell Carcinoma, Hypercalcemic Type
Age	Under 30 y	Mean 24 y
Location	Within ovary	Within ovary
Symptoms	Abdominal pain, swelling, dysmenorrhea	Abdominal pain and swelling
Signs	Pelvic/adnexal mass, isosexual precocity in 80%; 6% present with acute abdomen	Hypercalcemia in two-thirds; pelvic or abdominal mass
Etiology	Associations with Ollier disease and Maffucci syndrome (somatic mosaic *IDH1* and *IDH2* mutations reported in these syndromes); activating alterations in *AKT1* and *GNAS*; *FOXL2* mutation in a small subset; rare *DICER1* mutations; rare association with tuberous sclerosis and germline *TP53* and *PTEN* mutations	*SMARCA4* mutation (encodes BRG1)
Gross and histology	1. Mean 12.5 cm, 2% bilateral, 10% ruptured, nearly always stage I; solid and cystic, multilocular, often hemorrhagic 2. Solid cellular sheets with scattered well-defined follicle formation; may be pure solid or pure follicular; follicles vary in size and shape and often have blue secretions; linings of follicles tend to be smoother and with more cellular cohesion than in small cell carcinoma, hypercalcemic type *(Figs. 5.32.1-5.32.4)*; rare foci may resemble thecoma 3. Round hyperchromatic nuclei usually without grooves, abundant eosinophilic cytoplasm *(Figs. 5.32.5 and 5.32.6)*, often with a luteinized appearance; spindled theca cells usually luteinized; 10%-15% have severe atypia; mitoses variable 4. No mucinous component	1. Unilateral, stage I in 50%, mean 15 cm; usually solid but may have cystic component; soft gray-tan cut surface with hemorrhage and necrosis 2. Diffuse growth pattern of closely packed small cells *(Figs. 5.32.7 and 5.32.8)*; solid sheets, nests, cords, and spindle cell patterns may be present; most tumors display round follicle-like spaces containing eosinophilic secretions *(Fig. 5.32.9)*; lining of follicle-like spaces tends to be slightly irregular with cellular discohesion; lacks the well-defined follicular architecture of JGCT; geographic necrosis frequently present 3. Small cells with scanty cytoplasm, oval-round nuclei with coarsely clumped chromatin and small nucleoli, indistinct cell borders; large cells seen in 50% but rarely predominate (large cell variant); high mitotic index *(Fig. 5.32.10)* 4. Mucinous differentiation in 8%-15%
Special studies	• Inhibin+, calretinin+, SF-1+ • Cytokeratins and EMA usually (−) • No loss of BRG1 expression	• Inhibin−, calretinin−, SF-1− • Cytokeratins and EMA may be negative or have limited/focal expression • Loss of BRG1 expression
Treatment	Unilateral salpingo-oophorectomy	Hysterectomy and bilateral salpingo-oophorectomy, staging, and debulking; limited data on chemotherapy
Prognosis	97% of stage I are cured	Poor, with <10% survival; stage I has 33% survival

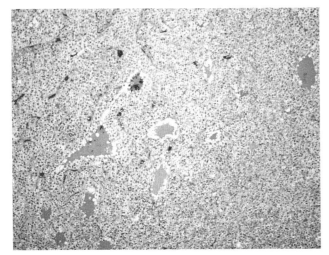

Figure 5.32.1   Juvenile granulosa cell tumor displaying diffuse sheets of granulosa cells with cysts containing blue to eosinophilic fluid.

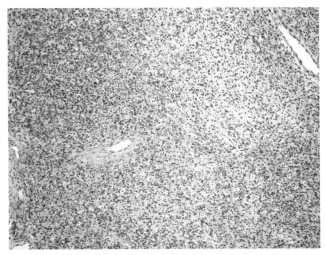

Figure 5.32.2   Juvenile granulosa cell tumor with diffuse sheet-like architecture, which can resemble small cell carcinoma, hypercalcemic type.

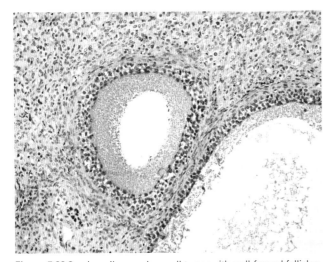

Figure 5.32.3   Juvenile granulosa cell tumor with well-formed follicles containing blue secretions.

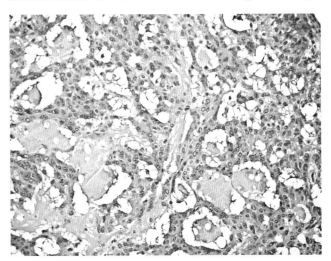

Figure 5.32.4   Juvenile granulosa cell tumor with small follicle-like spaces containing pale blue secretions, granulosa cells with bland nuclei, and abundant eosinophilic cytoplasm.

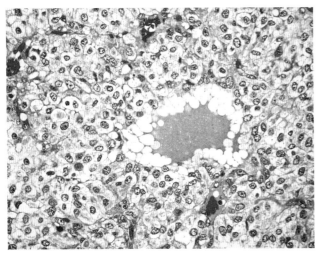

Figure 5.32.5   Juvenile granulosa cell tumor, same case as *Figure 5.32.1,* with round to polygonal cells showing abundant pale to eosinophilic cytoplasm, round nuclei with small nucleoli, and no nuclear grooves.

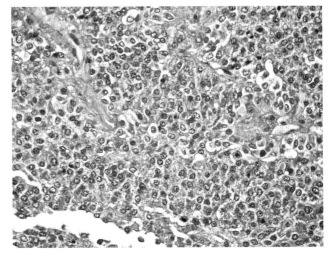

Figure 5.32.6   Juvenile granulosa cell tumor with polygonal cells containing moderate amounts of cytoplasm and round bland nuclei with only occasional grooves.

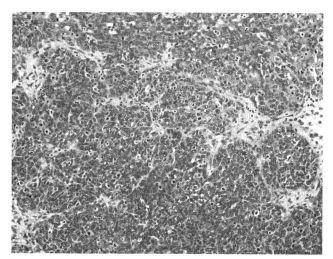

Figure 5.32.7   Small cell carcinoma, hypercalcemic type, composed of diffuse sheets of poorly differentiated cells with high-grade nuclei and scanty cytoplasm.

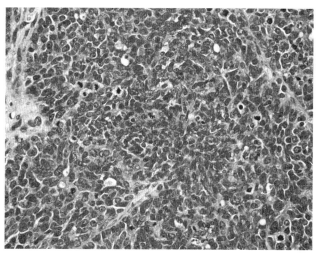

Figure 5.32.8   Small cell carcinoma, hypercalcemic type, same case as *Figure 5.32.7*, with diffuse growth of high-grade nuclei and hyperchromasia; mitotic figures are present.

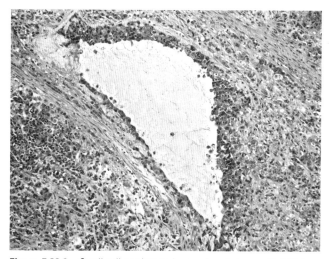

Figure 5.32.9   Small cell carcinoma, hypercalcemic type, with follicle-like space containing eosinophilic fluid and surrounded by diffuse growth of poorly differentiated carcinoma.

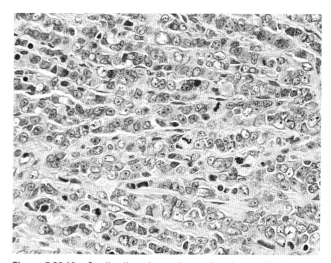

Figure 5.32.10   Small cell carcinoma, hypercalcemic type, displays high-grade nuclear features and mitotic figures; the cells in this example are large with vesicular nuclei and evident nucleoli reflecting a large cell component.

	Juvenile Granulosa Cell Tumor	Adult Granulosa Cell Tumor
Age	Under 30 y	Mean 50-55 y
Location	Within ovary	Within ovary
Symptoms	Abdominal pain, swelling, dysmenorrhea	Pelvic/lower abdominal pain; postmenopausal bleeding; 10% have acute abdomen with hemoperitoneum
Signs	Pelvic/adnexal mass, isosexual precocity in 80%; 6% present with acute abdomen	Pelvic/lower abdominal mass; may have estrogenic manifestations
Etiology	Associations with Ollier disease and Maffucci syndrome (somatic mosaic *IDH1* and *IDH2* mutations reported in these syndromes); activating alterations in *AKT1* and *GNAS*; *FOXL2* mutation in a small subset; rare *DICER1* mutations; rare association with tuberous sclerosis and germline *TP53* and *PTEN* mutations	*FOXL2* mutations
Gross and histology	1. Mean 12.5 cm, 2% bilateral, 10% ruptured, nearly always stage I; solid and cystic, multilocular, often hemorrhagic 2. Solid cellular sheets with scattered well-defined follicle formation *(Figs. 5.33.1-5.33.4)*; may be pure solid or pure follicular; follicles vary in size and shape and often have basophilic or eosinophilic secretions; *(Figs. 5.33.1, 5.33.3, and 5.33.4)*; rare foci may resemble thecoma 3. Round hyperchromatic nuclei usually without grooves, abundant eosinophilic cytoplasm *(Figs. 5.33.2 and 5.33.5)*, often with a luteinized appearance; spindled theca cells usually luteinized; 10%-15% have focal severe atypia *(Fig. 5.33.4)*; mitoses variable *(Fig. 5.33.5)*	1. Solid and cystic, hemorrhagic; mean size 10-12 cm; <5% bilateral; >90% stage I; solid and cystic with tan or yellow cut surfaces, hemorrhage with clotted blood within cysts common 2. Solid pattern *(Fig. 5.33.6)*, microfollicular (cribriform) pattern +/− Call-Exner bodies (eosinophilic luminal concretions) *(Figs. 5.33.7-5.33.9)*; insular pattern is characterized by islands and nests of granulosa cells divided into lobules by fibrothecomatous stroma, but cords of tumor cells may be admixed; solid tubular pattern mimics Sertoli tumor; wide variety of other architectural patterns: diffuse, microfollicular, macrofollicular, trabecular, tubular, and combinations; microfollicular pattern may have Call-Exner bodies 3. Small cells with ovoid or angulated/folded uniform nuclei, often with grooves *(Figs. 5.33.8 and 5.33.9)*; peripheral palisading of nuclei may be seen at edge of nests and islands; mitoses rare or absent; 2% contain bizarre nuclei
Special studies	Immunohistochemistry not useful in this differential	Immunohistochemistry not useful in this differential
Treatment	Unilateral salpingo-oophorectomy	Hysterectomy and bilateral salpingo-oophorectomy; unilateral salpingo-oophorectomy if fertility desired
Prognosis	97% of stage I are cured	Those with recurrent disease or tumors of advanced stage may be indolent, some with late recurrences after 5-10 y or more; stage I has about 90% survival at 10 y

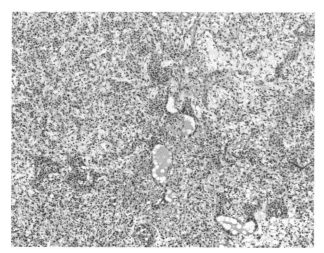

Figure 5.33.1 Juvenile granulosa cell tumor with small follicle-like spaces within an edematous stroma containing polygonal cells with round nuclei and abundant cytoplasm.

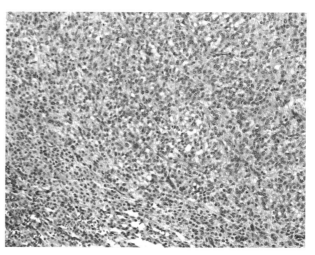

Figure 5.33.2 Juvenile granulosa cell tumor with ovoid to polygonal cells with round to ovoid nuclei lacking grooves and pale eosinophilic cytoplasm.

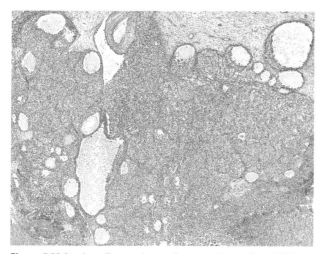

Figure 5.33.3 Juvenile granulosa cell tumor with prominent follicle-like spaces containing secretions.

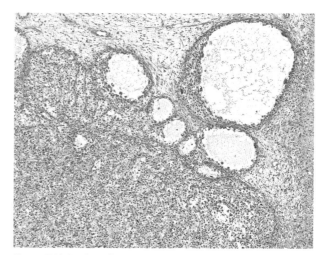

Figure 5.33.4 Juvenile granulosa cell tumor with follicle-like spaces, cords and gland-like structures and a few scattered bizarre nuclei (same case as *Fig. 5.33.3*).

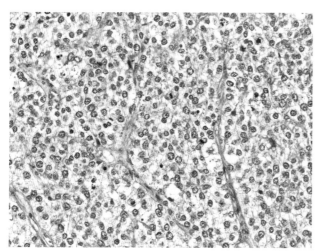

Figure 5.33.5 Juvenile granulosa cell tumor with polygonal cells with round nuclei lacking grooves, and abundant pale cytoplasm; a few mitotic figures are present (same case as *Fig. 5.33.3*).

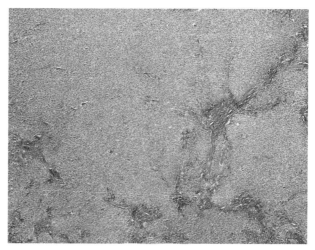

Figure 5.33.6 Adult granulosa cell tumor with solid cellular growth.

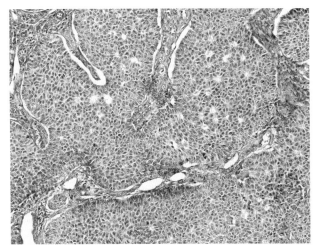

Figure 5.33.7   Adult granulosa cell tumor with microfollicular/cribriform pattern displaying nuclear grooves.

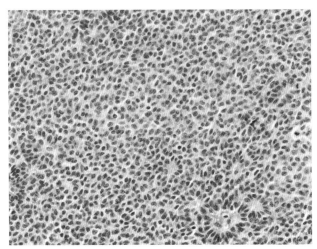

Figure 5.33.8   Adult granulosa cell tumor with bland ovoid nuclei displaying nuclear grooves.

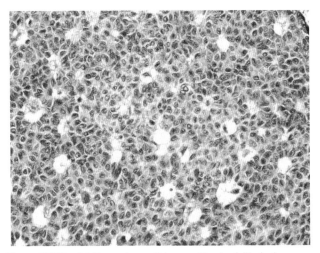

Figure 5.33.9   Adult granulosa cell tumor with microfollicular/cribriform pattern displaying nuclear grooves (same case as *Fig. 5.33.7*).

	Pseudoendometrioid Well-Differentiated Sertoli-Leydig Cell Tumor	Endometrioid Carcinoma
Age	Mean 34 y	Mean 55-58 y
Location	Within ovary	Within ovary
Symptoms	Irregular vaginal bleeding, amenorrhea	Pelvic pain, increasing abdominal girth, bloating, early satiety, vaginal bleeding, urinary symptoms
Signs	Pelvic/lower abdominal mass; menstrual irregularities, rarely virilization	Pelvic/abdominal mass, ascites
Etiology	*DICER1* and *FOXL2* mutations usually absent	Endometriosis; germline *MLH1, MSH2, PMS2,* or *MSH6* mutation (Lynch syndrome) in a subset of cases; *PTEN,* β-*catenin* (*CTNNB1*), *KRAS, ARID1A,* and *PIK3CA* mutations
Gross and histology	1. One of eight reported cases was bilateral; stage I, mean 7 cm; half are purely solid; others may be focally cystic 2. Sertoli cell pattern with hollow or solid tubules/cords; cuboidal to columnar cells, round-ovoid nuclei, minimal atypia, low mitotic activity; intermixed Leydig cells with small round nuclei and abundant eosinophilic cytoplasm may be inconspicuous 3. Pseudoendometrioid patterns occur in well- and intermediate-differentiated and retiform tumors, occupying >10% of the tumor; tubules are large and often dilated and may contain eosinophilic secretions; may be closely packed or separated by fibrous stroma; may be intermixed with typical Sertoli tubules *(Figs. 5.34.1-5.34.4)* 4. Cytologic features lining tubules are identical to the typical Sertoli component; occasionally with clear cytoplasm *(Figs. 5.34.5 and 5.34.6)* 5. Focal heterologous mucinous epithelium was present in one of nine reported cases	1. Usually unilateral, stage I in almost half; mean 15 cm; cystic or cystic and solid; cysts contain dark brown viscous fluid (old blood +/− mucus); papillary or nodular growths arise from cyst lining 2. Most are architecturally well differentiated with confluent glandular epithelial proliferation resembling endometrial endometrioid carcinoma; cribriform, papillary, glandular, and occasionally solid patterns; less commonly with infiltrative pattern of glands, nests, and solid masses with jagged edges *(Figs. 5.34.7-5.34.10)* 3. Tall columnar epithelium with sharp luminal gland margins, round to ovoid nuclei with hyperchromasia, and prominent nucleoli *(Fig. 5.34.10)*; mitotic activity variable, often high 4. Squamous differentiation in half; adenofibromatous component often present; associated endometriosis is present in majority and often shows atypia, hyperplasia, and other features reflecting origin within endometriotic cyst or associated endometrioid borderline tumor 5. Secretory, ciliated, and sertoliform variants can occur

	Pseudoendometrioid Well-Differentiated Sertoli-Leydig Cell Tumor	Endometrioid Carcinoma
Special studies	• Limited data suggest same immunoprofile as typical Sertoli-Leydig cell tumor: inhibin+, calretinin+, SF-1+; EMA−, CK7−; ER/PR+; PAX8−; WT-1+; other cytokeratin stains are nonspecific as they may be positive in Sertoli-Leydig cell tumors	• CK7+, ER/PR+, EMA+; usually PAX8+; WT1, inhibin, and calretinin usually (−) but may be focally or strongly (+) in small minority; SF-1−
		• Loss of staining for DNA mismatch repair proteins (MLH1, MSH2, PMS2, MSH6) in a subset of cases
Treatment	Unilateral salpingo-oophorectomy	Hysterectomy and bilateral salpingo-oophorectomy, staging (with debulking when indicated); chemotherapy (in adjuvant or neoadjuvant setting) except for low-grade stage IA/B; hormonal suppression may be used for recurrence
Prognosis	Limited data; presumed same as typical well- or intermediate-differentiated Sertoli-Leydig cell tumors, which are nearly always stage I and cured by unilateral salpingo-oophorectomy	Stage I >90% survival

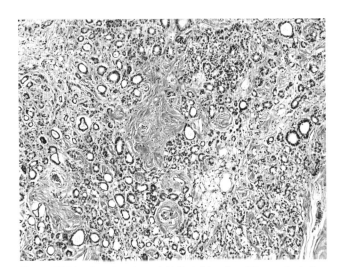

Figure 5.34.1   Pseudoendometrioid Sertoli-Leydig cell tumor displaying crowded and round tubules resembling invasive endometrioid carcinoma.

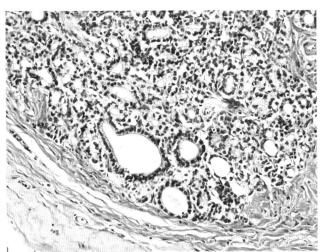

Figure 5.34.2   Pseudoendometrioid Sertoli-Leydig cell tumor displaying back-to-back Sertoli tubules intermixed with several larger ones resembling endometrioid carcinoma.

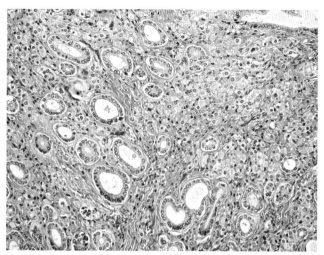

Figure 5.34.3 Pseudoendometrioid Sertoli-Leydig cell tumor displaying crowded variably sized open tubules with intervening Leydig cells.

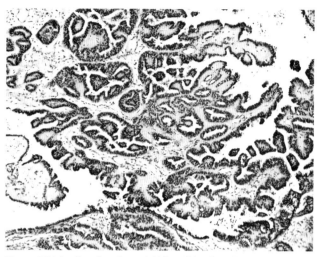

Figure 5.34.4 Pseudoendometrioid Sertoli-Leydig cell tumor displaying retiform architecture resembling endometrioid adenocarcinoma with papillary features.

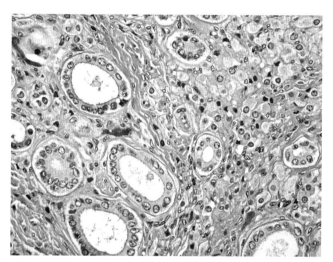

Figure 5.34.5 Same case as *Figure 5.34.3* with tubules lined by cuboidal cells with sharp luminal margins; Leydig cells are present in between the tubules.

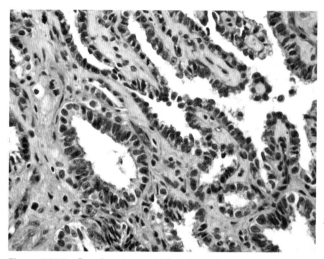

Figure 5.34.6 Pseudoendometrioid Sertoli-Leydig cell tumor displaying retiform Sertoli differentiation with tubule at **left** showing columnar cells with sharp luminal margin.

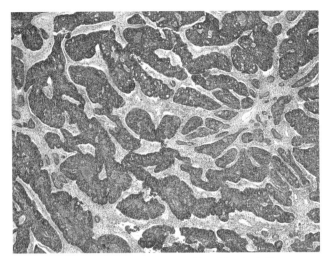

Figure 5.34.7 Endometrioid carcinoma with solid and cribriform interanastomosing and infiltrative masses.

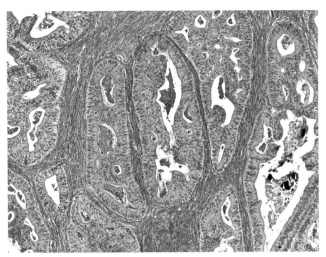

Figure 5.34.8 Endometrioid carcinoma with infiltrative cribriform glands lined by tall columnar epithelium.

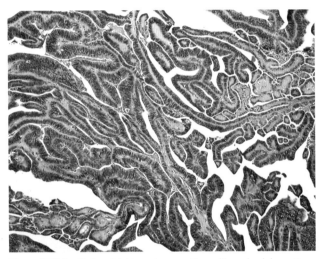

Figure 5.34.9 Endometrioid carcinoma with papillary glandular pattern resembling retiform Sertoli-Leydig cell tumor.

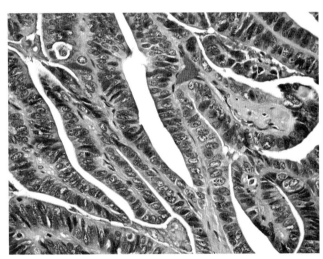

Figure 5.34.10 Endometrioid carcinoma (same case as *Fig. 5.34.9*) with cytologic atypia.

	Sertoli Cell Tumor	Carcinoid Tumor, Primary Ovarian
Age	Mean 30 y	Mean 51-53 y
Location	Within ovary	Within ovary
Symptoms	Pelvic/abdominal pain, swelling, vaginal bleeding	Pelvic/abdominal pain, abdominal enlargement, abnormal vaginal bleeding; flushing, diarrhea, wheezing (carcinoid syndrome)
Signs	40% have estrogenic manifestations	Pelvic or abdominal mass; one-third to one-fourth have carcinoid syndrome
Etiology	Rarely seen in patients with Peutz-Jeghers syndrome; *DICER1* mutations	Arise in mature cystic teratoma
Gross and histology	1. Unilateral, stage I, mean 8-9 cm	1. Unilateral, confined to ovary in >90%; peritoneal dissemination in 6%; median 4-5 cm; majority in cystic teratoma with solid nodule within wall; may be pure solid without associated dermoid, which may have been overgrown; contralateral teratoma in 10%-15%; bilateral carcinoid in 1%
	2. Uniform tubular pattern; hollow tubules lined by tall cuboidal or columnar cells; solid tubules may be elongated, round, or ovoid; closely packed solid tubules may mimic sheets; less commonly cords, trabecular, and spindled patterns *(Figs. 5.35.1-5.35.4)*	2. Discrete cellular nests, often with small round acini (insular pattern); trabecular carcinoid shows ribbons and trabeculae with columnar cells *(Figs. 5.35.5-5.35.8)*
	3. Bland round to ovoid uniform nuclei, pale to eosinophilic cytoplasm, mitotically inactive *(Figs. 5.35.3 and 5.35.4)*; rare lipid-rich and oxyphilic variants	3. Small rounded nuclei with neuroendocrine features, that is, salt and pepper stippled chromatin; uniform polygonal cells with moderate to abundant eosinophilic cytoplasm *(Figs. 5.35.6-5.35.8)*; reddish brown argentaffin granules often present
	4. No strumal or mucinous component	4. Strumal carcinoid variant displays thyroid follicular differentiation discretely or admixed with carcinoid component; 40% display mucinous epithelial glands and cysts; mucinous carcinoid is uncommon variant
	5. No teratomatous elements present	5. Multinodularity, bilaterality, and absence of teratoma suggest extraovarian primary
Special studies	• WT1+, SF-1+, inhibin+, calretinin+, ER/PR+ • Synaptophysin and chromogranin may be (+) uncommonly but should have limited expression if staining is present; CD56 is nonspecific as it may be (+) in either Sertoli cell tumor or carcinoid • CK7−, EMA−; other cytokeratins are nonspecific as they may be (+) in Sertoli cell tumor	• WT1−, SF-1−, inhibin−, calretinin−, ER/PR− • Synaptophysin+, chromogranin+; CD56 is nonspecific as it may be (+) in either Sertoli cell tumor or carcinoid • Limited CK7 staining may be present in a subset of cases; EMA−

	Sertoli Cell Tumor	**Carcinoid Tumor, Primary Ovarian**
Treatment	Unilateral salpingo-oophorectomy	Unilateral salpingo-oophorectomy or Hysterectomy and bilateral salpingo-oophorectomy
Prognosis	Usually benign; rare abdominopelvic recurrences	Survival >90%; teratoma-associated cases have better prognosis

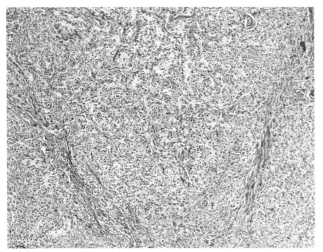

Figure 5.35.1   Sertoli cell tumor with closely packed back-to-back tubules.

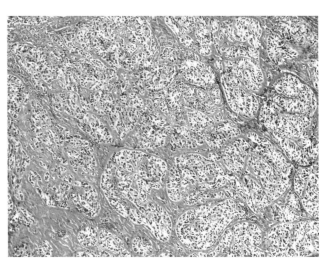

Figure 5.35.2   Sertoli cell tumor with well-formed tubules within a fibrous ovarian stroma.

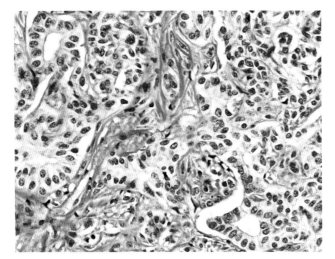

Figure 5.35.3   Sertoli cell tumor with cuboidal cells displaying pale to clear cytoplasm and ovoid bland nuclei.

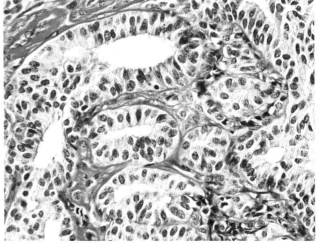

Figure 5.35.4   Sertoli cell tumor with cuboidal to columnar cells, pale cytoplasm, and ovoid nuclei.

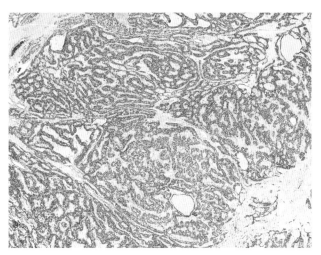

Figure 5.35.5   Carcinoid tumor with trabecular pattern of interanastomosing cords in a fibrous stroma.

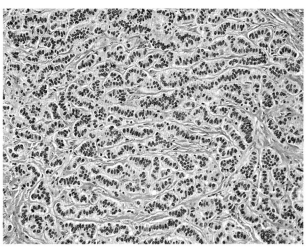

Figure 5.35.6   Carcinoid tumor with ramifying cords of tumor cells in a fibrous stroma.

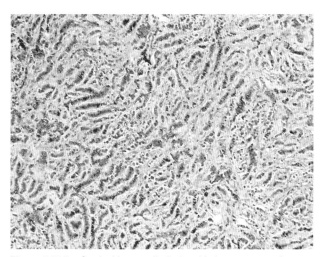

Figure 5.35.7   Carcinoid tumor displaying thin interanastomosing columns and cords.

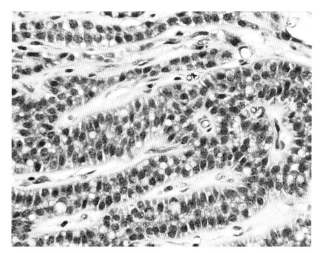

Figure 5.35.8   Carcinoid tumor displaying cords resembling tubules of Sertoli differentiation, with round to ovoid evenly distributed nuclei and finely stippled chromatin pattern.

	Adult Granulosa Cell Tumor	Carcinoid Tumor, Primary Ovarian
Age	Mean 50-55 y	Mean 51-53 y
Location	Within ovary	Within ovary
Symptoms	Pelvic/lower abdominal pain; postmenopausal bleeding; 10% have acute abdomen with hemoperitoneum	Pelvic/abdominal pain, abdominal enlargement, abnormal vaginal bleeding; flushing, diarrhea, wheezing (carcinoid syndrome)
Signs	Pelvic/lower abdominal mass; may have estrogenic manifestations	Pelvic or abdominal mass; one-third have carcinoid syndrome
Etiology	*FOXL2* mutations	Arise in mature cystic teratoma; rare association with MEN Type I
Gross and histology	1. Solid and cystic, hemorrhagic; mean size 10-12 cm; <5% bilateral; >90% stage I; solid and cystic with tan or yellow cut surfaces, hemorrhage with clotted blood within cysts common	1. Unilateral, confined to ovary in >90%; peritoneal dissemination in 6%; median 4-5 cm; majority in cystic teratoma with solid nodule within wall; may be pure solid without associated dermoid, which may have been overgrown; contralateral teratoma in 10%-15%; bilateral in 1%
	2. Microfollicular (cribriform) pattern +/− Call-Exner bodies (eosinophilic luminal concretions) *(Figs. 5.36.1-5.36.3)*; insular pattern is characterized by islands and nests of granulosa cells divided into lobules by fibrothecomatous stroma, but cords of tumor cells may be admixed; solid tubular pattern mimics Sertoli tumor; wide variety of other architectural patterns: diffuse, microfollicular, macrofollicular, trabecular, tubular, and combinations	2. Broad sheets and discrete islands with cribriform pattern of small round acini *(Figs. 5.36.5 and 5.36.6)*; discrete cellular nests with acini (insular pattern); trabecular carcinoid shows ribbons and trabeculae with columnar cells
	3. Small cells with ovoid or angulated/folded uniform nuclei, often with grooves *(Figs. 5.36.3 and 5.36.4)*; peripheral palisading of nuclei may be seen at edge of nests and islands; mitoses rare or absent; 2% contain bizarre nuclei	3. Small rounded nuclei with neuroendocrine features, that is, salt and pepper stippled chromatin; uniform polygonal cells with moderate to abundant eosinophilic cytoplasm *(Figs. 5.36.7-5.36.9)*; reddish pink neuroendocrine granules often present *(Fig. 5.36.7)*
	4. No mucinous epithelium or thyroid-like patterns	4. Strumal carcinoid variant displays thyroid follicular differentiation discretely or ad-mixed with carcinoid component; 40% display mucinous epithelial glands and cysts; mucinous carcinoid is uncommon variant

	Adult Granulosa Cell Tumor	**Carcinoid Tumor, Primary Ovarian**
Special studies	• Calretinin+, inhibin+, SF-1+, WT-1+, and ER/PR+ • Usually CK7−, synaptophysin and chromogranin usually negative • Other types of cytokeratins are nonspecific as they can be positive in adult granulosa cell tumor	• WT1−, SF-1−, inhibin−, calretinin−, ER/PR− • Synaptophysin+, chromogranin+ • Limited CK7 staining may be present in a subset of cases
Treatment	Hysterectomy and bilateral salpingo-oophorectomy; unilateral salpingo-oophorectomy if fertility desired	Unilateral salpingo-oophorectomy or hysterectomy and bilateral salpingo-oophorectomy
Prognosis	Those with recurrent disease or tumors of advanced stage may be indolent, some with late recurrences after 5-10 y or more; stage I has about 90% survival at 10 y	Survival >90%; teratoma-associated cases have better prognosis

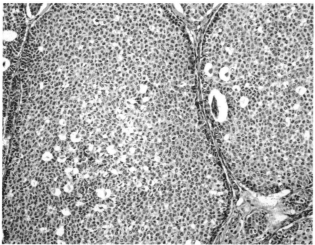

Figure 5.36.1   Granulosa cell tumor with microfollicular pattern and a few Call-Exner bodies.

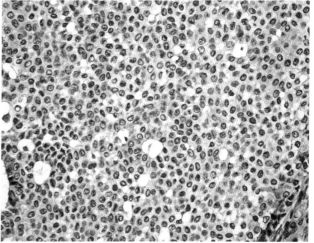

Figure 5.36.2   Granulosa cell tumor with microfollicular pattern and a few Call-Exner bodies. Nuclear grooves are present (same case as *Fig. 5.36.1*).

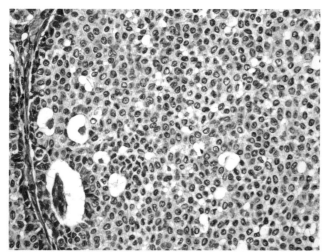

Figure 5.36.3   Granulosa cell tumor with microfollicular pattern and a few Call-Exner bodies. Nuclear grooves are present (same case as *Fig. 5.36.1*).

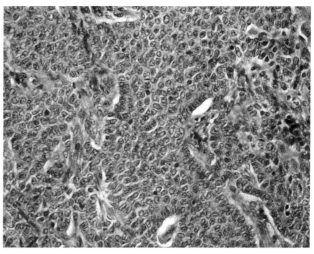

Figure 5.36.4   Granulosa cell tumor with trabeculae showing prominent nuclear grooves.

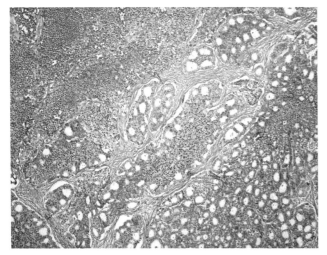

Figure 5.36.5   Carcinoid tumor with infiltrative pattern of solid and cribriform islands.

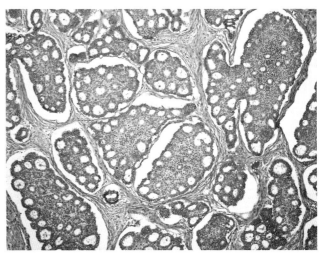

Figure 5.36.6   Carcinoid tumor with insular pattern of cribriform islands resembling the microfollicular pattern of granulosa cell tumor.

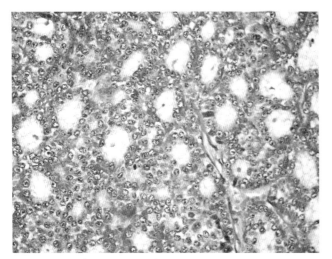

Figure 5.36.7   Carcinoid tumor. Same case as *Figure 5.36.5* with round evenly distributed nuclei and finely stippled chromatin pattern. Note presence of fine pink neuroendocrine granules at periphery of cytoplasm.

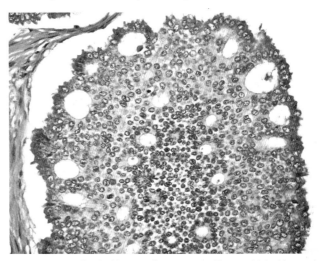

Figure 5.36.8   Carcinoid tumor. Same case as *Figure 5.36.6* with round evenly distributed nuclei and finely stippled chromatin pattern. Note presence of fine pink neuroendocrine granules at periphery of cytoplasm.

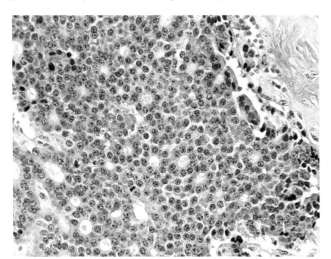

Figure 5.36.9   Carcinoid tumor with a cribriform pattern resembling the microfollicular pattern of granulosa cell tumor, with evenly distributed smooth round nuclei with finely stippled chromatin.

	Sex Cord Tumor with Annular Tubules (SCTAT)	Adult Granulosa Cell Tumor with Microfollicular Pattern
Age	Mean 27 y (with Peutz-Jeghers syndrome)	Mean 50-55 y
	Mean 34-36 y (without Peutz-Jeghers syndrome)	
Location	Within ovary	Within ovary
Symptoms	Incidental finding (with Peutz-Jeghers syndrome); pelvic pain/discomfort in others	Pelvic/lower abdominal pain; postmenopausal bleeding; 10% have acute abdomen with hemoperitoneum
Signs	One-third have Peutz-Jeghers syndrome; others have palpable pelvic mass and estrogenic or progestogenic manifestations	Pelvic/lower abdominal mass; may have estrogenic manifestations
Etiology	*STK11/LKB1* (Peutz-Jeghers syndrome gene) germline mutations in Peutz-Jeghers syndrome patients	*FOXL2* mutations
Gross and histology	1. With Peutz-Jeghers syndrome, bilateral, multiple, small yellowish nodules, <3 cm, may be microscopic only; without Peutz-Jeghers syndrome, unilateral, >3 cm large solid mass, rarely cystic, with yellowish cut surface 2. Simple and complex (cribriform) annular tubules; simple tubules are ring shaped; complex tubules feature intercommunicating rings; peripherally oriented nuclei around central rounded hyaline masses (antipodal or paired cell arrangement) *(Figs. 5.37.1-5.37.6)*; resemble Sertoli or granulosa cell tumor with microfollicular pattern; may show diffuse growth; calcification in syndromic tumors 3. Tall columnar cells with pale cytoplasm and small round-oval nuclei with small nucleoli; no nuclear grooves; minimal mitotic activity *(Figs. 5.37.4-5.37.6)*; marked nuclear atypia and mitotic activity may be present in nonsyndromic cases	1. Solid and cystic, hemorrhagic; mean 10-12 cm; <5% bilateral; >90% stage I; solid and cystic with tan or yellow cut surfaces and hemorrhage with clotted blood within cysts common 2. Microfollicular pattern resembling cribriform pattern where neoplastic cells surround small round regularly distributed spaces containing eosinophilic secretion, debris, or hyaline material (Call-Exner bodies) *(Figs. 5.37.7-5.37.10)*; wide variety of other architectural patterns: diffuse, macrofollicular, insular, trabecular, tubular, and combinations 3. Small cells with ovoid to angulated/folded uniform nuclei, often with grooves *(Figs. 5.37.8-5.37.10)*; high mitotic activity is rare or absent; 2% contain bizarre nuclei
Special studies	Not useful in this differential	Not useful in this differential
Treatment	Bilateral salpingo-oophorectomy or hysterectomy and bilateral salpingo-oophorectomy	Hysterectomy and bilateral salpingo-oophorectomy; unilateral salpingo-oophorectomy if fertility desired
Prognosis	Peutz-Jeghers syndrome–associated tumors are benign; 20% of nonsyndromic tumors have malignant behavior	Those with malignant behavior may be indolent, some with late recurrences after 5-10 y or more; stage I has about 90% survival at 10 y

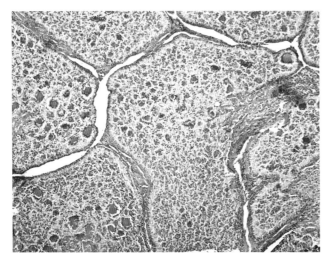

Figure 5.37.1   Sex cord tumor with annular tubules (SCTAT) displaying cribriform (complex tubular) islands with gland-like spaces containing eosinophilic concretions.

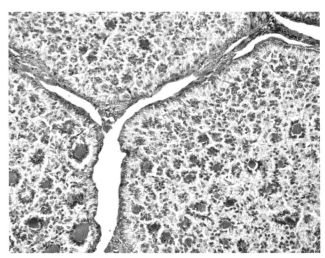

Figure 5.37.2   SCTAT, same case as *Figure 5.37.1*, with cribriform masses of Sertoli-like cells with basally oriented nuclei palisaded around the eosinophilic concretions.

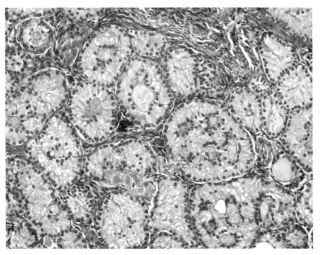

Figure 5.37.3   SCTAT islands with complex tubular pattern composed of tall columnar cells resembling Sertoli cells.

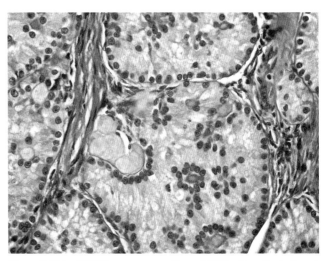

Figure 5.37.4   SCTAT, same case as *Figure 5.37.3*, with palisaded basal nuclei and dense, eosinophilic hyalinized nodule.

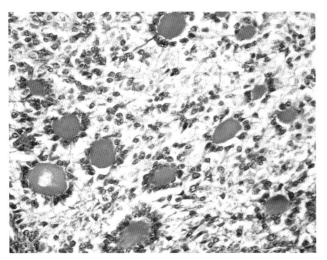

Figure 5.37.5   SCTAT, same case as *Figure 5.37.1*, with nuclei palisaded around eosinophilic concretions.

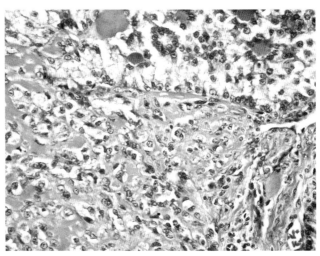

Figure 5.37.6   SCTAT with cribriform island at **top** and hyalinized material compressing tumor cells with loss of cribriform pattern at **bottom**.

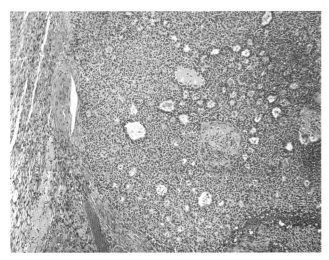

Figure 5.37.7   Granulosa cell tumor with microfollicular pattern; note smooth interface with surrounding ovarian stroma at **left**.

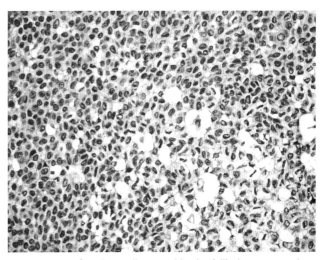

Figure 5.37.8   Granulosa cell tumor with microfollicular pattern and ovoid bland nuclei displaying grooves.

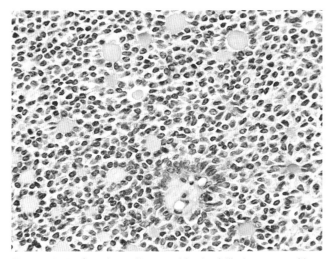

Figure 5.37.9   Granulosa cell tumor with microfollicular pattern with eosinophilic concretions (Call-Exner bodies) resembling similar structures in SCTAT.

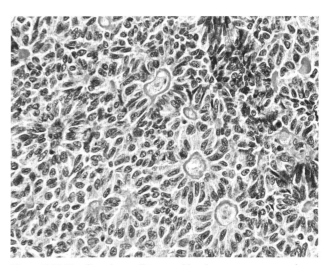

Figure 5.37.10   Granulosa cell tumor with columnar appearance of neoplastic cells with ovoid to spindled grooved nuclei and developing eosinophilic material at apical cell borders.

	Steroid (Lipid) Cell Tumor	Dysgerminoma
Age	Mean 43 y	Median in early 20s
Location	Within ovary	Within ovarian stroma; rarely in other midline sites (ie, retroperitoneum)
Symptoms	Pelvic pain, dysmenorrhea	Abdominal enlargement, pain
Signs	Estrogenic in 50%; virilization in 10%; rarely Cushing syndrome, hypercalcemia	Lower abdominal mass
Etiology	Likely derive from luteinized ovarian stromal cells; occasional association with von Hippel-Lindau syndrome	Derive from primordial germ cells at early arrested stage of development; may arise in gonadoblastoma in dysgenetic gonad (Denys-Drash syndrome, Frasier syndrome, and Swyer syndrome); Turner syndrome and androgen insensitivity syndrome also associated with gonadoblastoma; small isochromosome i(12p) and DNA copy number gains (12p, 12q, 21q, 22q) and loss (13q); some have *KIT* mutation (exon 17)
Gross and histology	1. Unilateral; extraovarian spread in 20%; mean 8.4 cm; solid, often yellow cut surface 2. Sheets to nested arrangement of large, rounded to polygonal cells with abundant vacuolated clear or eosinophilic cytoplasm; often resembles normal adrenal cortex; central round nucleus with minimal atypia and variably sized nucleoli, occasionally more marked atypia; typically mitotically inactive *(Figs. 5.38.1-5.38.4)*; 40% contain cytoplasmic lipofuscin; may have sparse stroma with prominent vasculature; edema and fibrosis may be present *(Fig. 5.38.5)* 3. Variants include stromal luteoma and stromal Leydig cell tumor	1. Solid fleshy mass >10 cm 2. Aggregates/islands and diffuse sheets of polygonal cells with eosinophilic or clear cytoplasm; distinct cell membranes; central, large primitive nucleus with coarse or vesicular chromatin and prominent nucleoli *(Figs. 5.38.6-5.38.9)* 3. Dense fibrous stroma *(Figs. 5.38.9 and 5.38.10)* often with dense lymphocytic infiltrate, sometimes with plasma cells and eosinophils; occasional granulomas; 3%-6% with syncytiotrophoblastic giant cells; identical to testicular seminoma
Special studies	• Inhibin+, calretinin+, SF-1+, Melan-A/MART1+ • SALL4−, CD117(c-kit)−, OCT-4−, D2-40−	• Inhibin−, calretinin−, SF-1−, Melan-A/MART1− • SALL4+, CD117(c-kit)+, OCT-4+, D2-40+
Treatment	Unilateral salpingo-oophorectomy	Stage-dependent: surgery, +/− combination chemotherapy
Prognosis	Malignant in approximately one-third; size >7 cm, necrosis, atypia, and mitoses >2/10 hpf correlate with malignancy	5-y survival 90% or higher

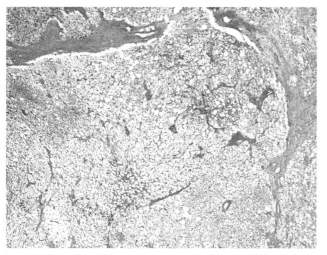

Figure 5.38.1 Steroid cell tumor composed of large smoothly contoured sheets of polygonal cells with clear cytoplasm.

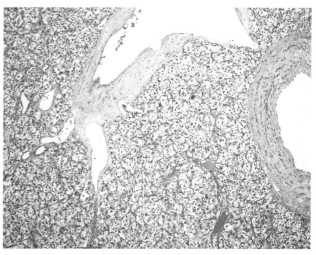

Figure 5.38.2 Steroid cell tumor with solid pattern. Large thick-walled vessels and smaller branching vessels divide the tumor into lobules.

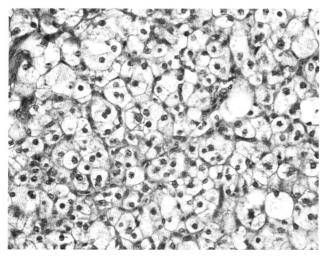

Figure 5.38.3 Same case as *Figure 5.38.1* displaying finely vacuolated clear cytoplasm, round bland nuclei, and prominent cell borders. Tumor cells are arranged in solid alveolar pattern.

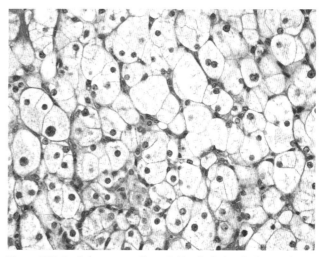

Figure 5.38.4 Same case as *Figure 5.38.1* displaying finely vacuolated clear cytoplasm, round bland nuclei, and prominent cell borders. Note the presence of occasional nucleoli.

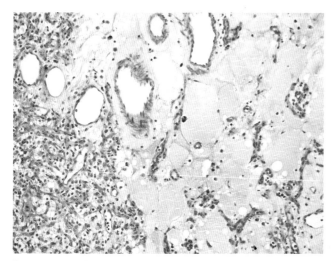

Figure 5.38.5 Steroid cell tumor with patchy edema and prominent fine capillary vascular network.

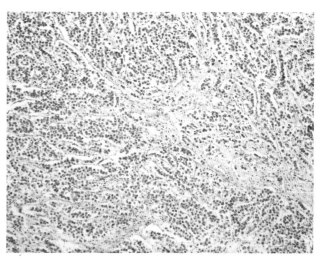

Figure 5.38.6 Dysgerminoma characterized by cells infiltrating in linear and narrow corded patterns.

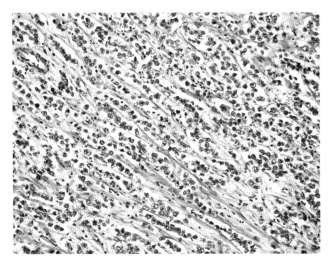

Figure 5.38.7   Dysgerminoma infiltrates linearly in single file and cords two to three cells thick.

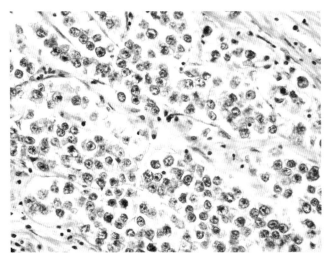

Figure 5.38.8   Dysgerminoma, same case as in *Figure 5.38.6*, with smooth round primitive nuclei, prominent nucleoli, and a nested pattern. Note the abundant clear cytoplasm.

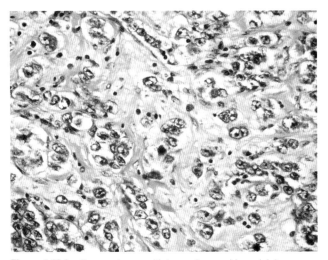

Figure 5.38.9   Dysgerminoma with large pleomorphic nuclei, large prominent nucleoli, and a dense fibrous stroma.

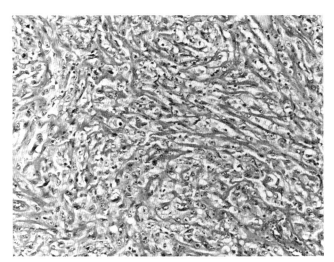

Figure 5.38.10   Dysgerminoma with dense collagenous stroma.

	Steroid (Lipid) Cell Tumor	Clear Cell Carcinoma
Age	Mean 43 y	Mean 50-53 y
Location	Within ovary	Within ovary; rarely arises in extraovarian sites from endometriosis
Symptoms	Pelvic pain, dysmenorrhea	Pelvic pain, increasing abdominal girth, bloating, early satiety, vaginal bleeding, urinary symptoms
Signs	Estrogenic manifestations in 50%; virilization in 10%; rarely Cushing syndrome, hypercalcemia	Pelvic/adnexal mass; rarely thromboembolic events or paraneoplastic hypercalcemia
Etiology	Likely derived from luteinized ovarian stromal cells; occasional cases associated with von Hippel-Lindau syndrome	Vast majority arise in endometriosis; *ARID1A, PIK3CA, PTEN, KRAS, TGF-βII* mutations, *TERT* promoter mutations; germline *MLH1, MSH2, PMS2, or MSH6* mutations (Lynch syndrome) in a small subset of cases
Gross and histology	1. Unilateral; extraovarian spread in 20%; mean 8.4 cm; size >7 cm correlates with malignancy 2. Diffuse sheets of large eosinophilic cells, generally without nodularity *(Figs. 5.39.1-5.39.3)*; smooth interface with surrounding ovarian stroma *(Figs. 5.39.1 and 5.39.4)* 3. Solid, highly vascularized pattern often resembling normal adrenal cortex; 40% contain cytoplasmic lipofuscin; sparse stroma with prominent vasculature *(Figs. 5.39.1-5.39.4)*; fibrosis may be present; variants include stromal luteoma, stromal Leydig cell tumor, and hilar Leydig cell tumor 4. Large, rounded to polygonal cells with abundant vacuolated clear or eosinophilic cytoplasm; typically have central round nucleus with small nucleoli and minimal atypia; mitotically inactive *(Figs. 5.39.3, 5.39.5, and 5.39.6)*	1. One-third to one-half are stage I; endometriosis and adhesions often present; high incidence of tumor rupture; <10% bilateral; mean 13-15 cm 2. Two-thirds arise in endometriotic cysts as a nodular or polypoid growth of the cyst wall; one-third have adenofibromatous architecture, often with yellow-white honeycomb cut surface 3. Characteristic architectural patterns are papillary, tubulocystic, tubulopapillary (including ring-like structures) and hobnail. Infiltrative small glands and solid growth may also occur *(Figs. 5.39.7-5.39.9)*; adenofibromatous background in one-third; stroma often dense, eosinophilic, and hyalinized (particularly evident in some papillary patterns) *(Fig. 5.39.10)* 4. Range of nuclear atypia from mild to severe (generally, not as marked as in high-grade serous carcinoma) *(Figs. 5.39.8-5.39.11)*; nucleoli often prominent and enlarged; cytoplasm is often but not always clear; abundant eosinophilic cytoplasm also commonly seen; hyaline globules may be present *(Fig. 5.39.11)*; mitotic figures very scant in most cases but occasionally over 10/10 hpf
Special studies	Inhibin+, calretinin+, SF-1+, CK7−, EMA−	CK7+, EMA+, SF-1−, inhibin−, calretinin−

	Steroid (Lipid) Cell Tumor	Clear Cell Carcinoma
Treatment	Unilateral salpingo-oophorectomy or hysterectomy and bilateral oophorectomy +/− staging	Staging (with debulking when indicated); chemotherapy (in neoadjuvant or adjuvant setting)
Prognosis	Malignant in approximately one-third of cases	Stage I has 90% survival; advanced stage appears to have worse prognosis as compared to high-grade serous carcinoma

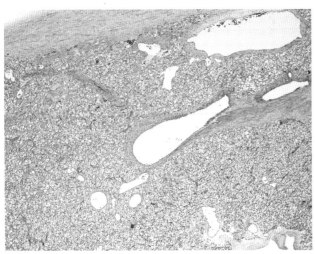

Figure 5.39.1   Steroid cell tumor with lobulated architecture, smooth border with surrounding ovarian stroma at **top**, and delicate vascular network.

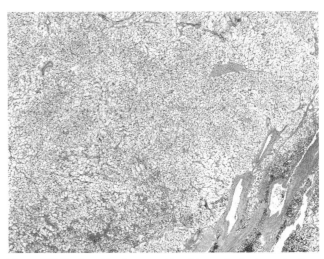

Figure 5.39.2   Steroid cell tumor with solid growth of polygonal cells with abundant clear cytoplasm

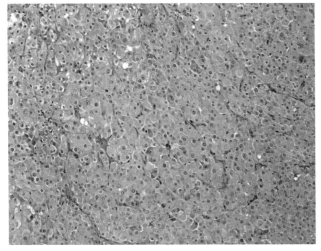

Figure 5.39.3   Steroid cell tumor with bland, round nuclei, brightly eosinophilic cytoplasm, and prominent capillary network.

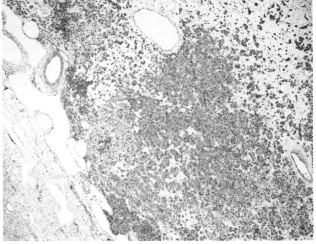

Figure 5.39.4   Steroid cell tumor with circumscribed and vascular border with surrounding ovarian stroma at **left**, and polygonal eosinophilic and clear cells with areas of edema.

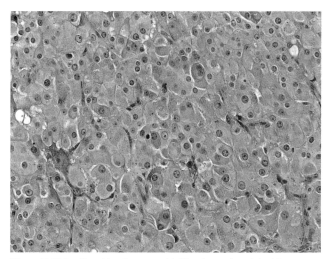

Figure 5.39.5 Steroid cell tumor with bland, round nuclei with prominent nucleoli, brightly eosinophilic cytoplasm, and prominent capillary network (same case as *Fig. 5.39.3*).

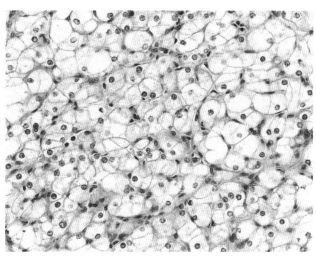

Figure 5.39.6 Steroid cell tumor with bland, round nuclei with prominent nucleoli, clear vacuolated cytoplasm, and prominent capillary network.

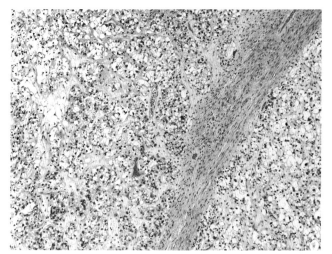

Figure 5.39.7 Clear cell carcinoma displaying a somewhat lobulated growth pattern of clear cells with moderate to severe nuclear atypia.

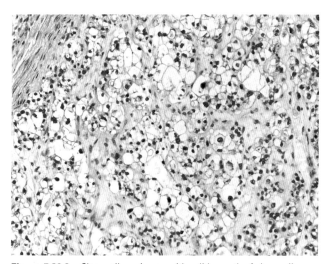

Figure 5.39.8 Clear cell carcinoma with solid growth of clear cells with severe nuclear atypia (same case as *Fig. 5.39.7*).

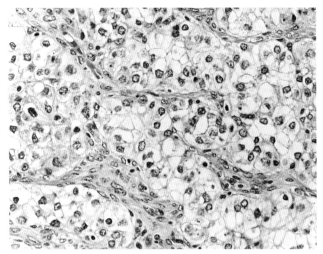

Figure 5.39.9 Clear cell carcinoma with solid and glandular pattern of clear cells with severe nuclear atypia.

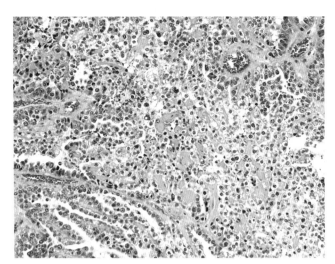

Figure 5.39.10 Clear cell carcinoma with papillary pattern, focal hobnail pattern, severe nuclear atypia, clear to eosinophilic cytoplasm, and prominent hyalinized fibrous stroma.

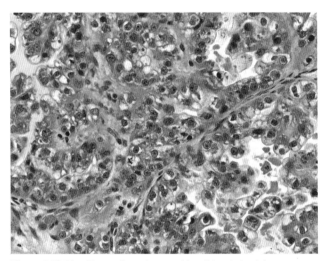

Figure 5.39.11 Clear cell carcinoma with solid and glandular pattern of cells with abundant eosinophilic cytoplasm and severe nuclear atypia. Occasional hyaline globules are noted.

	Small Cell Carcinoma, Hypercalcemic Type	Lymphoma, Diffuse Large B Cell, Primary Ovarian
Age	Mean 24 y	Mean 48 y
Location	Within ovary	Diffuse ovarian involvement
Symptoms	Abdominal pain and swelling	Pelvic pain, urinary symptoms
Signs	Hypercalcemia in two-thirds; pelvic or abdominal mass	Pelvic mass
Etiology	*SMARCA4* mutation (encodes BRG1)	No data specific for ovarian primary site
Gross and histology	1. Unilateral, stage I in 50%, mean 15 cm; usually solid but may have cystic component; soft gray-tan cut surface with hemorrhage and necrosis 2. Diffuse growth pattern of closely packed small cells; nests, cords, and spindle cell patterns may be present; most tumors display round follicle-like spaces containing eosinophilic secretions *(Figs. 5.40.1-5.40.3)*; frequent geographic necrosis 3. Small cells with scanty cytoplasm, oval-round nuclei with coarsely clumped chromatin and small nucleoli, and indistinct cell borders *(Figs. 5.40.4 and 5.40.5)*; large cells seen in 50% but rarely predominate (large cell variant); high mitotic index 4. Mucinous differentiation in 8%-15%	1. Unilateral, 11 cm 2. Usually diffuse architecture, may occasionally contain follicular areas; necrosis and sclerosis often present 3. Sheets of discohesive large lymphoid cells with moderate amounts of pale cytoplasm; round or irregular nuclear contours, prominent nucleoli, and high mitotic index *(Figs. 5.40.6-5.40.10)* 4. No mucinous differentiation
Special studies	• WT1+, cytokeratins and EMA may be negative or have limited/focal expression • Loss of BRG1 (SMARCA4) expression • Negative for hematolymphoid markers including CD10	• Negative for cytokeratins or EMA • Insufficient BRG1 data for lymphomas but no loss of expression would be expected • CD20+ *(Fig. 5.40.11,* **left***)*, CD45+ *(Fig. 5.40.11,* **right***)*, bcl-6+, bcl-2+, and CD10+
Treatment	Hysterectomy and bilateral salpingo-oophorectomy, staging, and debulking; limited data on chemotherapy	Chemotherapy as per standards for lymphoma
Prognosis	Poor, with <10% survival; stage I has 33% survival	Limited data suggest 80%-100% 5-y survival

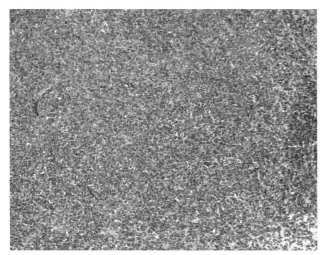

Figure 5.40.1   Small cell carcinoma, hypercalcemic type, displays diffuse patternless sheets of round cells.

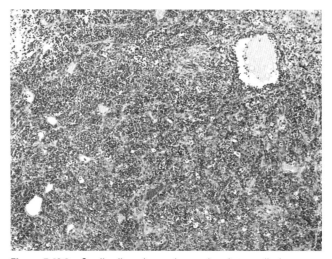

Figure 5.40.2   Small cell carcinoma, hypercalcemic type, displays diffuse sheets of round cells with a follicle-like space containing eosinophilic fluid at **top right**.

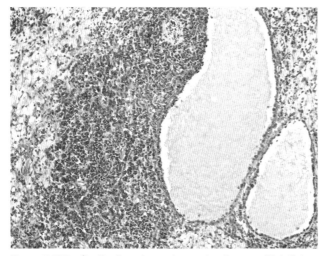

Figure 5.40.3   Small cell carcinoma, hypercalcemic type, with follicle-like spaces containing eosinophilic fluid.

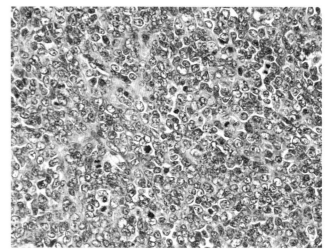

Figure 5.40.4   Small cell carcinoma, hypercalcemic type, with high-grade malignant nuclei, scanty cytoplasm, and mitotic activity.

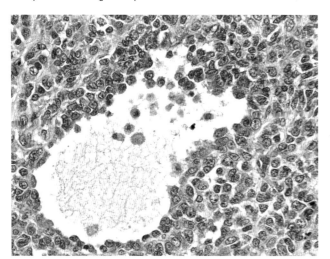

Figure 5.40.5   Small cell carcinoma, hypercalcemic type, with irregular lining of follicle-like space showing exfoliation of tumor cells.

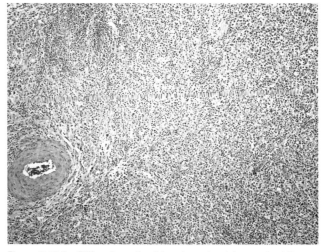

Figure 5.40.6   Diffuse large B-cell lymphoma involving ovarian hilum with entrapment of large thick-walled artery.

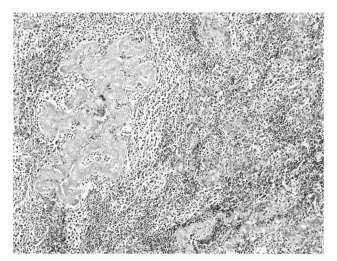

Figure 5.40.7   Diffuse large B-cell lymphoma surrounding and infiltrating a corpus fibrosum.

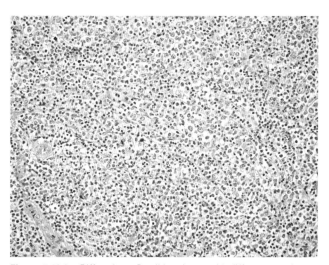

Figure 5.40.8   Diffuse large B-cell lymphoma with diffuse patternless sheets of round lymphoid cells.

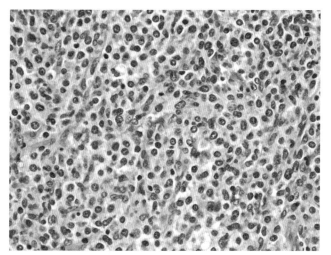

Figure 5.40.9   Diffuse large B-cell lymphoma with round to ovoid nuclei and moderate amounts of eosinophilic cytoplasm.

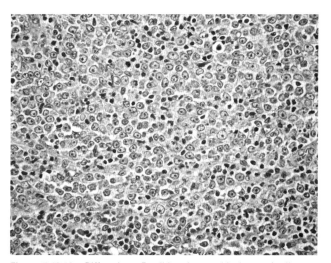

Figure 5.40.10   Diffuse large B-cell lymphoma with sheets of cells showing round nuclei, vesicular chromatin, and prominent nucleoli.

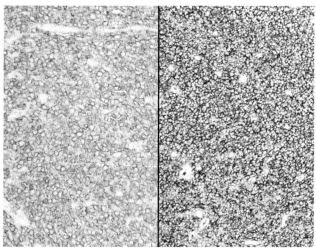

Figure 5.40.11   Diffuse large B-cell lymphoma: immunohistochemical stains for CD20 **(left)** and CD45 **(right)** show diffuse expression.

	Metastatic Endometrioid Adenocarcinoma of Endometrial Origin	Endometrioid Carcinoma, Primary Ovarian
Age	Mean 55-60 y	Mean 55-58 y
Location	Within ovary and on ovarian surface	Within ovary
Symptoms	Dysmenorrhea, postmenopausal bleeding, pelvic pain	Pelvic pain, increasing abdominal girth, bloating, early satiety, vaginal bleeding, urinary symptoms
Signs	Pelvic/abdominal mass	Pelvic/abdominal mass, ascites
Etiology	Primary uterine endometrial adenocarcinoma with ovarian metastasis	Synchronous independent primary endometrial and ovarian adenocarcinomas
	Germline *MSH6, MSH2, MLH1,* or *PMS2* mutation (Lynch syndrome) (~2%-5% of cases) or inactivation due to *MLH1* promoter hypermethylation; *PTEN,* β-*catenin* (*CTNNB1*), and *PIK3CA* mutations; occasionally *KRAS* mutation	Ovarian tumor: endometriosis as precursor lesion; germline *MSH6, MSH2, MLH1* or *PMS2* mutation (Lynch syndrome) in a small subset of cases; *PTEN,* β-*catenin* (*CTNNB1*), *KRAS, ARID1A,* and *PIK3CA* mutations
Gross and histology	1. Often bilateral, small, and multinodular and may be cystic and/or solid; usually <5 cm	1. Usually unilateral, stage I in almost half; mean 15 cm; cystic or cystic and solid; cysts contain dark brown viscous fluid (old blood +/− mucus); papillary or nodular growths arise from cyst lining
	2. Nodular pattern of ovarian involvement *(Figs. 5.41.1 and 5.41.2)*; resembles eutopic endometrial adenocarcinoma, endometrioid type, often high grade; cribriform and solid patterns common with high nuclear grade, often with infiltrative glandular pattern and notable mitotic activity; may involve ovarian surface or superficial ovarian cortex *(Figs. 5.41.1-5.41.3)*; tall columnar epithelium with sharp luminal gland margins, round to ovoid nuclei with hyperchromasia, and prominent nucleoli *(Fig. 5.41.4)*	2. Most are architecturally well differentiated with confluent glandular epithelial proliferation resembling endometrial endometrioid carcinoma; cribriform, papillary, confluent glandular, and occasionally solid patterns *(Figs. 5.41.5 and 5.41.6)*; garland pattern necrosis occasionally present *(Fig. 5.41.7)*; less commonly with infiltrative pattern of glands, nests, and solid masses with jagged edges; tall columnar epithelium with sharp luminal gland margins, round to ovoid nuclei with hyperchromasia, and prominent nucleoli *(Fig. 5.41.8)*; mitotic activity variable, often high
	3. Endometriosis and adenofibromatous endometrioid borderline tumor component absent; squamous differentiation may be present	3. Squamous differentiation in half; adenofibromatous component often present; associated endometriosis is present in majority and often shows atypia, hyperplasia, and other features reflecting origin within endometriotic cyst or associated endometrioid borderline tumor

	Metastatic Endometrioid Adenocarcinoma of Endometrial Origin	**Endometrioid Carcinoma, Primary Ovarian**
	4. Endometrial carcinoma likely to be high grade and/or deeply myoinvasive; lymphovascular space invasion may be present; endometrial and ovarian tumors usually histologically similar; may have extrauterine/extraovarian disease; some synchronous endometrial/ovarian tumors that show traditional clinicopathologic features of independent endometrial and ovarian primaries have been shown to be clonally related (and consistent with an endometrial primary with metastasis to the ovary) based on molecular studies; thus, traditional clinicopathologic features are imperfect	**4.** Associated endometrial tumor usually non-myoinvasive or invasive into the inner half of myometrium; no lymphovascular space invasion; endometrial and ovarian tumors may have some dissimilar histologic features
Special studies	Immunohistochemistry not useful in this differential	Immunohistochemistry not useful in this differential
Treatment	Hysterectomy and bilateral salpingo-oophorectomy; may add chemotherapy and/or pelvic radiation, as for FIGO stage III endometrial carcinoma; hormonal suppression and/or immunotherapy may be used for recurrence	Staging (with debulking when indicated); chemotherapy (in adjuvant or neoadjuvant setting) except for low-grade stage IA/B; hormonal suppression may be used for recurrence; further treatment based on features of synchronous independent uterine tumor
Prognosis	As for stage III endometrial carcinoma; recurrence rate of ~50%	Stage I ovarian tumors associated with >90% survival

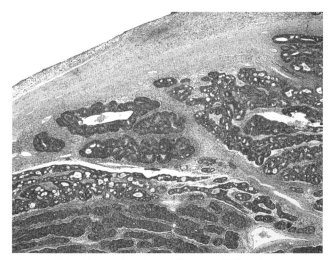

Figure 5.41.1 Metastatic endometrial endometrioid carcinoma displaying a nodular pattern of ovarian cortical involvement. The ovarian surface is seen at the **upper left**.

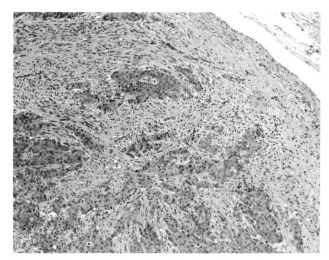

Figure 5.41.2 Metastatic endometrial endometrioid carcinoma. This focus is vaguely nodular but shows an infiltrating pattern with desmoplasia. The ovarian surface is seen at the **upper right**.

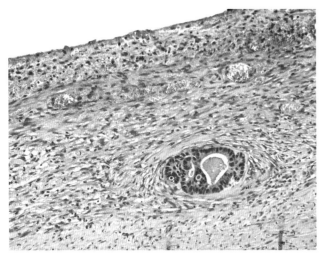

Figure 5.41.3 Metastatic endometrial endometrioid carcinoma embedded in adhesions on the ovarian surface.

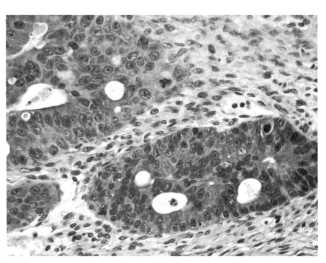

Figure 5.41.4 Metastatic endometrial endometrioid carcinoma with cribriform glands showing high-grade atypia and mitotic activity.

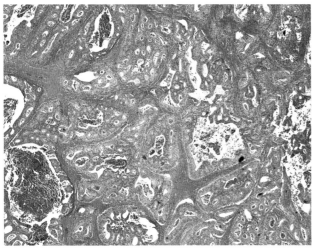

Figure 5.41.5 Primary ovarian endometrioid carcinoma displaying an infiltrative pattern of predominantly smoothly contoured but focally angulated islands of cribriform glands.

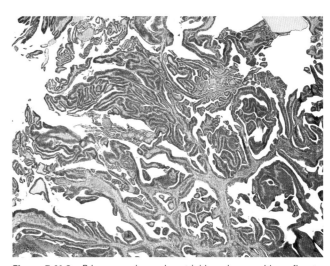

Figure 5.41.6 Primary ovarian endometrioid carcinoma with confluent papillary and glandular pattern.

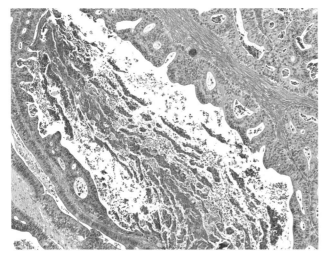

Figure 5.41.7 Primary ovarian endometrioid carcinoma with garland formation with central necrosis resembling metastatic colonic carcinoma (see Sections 5.14 and 5.42).

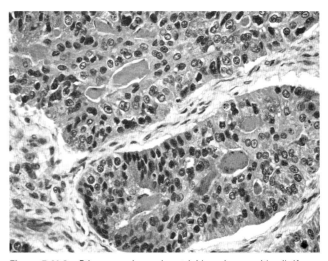

Figure 5.41.8 Primary ovarian endometrioid carcinoma with cribriform glands and moderate cytologic atypia.

	Metastatic Mucinous Carcinoma of Colonic Origin	Mucinous Carcinoma, Primary Ovarian
Age	Mean in 60s	Mean 50 y
Location	Within ovaries and on ovarian surface	Within ovary
Symptoms	Pelvic/abdominal pain	Pelvic/abdominal pain, increasing abdominal girth
Signs	Pelvic/abdominal mass	Large pelvic/abdominal mass
Etiology	Metastasis from primary colorectal carcinoma with secondary involvement of ovary	Arise from mucinous cystadenomas through mucinous borderline tumor (*MBT*); majority have *KRAS* and *TP53* mutations; rarely *BRAF* mutations; majority have copy number loss of *CDKN2A*; no association with Lynch syndrome
	Colorectal mucinous adenocarcinoma; more common in right colon; *KRAS, BRAF, APC* and *CTNNB1* mutations; may have *TP53* mutation; high microsatellite instability in one-third; subset can be associated with Lynch syndrome (germline *MLH1, MSH2, PMS2,* or *MSH6* mutation)	
Gross and histology	1. 60% bilateral, mean 13 cm, typically cystic, less commonly solid and cystic	1. Nearly always unilateral, mean size 21 cm; 90% stage I; grossly similar to mucinous cystadenomas and MBT, with large, mucin-filled cysts; papillary growths sometimes arise in cyst walls
	2. Low magnification commonly reveals nodular pattern, with 2-4 mm nodules compressing intervening stroma; garlands with cribriform glands surrounding areas of dirty necrosis may be present; confluent growth or diffuse, haphazard infiltrative pattern of small- and medium-sized round and angulated mucinous glands may be seen; rupture of mucinous glands/cysts may produce pseudomyxoma ovarii; may have tumor involving hilus (particularly, with lymphovascular invasion) *(Figs. 5.42.1-5.42.5)*	2. Mucinous epithelial lining displays abundant basophilic or eosinophilic cytoplasm; complex papillary and glandular growth reflects invasion in the confluent/expansile pattern *(Figs. 5.42.6-5.42.9)*; less commonly, a haphazard infiltrative pattern of small and moderately sized mucinous glands, nests, and single cells reflects destructive stromal invasion; ≥5 mm of confluent or invasive growth is required for a diagnosis of carcinoma; may have background of MBT; should not have pseudomyxoma ovarii (gland rupture can be present)
	3. Cytologic atypia is variable depending on appearance of the primary tumor; non–invasive-appearing cysts may display cytologically bland mucinous epithelium; severe atypia in architecturally simple and minimally proliferative mucinous epithelium suggests metastasis; signet ring cell component in 5%	3. Cytologically, areas of cystadenoma display small basal nuclei; in other areas, there is a spectrum of atypia present from mild to severe, with nuclear enlargement, hyperchromasia, prominent nucleoli, and pseudostratification and often with numerous mitotic figures
	4. Primary colon tumor displays abundant extra-cellular mucin (>50% of tumor) with dissection	4. No synchronous colonic primary

	Metastatic Mucinous Carcinoma of Colonic Origin	Mucinous Carcinoma, Primary Ovarian
Special studies	• CK7 negative or focal expression; CK20 patchy or diffuse expression; extent of expression: CK7 < CK20; SATB2+ • Caveat: rare primary ovarian mucinous carcinomas arising from teratomas may share histologic and immunohistochemical features of colonic adenocarcinomas	• CK7 patchy or diffuse expression; CK20 negative, focal, or patchy expression; extent of expression: CK7 > CK20; SATB2−
Treatment	As per stage IV colorectal carcinoma	Staging (with debulking when indicated) (omission of lymph nodes acceptable); +/− appendectomy; chemotherapy (in neoadjuvant or adjuvant setting) except for low-grade stages IA and IB
Prognosis	5-y survival for stage IV ~10%	95% survival for stage I; advanced stage, which is rare, has dismal prognosis

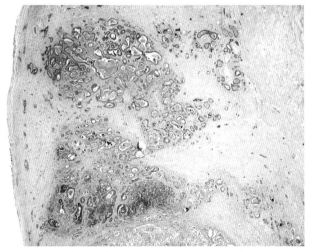

Figure 5.42.1 Metastatic colonic mucinous carcinoma displaying nodular pattern of ovarian involvement.

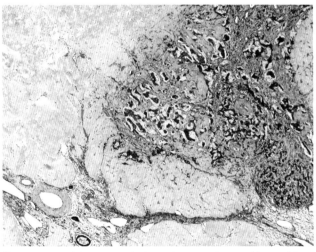

Figure 5.42.2 Metastatic colonic mucinous carcinoma with a nodular configuration infiltrating a corpus albicans.

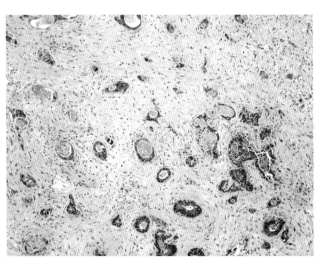

Figure 5.42.3 Metastatic colonic mucinous carcinoma with infiltrative pattern and desmoplasia.

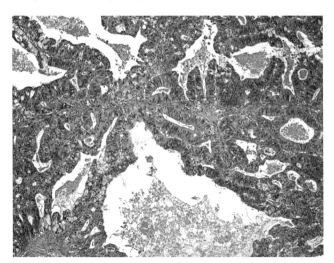

Figure 5.42.4 Metastatic colonic mucinous carcinoma with confluent pattern of interconnecting cribriform glands lined by intestinal-type epithelium with goblet cells. This pattern can simulate a primary ovarian mucinous tumor.

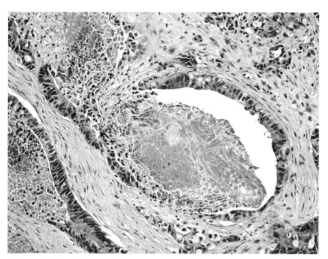

Figure 5.42.5 Metastatic colonic mucinous carcinoma with incomplete and necrotic glands.

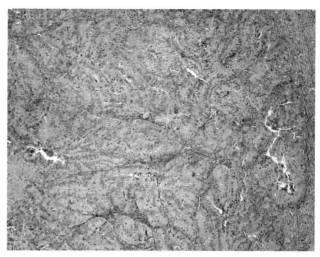

Figure 5.42.6 Mucinous ovarian carcinoma with confluent glandular growth. The glands are back-to-back and lack intervening stroma in many areas.

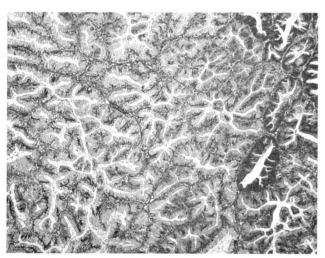

Figure 5.42.7 Mucinous ovarian carcinoma with confluent and complex glandular and papillary pattern and anastomosing epithelium.

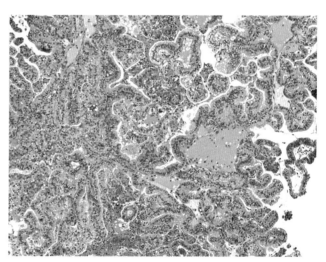

Figure 5.42.8 Mucinous ovarian carcinoma with confluent papillary pattern.

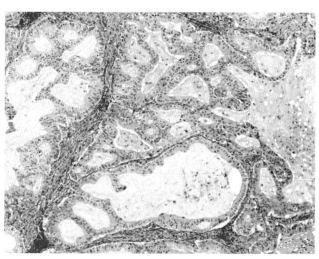

Figure 5.42.9 Mucinous ovarian carcinoma with confluent/expansile glandular pattern of invasion.

5.43

METASTATIC ENDOCERVICAL ADENOCARCINOMA, USUAL TYPE VS MUCINOUS BORDERLINE TUMOR (MBT) WITH INTRAEPITHELIAL CARCINOMA

	Metastatic Endocervical Adenocarcinoma, Usual Type	Mucinous Borderline Tumor (MBT) with Intraepithelial Carcinoma
Age	Mean 43 y	Mean 50 y
Location	Within ovary	Within ovary
Symptoms	Pelvic/abdominal pain and increasing abdominal girth	Pelvic/abdominal pain and increasing abdominal girth
Signs	Adnexal or pelvic mass; 17% have prior established diagnosis of endocervical adenocarcinoma	Large pelvic/abdominal mass
Etiology	Metastasis from primary endocervical carcinoma with secondary involvement of ovary HPV-related, usually HPV 16 or 18; Possibly due to transtubal/retrograde spread in some cases	Arise in mucinous cystadenomas; *KRAS* mutations, rarely *BRAF* mutations; low frequency of *TP53* mutations
Gross and histology	1. Two-thirds unilateral, mean 13 cm; majority of unilateral tumors >10 cm; usually multicystic, sometimes with solid or papillary areas 2. One or more patterns of primary ovarian epithelial tumors, that is, borderline-like, confluent glandular or cribriform, and papillary, glandular patterns; may simulate MBT or invasive mucinous carcinoma; invasive pattern usually focal; predominance of infiltrative pattern in 10% of cases *(Figs. 5.43.1-5.43.3)* 3. Often hybrid endometrioid-mucinous appearance, that is, endometrioid patterns at low-power magnification, and apical mucin seen at high-power magnification; nuclei enlarged, elongated, and hyperchromatic; basal apoptotic bodies and high mitotic index *(Fig. 5.43.3)*; mitotic figures are especially noticeable in the luminal half of the cell 4. Endocervical tumor usually clearly invasive but occasionally may appear to be adenocarcinoma *in situ* with minimal invasion; often extends into lower uterine segment/corpus endometrium	1. Nearly always unilateral, mean size 22 cm; grossly similar to mucinous cystadenomas, with large, mucin-filled cysts; papillary growths sometimes arise in cyst walls 2. Complex glandular and papillary architecture without confluent growth pattern; epithelium is stratified with exfoliated epithelial clusters in cystic or glandular spaces; no anastomosing or cribriform architecture; no nodular growth patterns or surface or hilum involvement *(Figs. 5.43.5 and 5.43.6)* 3. Mucinous epithelial lining displays abundant basophilic or eosinophilic cytoplasm; areas of cystadenoma with small basal nuclei; areas of grade 3 atypia are present, displaying unequivocal cytologic features of malignancy with nuclear enlargement, hyperchromasia, prominent nucleoli, and pseudostratification; mitotic figures can be seen but not very common *(Fig. 5.43.7)* 4. Tumors should be well sampled to exclude invasion
Special studies	p16+ (diffuse pattern, usually >90% positive cells) *(Fig. 5.43.4)*, HPV *in situ* hybridization usually (+) (most HPV 16 or 18) *(Fig. 5.43.4,* **inset***)*, but sensitivity of *in situ* hybridization is <100%; CK7, CK20, and ER/PR of no help in this differential diagnosis	p16− (nondiffuse pattern); no definite detectable HPV by *in situ* hybridization; CK7, CK20, and ER/PR of no help in this differential diagnosis

	Metastatic Endocervical Adenocarcinoma, Usual Type	Mucinous Borderline Tumor (MBT) with Intraepithelial Carcinoma
Treatment	Insufficient data; may be treated as per advanced stage cervical carcinoma	Unilateral salpingo-oophorectomy +/− staging, +/− appendectomy
Prognosis	3-y disease-free survival ~75%	Nearly 100% survival if well sampled and metastatic carcinoma to the ovary is rigorously excluded

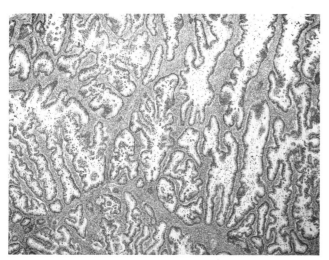

Figure 5.43.1 Metastatic endocervical adenocarcinoma simulating an ovarian mucinous borderline tumor.

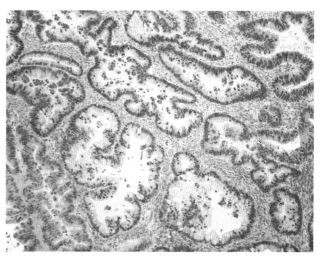

Figure 5.43.2 Metastatic endocervical adenocarcinoma, same case as *Figure 5.43.1*, with branching and irregular glands, lined by mucinous epithelium with stratified hyperchromatic nuclei and numerous mitotic figures.

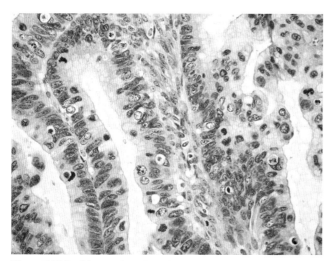

Figure 5.43.3 Metastatic endocervical adenocarcinoma, same case as *Figure 5.43.1*, with severely atypical mucinous epithelium, high mitotic activity, and apoptotic bodies.

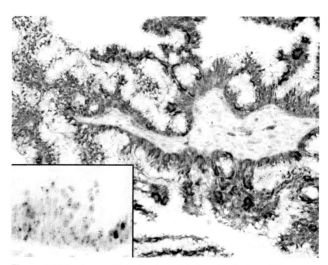

Figure 5.43.4 Immunohistochemical stain for p16 displays diffuse positive nuclear and cytoplasmic staining; *in situ* hybridization for HPV 16 displays positivity in the tumor cell nuclei **(inset)**.

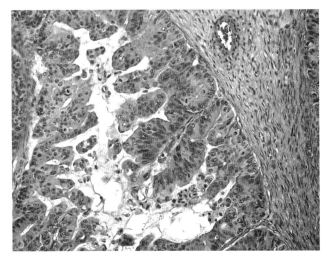

Figure 5.43.5 Mucinous borderline tumor with intraepithelial carcinoma displays intraglandular papillary proliferation with marked cytologic atypia.

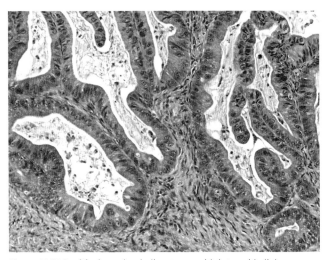

Figure 5.43.6 Mucinous borderline tumor with intraepithelial carcinoma displays nuclear enlargement and prominent nucleoli.

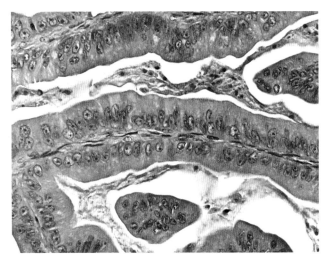

Figure 5.43.7 Mucinous borderline tumor with intraepithelial carcinoma showing severe atypia and large, prominent nucleoli.

	Metastatic Pancreatic Adenocarcinoma	Mucinous Borderline Tumor (MBT)
Age	Mean 56-63 y	Mean 50 y
Location	Ovarian stroma and surface; often bilateral	Within ovary
Symptoms	Abdominal pain, vomiting, fever, jaundice, weight loss	Pelvic/abdominal pain, increasing abdominal girth
Signs	Pelvic/adnexal mass may be the presenting manifestation	Large pelvic/abdominal mass
Etiology	Metastasis from primary pancreatic carcinoma with secondary involvement of ovary	Arise in mucinous cystadenomas; *KRAS* mutations, rarely *BRAF* mutations; low frequency of *TP53* mutations
Gross and histology	1. Solid or large, cystic, and multiloculated; mean/median size 9.0/7.4 cm; surface involvement is common; extraovarian/abdominal spread is often seen but not always present; bilaterality is consistent with metastatic origin but rarely can be unilateral 2. In solid nodular pattern, small angulated glands haphazardly infiltrate desmoplastic stroma *(Figs. 5.44.1-5.44.3)*; cystic tumors may resemble mucinous cystadenoma and MBT *(Figs. 5.44.4 and 5.44.5)*; areas of obvious invasive carcinoma may be minor; mucin granulomas less commonly seen as compared to primary mucinous tumors 3. Cytologic atypia is often high *(Fig. 5.44.6)*, but nuclei may be deceptively bland *(Fig. 5.44.4)* 4. Extensive sampling in difficult cases may be useful to reveal more obvious patterns suggestive of metastasis	1. Nearly always unilateral, mean size 22 cm; grossly similar to mucinous cystadenomas, with large, mucin-filled cysts; papillary growths sometimes arise in cyst walls 2. Architectural complexity with glandular crowding and cystic areas with epithelial stratification, intraglandular papillary growth, and detached epithelial clusters *(Figs. 5.44.7 and 5.44.8)* 3. Mucinous epithelial lining displays abundant basophilic or eosinophilic cytoplasm with grade 1-2 atypia *(Figs. 5.44.9 and 5.44.10)* (grade 3 atypia warrants a designation of intraepithelial carcinoma [see Section 5.43], with marked nuclear enlargement, hyperchromasia, and prominent nucleoli, often with mitotic figures); proliferative areas with atypical architecture and cytology constitute >10% of the tumor; areas of cystadenoma with small basal nuclei may be present 4. Tumors should be well sampled to exclude invasion
Special studies	• Loss of Dpc4 expression in half of cases • CK7/CK20 coordinate expression patterns of no help for distinguishing from primary ovarian origin (extent of expression: CK7 > CK20); ER/PR− • PAX8−	• No loss of Dpc4 expression • CK7/CK20 coordinate expression patterns of no help for distinguishing from pancreatic origin (extent of expression: CK7 > CK20); ER/PR− (weak and focal expression can be seen) • PAX8 often (−) but may be (+) in a subset of cases

	Metastatic Pancreatic Adenocarcinoma	Mucinous Borderline Tumor (MBT)
Treatment	Chemotherapy as for stage IV pancreatic carcinoma	Unilateral salpingo-oophorectomy +/− appendectomy, +/− staging
Prognosis	Median survival for stage IV with best current therapy is 11 mo	Benign

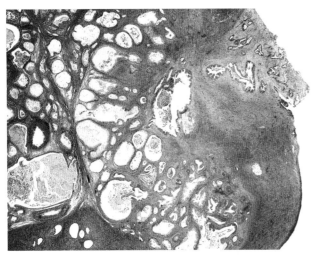

Figure 5.44.1 Metastatic pancreatic carcinoma displays nodular pattern of invasion of ovarian stroma seen at low magnification. Surface involvement is present at the **upper right**.

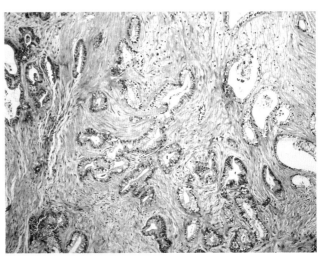

Figure 5.44.2 Metastatic pancreatic carcinoma with haphazard infiltrative pattern of medium-sized glands associated with reactive, edematous fibroblastic stroma.

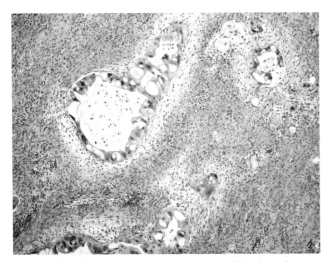

Figure 5.44.3 Metastatic pancreatic carcinoma with haphazard infiltrative pattern of variably sized glands as well as single cells and small cell clusters and nests.

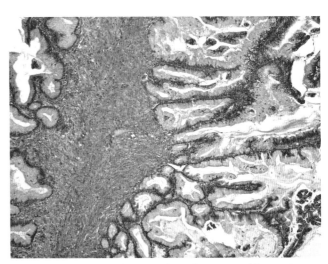

Figure 5.44.4 Metastatic pancreatic carcinoma resembling mucinous borderline tumor with an orderly glandular and papillary pattern without infiltrative features.

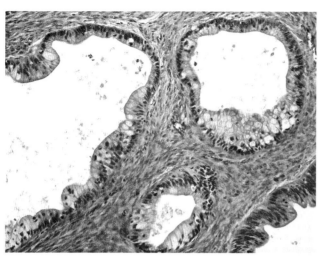

Figure 5.44.5 Metastatic pancreatic carcinoma resembling mucinous borderline tumor showing glands without infiltrative features and with mild to moderate cytologic atypia.

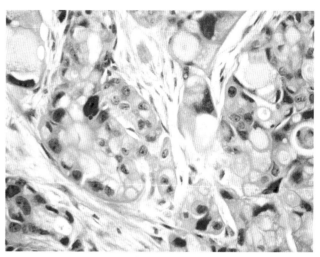

Figure 5.44.6 Metastatic pancreatic carcinoma with angulated, infiltrative glands with severe cytologic atypia and occasional signet ring–like cells.

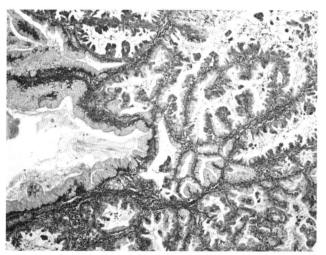

Figure 5.44.7 Mucinous borderline tumor with cystic, glandular, and papillary pattern with epithelial stratification and tufting.

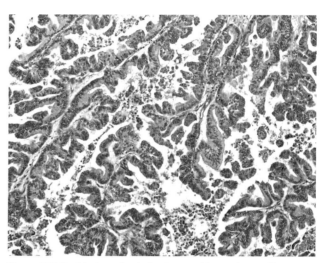

Figure 5.44.8 Mucinous borderline tumor with complex papillary proliferation with epithelial stratification and tufting.

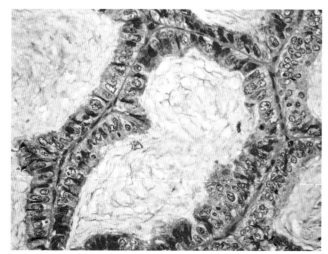

Figure 5.44.9 Mucinous borderline tumor with moderate cytologic atypia.

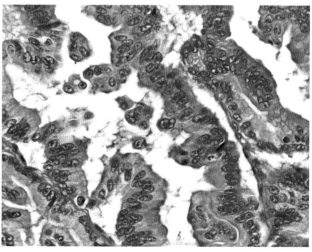

Figure 5.44.10 Mucinous borderline tumor with stratification and mild to moderate cytologic atypia.

5 OVARY

	Metastatic Breast Carcinoma	Endometrioid Carcinoma
Age	Mean 49 y	Mean 55-58 y
Location	Within ovaries	Within ovary
Symptoms	Usually asymptomatic with reference to the ovarian lesions	Pelvic pain, increasing abdominal girth, bloating, early satiety, vaginal bleeding, urinary symptoms
Signs	Majority are incidental findings at therapeutic oophorectomy; pelvic mass in 10%-15%; presents at mean of 1 y after diagnosis of breast carcinoma	Pelvic/abdominal mass, ascites
Etiology	Metastasis from primary breast carcinoma with secondary involvement of ovary	Endometriosis; germline *MLH1, MSH2, PMS2, or MSH6* mutation (Lynch syndrome) in a subset of cases; *PTEN*, β-catenin (*CTNNB1*), *KRAS, ARID1A,* and *PIK3CA* mutations
Gross and histology	1. Two-thirds bilateral; half of ovaries grossly normal; one-third of ovaries solid and diffusely enlarged; one-third of metastatic lesions microscopic (<1 mm); half of tumor nodules <1 cm	1. Usually unilateral, stage I in almost half; mean 15 cm; cystic or cystic and solid; cysts contain dark brown viscous fluid (old blood +/− mucus); papillary or nodular growths arise from cyst lining
	2. Ductal and lobular (single file) patterns most common; less commonly solid and diffuse, and single cell infiltration; occasionally signet ring cells and cribriform pattern may be present *(Figs. 5.45.1-5.45.4)*	2. Most are architecturally well differentiated with confluent glandular epithelial proliferation resembling endometrial endometrioid carcinoma *(Figs. 5.45.6 and 5.45.7)*; cribriform, papillary, glandular *(Fig. 5.45.8)*, and occasionally solid patterns; less commonly with infiltrative pattern of glands, nests, and solid masses with jagged edges
	3. Epithelium may be low grade with monomorphous round bland nuclei as seen in low-grade ductal carcinoma of breast *(Figs. 5.45.4 and 5.45.5)*; ovarian stroma occasionally luteinized	3. Tall columnar epithelium with sharp luminal gland margins, round to ovoid nuclei with hyperchromasia, and prominent nucleoli; mitotic activity variable, often high *(Figs. 5.45.7 and 5.45.9)*
	4. No squamous differentiation or endometriosis	4. Squamous differentiation in half; adenofibromatous component often present; associated endometriosis is present in majority and often shows atypia, hyperplasia, and other features reflecting origin within endometriotic cyst or associated endometrioid borderline tumor
	5. No secretory, ciliated, or sertoliform differentiation	5. Secretory, ciliated, and sertoliform variants can be seen
Special studies	• GATA-3+; GCDFP-15+ in a subset of cases; PAX8−; depending on primary tumor characteristics, may be ER/PR+	• GATA-3−; GCDFP-15−; usually PAX8+; ER/PR (+) or (−) • Loss of staining for DNA mismatch repair proteins (MLH1, MSH2, PMS2, MSH6) in a subset of cases

	Metastatic Breast Carcinoma	Endometrioid Carcinoma
Treatment	As per advanced stage breast carcinoma, depending on HER2 and ER/PR status	Staging (with debulking when indicated); chemotherapy (in neoadjuvant or adjuvant setting) except for low-grade stage IA/B; hormonal suppression may be used for recurrence
Prognosis	As per advanced stage breast carcinoma, depending on HER2 and ER/PR status	Stage I >90% survival

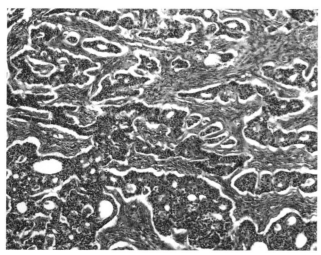

Figure 5.45.1   Metastatic breast ductal carcinoma with haphazard infiltrative pattern.

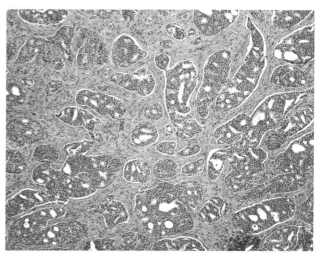

Figure 5.45.2   Metastatic breast carcinoma with smoothly contoured and focally angulated islands and nests of cribriform epithelium with an infiltrative pattern simulating an endometrioid carcinoma.

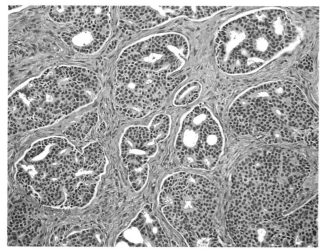

Figure 5.45.3   Metastatic breast carcinoma. Same case as *Figure 5.45.2* displaying cribriform pattern with monotonous round, bland evenly spaced nuclei characteristic of low-grade ductal carcinoma of breast.

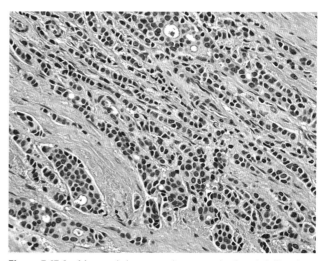

Figure 5.45.4   Metastatic breast carcinoma, predominantly infiltrating lobular type, with single file infiltration of small cells with angular nuclei characteristic of invasive lobular carcinoma; note glands reflecting focal ductal features toward **bottom left and top center**.

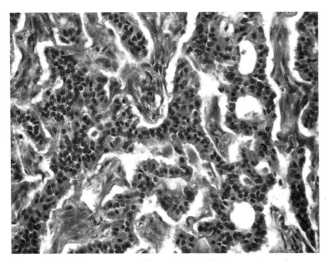

Figure 5.45.5   Same case as *Figure 5.45.1* with interanastomosing cords and glands of low-grade ductal carcinoma of breast; note minimal atypia with small round evenly spaced nuclei.

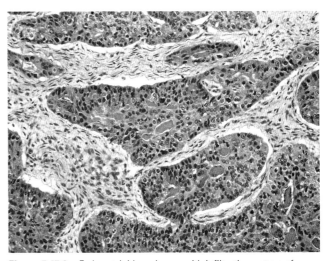

Figure 5.45.6   Endometrioid carcinoma with infiltrative pattern of cribriform islands of epithelium.

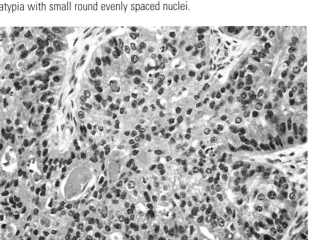

Figure 5.45.7   Ovarian endometrioid carcinoma with low-grade nuclear features of columnar epithelium resembling endometrial endometrioid adenocarcinoma.

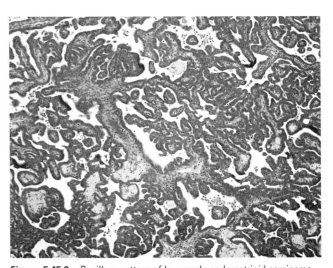

Figure 5.45.8   Papillary pattern of low-grade endometrioid carcinoma with complex and confluent architecture.

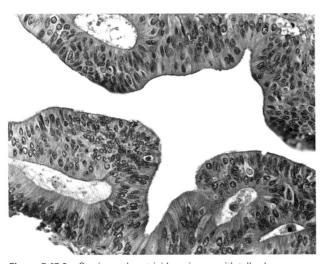

Figure 5.45.9   Ovarian endometrioid carcinoma with tall columnar epithelium and sharp luminal margins resembling endometrial endometrioid carcinoma.

5.46

METASTATIC CERVICAL HPV-UNRELATED ADENOCARCINOMA (ADENOMA MALIGNUM/MINIMAL DEVIATION ADENOCARCINOMA/GASTRIC-TYPE ADENOCARCINOMA) VS MUCINOUS BORDERLINE TUMOR (MBT)

	Metastatic Cervical HPV-Unrelated Adenocarcinoma (Adenoma Malignum/Minimal Deviation Adenocarcinoma/Gastric-Type Adenocarcinoma)	**Mucinous Borderline Tumor (MBT)**
Age	40-60 y	Mean 50 y
Location	Within ovary and on ovarian surface	Within ovary
Symptoms	Pelvic/abdominal pain; some patients may have history of Peutz-Jeghers syndrome (adenoma malignum/minimal deviation adenocarcinoma); the ovarian tumor can be the first manifestation of disease, and a prior cervical tumor may not be known; some patients may have had a prior hysterectomy with "benign" findings per report in cases for which a cervical tumor was not recognized or misclassified as benign	Pelvic/abdominal pain, increasing abdominal girth
Signs	Pelvic mass; cervical cytology generally unrevealing	Large pelvic/abdominal mass
Etiology	Metastasis from primary HPV-unrelated cervical adenocarcinoma with secondary involvement of ovary	Arise in mucinous cystadenomas; *KRAS* mutations, rarely *BRAF* mutations; low frequency of *TP53* mutations
	Associated with Peutz-Jeghers syndrome (*STK11/LKB1* mutation) (adenoma malignum/minimal deviation adenocarcinoma)	
Gross and histology	1. Bilateral, with peritoneal metastases	1. Nearly always unilateral, mean size 22 cm; grossly similar to mucinous cystadenomas, with large, mucin-filled cysts; papillary growths sometimes arise in cyst walls
	2. Nodular pattern and ovarian surface involvement may be present; infiltrative pattern generally absent; some cases may be deceptively cystic and mimic primary ovarian mucinous cystadenoma *(Figs. 5.46.1 and 5.46.2)* or MBT without classic histologic features seen in metastases secondarily involving the ovary	2. Architectural complexity with glandular crowding and cystic areas with epithelial stratification, intraglandular papillary growth, and detached epithelial clusters *(Figs. 5.46.4-5.46.6)*
	3. Well-differentiated mucinous glands with no to minimal atypia *(Fig. 5.46.3)*; cytologic features classic for adenoma malignum as seen in the cervix may be present within the epithelial component in the ovary (columnar cells with abundant mucin and basally situated medium-sized round nuclei with slightly pale chromatin and small nucleoli; low mitotic index); intestinal differentiation with goblet and Paneth cells may be present	3. Mucinous epithelial lining displays abundant basophilic or eosinophilic cytoplasm with grade 1-2 atypia *(Fig. 5.46.7)* (grade 3 atypia warrants a designation of MBT with intraepithelial carcinoma [see Section 5.43], with marked nuclear enlargement, hyperchromasia, and prominent nucleoli, often with mitotic figures). Proliferative areas with atypical architecture and cytology constitute >10% of the tumor. Areas of cystadenoma with small basal nuclei may be present

Metastatic Cervical HPV-Unrelated Adenocarcinoma (Adenoma Malignum/Minimal Deviation Adenocarcinoma/Gastric-Type Adenocarcinoma)	Mucinous Borderline Tumor (MBT)
4. Extensive sampling of the ovarian tumor may be necessary to reveal more obvious patterns of a metastasis; other associated findings, which can raise the possibility of metastatic adenoma malignum in syndromic cases, are SCTAT (sex cord tumor with annular tubules; see Section 5.37) tumorlets in the ovary and mucinous metaplasia in the fallopian tube mucosa; if a concurrent hysterectomy specimen is available, submitting all cervical tissue for histologic examination is helpful	**4.** Tumors should be well sampled to exclude invasion

	Metastatic Cervical HPV-Unrelated Adenocarcinoma	Mucinous Borderline Tumor (MBT)
Special studies	P53 can be aberrant in about half; ER/PR and p16 of limited use *In situ* hybridization for HPV of no use for this differential diagnosis	P53 usually wild-type staining; ER/PR and p16 of limited use *In situ* hybridization for HPV of no use for this differential diagnosis
Treatment	Limited data; may be treated as per advanced-stage cervical carcinoma	Unilateral salpingo-oophorectomy +/− appendectomy, +/− staging
Prognosis	Prognosis appears poor based on limited data	Benign

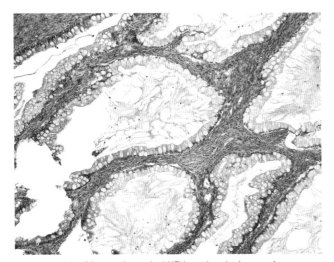

Figure 5.46.1 Metastatic cervical HPV-unrelated adenocarcinoma characterized by large dilated mucinous glands lacking overtly infiltrative features. The low-power appearance can easily simulate a primary ovarian mucinous tumor.

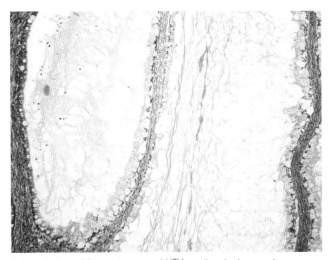

Figure 5.46.2 Metastatic cervical HPV-unrelated adenocarcinoma. Same case as *Figure 5.46.1*, with dilated mucinous glands.

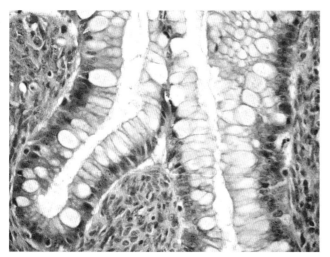

Figure 5.46.3   Metastatic cervical HPV-unrelated adenocarcinoma with goblet cells and deceptively bland nuclei with only mild atypia.

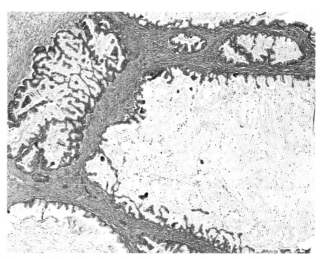

Figure 5.46.4   Mucinous borderline tumor with cystic architecture and epithelial stratification.

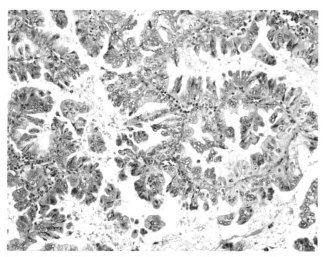

Figure 5.46.5   Mucinous borderline tumor with papillary architecture, stratification, and tufting.

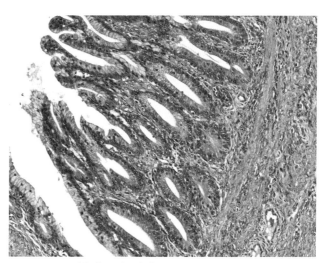

Figure 5.46.6   Mucinous borderline tumor with crowded basally oriented mucinous glands and small papillae at the surface.

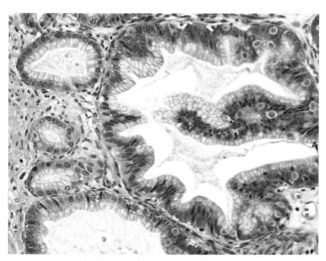

Figure 5.46.7   Mucinous borderline tumor with crowded glands and bland nuclei.

	Secondary Ovarian Involvement by Low-Grade Mucinous Neoplasm of Appendix	Mucinous Borderline Tumor (MBT)
Age	Mean 45 y	Mean 50 y
Location	Ovarian surface and within superficial and deep cortical stroma	Within ovary
Symptoms	Abdominal distension and pain	Pelvic/abdominal pain and increasing abdominal girth
Signs	Pelvic/abdominal mass, ascites; pseudomyxoma peritonei may be present	Large pelvic/abdominal mass
Etiology	Ruptured low-grade appendiceal mucinous neoplasm with secondary involvement of ovary	Arise in mucinous cystadenomas; *KRAS* mutations; low frequency of *TP53* mutations; rarely *BRAF* mutations
Gross and histology	1. Mean 7-16 cm, 75%-80% bilateral; slight right-sided predominance for unilateral tumors; mucinous nodules involving ovarian surface and stroma; appendix typically ruptured and/or dilated 2. Ovarian surface involvement, superficial and deep cortical involvement, and mucin dissection through ovarian stroma (pseudomyxoma ovarii) in two-thirds, extensive in majority of these *(Figs. 5.47.1 and 5.47.2)* 3. Mucin lakes containing scant strips of simple, focally proliferative mucinous epithelium with mild nuclear atypia and minimal mitotic activity *(Fig. 5.47.3)*; cells may have hypermucinous appearance with tufting and small papillae *(Figs. 5.47.4 and 5.47.5)*; peritoneal lesions have similar appearance 4. Primary appendiceal tumor typically ruptured with extensive mucin dissection through wall and similar epithelium as in ovarian lesions	1. Nearly always unilateral, mean size 22 cm; grossly similar to mucinous cystadenomas, with large, mucin-filled cysts; papillary growths sometimes arise in cyst walls 2. Cystic and glandular growth pattern with areas of complex papillary or intraglandular growth *(Figs. 5.47.6 and 5.47.7)*; pseudomyxoma ovarii usually absent; focal when present 3. Mucinous epithelial lining displays abundant basophilic or eosinophilic cytoplasm with grade 1-2 atypia *(Figs. 5.47.8 and 5.47.9)* (grade 3 atypia warrants a designation of MBT with intraepithelial carcinoma [see Section 5.43], with marked nuclear enlargement, hyperchromasia, prominent nucleoli, pseudostratification, often with mitotic figures); proliferative areas with atypical architecture and cytology constitute >10% of the tumor; areas of cystadenoma with small basal nuclei may be present 4. Tumors should be well sampled to exclude invasion
Special studies	• CK7 negative or focal expression; CK20 patchy or diffuse expression; extent of expression: CK7 < CK20; SATB2+ • Caveat: rare primary ovarian low-grade (adenomatous) mucinous neoplasms arising from teratomas may share histologic and immunohistochemical features of low-grade appendiceal mucinous neoplasms	• CK7 patchy or diffuse expression; CK20 negative, focal, or patchy expression; extent of expression: CK7 > CK20; SATB2−

	Secondary Ovarian Involvement by Low-Grade Mucinous Neoplasm of Appendix	**Mucinous Borderline Tumor (MBT)**
Treatment	Hysterectomy and bilateral salpingo-oophorectomy, appendectomy, debulking of abdominal and pelvic tumor; heated intraperitoneal chemotherapy commonly used but limited data on its efficacy	Unilateral salpingo-oophorectomy +/− appendectomy +/− staging
Prognosis	Indolent course with 10-y survival approaching 50%	Benign

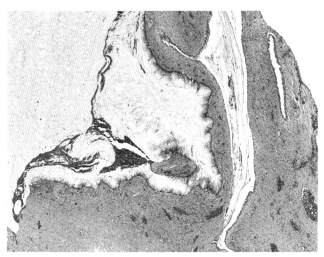

Figure 5.47.1 Secondary ovarian involvement by low-grade appendiceal mucinous neoplasm characterized by large mucinous epithelial-lined cysts and extracellular mucin lakes dissecting through ovarian stroma (pseudomyxoma ovarii).

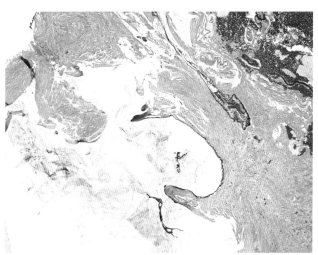

Figure 5.47.2 Secondary ovarian involvement by low-grade appendiceal mucinous neoplasm with disrupted mucinous glands, large mucin-containing cysts partially lined by mucinous epithelium, and extracellular mucin lakes dissecting through dense fibrotic tissue (pseudomyxoma ovarii).

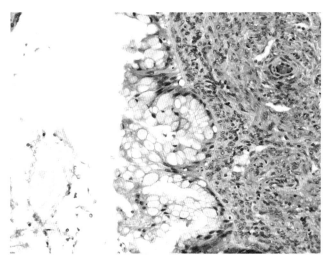

Figure 5.47.3 Secondary ovarian involvement by low-grade appendiceal mucinous neoplasm with abundant cytoplasmic mucin, prominent goblet cells, and minimal nuclear atypia.

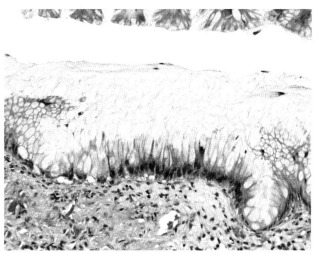

Figure 5.47.4 Secondary ovarian involvement by low-grade appendiceal mucinous neoplasm with "hypermucinous" appearance of the epithelium with large quantities of mucin being produced and extruded into glandular spaces.

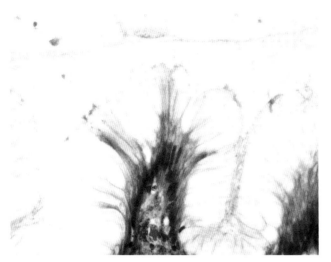

Figure 5.47.5   Secondary ovarian involvement by low-grade appendiceal mucinous neoplasm with "hypermucinous" appearance of the epithelium with bland basal nuclei.

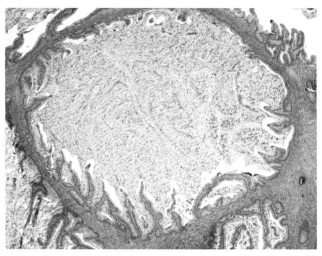

Figure 5.47.6   Mucinous borderline tumor with epithelial stratification and villous architecture.

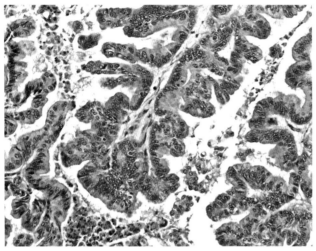

Figure 5.47.7   Mucinous borderline tumor with epithelial stratification, tufting, and moderate cytologic atypia.

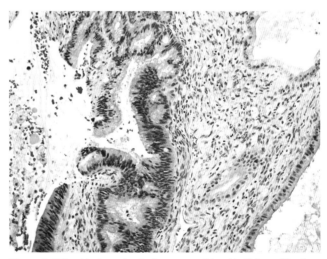

Figure 5.47.8   Mucinous borderline tumor with epithelial stratification and mild atypia on the **left side**; compare to mucinous cystadenoma component at **right** with no proliferation and minimal atypia.

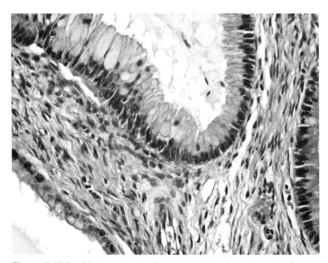

Figure 5.47.9   Mucinous borderline tumor with minimal atypia of mucinous epithelium. Note difference in cytologic appearance compared with secondary ovarian involvement by low-grade appendiceal mucinous neoplasm.

5.48

ENDOMETRIOTIC CYST WITH EPITHELIAL ATYPIA VS ENDOMETRIOTIC CYST WITH EARLY CLEAR CELL CARCINOMA/ INTRAEPITHELIAL CLEAR CELL CARCINOMA

	Endometriotic Cyst with Epithelial Atypia	Endometriotic Cyst with Early Clear Cell Carcinoma/Intraepithelial Clear Cell Carcinoma
Age	Mean 35 y	40-50 y
Location	Usually ovarian, occasionally pelvic peritoneum, or less common sites of endometriosis	Usually ovarian, occasionally pelvic peritoneum, or less common sites of endometriosis
Symptoms	Pelvic pain, dysmenorrhea	Pelvic pain, dysmenorrhea
Signs	Pelvic mass	Pelvic mass
Etiology	Arise in endometriosis, which is often neoplastic; multifocal lesions often clonally related, including some lesions without atypia; may have loss of *ARID1A* expression, suggesting mutation	*ARID1A* and *PIK3CA* mutations usually present in carcinoma-associated lesions arising from endometriosis; same mutations may be present in associated noncontiguous endometriotic lesions without atypia; *MET* amplification sometimes present
Gross and histology	1. Chocolate cyst typical of endometriosis; usually unilateral 2. Cyst lining epithelium usually flattened or cuboidal; acute inflammation commonly present; nuclear atypia characterized by enlarged nuclei with prominent nucleoli, often smudged chromatin, mitotically inactive *(Figs. 5.48.1-5.48.3)*; morphologic features are suggestive of reparative/ reactive changes; level of atypia not as marked as in clear cell carcinoma; areas denuded of epithelium commonly seen; hemosiderin or pseudoxanthoma cells often underlie epithelium; endometriotic-type stroma often present *(Fig. 5.48.4)* 3. Limited epithelial stratification may be present, with mild tufting, occasionally with small papillae and often with mucinous metaplasia; lacks other architectural patterns typical of clear cell carcinoma; in worrisome cases, submitting the entire specimen for histologic examination is advised	1. Chocolate cyst typical of endometriosis; usually unilateral 2. Mostly single layer of cyst lining, but focal stratification and epithelial complexity may be evident *(Figs. 5.48.5 and 5.48.6)*; epithelium displays range of nuclear atypia *(Figs. 5.48.7-5.48.9)*, which may be mild, characterized by enlarged nuclei with prominent nucleoli but can exhibit notable pleomorphism; level of atypia generally greater than that encountered in atypical endometriosis without clear cell carcinoma; hobnail features and clear or pale, eosinophilic cytoplasm present; mitotically inactive; pseudoxanthoma cells often present in underlying reactive endometriotic-type stroma Note: The criteria for early clear cell carcinoma and intraepithelial clear cell carcinoma are not well-defined 3. This lesion is rarely seen alone; more commonly associated with invasive clear cell carcinoma, which may be evident with extensive sampling; in some cases, the level of atypia seen in atypical endometriosis without clear cell carcinoma may significantly overlap that of endometriosis with early clear cell carcinoma, precluding a definitive diagnosis (in worrisome cases, submitting the entire specimen for histologic examination is advised)

	Endometriotic Cyst with Epithelial Atypia	**Endometriotic Cyst with Early Clear Cell Carcinoma/Intraepithelial Clear Cell Carcinoma**
Special studies	Immunohistochemistry is of limited use in this differential	Immunohistochemistry is of limited use in this differential
Treatment	Hormonal suppression or bilateral salpingo-oophorectomy as for usual endometriosis; for oophorectomy specimens with equivocal histologic findings, additional follow-up is recommended; for cystectomy specimens with equivocal histologic findings, clinical correlation is suggested to assess the completeness of excision and need for oophorectomy	Insufficient data; consider staging
Prognosis	Benign; endometriosis may persist	In stage IA (comprehensively staged), 5 y survival ~90% (limited data)

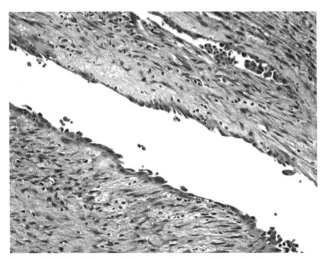

Figure 5.48.1 Endometriotic cyst with atypia. The lesion shows a flattened cyst lining with atypia and focal hobnail features; scant lymphocytes and neutrophils are present in the stroma.

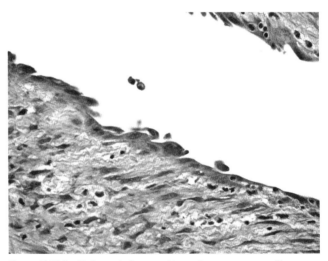

Figure 5.48.2 Endometriotic cyst with atypia, same case as *Figure 5.48.1*. The lesion shows focal nuclear atypia with smudgy chromatin; note scattered inflammatory cells in underlying stroma.

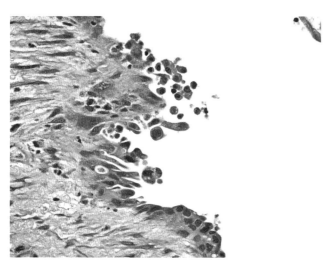

Figure 5.48.3 Endometriotic cyst with atypia. The lesion shows minimal stratification and some cellular discohesion, atypia with smudged chromatin, and few neutrophils and nuclear debris within underlying fibrous reactive stroma.

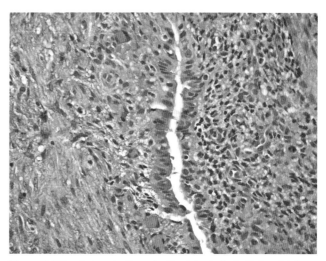

Figure 5.48.4 Endometriotic cyst with minimal atypia. Endometriotic stroma is present.

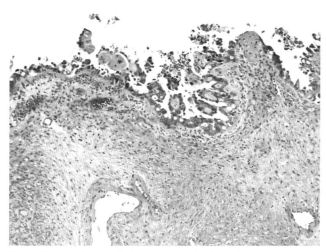

Figure 5.48.5 Endometriotic cyst with early clear cell carcinoma. Note early papillary formation with hyalinized stromal cores within the papillae.

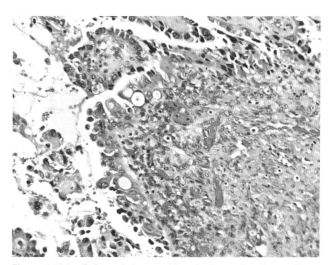

Figure 5.48.6 Endometriotic cyst with early clear cell carcinoma. Note early papillary formation and underlying endometriotic stroma.

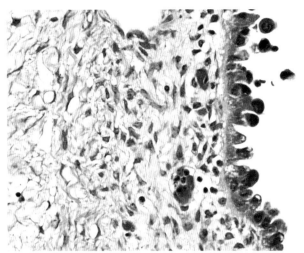

Figure 5.48.7 Endometriotic cyst with marked nuclear atypia adjacent to early clear cell carcinoma (not shown). The cells display hobnail features, nuclear enlargement and rounding, and hyperchromasia. These features are highly concerning for clear cell carcinoma but are insufficient for an unequivocal diagnosis in isolation.

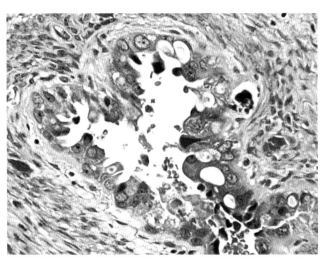

Figure 5.48.8 Endometriotic cyst with intraepithelial clear cell carcinoma.

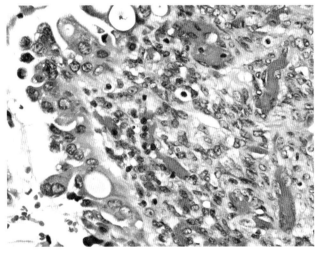

Figure 5.48.9 Endometriotic cyst with intraepithelial clear cell carcinoma. Note underlying endometriotic stroma (same focus as in *Fig. 5.48.6*).

	Pregnancy Luteoma	Steroid (Lipid) Cell Tumor
Age	Mean about 30 y	Mean 43 y
Location	Within ovarian stroma	Within ovary
Symptoms	Occurs in late pregnancy	Pelvic pain, dysmenorrhea
Signs	Androgenic manifestations in 25%; often incidental finding at cesarean section	Estrogenic manifestations in 50%; virilization in 10%; rarely Cushing syndrome, hypercalcemia
Etiology	A pseudoneoplastic condition, which may be derived from hCG-induced proliferation of luteinized stromal cells; origin from luteinized granulosa and theca cells is an alternative hypothesis	Likely derived from luteinized ovarian stromal cells; occasional association with von Hippel-Lindau syndrome
Gross and histology	1. Multifocal and bilateral in 30%; multinodular cut surface with red-brown nodules; occasionally may be solitary; mean 6-7 cm 2. Luteinized cells in diffuse sheets constituting nodules that compress intervening ovarian stroma (Figs. 5.49.1 and 5.49.2); may form follicle-like spaces 3. Large polygonal cells have small round nuclei, abundant eosinophilic cytoplasm, and small prominent nucleoli (Figs. 5.49.3-5.49.5); occasional mild nuclear atypia; mitotic figures may be present; in the setting of a unilateral solitary lesion during pregnancy, unequivocal distinction from an ovarian steroid cell tumor arising in a pregnant woman may not be possible	1. Unilateral; extraovarian spread in 20%; mean 8.4 cm; size >7 cm correlates with malignancy 2. Diffuse sheets of large eosinophilic cells, generally without nodularity (Figs. 5.49.6 and 5.49.7); smooth interface with surrounding ovarian stroma; no follicle-like spaces 3. Large, rounded to polygonal cells with abundant vacuolated clear or eosinophilic cytoplasm (Figs. 5.49.7 and 5.49.8); may resemble normal adrenal cortex; central round nucleus with small nucleoli and minimal atypia; mitotically inactive; 40% contain cytoplasmic lipofuscin; sparse stroma with prominent vasculature (Figs. 5.49.7 and 5.49.8); fibrosis may be present; variants include stromal luteoma, stromal Leydig cell tumor, and hilar Leydig cell tumor
Special studies	Not useful in this differential	Not useful in this differential
Treatment	None needed	Unilateral salpingo-oophorectomy or hysterectomy and bilateral salpingo-oophorectomy; staging
Prognosis	Usually regresses spontaneously after pregnancy	Malignant in approximately one-third

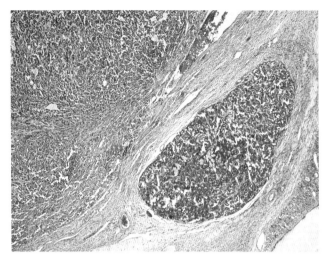

Figure 5.49.1   Pregnancy luteoma at low magnification displays a nodular appearance with variably sized smoothly contoured nodules of solid sheets of eosinophilic cells within the ovarian stroma.

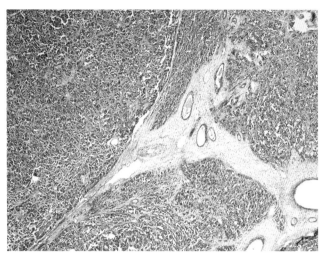

Figure 5.49.2   Pregnancy luteoma at low magnification displays a nodular appearance with variably sized smoothly contoured nodules of solid sheets of eosinophilic cells within the ovarian stroma; note edema of ovarian stroma between the nodules.

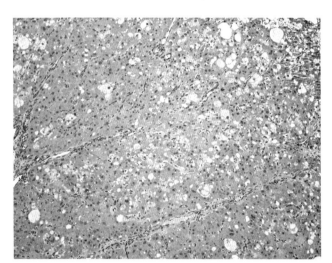

Figure 5.49.3   Pregnancy luteoma with sheets of cells with small nuclei and abundant eosinophilic or clear and vacuolated cytoplasm. Some of the microcystic change represents early follicle-like space formation.

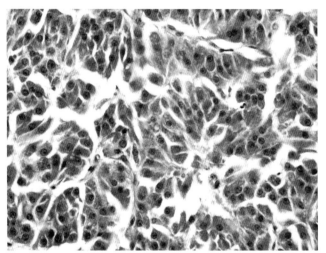

Figure 5.49.4   Pregnancy luteoma displays small round nuclei with evenly dispersed and slightly pale chromatin, small nucleoli, and abundant eosinophilic granular cytoplasm.

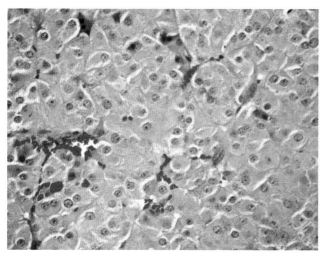

Figure 5.49.5 Pregnancy luteoma displays small round nuclei with small prominent nucleoli, evenly dispersed chromatin, and abundant eosinophilic cytoplasm; note fine capillary vascular network between tumor cell aggregates.

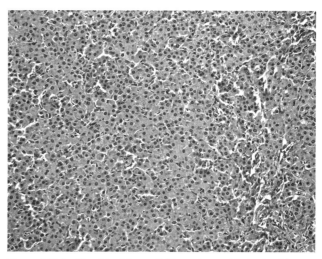

Figure 5.49.6 Steroid cell tumor, lipid-poor type, with sheets of large eosinophilic cells.

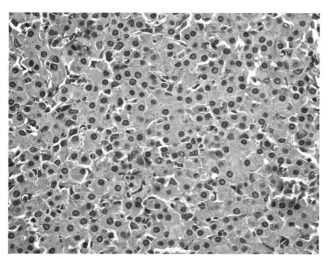

Figure 5.49.7 Steroid cell tumor, lipid-poor type, higher magnification of *Figure 5.49.6*, with large polygonal cells with round nuclei and evenly dispersed chromatin; note fine capillary vascular network.

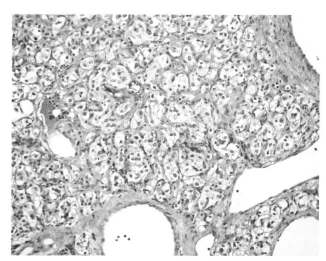

Figure 5.49.8 Steroid cell tumor, lipid-rich type, with nested pattern of large polygonal cells with clear vacuolated cytoplasm; note prominent vasculature.

	Stromal Hyperthecosis	Metastatic Signet Ring Cell Carcinoma
Age	Postmenopausal	Mean 45 y
Location	Ovarian stroma	Ovarian stroma
Symptoms	Asymptomatic; may present with endocrine manifestations	Abdominal swelling/pain
Signs	Often virilizing	Primary tumor diagnosed prior to ovarian involvement in one-third; ascites in 43%; 12% asymptomatic; 10% pregnant
Etiology	Common accompaniment of aging (seen in one-third of women >65 y); hyperinsulinism and overproduction of androgens may play a role; associated with HAIR-AN syndrome (hyperandrogenism, insulin resistance, diabetes, acanthosis nigricans)	Secondary ovarian involvement by signet ring cell carcinoma; primary carcinoma of stomach, appendix, or breast are most common but may also be from a variety of other gastrointestinal sites
Gross and histology	1. Bilateral ovaries normal sized or moderately enlarged (up to 7 cm), yellow-white cut surface 2. Highly cellular spindle cell ovarian stroma with luteinized cells diffusely scattered singly or in small aggregates *(Figs. 5.50.1-5.50.3)*	1. Bilateral in three-fourths; mean 10.4 cm; nodular, solid cut surface, with small cysts in one-third; hemorrhage or necrosis often seen 2. Diffuse cellular sheets, nodular aggregates, compact and hypocellular areas; intervening ovarian stroma may appear normal or may be luteinized, edematous, and fibrotic or contain extracellular mucin dissecting or in pools; carcinoma cells on occasion are sparsely distributed *(Figs. 5.50.4 and 5.50.5)*; thus, the low-power magnification appearance can resemble stromal hyperplasia/hyperthecosis (particularly, at the time of frozen section) because of predominance of abundant reactive stromal proliferation and scattered distribution of individual tumor cells without obvious nest or gland formation
	3. Absence of gland formation	3. Signet ring cells occur singly, in small groups, as larger closely packed aggregates, or as single files *(Figs. 5.50.6-5.50.8)*; tubular-glandular pattern displays small- to medium-sized glands, sometimes with flattened lining cells; solid cords or intestinal-like glands also occur
	4. Proliferating stromal cells have ovoid nuclei and scant cytoplasm; luteinized cells display small round nuclei (without atypia) and abundant pale, clear, or eosinophilic cytoplasm *(Figs. 5.50.2 and 5.50.3)*; if luteinized stromal cells show signet ring–like change, then intracellular mucin will be absent	4. Nuclei are often crescent shaped and may be small and pale with deceptively bland features *(Figs. 5.50.7 and 5.50.8)* or hyperchromatic and moderately pleomorphic; cytoplasmic mucin *(Fig. 5.50.8)* may appear as a clear or basophilic vacuole, occasionally eosinophilic; pale cytoplasm and basal nuclei may mimic Sertoli differentiation in tubular pattern; poorly differentiated cells without obvious mucin often are present and occasionally predominate *(Fig. 5.50.6)*

	Stromal Hyperthecosis	**Metastatic Signet Ring Cell Carcinoma**
Special studies	• Luteinized cells are negative for EMA and cytokeratins; positive for inhibin, calretinin, and SF-1 • Mucin and PAS negative	• Positive for cytokeratins and EMA; negative for inhibin, calretinin, and SF-1 • For breast, GATA3, GCDFP, mammaglobin may be useful • For lower GI, CK7/CK20 and SATB2 may be useful • Mucin and PAS can highlight mucin within signet ring cells
Treatment	None	As per advanced stage/metastatic carcinoma of the respective sites
Prognosis	Benign	Generally poor; majority die within 1 y, as per advanced stage/metastatic carcinoma of the respective sites

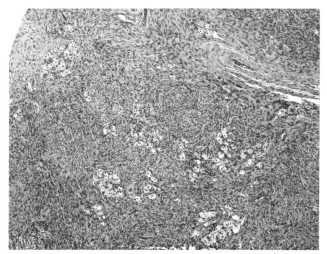

Figure 5.50.1 Stromal hyperthecosis displays hypercellular ovarian stroma with scattered clusters of pale luteinized stromal cells.

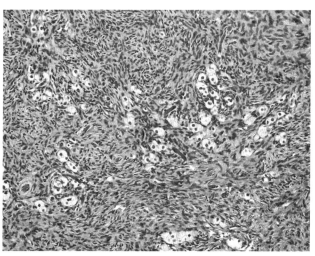

Figure 5.50.2 Stromal hyperthecosis with highly cellular ovarian stroma containing clustered luteinized stromal cells with abundant pale to clear vacuolated cytoplasm (higher magnification of *Fig. 5.50.1*).

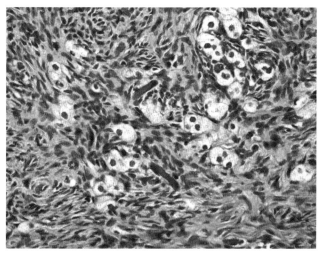

Figure 5.50.3 Stromal hyperthecosis with luteinized stromal cells with small round bland nuclei and abundant vacuolated cytoplasm (higher magnification of *Fig. 5.50.2*).

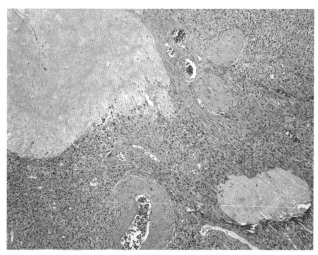

Figure 5.50.4 Metastatic signet ring cell carcinoma at low magnification displays preservation of ovarian architecture with tumor cells permeating between intact corpora albicantia and large thick-walled vessels.

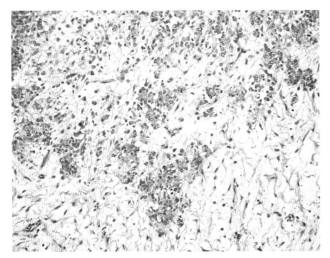

Figure 5.50.5   Metastatic signet ring cell carcinoma with clusters of infiltrating carcinoma cells in a background of edematous ovarian stroma.

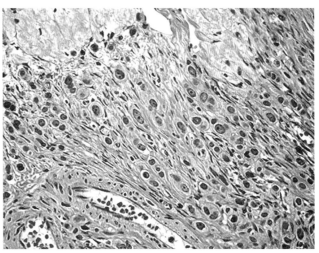

Figure 5.50.6   Same case as *Figure 5.50.4* with tumor cells infiltrating the ovarian stroma singly and showing enlarged, hyperchromatic, and atypical nuclei. Classic intracytoplasmic mucin-filled vacuoles are not shown in this photograph, but some of these morphologic features can resemble stromal hyperthecosis.

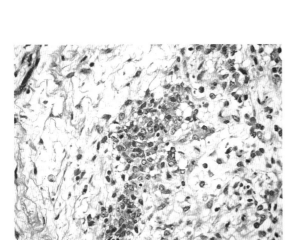

Figure 5.50.7   Same case as *Figure 5.50.5* with clustered infiltrating carcinoma cells with deceptively bland nuclear features in an edematous background.

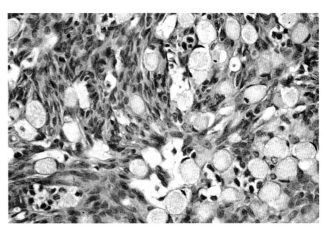

Figure 5.50.8   Metastatic signet ring cell carcinoma with individual cells in fibromatous stroma. Note the presence of intracytoplasmic mucin and deceptively bland peripheral nuclei.

	Mesonephric-like Carcinoma	Endometrioid Carcinoma
Age	Mean/median 60-62 y	Mean 55-58 y
Location	Within ovary	Within ovary
Symptoms	Pelvic pain, abdominal distention, abnormal uterine bleeding	Pelvic pain, increasing abdominal girth, bloating, early satiety, vaginal bleeding, urinary symptoms
Signs	Pelvic/abdominal mass	Pelvic/abdominal mass, ascites
Etiology	KRAS and NRAS mutations; subset with PIK3CA and ARID1A mutations; rare case with CTNNB1 mutation; no KIT mutations; associated with endometriosis, which may be admixed with tumor, and adenofibromas; minority associated with serous borderline tumor, mucinous borderline tumor (MBT), endometrioid borderline tumor, or low-grade serous carcinoma; histogenesis unclear but appears more likely to reflect aberrant differentiation of a müllerian tumor rather than true mesonephric origin	Endometriosis; germline MLH1, MSH2, PMS2, or MSH6 mutation (Lynch syndrome); PTEN, β-catenin (CTNNB1), KRAS, ARID1A, and PIK3CA mutations
Gross and histology	1. About two-thirds present in stage I; about one-third bilateral; mean/median size 10-11 cm; solid and cystic, papillary excrescences may be seen 2. Confluent invasive well-differentiated glandular architecture *(Figs. 5.51.1-5.51.5)* with ductal, tubular *(Figs. 5.51.1-5.51.3)*, papillary *(Figs. 5.51.1 and 5.51.6)*, and less commonly retiform, sieve-like and solid patterns; spindle cell, glomeruloid and sex cord–like elements may be seen *(Figs. 5.51.4 and 5.51.5)*; features overlap with female adnexal tumor of wolffian origin (see Section 7.10) and endometrioid carcinoma; may be mixed with more typical müllerian neoplasms of mucinous, endometrioid, or serous type; rarely contain a sarcomatous component ("mesonephric-like carcinosarcoma"); mesonephric remnants not usually identified *(Fig. 5.51.1)*	1. Usually unilateral, stage I in almost half; mean 15 cm; cystic or cystic and solid; cysts contain dark brown viscous fluid (old blood with mucus); papillary or nodular growths arise from cyst lining 2. Most are architecturally well differentiated with confluent glandular epithelial proliferation resembling endometrial endometrioid carcinoma; cribriform, papillary, glandular, and occasionally solid patterns *(Figs. 5.51.8-5.51.10)*; less commonly with infiltrative pattern of glands, nests, and solid masses with jagged edges

Mesonephric-like Carcinoma	Endometrioid Carcinoma
3. Cuboidal to columnar cells, minimal cytoplasm *(Figs. 5.51.4-5.51.6)*; nuclei may have atypia, grooves, or pseudoinclusions creating a resemblance to thyroid papillary carcinoma *(Fig. 5.51.7)*; eosinophilic colloid-like material may be seen in lumen *(Fig. 5.51.3)*; no mucinous differentiation (although MBT may be associated)	3. Tall columnar epithelium with sharp luminal gland margins, round to ovoid nuclei with hyperchromasia, prominent nucleoli *(Fig. 5.51.10)*; mitotic activity variable, often high; necrosis may occasionally be present; mucinous differentiation can be present
4. Squamous differentiation not reported but may be present in an associated endometrioid component; endometriosis commonly present	4. Squamous differentiation in half; adenofibromatous component often present; associated endometriosis is present in majority and often shows atypia, hyperplasia, and other features reflecting origin within endometriotic cyst or associated endometrioid borderline tumor
5. No secretory or ciliated differentiation; sex cord–like elements may occasionally be seen *(Fig. 5.51.5)*	5. Secretory, ciliated, and sertoliform variants may occur
Special studies	GATA3+, TTF1+, calretinin+, CD10+ (luminal staining), PAX8+, CK7+; often c-KIT+ (limited data); usually ER/PR–, WT1–, CEA–, p16–	GATA3–, TTF1–, calretinin variable, CD10 variable; CK7 patchy or diffuse; CK20 negative, focal, or patchy (extent of CK7 > CK20); CDX-2 negative (may be [+] in a component with mucinous differentiation); SATB2–; ER/PR+; usually PAX8+
Treatment	Insufficient data to treat differently from endometrioid carcinoma	Staging (with debulking when indicated); chemotherapy (in neoadjuvant or adjuvant setting) except for low-grade stage IA/B; hormonal suppression often used for recurrence
Prognosis	71% 5-y disease-specific survival based on limited data	Stage I >90% survival

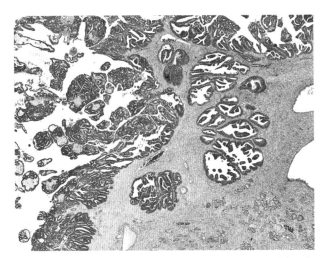

Figure 5.51.1 Mesonephric-like carcinoma with papillary and ductal patterns; note mesonephric-like remnants at **lower right**.

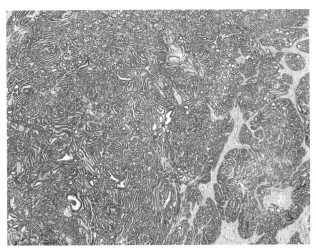

Figure 5.51.2 Same case as *Figure 5.51.1* with tubular pattern.

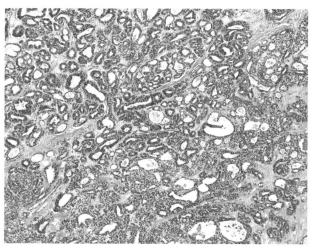

Figure 5.51.3 Same case as *Figure 5.51.1* with tubular pattern and foci of solid growth toward **bottom left**. Note occasional tubules containing eosinophilic material.

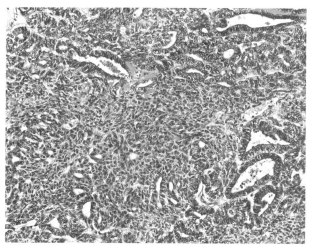

Figure 5.51.4 Same case as *Figure 5.51.1* with solid and spindle cell growth in **center** and tubules toward periphery. Note sharp luminal borders, ovoid nuclei, and high nuclear-to-cytoplasmic ratio.

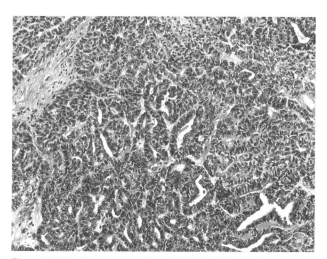

Figure 5.51.5 Same case as *Figure 5.51.1* displaying hollow and solid tubules with sex cord–like pattern.

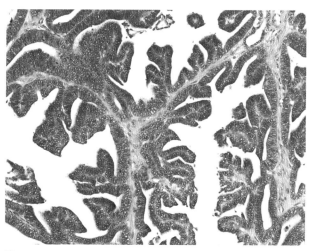

Figure 5.51.6 Same case as *Figure 5.51.1* with papillary pattern lined by cuboidal to columnar cells displaying ovoid nuclei and high nuclear-to-cytoplasmic ratio.

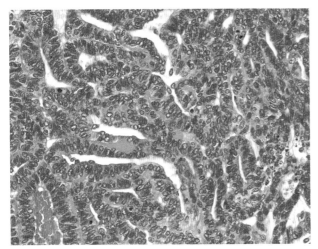

Figure 5.51.7   Same case as *Figure 5.51.1* with tubules lined by columnar cells with ovoid nuclei displaying chromatin clearing and occasional pseudoinclusions creating a resemblance to papillary thyroid carcinoma.

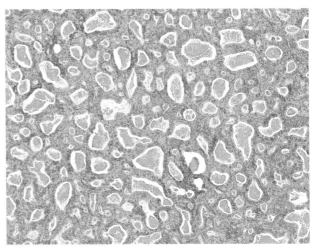

Figure 5.51.8   Endometrioid carcinoma with confluent glandular pattern resembling the tubular pattern of mesonephric-like carcinoma. Note eosinophilic material within glands.

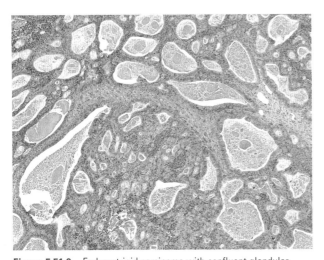

Figure 5.51.9   Endometrioid carcinoma with confluent glandular pattern and areas of cribriform growth.

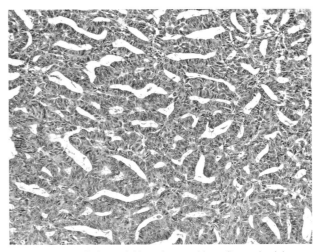

Figure 5.51.10   Endometrioid carcinoma with confluent glandular pattern, tall columnar epithelium, and sharp luminal margins.

SUGGESTED READINGS

5.1-5.5

Birge O, Bakir MS, Karadag C, et al. Risk factors that increase recurrence in borderline ovarian cancers. *Am J Transl Res.* 2021;13:8438-8449.

Camatte S, Morice P, Atallah D, et al. Lymph node disorders and prognostic value of nodal involvement in patients treated for a borderline ovarian tumor: an analysis of a series of 42 lymphadenectomies. *J Am Coll Surg.* 2002;195:332-338.

Cheng EJ, Kurman RJ, Wang M, et al. Molecular genetic analysis of ovarian serous cystadenomas. *Lab Invest.* 2004;84:778-784.

Cheung AN, Ellenson LH, Gilks CB, et al. Tumours of the ovary. In: WHO Classification of Tumours Editorial Board, eds. *Female Genital Tumours, WHO Classification of Tumours.* 5th ed. International Agency for Research on Cancer; 2020:31-167.

Chui MH, Xing D, Zeppernick F, et al. Clinicopathologic and molecular features of paired cases of metachronous ovarian serous borderline tumor and subsequent serous carcinoma. *Am J Surg Pathol.* 2019;43.1402-1472.

Djordjevic B, Clement-Kruzel S, Atkinson NE, Malpica A. Nodal endosalpingiosis in ovarian serous tumors of low malignant potential with lymph node involvement: a case for a precursor lesion. *Am J Surg Pathol.* 2010;34:1442-1448.

Djordjevic B, Malpica A. Lymph node involvement in ovarian serous tumors of low malignant potential: a clinicopathologic study of thirty-six cases. *Am J Surg Pathol.* 2010;34:1-9.

Dube V, Roy M, Plante M, et al. Mucinous ovarian tumors of mullerian type: an analysis of 17 cases including borderline tumors and intraepithelial, microinvasive, and invasive carcinomas. *Int J Gynecol Pathol.* 2005;24:138-146.

Esselen KM, Ng S-K, Hua Y, et al. Endosalpingiosis as it relates to tubal, ovarian and serous neoplastic tissues: an immunohistochemical study of tubal and Mullerian antigens. *Gynecol Oncol.* 2014;132:316-321.

Fan Y, Zhang YF, Wang MY, et al. Influence of lymph node involvement or lymphadenectomy on prognosis of patients with borderline ovarian tumors: a systematic review and meta-analysis. *Gynecol Oncol.* 2021;162:797-803.

Hannibal CG, Vang R, Junge J, et al. A nationwide study of serous "borderline" ovarian tumors in Denmark 1978–2002: centralized pathology review and overall survival compared with the general population. *Gynecol Oncol.* 2014;134:267-273.

Hannibal CG, Frederiksen K, Vang R, et al. Risk of specific types of ovarian cancer after borderline ovarian tumors in Denmark: a nationwide study. *Int J Cancer.* 2020;147:990-995.

Hannibal CG, Vang R, Junge J, et al. A nationwide study of ovarian serous borderline tumors in Denmark 1978–2002. Risk of recurrence, and development of ovarian serous carcinoma. *Gynecol Oncol.* 2017;144:174-180.

Hogg R, Scurry J, Kim S-N, et al. Microinvasion links ovarian serous borderline tumor and grade 1 invasive carcinoma. *Gynecol Oncol.* 2007;106:44-51.

Hunter SM, Anglesio MS, Sharma R, et al. Copy number aberrations in benign ovarian serous tumors: a case for reclassification? *Clin Cancer Res.* 2011;17:7273-7282.

Kobel M, Bak J, Bertelsen BI, et al. Ovarian carcinoma histotype determination is highly reproducible and is improved through the use of immunohistochemistry. *Histopathology.* 2014;64:1004-1013.

Kraus JA, Seidman JD. The relationship between papillary infarction and microinvasion in ovarian atypical proliferative ("borderline") serous and seromucinous tumors. *Int J Gynecol Pathol.* 2010;29:303-309.

Maniar KP, Wang Y, Visvanathan K, et al. Evaluation of microinvasion and lymph node involvement in ovarian serous borderline/atypical proliferative serous tumors: a morphologic and immunohistochemical analysis of 37 cases. *Am J Surg Pathol.* 2014;38:743-755.

McKenney JK, Balzer BL, Longacre TA. Lymph node involvement in ovarian serous tumors of low malignant potential (borderline tumors): pathology, prognosis and proposed classification. *Am J Surg Pathol.* 2006;30:614-624.

McKenney JK, Balzer BL, Longacre TA. Patterns of stromal invasion in ovarian serous tumors of low malignant potential (borderline tumors): a reevaluation of the concept of stromal microinvasion. *Am J Surg Pathol.* 2006;30:1209-1221.

Nagamine M, Mikami Y. Ovarian seromucinous tumors: pathogenesis, morphologic spectrum, and clinical issues. *Diagnostics (Basel).* 2020;10:77.

Rambau PF, McIntyre JB, Taylor J, et al. Morphologic reproducibility, genotyping, and immunohistochemical profiling do not support a category of seromucinous carcinoma of the ovary. *Am J Surg Pathol.* 2017;41:685-695.

Rollins SE, Young RH, Bell DA. Autoimplants in serous borderline tumors of the ovary: a clinicopathologic study of 30 cases of a process to be distinguished from serous adenocarcinoma. *Am J Surg Pathol.* 2006;30:457-462.

Rutgers JL, Scully RE. Ovarian mullerian mucinous papillary cystadenomas of borderline malignancy: a clinicopathologic analysis. *Cancer.* 1988;61:340-348.

Seidman JD, Bell D, Gilks CB, et al. Tumours of the ovary: serous tumours. In: Kurman RJ, Carcangiu ML, Herrington S, et al., eds. *WHO Classification of Tumours of the Female Reproductive Organs.* IUCC; 2014:17-24.

Seidman JD, Mehrotra A. Benign ovarian serous tumors: a re-evaluation and proposed reclassification of serous "cystadenomas" and "cystadenofibromas." *Gynecol Oncol.* 2005;96:395-401.

Seidman JD, Ronnett BM, Shih IM, Cho KR, Kurman RJ. Epithelial tumors of the ovary. In: Kurman RJ, Ellenson LH, Ronnett BM, eds. *Blaustein's Pathology of the Female Genital Tract.* 7th ed. Springer; 2019:841-966.

Seidman JD, Soslow RA, Vang R, et al. Borderline ovarian tumors: diverse contemporary viewpoints on terminology and diagnostic criteria with illustrative images. *Hum Pathol.* 2004;35:918-933.

Shappell HW, Riopel MA, Smith Sehdev AE, et al. Diagnostic criteria and behavior of ovarian seromucinous (endocervical-type mucinous and mixed cell-type) tumors: atypical proliferative (borderline) tumors, intraepithelial, microinvasive, and invasive carcinomas. *Am J Surg Pathol.* 2002;26:1529-1541.

Talia KL, Parra-Herran C, McCluggage WG. Ovarian mucinous and seromucinous neoplasms: problematic aspects and modern diagnostic approach. *Histopathology.* 2022;80(2):255-278. doi.org/10.1111/his.14399

Taylor J, McCluggage WG. Ovarian seromucinous carcinoma: report of a series of a newly categorized and uncommon neoplasm. *Am J Surg Pathol.* 2015;39:983-992.

Tsang YT, Deavers MT, Sun CC, et al. KRAS (but not BRAF) mutations in ovarian serous borderline tumour are associated with recurrent low-grade serous carcinoma. *J Pathol.* 2013;231:449-456.

Vang R, Hannibal CG, Junge J, et al. Long-term behavior of serous borderline tumors subdivided into atypical proliferative tumors and non-invasive low-grade carcinomas: a population-based clinicopathologic study of 942 cases. *Am J Surg Pathol.* 2017;41:725-737.

Vang R, Shih IM, Kurman RJ. Ovarian low grade and high grade serous carcinoma: pathogenesis, clinicopathologic and molecular biological features, and diagnostic problems. *Adv Anat Pathol.* 2009;16:267-282.

Yemelyanova A, Mao TL, Nakayama N, et al. Low-grade serous carcinoma of the ovary displaying a macropapillary pattern of invasion. *Am J Surg Pathol.* 2008;32:1800-1806.

5.6-5.9 (See also references for sections 5.1-5.5)

Ahn G, Folkins AK, McKenney JK, Longacre TA. Low-grade serous carcinoma of the ovary. *Am J Surg Pathol.* 2016;40:1165-1176.

Assem H, Rambau PF, Lee S, et al. High grade endometrioid carcinoma of the ovary. *Am J Surg Pathol.* 2018;42:534-544.

Bell DA. Low grade serous tumors of ovary. *Int J Gynecol Pathol.* 2014;33:348-356.

Bodurka DC, Deavers MT, Tian C, et al. Reclassification of serous ovarian carcinoma by a 2-tier system. *Cancer.* 2012;118:3087-3094.

Cancer Genome Atlas Research Network. Integrated genomic analyses of ovarian carcinoma. *Nature.* 2011;474:609-615.

El Hallani S, Arora R, Lin DI, et al. Mixed endometrioid adenocarcinoma and müllerian adenosarcoma of the uterus and ovary: clinicopathologic characterization with emphasis on its distinction from carcinosarcoma. *Am J Surg Pathol.* 2021;45:374-383.

Espinosa I, Gallardo A, D'Angelo E, et al. Simultaneous carcinomas of the breast and ovary: utility of PAX-8, WT-1, and GATA3 for distinguishing independent primary tumors from metastases. *Int J Gynecol Pathol.* 2015;34:257-265.

Fader AN, Java J, Ueda S, et al. Survival in women with grade 1 serous ovarian carcinoma. *Obstet Gynecol.* 2013;122:225-232.

Garg K, Levine DA, Olvera N, et al. BRCA1 immunohistochemistry in a molecularly characterized cohort of ovarian high-grade serous carcinomas. *Am J Surg Pathol.* 2013;37:138-146.

Geyer JT, Lopez-Garcia M, Sanchez-Estevez C, et al. Pathogenetic pathways in ovarian endometrioid adenocarcinoma: a molecular study of 29 cases. *Am J Surg Pathol.* 2009;33:1157-1163.

Hollis RL, Thomson JP, Stenley B, et al. Molecular stratification of endometrioid ovarian carcinoma predicts clinical outcome. *Nat Commun.* 2020;11:4995.

Imamura H, Ohishi Y, Aman M, et al. Ovarian high grade serous carcinoma with a noninvasive growth pattern simulating a serous borderline tumor. *Hum Pathol.* 2015;46:1455-1463.

Lim D, Murali R, Murray MP, et al. Morphological and immunohistochemical reevaluation of tumors initially diagnosed as ovarian endometrioid carcinoma with emphasis on high-grade tumors. *Am J Surg Pathol.* 2016;40:302-312.

Malpica A, Deavers MT, Lu K, et al. Grading ovarian serous carcinoma using a two-tier system. *Am J Surg Pathol.* 2004;28:496-504.

Malpica A, Deavers MT, Tornos C, et al. Interobserver and intraobserver variability of a two-tier system for grading ovarian serous carcinoma. *Am J Surg Pathol.* 2007;31:1168-1174.

Rauh-Hain J, Diver EJ, Clemmer JT, et al. Carcinosarcoma of the ovary compared to papillary serous ovarian carcinoma: a SEER analysis. *Gynecol Oncol.* 2013;131:46-51.

Schlosshauer PW, Deligdish L, Penault-Llorca F, et al. Loss of p16 INK4A expression in low grade ovarian serous carcinomas. *Int J Gynecol Pathol.* 2011;30:22-29.

Seidman JD, Savage J, Krishnan J, Vang R, Kurman RJ. Intratumoral heterogeneity accounts for apparent progression of noninvasive serous tumors to invasive low-grade serous carcinoma: a study of 30 low-grade serous tumors of the ovary in 18 patients with peritoneal carcinomatosis. *Int J Gynecol Pathol.* 2020;39:43-54.

Silva EG, Deavers MT, Malpica A. Patterns of low-grade serous carcinoma with emphasis on the nonepithelial-lined spaces pattern of invasion and the disorganized orphan papillae. *Int J Gynecol Pathol.* 2010;29:507-512.

Slomovitz B, Gourley C, Carey MS, et al. Low-grade serous ovarian cancer: state of the science. *Gynecol Oncol.* 2020;156:715-725.

Soslow RA, Han G, Park KJ, et al. Morphologic patterns associated with BRCA1 and BRCA2 genotype in ovarian carcinoma. *Mod Pathol.* 2012;25:625-636.

Storey DJ, Rush R, Stewart M, et al. Endometrioid epithelial ovarian cancer: 20 years of prospectively collected data from a single center. *Cancer.* 2008;112:2211-2220.

Vang R, Gown AM, Farinola M, et al. p16 expression in primary ovarian mucinous and endometrioid tumors and metastatic adenocarcinomas in the ovary: utility for identification of metastatic HPV-related endocervical adenocarcinomas. *Am J Surg Pathol.* 2007;31:653-663.

Vang R, Levine DA, Soslow RA, et al. Molecular alterations of TP53 are a defining feature of ovarian high-grade serous carcinoma: a rereview of cases lacking TP53 mutations in The Cancer Genome Atlas Ovarian Study. *Int J Gynecol Pathol.* 2016;35:48-55.

Vang R, Shih IM, Kurman RJ. Ovarian low grade and high grade serous carcinoma: pathogenesis, clinicopathologic and molecular biological features, and diagnostic problems. *Adv Anat Pathol.* 2009;16:267-282.

Zarei S, Wang Y, Jenkins SM, et al. Clinicopathologic, immunohistochemical, and molecular characteristics of ovarian serous carcinoma with mixed morphologic features of high-grade and low-grade serous carcinoma. *Am J Surg Pathol.* 2020;44:316-328.

Zhao C, Bratthauer GL, Barner R, et al. Comparative analysis of alternative and traditional immunohistochemical markers for the distinction of ovarian sertoli cell tumor from endometrioid tumors and carcinoid tumor: a study of 160 cases. *Am J Surg Pathol.* 2007;31:255-266.

5.10-5.12

Hada T, Miyamoto M, Ishibashi H, et al. Prognostic similarity between ovarian mucinous carcinoma with expansile invasion and ovarian mucinous borderline tumor: a retrospective analysis. *Medicine.* 2021;100:e26895.

Irving JA, Clement PB. Recurrent intestinal mucinous borderline tumors of the ovary: a report of 5 cases causing problems in diagnosis, including distinction from mucinous carcinoma. *Int J Gynecol Pathol.* 2014;33:156-165.

Khunamornpong S, Settakorn J, Sukpan K, et al. Mucinous tumor of low malignant potential ("borderline" or "atypical proliferative" tumor) of the ovary: a study of 171 cases with the assessment of intraepithelial carcinoma and microinvasion. *Int J Gynecol Pathol.* 2011;30:218-230.

Khunamornpong S, Settakorn J, Sukpan K, et al. Primary ovarian mucinous adenocarcinoma of intestinal type: a clinicopathologic study of 46 cases. *Int J Gynecol Pathol.* 2014;33:176-185.

Kim K-R, Lee H-I, Lee S-K, et al. Is stromal microinvasion in primary mucinous ovarian tumors with "mucin granuloma" true invasion? *Am J Surg Pathol.* 2007;31:546-554.

Matsuo K, Machida H, Mandelbaum RS, et al. Mucinous borderline ovarian tumor versus invasive well-differentiated mucinous ovarian cancer: difference in characteristics and outcomes. *Gynecol Oncol.* 2019;153:230-237.

Ronnett BM, Kajdacsy-Balla A, Gilks CB, et al. Mucinous borderline tumors: points of general agreement, and persistent controversies regarding nomenclature, diagnostic criteria and behavior. *Hum Pathol.* 2004;35:949-960.

Tabrizi AD, Kalloger SE, Kobel M, et al. Primary ovarian mucinous carcinoma of intestinal type: significance of pattern of invasion and immunohistochemical expression profile in a series of 31 cases. *Int J Gynecol Pathol.* 2010;29:99-107.

Vang R, Gown AM, Barry TS, et al. Cytokeratins 7 and 20 in primary and metastatic mucinous tumors of the ovary: analysis of coordinate immunohistochemical expression profiles and staining distribution in 179 cases. *Am J Surg Pathol.* 2006;30:1130-1139.

Vang R, Gown AM, Wu LSF, et al. Immunohistochemical expression of CDX2 in primary ovarian mucinous tumors and metastatic mucinous carcinomas involving the ovary: comparison with CK20 and correlation with coordinate expression of CK7. *Mod Pathol.* 2006;19:1421-1428.

Zaino RJ, Brady MF, Lele SM, et al. Advanced stage mucinous adenocarcinoma is both rare and highly lethal: a Gynecologic Oncology Group study. *Cancer.* 2011;117:554-562.

5.13-5.18

Bell KA, Kurman RJ. A clinicopathologic analysis of atypical proliferative (borderline) tumors and well-differentiated endometrioid adenocarcinomas of the ovary. *Am J Surg Pathol.* 2000;24:1465-1479.

Chen S, Leitao MM, Tornos C, et al. Invasion patterns in stage I endometrioid and mucinous ovarian carcinomas: a clinicopathologic analysis emphasizing favorable outcomes in carcinomas without destructive stromal invasion and the occasional malignant course of carcinomas with limited destructive stromal invasion. *Mod Pathol.* 2005;18:903-911.

Conlon N, Schultheis AM, Piscuoglio S, et al. A survey of DICER1 hotspot mutations in ovarian and testicular sex cord-stromal tumors. *Mod Pathol.* 2015;28:1603-1612.

De Paolis ED, Paragliola RM, Concolino P. Spectrum of DICER1 germline pathogenic variants in ovarian Sertoli–Leydig cell tumor. *J Clin Med.* 2021;10:1845.

Farinola MA, Gown AM, Judson K, et al. Estrogen receptor alpha and progesterone receptor expression in ovarian adult granulosa cell tumors and Sertoli-Leydig cell tumors. *Int J Gynecol Pathol.* 2007;26:375-382.

Gavrielides MA, Ronnett BM, Vang R, Sheikhzadeh F, Seidman JD. Selection of representative histologic slides in interobserver reproducibility studies: insights from expert review for ovarian carcinoma subtype classification. *J Pathol Inform.* 2021;12:15.

Geyer JT, López-García MA, Sánchez-Estevez C, et al. Pathogenetic pathways in ovarian endometrioid adenocarcinoma: a molecular study of 29 cases. *Am J Surg Pathol.* 2009;33:1157-1163.

Judson K, McCormick C, Vang R, et al. Women with undiagnosed colorectal adenocarcinomas presenting with ovarian metastases: clinicopathologic features and comparison with women having known colorectal adenocarcinomas and ovarian involvement. *Int J Gynecol Pathol.* 2008;27:182-190.

Kubecek O, Laco J, Petera J, et al. The pathogenesis, diagnosis, and management of metastatic tumors to the ovary: a comprehensive review. *Clin Exp Metastasis.* 2017;34:295-307.

Lewis MR, Deavers MT, Silva EG, et al. Ovarian involvement by metastatic colorectal adenocarcinoma: still a diagnostic challenge. *Am J Surg Pathol.* 2006;30:177-184.

Meagher NS, Wang L, Rambau PF, et al. A combination of the immunohistochemical markers CK7 and SATB2 is highly sensitive and specific for distinguishing primary ovarian mucinous tumors from colorectal and appendiceal metastases. *Mod Pathol.* 2019;32:1834-1846.

Misir A, Sur M. Sertoliform endometrioid carcinoma of the ovary: a potential diagnostic pitfall. *Arch Pathol Lab Med.* 2007;131:979-981.

Oliva E, Alvarez T, Young RH. Sertoli cell tumors of the ovary: a clinicopathologic and immunohistochemical study of 54 cases. *Am J Surg Pathol.* 2005;29:143-156.

Ordi J, Schammel DP, Rasekh L, et al. Sertoliform endometrioid carcinomas of the ovary: a clinicopathologic and immunohistochemical study of 13 cases. *Mod Pathol.* 1999;12:933-940.

Paula ADC, da Silva EM, Segura SE, et al. Genomic profiling of primary and recurrent adult granulosa cell tumors of the ovary. *Mod Pathol.* 2020;33:1606-1617.

Roze J, Monroe G, Kutzera J, et al. Whole genome analysis of ovarian granulosa cell tumors reveals tumor heterogeneity and a high-grade TP53-specific subgroup. *Cancers (Basel).* 2020;12:1308.

Shah SP, Kobel M, Senz J, et al. Mutation of FOXL2 in granulosa-cell tumors of the ovary. *N Engl J Med.* 2009;360:2719-2729.

Tornos C, Silva EG, Ordonez NG, et al. Endometrioid carcinoma of the ovary with a prominent spindle-cell component, a source of diagnostic confusion: a report of 14 cases. *Am J Surg Pathol.* 1995;19:1343-1353.

Uzan C, Berretta R, Rolla M, et al. Management and prognosis of endometrioid borderline tumors of the ovary. *Surg Oncol.* 2012;21:178-184.

Vang R, Gown AM, Barry TS, et al. Cytokeratins 7 and 20 in primary and metastatic mucinous tumors of the ovary: analysis of coordinate immunohistochemical expression profiles and staining distribution in 179 cases. *Am J Surg Pathol.* 2006;30:1130-1139.

Vang R, Ronnett BM. A practical approach to mucinous tumors involving the ovary: distinction of primary from metastatic tumors and prediction of site of origin for metastases of uncertain origin. *Pathol Case Rev.* 2006;11:18-30.

Wang WC, Lai YC. Molecular pathogenesis in granulosa cell tumor is not only due to somatic FOX L2 mutation. *J Ovarian Res.* 2014;7:88.

Woodbeck R, Kelemen LE, Kobel M. Ovarian endometrioid carcinoma misdiagnosed as mucinous carcinoma: an underrecognized problem. *Int J Gynecol Pathol.* 2019;38:568-575.

Yemelyanova AV, Vang R, Judson K, et al. Distinction of primary and metastatic mucinous tumors involving the ovary: analysis of size and laterality data by primary site with reevaluation of an algorithm for tumor classification. *Am J Surg Pathol.* 2008;32:128-138.

5   OVARY

Young RH, Prat J, Scully RE. Ovarian endometrioid carcinomas resembling sex cord-stromal tumors. A clinicopathological analysis of 13 cases. *Am J Surg Pathol.* 1982;6:513-522.

Zhao C, Barner R, Vinh TN, et al. SF-1 is a diagnostically useful immunohistochemical marker and comparable to other sex cord-stromal tumor markers for the differential diagnosis of ovarian sertoli cell tumor. *Int J Gynecol Pathol.* 2008;27:507-514.

Zhao C, Bratthauer G, Barner R, et al. Comparative analysis of alternative and traditional immunohistochemical markers for the distinction of ovarian Sertoli cell tumor from endometrioid tumors and carcinoid tumor: a study of 160 cases. *Am J Surg Pathol.* 2007;31:255-266.

Zhao C, Bratthauer GL, Barner R, et al. Diagnostic utility of WT1 immunostaining in ovarian Sertoli cell tumor. *Am J Surg Pathol.* 2007;31:1378-1386.

5.19-5.23

Anglesio MS, Bashashati A, Wang YK, et al. Multifocal endometriotic lesions associated with cancer are clonal and carry a high mutation burden. *J Pathol.* 2015;236:201-209.

Bennett JA, Dong F, Young RH, et al. Clear cell carcinoma of the ovary: evaluation of prognostic parameters based on a clinicopathological analysis of 100 cases. *Histopathology.* 2015;66:808-815.

Delair D, Han G, Irving JA, et al. HNF1-beta in ovarian carcinomas with serous and clear cell change. *Int J Gynecol Pathol.* 2013;32:541-546.

DeLair D, Oliva E, Köbel M, et al. Morphologic spectrum of immunohistochemically characterized clear cell carcinoma of the ovary: a study of 155 cases. *Am J Surg Pathol.* 2011;35:36-44.

Han G, Gilks CB, Leung S, et al. Mixed ovarian epithelial carcinomas with clear cell and serous components are variants of high-grade serous carcinoma: an interobserver correlative and immunohistochemical study of 32 cases. *Am J Surg Pathol.* 2008;32:955-964.

Hodroj K, Stevovic A, Attignon V, et al. Molecular characterization of ovarian yolk sac tumor (OYST). *Cancers (Basel).* 2021;13:220.

Lim D, Ip PPC, Cheung ANY, et al. Immunohistochemical comparison of ovarian and uterine endometrioid carcinoma, endometrioid carcinoma with clear cell change, and clear cell carcinoma. *Am J Surg Pathol.* 2015;39:1061-1069.

Nogales FF, Prat J, Schuldt M, et al. Germ cell tumour growth patterns originating from clear cell carcinomas of the ovary and endometrium: a comparative immunohistochemical study favouring their origin from somatic stem cells. *Histopathology.* 2018;72:634-647.

Oliver KE, Brady WE, Birrer M, et al. An evaluation of progression free survival and overall survival of ovarian cancer patients with clear cell carcinoma versus serous carcinoma treated with platinum therapy: an NRG Oncology/Gynecologic Oncology Group experience. *Gynecol Oncol.* 2017;147:243-249.

Ramalingam P, Malpica A, Silva EG, et al. The use of cytokeratin 7 and EMA in differentiating ovarian yolk sac tumors from endometrioid and clear cell carcinomas. *Am J Surg Pathol.* 2004;28:1499-1505.

Sangoi AR, Soslow RA, Teng NN, et al. Ovarian clear cell carcinoma with papillary features: a potential mimic of serous tumor of low malignant potential. *Am J Surg Pathol.* 2008;32:269-274.

Veras E, Mao TL, Ayhan A, et al. Cystic and adenofibromatous clear cell carcinomas of the ovary: distinctive tumors that differ in their pathogenesis and behavior: a clinicopathologic analysis of 122 cases. *Am J Surg Pathol.* 2009;33:844-853.

Willis BC, Sloan EA, Atkins KA, Stoler MH, Mills AM. Mismatch repair status and PD-L1 expression in clear cell carcinomas of the ovary and endometrium. *Mod Pathol.* 2017;30:1622-1632.

Young RH, Wong A, Stall JN. Yolk sac tumor of the ovary: a report of 150 cases and review of the literature. *Am J Surg Pathol.* 2022;46(3):309-325.

Zhao C, Wu LS, Barner R. Pathogenesis of ovarian clear cell adenofibroma, atypical proliferative (borderline) tumor, and carcinoma: clinicopathologic features of tumors with endometriosis or adenofibromatous components support two related pathways of tumor development. *J Cancer.* 2011;2:94-106.

5.24 and 5.25

Austin RM, Norris HJ. Malignant Brenner tumor and transitional cell carcinoma of the ovary: a comparison. *Int J Gynecol Pathol.* 1987;6:29-39.

Cuatrecasas M, Catasus L, Palacios J, et al. Transitional cell tumors of the ovary: a comparative clinicopathologic, immunohistochemical, and molecular genetic analysis of Brenner tumors and transitional cell carcinomas. *Am J Surg Pathol.* 2009;33:556-567.

Hallgrimsson J, Scully RE. Borderline and malignant Brenner tumours of the ovary. A report of 15 cases. *Acta Pathol Microbiol Scand A.* 1972;233:56-66.

Khedmati F. Exploring the histogenesis of ovarian mucinous and transitional cell (Brenner) tumors: a study of 120 tumors. *Arch Pathol Lab Med.* 2008;132:1753-1760.

Kuhn E, Ayhan A, Shih I-M, et al. Ovarian Brenner tumor: a morphologic and immunohistochemical analysis suggesting an origin from fallopian tube epithelium. *Eur J Cancer.* 2013;49:3839-3849.

Kuhn E, Ayhan A, Shih I-M, et al. The pathogenesis of atypical proliferative Brenner tumor: an immunohistochemical and molecular genetic analysis. *Mod Pathol.* 2014;27:231-237.

Lin DI, Killian JK, Venstrom JM, Ramkissoon SH, Ross JS, Elvin JA. Recurrent urothelial carcinoma-like FGFR3 genomic alterations in malignant Brenner tumors of the ovary. *Mod Pathol.* 2021;34:983-993.

Miles PA, Norris HJ. Proliferative and malignant Brenner tumors of the ovary. *Cancer.* 1972;30:174-186.

Ricotta G, Maulard A, Genestie C, et al. Brenner borderline ovarian tumor: a case series and literature review. *Ann Surg Oncol.* 2021;28:6714-6720.

Roth LM, Dallenbach-Hellweg G, Czernobilsky B. Ovarian Brenner tumors. I. Metaplastic, proliferating, and of low malignant potential. *Cancer.* 1985;56:582-591.

Seidman JD, Yemelyanova A, Zaino RJ, et al. The fallopian tube-peritoneal junction: a potential site of carcinogenesis. *Int J Gynecol Pathol.* 2011;30:4-11.

Uzan C, Dufeau-Lefebvre M, Fauvet R, et al. Management and prognosis of borderline ovarian Brenner tumors. *Int J Gynecol Cancer.* 2012;22:1332-1336.

5.26

Alwazzan AB, Popowich S, Dean E, et al. Pure immature teratoma of the ovary in adults: thirty year experience of a single tertiary care center. *Int J Gynecol Cancer.* 2015;25:1616-1622.

Heskett MB, Sanborn JZ, Boniface C, et al. Multiregion exome sequencing of ovarian immature teratomas reveals 2N near-diploid genomes, paucity of somatic mutations, and extensive allelic imbalances shared across mature, immature, and disseminated components. *Mod Pathol.* 2020;33:1193-1206.

Norris HJ, Zirkin HJ, Benson WL. Immature (malignant) teratoma of the ovary: a clinical and pathologic study of 58 cases. *Cancer.* 1976;37:2359-2372.

O'Connor DM, Norris HJ. The influence of grade on the outcome of stage I ovarian immature (malignant) teratomas and the reproducibility of grading. *Int J Gynecol Pathol.* 1994;13:283-289.

Poulos C, Cheng L, Zhang S, et al. Analysis of ovarian teratomas for isochromosome 12p: evidence supporting a dual histogenetic pathway for teratomatous elements. *Mod Pathol.* 2006;19:766-771.

Snir OL, DeJoseph M, Wong S, et al. Frequent homozygosity in both mature and immature teratomas: a shared genetic basis of tumorigenesis. *Mod Pathol.* 2017;30:1467-1475.

Zhao T, Liu Y, Wang X, et al. Ovarian cystectomy in the treatment of apparent early-stage immature. Teratoma. *J Int Med Res.* 2017;45:771-780.

5.27 and 5.28

Conlon N, Schultheis AM, Piscuoglio S, et al. A survey of DICER1 hotspot mutations in ovarian and testicular sex cord-stromal tumors. *Mod Pathol.* 2015;28:1603-1612.

Irving JA, et al. Cellular fibromas of the ovary: a report of 75 cases including 40 mitotically active tumors emphasizing their distinction from fibrosarcoma. *Am J Surg Pathol.* 2006;30:929-938.

Kim JY, Na K, Kim HS. Clinicopathological characteristics of mitotically-active cellular fibroma of the ovary: a single-institutional experience. *Anticancer Res.* 2017;37:2557-2564.

Nasioudis D, Mastroyannis SA, Haggerty AF, Ko EM, Latif NA. Ovarian Sertoli-Leydig and granulosa cell tumor: comparison of epidemiology and survival outcomes. *Arch Gynecol Obstet.* 2020;302:481-486.

Oost EE, Charles A, Choong CS, et al. Ovarian sex cord-stromal tumors in patients with probable or confirmed germline DICER1 mutations. *Int J Gynecol Pathol.* 2015;34:266-274.

Roth LM, Czernobilsky B. Perspectives on pure ovarian stromal neoplasms and tumor-like proliferations of the ovarian stroma. *Am J Surg Pathol.* 2011;35:e15-e33.

Schultz KAP, Harris A, Messinger Y, et al. Ovarian tumors related to intronic mutations in DICER1: a report from the international ovarian and testicular stromal tumor registry. *Fam Cancer.* 2016;15:105-110.

Seidman JD. Unclassified ovarian gonadal stromal tumors: a clinicopathologic study of 32 cases. *Am J Surg Pathol.* 1996;20:699-706.

Simpson JL, Michael H, Roth LM. Unclassified sex cord-stromal tumors of the ovary: a report of eight cases. *Arch Pathol Lab Med.* 1998;122:52-55.

Stewart CJR, Alexiadis M, Crook ML, et al. An immunohistochemical and molecular analysis of problematic and unclassified sex cord-stromal tumors. *Hum Pathol.* 2013;44:2774-2781.

Young RH, Scully RE. Ovarian Sertoli-Leydig cell tumors. A clinicopathological analysis of 207 cases. *Am J Surg Pathol.* 1985;9:543-569.

5.29-5.34

Ali RH, Seidman JD, Luk M, et al. Transitional cell carcinoma of the ovary is related to high grade serous carcinoma and is distinct from malignant Brenner tumor. *Int J Gynecol Pathol.* 2012;31:499-506.

Ganesan R, Hirschowitz L, Baltrušaitytė I, et al. Luteinized adult granulosa cell tumor—a series of 9 cases: revisiting a rare variant of adult granulosa cell tumor. *Int J Gynecol Pathol.* 2011;30:452-459.

Irving JA, Young RH. Granulosa cell tumors of the ovary with a pseudopapillary pattern: a study of 14 cases of an unusual morphologic variant emphasizing their distinction from transitional cell neoplasms and other papillary ovarian tumors. *Am J Surg Pathol.* 2008;32:581-586.

Jarboe EA, Hirschowitz SL, Geiersbach KB, et al. Juvenile granulosa cell tumors: immunoreactivity for CD99 and Fli-1 and EWSR1 translocation status: a study of 11 cases. *Int J Gynecol Pathol.* 2014;33:11-15.

Jelinic P, Ricca J, Oudenhove EV, et al. Immune-active microenvironment in small cell carcinoma of the ovary, hypercalcemic type: rationale for immune checkpoint blockade. *J Natl Cancer Inst.* 2018;110:787-790.

McCluggage WG, Young RH. Ovarian Sertoli Leydig cell tumors with pseudoendometrioid tubules (pseudoendometrioid Sertoli-Leydig cell tumors). *Am J Surg Pathol.* 2007;31:592-597.

Mulvany NJ, Riley CB. Granulosa cell tumors of unilocular cystic type. *Pathology.* 1997;29:348-353.

Nakashima N, Young RH, Scully RE. Androgenic granulosa cell tumors of the ovary. A clinicopathologic analysis of 17 cases and review of the literature. *Arch Pathol Lab Med.* 1984;108:786-791.

Parishaa G, Ariba Z, Pranab D, et al. Juvenile granulosa cell tumor of the ovary: a comprehensive clinicopathologic analysis of 15 cases. *Ann Diagn Pathol.* 2021;52:151721.

Seidman JD. Young RH, Dickersin GR, Scully RE. Juvenile granulosa cell tumor of the ovary. A clinicopathological analysis of 125 cases. *Am J Surg Pathol.* 1984;8:575-596.

Stall JN, Young RH. Granulosa cell tumors of the ovary with prominent thecoma-like foci: a report of 16 cases emphasizing the ongoing utility of the reticulin stain in the modern era. *Int J Gynecol Pathol.* 2019;38:143-150.

Watkins JC, Young RH. Follicle cysts of the ovary: a report of 30 cases of a common benign lesion emphasizing its unusual clinical and pathologic aspects. *Int J Gynecol Pathol.* 2021;40:359-368.

Young RH, Oliva E, Scully RE. Luteinized adult granulosa cell tumors of the ovary: a report of 4 cases. *Int J Gynecol Pathol.* 1994;13:302-310.

Young RH, Oliva E, Scully RE. Small cell carcinoma of the ovary, hypercalcemic type: a clinicopathological analysis of 150 cases. *Am J Surg Pathol.* 1994;18:1102-1116.

Zaloudek C, Norris HJ. Granulosa tumors of the ovary in children: a clinical and pathologic study of 32 cases. *Am J Surg Pathol.* 1982;6:503-512.

5.35-5.39 (See also references for sections 5.29-5.34)

Chang RJ, Reuther J, Gandhi I, et al. Sex cord tumor with annular tubules–like histologic pattern in adult granulosa cell tumor: case report of a hitherto unreported morphologic variant. *Int J Surg Pathol.* 2021;29:433-437.

Hayes MC, Scully RE. Ovarian steroid cell tumors (not otherwise specified). A clinicopathological analysis of 63 cases. *Am J Surg Pathol.* 1987;11:835-845.

Jones MW, Harri R, Dabbs DJ, et al. Immunohistochemical profile of steroid cell tumor of the ovary: a study of 14 cases and a review of the literature. *Int J Gynecol Pathol.* 2010;29:315-320.

Oliva E, Alvarez T, Young RH. Sertoli cell tumors of the ovary: a clinicopathologic and immunohistochemical study of 54 cases. *Am J Surg Pathol.* 2005;29:143-156.

Preda VA, Chitoni M, Talbot D, Reed N, Grossman AB. Primary ovarian carcinoid: extensive clinical experience with an underrecognized uncommon entity. *Int J Gynecol Cancer.* 2018; 28:466-471.

Scully RE. Sex cord tumor with annular tubules: a distinctive ovarian tumor of the Peutz-Jeghers syndrome. *Cancer.* 1970;25:1107-1121.

Soga J, Osaka M, Yakuwa Y. Carcinoids of the ovary: an analysis of 329 reported cases. *J Exp Clin Cancer Res.* 2000;19:271-280.

Warnnissorn M, Watkins JC, Young RH. Dysgerminoma of the ovary: an analysis of 140 cases emphasizing unusual microscopic findings and resultant diagnostic problems. *Am J Surg Pathol.* 2021;45:1009-1027.

Young RH, Welch WR, Dickersin GR, et al. Ovarian sex cord tumor with annular tubules: review of 74 cases including 27 with Peutz-Jeghers syndrome and four with adenoma malignum of the cervix. *Cancer.* 1982;50:1384-1402.

Zhao C, Bratthauer GL, Barner R, et al. Comparative analysis of alternative and traditional immunohistochemical markers for the distinction of ovarian Sertoli cell tumor from endometrioid tumors and carcinoid tumor: a study of 160 cases. *Am J Surg Pathol.* 2007;31:255-266.

5.40

Kosari F, Daneshbod Y, Parwaresch R, et al. Lymphomas of the female genital tract: a study of 186 cases and review of the literature. *Am J Surg Pathol.* 2005;29:1512-1520.

Vang R, Medeiros LJ, Fuller GN, et al. Non-Hodgkin's lymphoma involving the gynecologic tract. A review of 88 cases. *Adv Anat Pathol.* 2001;8:200-217.

Vang R, Medeiros LJ, Warnke RA, et al. Ovarian non-Hodgkin's lymphoma: a clinicopathologic study of eight primary cases. *Mod Pathol.* 2001;14:1093-1099.

Young RH, Oliva E, Scully RE. Small cell carcinoma of the ovary, hypercalcemic type: a clinicopathologic analysis of 150 cases. *Am J Surg Pathol.* 1994;18:1102-1116.

5.41-5.46

Anglesio MS, Wang YK, Maassen M, et al. Synchronous endometrial and ovarian carcinomas: evidence of clonality. *J Natl Cancer Inst.* 2016;108(6):djv428.

Bassiouny D, Ismiil N, Dube V, et al. Comprehensive clinicopathologic and updated immuno-histochemical characterization of primary ovarian mucinous carcinoma. *Int J Surg Pathol.* 2018;26:306-317.

Elishaev E, Gilks CB, Miller D, et al. Synchronous and metachronous endocervical and ovarian neoplasms: evidence supporting interpretation of the ovarian neoplasms as metastatic endocervical adenocarcinomas simulating primary ovarian surface epithelial neoplasms. *Am J Surg Pathol.* 2005;29:281-294.

Gagnon Y, Tetu B. Ovarian metastases of breast carcinoma: a clinicopathologic study of 59 cases. *Cancer.* 1989;64:892-898.

Kubecek O, Laco J, Spacek J, et al. The pathogenesis, diagnosis, and management of metastatic tumors to the ovary: a comprehensive review. *Clin Exp Metastasis.* 2017;34:295-307.

Lewis MR, Deavers MT, Silva EG, et al. Ovarian involvement by metastatic colorectal adenocarcinoma: still a diagnostic challenge. *Am J Surg Pathol.* 2006;30:177-184.

Lin KY, Miller DS, Bailey AA, et al. Ovarian involvement in endometrioid adenocarcinoma of the uterus. *Gynecol Oncol.* 2015;138:532-535.

Meriden Z, Yemelyanova AV, Vang R, et al. Ovarian metastases of pancreaticobiliary tract adenocarcinomas: analysis of 35 cases with emphasis on the ability of metastases to simulate primary ovarian mucinous tumors. *Am J Surg Pathol.* 2011;35:276-288.

Ramus SJ, Elmasry K, Luo Z, et al. Predicting clinical outcome in patients diagnosed with synchronous ovarian and endometrial cancer. *Clin Cancer Res.* 2008;14:5840-5848.

Ronnett BM, Yemelyanova AV, Vang R, et al. Endocervical adenocarcinomas with ovarian metastases: analysis of 29 cases with emphasis on minimally invasive cervical tumors and the ability of the metastases to simulate primary ovarian neoplasms. *Am J Surg Pathol.* 2008;32:1835-1853.

Soliman PT, Slomovitz BM, Broaddus RR, et al. Synchronous primary cancers of the endometrium and ovary: a single institution review of 84 cases. *Gynecol Oncol.* 2004;94:456-462.

Stewart CJR, Crum CP, McCluggage WG, et al. Guidelines to aid in the distinction of endometrial and endocervical carcinomas, and the distinction of independent primary carcinomas of the endometrium and adnexa from metastatic spread between these and other sites. *Int J Gynecol Pathol.* 2019;38(Suppl 1):S75-S92.

Tornos C, Soslow R, Chen S, et al. Expression of WT1, Ca 125, and GCDFP-15 as useful markers in the differential diagnosis of primary ovarian carcinoma versus metastatic breast cancer to the ovary. *Am J Surg Pathol.* 2005;29:1482-1489.

Vang R, Gown AM, Barry TS, et al. Cytokeratins 7 and 20 in primary and metastatic mucinous tumors of the ovary: analysis of coordinate immunohistochemical expression profiles and staining distribution in 179 cases. *Am J Surg Pathol.* 2006;30:1130-1139.

Vang R, Ronnett BM. A practical approach to mucinous tumors involving the ovary: distinction of primary from metastatic tumors and prediction of site of origin for metastases of uncertain origin. *Pathol Case Rev.* 2006;11:18-30.

Yemelyanova A, Vang R, Judson K, et al. Distinction of primary and metastatic tumors involving the ovary: analysis of size and laterality data by primary site with reevaluation of an algorithm for tumor classification. *Am J Surg Pathol.* 2008;32:128-138.

Zaino R, Whitney C, Brady MF, et al. Simultaneously detected endometrial and ovarian carcinomas—a prospective clinicopathologic study of 74 cases: a gynecologic oncology group study. *Gynecol Oncol.* 2001;83:355-362.

5.47

Bhatt A, Mishra S, Prabhu R, et al. Can low grade PMP be divided into prognostically distinct subgroups based on histological features? A retrospective study and the importance of using the appropriate classification. *Eur J Surg Oncol.* 2018;44:1105-1111.

Carr NJ, Cecil TD, Mohamed F, et al. A consensus for classification and pathologic reporting of pseudomyxoma peritonei and associated appendiceal neoplasia: the results of the Peritoneal Surface Oncology Group International (PSOGI) modified delphi process. *Am J Surg Pathol.* 2016;40:14-26.

Cheung AN, Kim K-R, Longacre TA, Malpica A, eds. Tumours of the peritoneum. In: WHO Classification of Tumours Editorial Board, eds. *Female Genital Tumours, WHO Classification of Tumours.* 5th ed. International Agency for Research on Cancer; 2020:175-214.

Ronnett BM, Kurman RJ, Zahn CM, et al. Pseudomyxoma peritonei in women: a clinicopathologic analysis of 30 cases with emphasis on site of origin, prognosis, and relationship to ovarian mucinous tumors of low malignant potential. *Hum Pathol.* 1995;26:509-524.

Rufian-Andujar B, Valanzuela-Molina F, Rufian-Pena S, et al. From the Ronnett to the PSOGI classification system for pseudomyxoma peritonei: a validation study. *Ann Surg Oncol.* 2021;28:2819-2827.

Vang R, Gown AM, Barry TS, et al. Cytokeratins 7 and 20 in primary and metastatic mucinous tumors of the ovary: analysis of coordinate immunohistochemical expression profiles and staining distribution in 179 cases. *Am J Surg Pathol.* 2006;30:1130-1139.

5.48 (See also references for sections 5.19-5.23)

Anglesio MS, Bashashati A, Wang YK, et al. Multifocal endometriotic lesions associated with cancer are clonal and carry a high mutation burden. *J Pathol.* 2015;236:201-209.

Maier IM, Maier AC, Crisan A, Puscasiu L. Clinical and pathological significance of cellular atypia in endometriosis. *Medicina.* 2021;57:453.

Samartzis EP, Noske A, Dedes KJ, et al. ARID1A mutations and PI3K/AKT pathway alterations in endometriosis and endometriosis associated ovarian carcinomas. *Int J Mol Sci.* 2013;14:18824-18849.

Seidman JD. Prognostic importance of hyperplasia and atypia in endometriosis. *Int J Gynecol Pathol.* 1996;15:1-9.

Sevilla IN, Linde FM, Sanchez MDPM, Arense JJ, Diaz AN, Ferrer MLS. Prognostic importance of atypical endometriosis with architectural hyperplasia versus cytologic atypia in endometriosis-associated ovarian cancer. *J Gynecol Oncol.* 2019;30:e63.

5.49-5.50

Burandt E, Young RH. Pregnancy luteoma: a study of 20 cases on the occasion of the 50th anniversary of its description by Dr. William H. Sternberg, with an emphasis on the common presence of follicle-like spaces and their diagnostic implications. *Am J Surg Pathol.* 2014;38:239-244.

Deavers MT, Malpica A, Ordonez NG, et al. Ovarian steroid cell tumors: an immunohistochemical study including a comparison of calretinin with inhibin. *Int J Gynecol Pathol.* 2003;22:162-167.

Hayes MC, Scully RE. Ovarian steroid cell tumors (not otherwise specified). A clinicopathological analysis of 63 cases. *Am J Surg Pathol.* 1987;11:835-845.

Kiyokawa T, Young RH, Scully RE. Krukenberg tumors of the ovary: a clinicopathologic analysis of 120 cases with emphasis on their variable pathologic manifestations. *Am J Surg Pathol.* 2006;30:277-299.

Roth LM, Czernobilsky B. Perspectives on pure ovarian stromal neoplasms and tumor-like proliferations of the ovarian stroma. *Am J Surg Pathol.* 2011;35:e15-e33.

Vang R, Ronnett BM. A practical approach to mucinous tumors involving the ovary: distinction of primary from metastatic tumors and prediction of site of origin for metastases of uncertain origin. *Pathol Case Rev.* 2006;11:18-30.

Young RH. From Krukenberg to today; the ever present problems posed by metastatic tumors in the ovary. Part I: historical perspective, general principles, mucinous tumors including the Krukenberg tumor. *Adv Anat Pathol.* 2006;13:205-227.

Young RH. From Krukenberg to today; the ever present problems posed by metastatic tumors in the ovary. Part II. *Adv Anat Pathol.* 2007;14:149-177.

5.51

DaSilva EM, Fix DJ, Senastiao APM, et al. Mesonephric and mesonephric-like carcinomas of the female genital tract:

molecular characterization including cases with mixed histology and matched metastases. *Mod Pathol.* 2021;34:1570-1587.

Deolet E, Arora I, Van Dorpe J, et al. Extrauterine mesonephric-like neoplasms: expanding the morphologic spectrum. *Am J Surg Pathol.* 2022;46:124-133.

McCluggage WG, Vosmikova H, Laco J. Ovarian combined low-grade serous and mesonephric-like adenocarcinoma: further evidence for a mullerian origin of mesonephric-like adenocarcinoma. *Int J Gynecol Pathol.* 2020;39:84-92.

McFarland M, Quick CM, McCluggage WG. Hormone receptor-negative, thyroid transcription factor 1-positive uterine and ovarian adenocarcinomas: report of a series of mesonephric-like adenocarcinomas. *Histopathology.* 2016;68:1013-1020.

Mirkovic J, McFarland M, Garcia E, et al. Targeted genomic profiling reveals recurrent KRAS mutations in mesonephric-like adenocarcinomas of the female genital tract. *Am J Surg Pathol.* 2018;42:227-233.

Pors J, Segura S, Chiu DS, et al. Clinicopathologic characteristics of mesonephric adenocarcinomas and mesonephric-like adenocarcinomas in the gynecologic tract: a multi-institutional study. *Am J Surg Pathol.* 2021;45:498-506.

6

Peritoneum/Omentum*

---

*Please refer to the Preface for the Ovary chapter regarding changes in serous borderline tumor terminology

	Noninvasive Implants Associated With Serous Borderline Tumor	Endosalpingiosis
Age	50 y (median)	Premenopausal
Location	Peritoneal surfaces, including omentum	Peritoneal surfaces (including omentum) and/or lymph nodes
Symptoms	Symptoms attributable to ovarian mass	Asymptomatic
Signs	May appear as small nodules on peritoneal surfaces or be a microscopic finding	No gross lesion; microscopic finding
Etiology	Data suggest that some implants may be clonally related to the primary ovarian tumor; they are thought to become detached from the tumor and directly implant onto peritoneal surfaces as opposed to being of independent primary peritoneal origin	Unknown; may be due to exfoliated fallopian tube epithelium that implants onto peritoneal surfaces (analogous to mechanism for endometriosis); a coexisting ovarian serous borderline tumor and/or implants can be present
Histology	1. Variable number of foci present on serosal surfaces or within septa between lobules of adipose tissue in the omentum *(Fig. 6.1.1)* 2. Lesional foci composed of glands, papillae, and/or solid nests *(Fig. 6.1.2)* 3. Lesional foci may be isolated or crowded 4. Lesional epithelium may display complexity with stratification and detached clusters; consists of bland tubal-type cells *(Figs. 6.1.3-6.1.6)* 5. Implants can be purely epithelial-type or have desmoplastic stroma (the latter often present as a plaque on surface of serosa) *(Fig. 6.1.1)* 6. Psammoma bodies can be present	1. Variable number of foci present on serosal surfaces or within septa between lobules of adipose tissue in the omentum 2. Lesional foci composed of only glands (rare limited intraglandular papillary formations can be seen) *(Fig. 6.1.7)* 3. Lesional foci usually isolated but occasionally can have some degree of crowding *(Fig. 6.1.8)* 4. No epithelial complexity; glands lined by single layer of bland tubal-type cells *(Fig. 6.1.9)* 5. No desmoplasia 6. Psammoma bodies can be present *(Fig. 6.1.10)*
Special studies	Of no use for this differential diagnosis	Of no use for this differential diagnosis
Treatment	Surgical excision, including debulking of all grossly visible disease	No therapy necessary
Prognosis	The presence of implants qualifies for advanced stage serous borderline tumor (usually stage II or III); women with noninvasive implants have a significantly higher risk for subsequent development of low-grade serous carcinoma compared with women who have serous borderline tumors without implants	Benign; in the setting of an ovarian serous borderline tumor, endosalpingiosis does not result in upstaging or affect prognosis

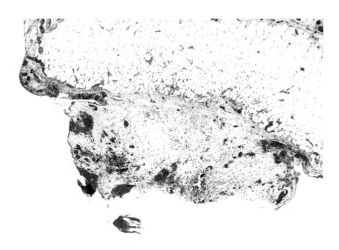

Figure 6.1.1   Desmoplastic noninvasive implant of serous borderline tumor with plaque-like involvement of surface of the omentum.

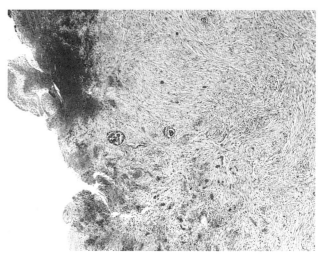

Figure 6.1.2   Desmoplastic noninvasive implant of serous borderline tumor. The glands at low-power magnification can resemble endosalpingiosis.

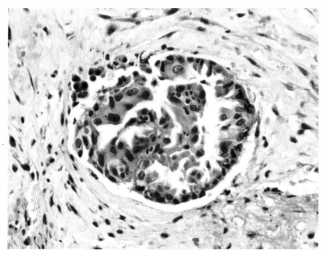

Figure 6.1.3   Desmoplastic noninvasive implant of serous borderline tumor. The glands exhibit some degree of epithelial stratification.

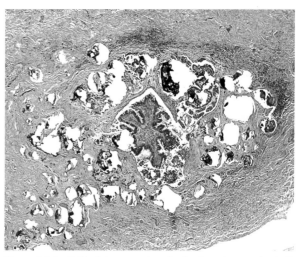

Figure 6.1.4   Epithelial-type noninvasive implant of serous borderline tumor with papillae.

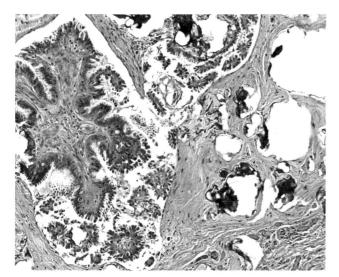

Figure 6.1.5   Epithelial-type noninvasive implant of serous borderline tumor with papillae (*higher-power magnification of Fig. 6.1.4*). Note the presence of psammoma bodies.

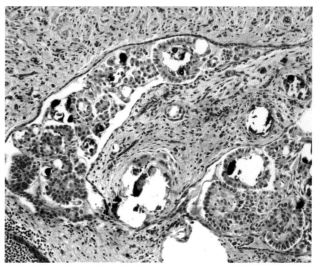

Figure 6.1.6   Epithelial-type noninvasive implant of serous borderline tumor with papillae and detached epithelial clusters.

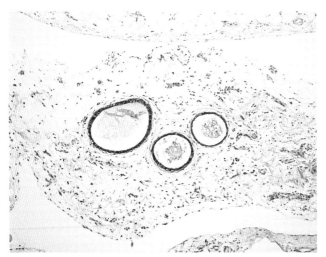

Figure 6.1.7   Endosalpingiosis with simple and cystically dilated glands.

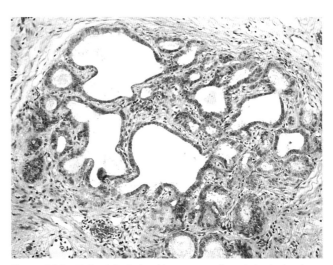

Figure 6.1.8   Endosalpingiosis with more crowding of glands than is typically seen.

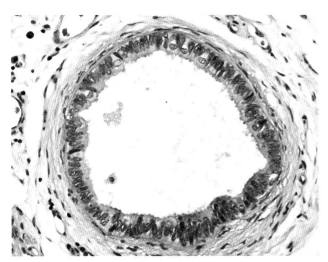

Figure 6.1.9   Endosalpingiosis composed of a single layer of tubal-type epithelium, including ciliated cells.

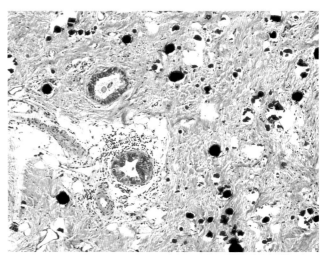

Figure 6.1.10   Endosalpingiosis with numerous psammoma bodies.

	Noninvasive Implants Associated With Serous Borderline Tumor	Low-Grade Serous Carcinoma (Invasive Implants)
Age	50 y (median)	50 y (median)
Location	Peritoneal surfaces, including omentum	Peritoneal surfaces, including omentum
Symptoms	Symptoms attributable to ovarian mass	Symptoms attributable to ovarian mass
Signs	May appear as small nodules on peritoneal surfaces or be a microscopic finding	May appear as small nodules on peritoneal surfaces or be a microscopic finding; some cases can have a grossly visible mass
Etiology	Data suggest that some implants may be clonally related to the primary ovarian tumor; they are thought to become detached from the tumor and directly implant onto peritoneal surfaces as opposed to being of independent primary peritoneal origin	"Invasive implants" may represent metastasis from occult invasion within the ovarian tumor, detachment from an exophytic ovarian micropapillary serous borderline tumor with direct implantation onto peritoneal surfaces, or transformation of a noninvasive implant as opposed to being of independent primary peritoneal origin; the primary designation for "invasive implants" is "low-grade serous carcinoma" in the 2020 WHO Classification
Histology	1. Variable number of foci present on serosal surfaces or within septa between lobules of adipose tissue in the omentum; no infiltration of underlying tissue	1. Variable number of foci present on serosal surfaces or within septa between lobules of adipose tissue in the omentum; invasive implants also infiltrate underlying tissues with a morphologic appearance identical to ovarian invasive low-grade serous carcinoma (nests, glands, and papillae with haphazard arrangements) *(Figs. 6.2.6 and 6.2.7)*
	2. No exophytic micropapillary pattern or small solid nests within clear lacunar spaces as seen in the expanded criteria for invasive implants (limited numbers of small solid nests within clear lacunar spaces without significant crowding are allowed within the spectrum of noninvasive implants)	2. Expanded criteria include exophytic micropapillary patterns (including cribriform architecture) identical to noninvasive low-grade serous carcinoma if in the ovary (micropapillary serous borderline tumor) and small solid nests within clear lacunar spaces (these should consist of numerous and significantly crowded nests within the same focus with a morphologic appearance similar to that of ovarian low-grade serous carcinoma) *(Figs. 6.2.8-6.2.10)*
	3. Lesional foci composed of glands, papillae, and/or solid nests *(Figs. 6.2.1 and 6.2.2)*	3. Lesional foci composed of glands, papillae, and/or solid nests; a background of coexisting noninvasive implants may be present
	4. Lesional foci may be isolated or crowded	4. Lesional foci may be isolated or crowded
	5. Lesional epithelium may display complexity with stratification and detached clusters *(Fig. 6.2.3)*	5. Lesional epithelium may display complexity with stratification and detached clusters

	Noninvasive Implants Associated With Serous Borderline Tumor	Low-Grade Serous Carcinoma (Invasive Implants)
	6. Implants can be purely epithelial-type or have desmoplastic stroma (the latter often present as a plaque on the surface of serosa) *(Fig. 6.2.4)*; individual epithelioid cells with abundant eosinophilic cytoplasm may be present *(Fig. 6.2.5)* **7.** Epithelial-to-stromal ratio in favor of stroma (for desmoplastic-type implants) **8.** Psammoma bodies can be present	**6.** Desmoplastic stroma can be present but is not necessary for classification as low-grade serous carcinoma (invasive implants); a background of coexisting noninvasive implants may be seen **7.** Epithelial-to-stromal ratio in favor of epithelium **8.** Psammoma bodies can be present
Special studies	Of no use for this differential diagnosis	Of no use for this differential diagnosis
Treatment	Surgical excision, including debulking of all grossly visible disease	Surgical excision, including debulking of all grossly visible disease; further management options include observation, chemotherapy, or hormonal therapy
Prognosis	Women with noninvasive implants have a significantly higher survival rate and lower risk for progressive disease compared with women who have "invasive implants"	Women with "invasive implants" have a significantly lower survival rate and higher risk for progressive disease compared with women who have noninvasive implants, supporting the classification as low-grade serous carcinoma

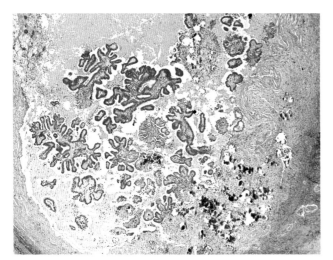

Figure 6.2.1 Epithelial-type noninvasive implant with complex papillary architecture.

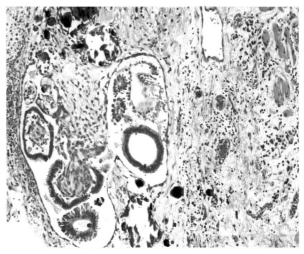

Figure 6.2.2 Epithelial-type noninvasive implant showing papillae with fibrous cores.

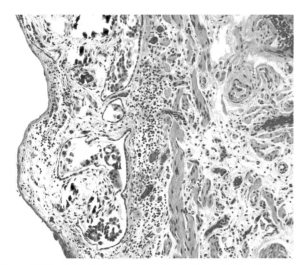

Figure 6.2.3 Epithelial-type noninvasive implant with detached epithelial clusters in mesothelial-lined spaces.

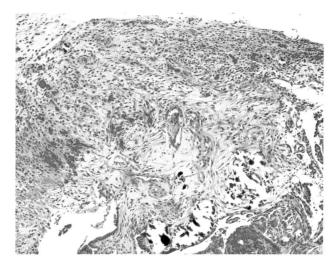

Figure 6.2.4 Desmoplastic noninvasive implant. Glands are embedded within desmoplastic stroma.

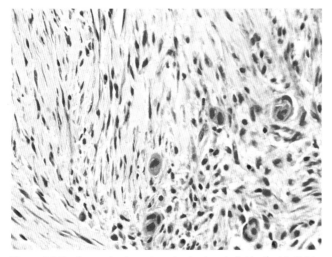

Figure 6.2.5 Desmoplastic noninvasive implant. Individual epithelioid cells with abundant eosinophilic cytoplasm are present within desmoplastic stroma.

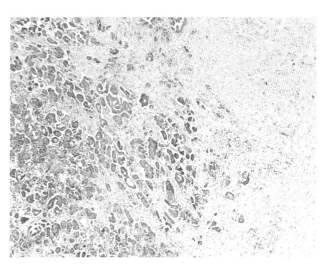

Figure 6.2.6 Low-grade serous carcinoma (invasive implant) with infiltrating pattern.

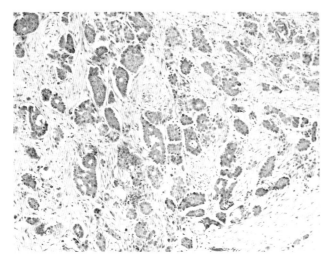

Figure 6.2.7   Low-grade serous carcinoma (invasive implant) with infiltrating pattern. Note the haphazard arrangements of nests.

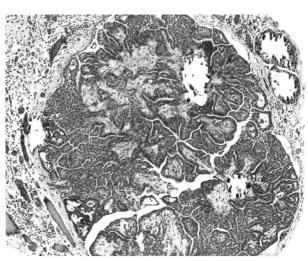

Figure 6.2.8   Low-grade serous carcinoma (invasive implant) with the same type of micropapillary pattern seen in an exophytic form of ovarian micropapillary serous borderline tumor. The interface between epithelium and stroma is smooth without infiltration, but this pattern is considered an "invasive implant" per expanded criteria.

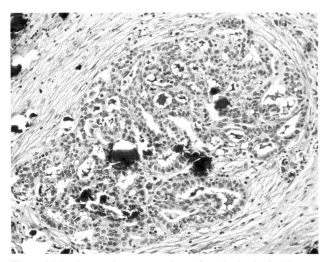

Figure 6.2.9   Low-grade serous carcinoma (invasive implant) with cribriform pattern.

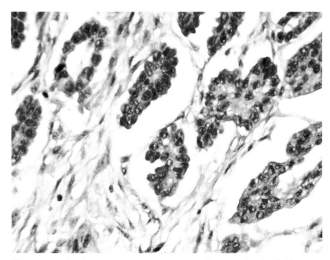

Figure 6.2.10   Low-grade serous carcinoma (invasive implant). These solid/micropapillary nests are present within clear lacunar spaces.

	Nondiagnostic Low-Grade Serous Proliferation	**Low-Grade Serous Carcinoma**
Age	Usually premenopausal	Most peri- or postmenopausal
Location	Intra-abdominal/pelvic serosal/peritoneal sites	Intra-abdominal/pelvic serosal/peritoneal sites; may have parenchymal involvement of intra-abdominal/pelvic organs or lymph nodes *(Figs. 6.3.7 and 6.3.8)*
Symptoms	May be incidental microscopic finding in specimens from surgeries performed for other indications, or patients may present with pelvic/abdominal pain	Abdominal pain, but may be incidental finding
Signs	May be incidental microscopic finding, or patients may have adhesions or peritoneal granules/nodules; however, a mass should not be present	Nodules, adhesions, and/or dominant mass
Etiology	"Low-grade serous proliferation" is a descriptive diagnosis for an ill-defined heterogeneous category that may represent either: **(A)** secondary microscopic peritoneal involvement by a low-grade serous tumor (borderline tumor or carcinoma), in which the low-grade serous tumor is only identified after the initial surgery, and that the peritoneal low-grade serous proliferation is insufficient for further classification by itself, or **(B)** a microscopic peritoneal lesion in which a low-grade serous tumor is not identified after further clinical evaluation and that the low-grade serous proliferation is insufficient for further classification This nondiagnostic lesion may resemble noninvasive implants, but there is no known serous borderline tumor elsewhere The lesion discussed herein is similar to what other authors have described as "peritoneal serous borderline tumor," "peritoneal serous micropapillomatosis of low malignant potential," and "atypical endosalpingiosis"; however, this nondiagnostic low-grade serous proliferation is insufficient for further classification as a serous borderline tumor or low-grade carcinoma (including the "serous psammocarcinoma" variant) as it lacks the diagnostic histologic features of either of those tumors	Derive from endosalpingiosis and serous borderline; *KRAS* and *BRAF* mutations

	Nondiagnostic Low-Grade Serous Proliferation	**Low-Grade Serous Carcinoma**
Histology	1. Lesion involves serosal/peritoneal surfaces without invasion of underlying tissue *(Figs. 6.3.1 and 6.3.2)*; expanded criteria for "invasive implants" (see Section 6.2) should also be absent; extensive sampling of the gross specimen is warranted	1. Lesion involves serosal/peritoneal surfaces, but invasion of underlying tissue (or expanded criteria for "invasive implants" [see Section 6.2]) should be present *(Figs. 6.3.9 and 6.3.10)*; criteria for the minimal diagnostic threshold for low-grade serous carcinoma may vary between gynecologic pathologists
	2. Lesion may be unifocal or multifocal	2. Lesion may be unifocal or multifocal, but many cases will have widespread disease
	3. Composed of mixture of glands, papillae, and/or solid nests; similar to noninvasive implants associated with serous borderline tumors *(Figs. 6.3.3 and 6.3.4)*; degree of crowding of epithelial structures not as great as in carcinoma *(Fig. 6.3.4)*; no haphazard arrangement; lesional epithelium may be embedded within adhesions and associated with psammoma bodies *(Figs. 6.3.5 and 6.3.6)*	3. Composed of mixture of glands, papillae, and/or solid nests with marked crowding of epithelial structures and haphazard arrangement; psammoma bodies may be present *(Figs. 6.3.7-6.3.10)*
	4. Lesional epithelium may have stratification and detached epithelial clusters *(Fig. 6.3.2)*	4. Lesional epithelium may have stratification and detached epithelial clusters
	5. Consists of bland tubal-type epithelium *(Figs. 6.3.4 and 6.3.6)*	5. Consists of bland tubal-type epithelium, although ciliated cells are scant to absent; atypia may be present but is low-grade
	6. A background of endosalpingiosis may be present	6. A background of endosalpingiosis may be present
Special studies	Of no use for this differential diagnosis	Of no use for this differential diagnosis
Treatment	Further clinical evaluation is necessary to exclude the possibility that this represents either noninvasive implants of a serous borderline tumor or subtle metastases of a low-grade serous carcinoma elsewhere	Hysterectomy and bilateral salpingo-oophorectomy, including debulking of all grossly visible disease; further management options include observation, chemotherapy, or hormonal therapy
Prognosis	Unknown; short-term follow-up based on relatively limited data for lesions with a histologic appearance similar to what has been reported in the literature as "peritoneal serous borderline tumor," "peritoneal serous micropapillomatosis of low malignant potential," and "atypical endosalpingiosis" (but without a serous borderline tumor elsewhere) suggest a generally favorable outcome, typically without progressive disease; in the absence of a coexisting borderline tumor or carcinoma detected upon further clinical investigation, it is unclear whether this lesion may (a) represent a precursor to a low-grade serous tumor that might take years to fully manifest as such or (b) be associated with an increased risk for a subsequent low-grade serous tumor; accordingly, long-term follow-up is suggested	Median survival, 48-82 mo (advanced stage ovarian low-grade serous carcinoma)

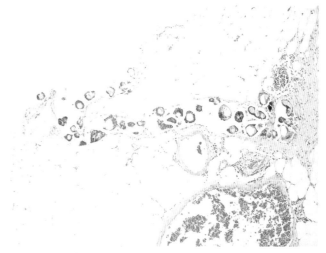

Figure 6.3.1   Nondiagnostic low-grade serous proliferation distributed along the septa of lobules of adipose tissue within the omentum. No invasion into underlying tissue is present.

Figure 6.3.2   Nondiagnostic low-grade serous proliferation with detached papillae on the surface of the omentum.

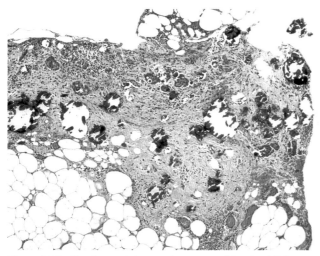

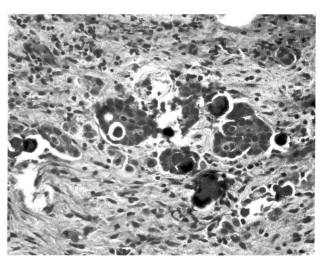

Figure 6.3.3   Nondiagnostic low-grade serous proliferation. While the histologic appearance can create concern for low-grade serous carcinoma, the limited anatomic distribution (*not shown*) and absence of a mass in this case are insufficient for that diagnosis. Also, note that epithelial clusters are present within adhesions on the surface of the omentum without invasion of underlying adipose tissue.

Figure 6.3.4   Nondiagnostic low-grade serous proliferation (*same focus shown in Fig. 6.3.3, higher-power magnification*). These histologic findings can be concerning for low-grade serous carcinoma but are insufficient for definitive diagnosis as such (see legend for *Fig. 6.3.3*).

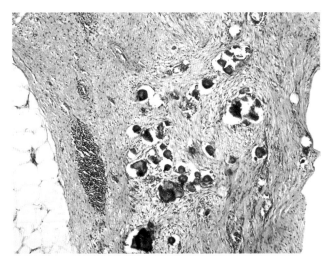

Figure 6.3.5   Numerous psammoma bodies within adhesions from a case of nondiagnostic low-grade serous proliferation (the epithelial component is not present in this field).

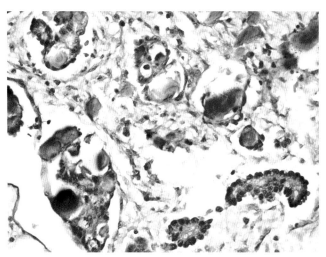

Figure 6.3.6   Nondiagnostic low-grade serous proliferation. Psammoma bodies are present within small papillae. The histologic appearance of this focus can create concern for low-grade serous carcinoma at high-power magnification. However, the combination of assessment of the anatomic distribution of disease to reveal a limited extent of proliferation, absence of a mass, and presence of these epithelial clusters within adhesions involving serosa without true invasion of underlying tissue in this case is insufficient for a diagnosis of low-grade serous carcinoma.

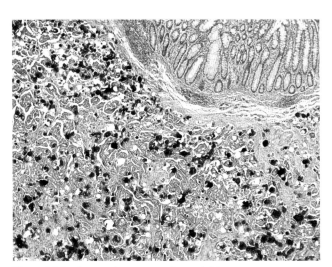

Figure 6.3.7   Low-grade serous carcinoma (with numerous psammoma bodies) invading the wall of the colon.

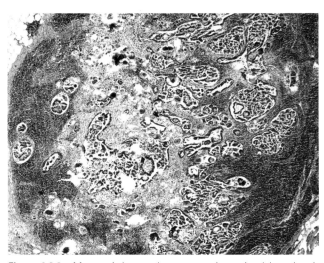

Figure 6.3.8   Metastatic low-grade serous carcinoma involving a lymph node.

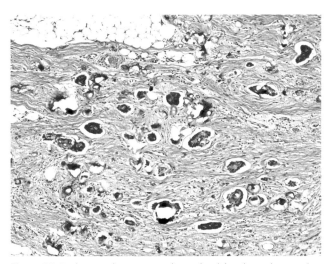

Figure 6.3.9　Low-grade serous carcinoma involving the peritoneum/omentum. Note the presence of solid nests within clear lacunar spaces.

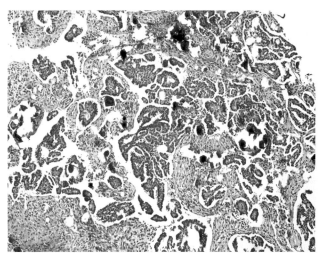

Figure 6.3.10　Low-grade serous carcinoma involving the peritoneum/omentum. Crowded micropapillae are arranged haphazardly with destructive stromal invasion.

6.4

WELL-DIFFERENTIATED PAPILLARY MESOTHELIAL TUMOR VS LOW-GRADE SEROUS NEOPLASMS (SEROUS BORDERLINE TUMOR/LOW-GRADE SEROUS CARCINOMA)

	Well-Differentiated Papillary Mesothelial Tumor	Low-Grade Serous Neoplasms (Serous Borderline Tumor/Low-Grade Serous Carcinoma)
Age	Mean, 49 y	Usually peri- or postmenopausal
Location	Intra-abdominal/pelvic serosal/peritoneal sites	Serosal/peritoneal sites, ovaries, and/or fallopian tubes
Symptoms	Typically incidental finding in specimens from surgery performed for other indications	Abdominal pain, but may be incidental finding
Signs	Single or multiple nodules, ranging from 0.1 to 2 cm with most <1 cm	Dominant mass, intra-abdominal/pelvic carcinomatosis, and/or implants/tumor nodules
Etiology	Unknown but does not appear to be related to asbestos exposure; mutations in either *TRAF7* or *CDC42*	Low-grade serous neoplasms (serous borderline tumor/low-grade serous carcinoma) often harbor *BRAF/KRAS* mutations
Histology	1. Predominantly papillary architecture; variably sized papillae with simple pattern and moderate to abundant fibrous stroma; no fine fibrovascular cores; no complex papillary branching *(Figs. 6.4.1-6.4.3)*; this neoplasm was previously designated well-differentiated papillary mesothelioma 2. Focal tubules may be present *(Fig. 6.4.4)* 3. No stromal invasion (cases with small foci of invasion within papillae have been described but are considered within the spectrum of well-differentiated papillary mesothelioma) 4. No epithelial stratification *(Fig. 6.4.5)* 5. Epithelial structures lined by mostly low-cuboidal cells *(Fig. 6.4.5)* 6. No ciliated cells 7. Bland nuclei 8. No psammoma bodies	1. Simple to complex papillary architecture with hierarchical branching of variably sized papillae, variable amount of fibrous stroma, and fine fibrovascular cores without invasion (atypical proliferative [borderline] serous tumor) *(Figs. 6.4.6 and 6.4.7)* 2. Papillary (including micropapillary features [*Fig. 6.4.8*]), glandular, and nested patterns may be present with haphazard orientation (low-grade serous carcinoma) 3. Stromal invasion present (low-grade serous carcinoma) *(Fig. 6.4.9)* 4. Epithelial stratification, including detached clusters of cells *(Fig. 6.4.10)* 5. Epithelial structures lined by mostly columnar cells 6. +/− Ciliated cells *(Fig. 6.4.11)* 7. Bland nuclei (atypia in carcinoma may be present but is low-grade) 8. +/− Psammoma bodies
Special studies	• Calretinin: diffuse expression • PAX8: +/− • WT-1: positive • MOC-31/Ber-EP4/Claudin-4: negative • ER/PR: negative	• Calretinin: negative or nondiffuse expression • PAX8: positive • WT-1: positive • MOC-31/Ber-EP4/Claudin-4: positive • ER/PR: positive

	Well-Differentiated Papillary Mesothelial Tumor	**Low-Grade Serous Neoplasms (Serous Borderline Tumor/Low-Grade Serous Carcinoma)**
Treatment	Surgical excision with careful exploration to exclude the possibility of undersampled malignant mesothelioma	Surgical excision, including debulking of all grossly visible disease; further management options for low-grade serous carcinoma include observation, chemotherapy, or hormonal therapy
Prognosis	The 2020 WHO considers these tumors benign. However, follow-up is warranted because of recurrences in a small subset of patients	Serous borderline tumor with noninvasive implants: overall favorable outcome, but a subset will develop subsequent low-grade serous carcinoma; low-grade serous carcinoma: indolent with 5-/10-y survival ~75%/45%, respectively, for stage III

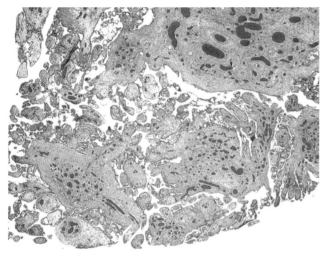

Figure 6.4.1 Well-differentiated papillary mesothelial tumor with prominent papillary architecture.

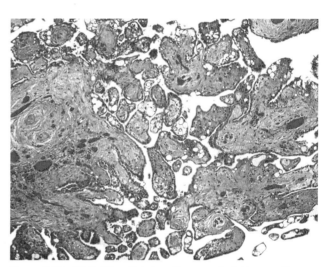

Figure 6.4.2 Well-differentiated papillary mesothelial tumor with numerous crowded papillae.

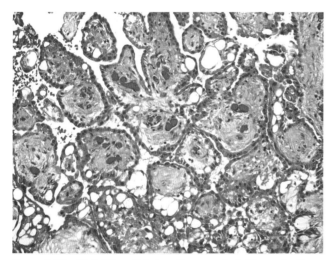

Figure 6.4.3 Well-differentiated papillary mesothelial tumor. Papillae are simple with abundant fibrous stroma.

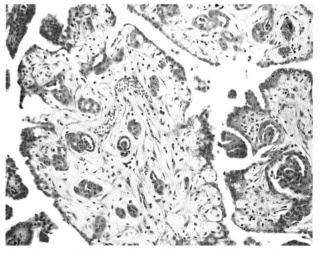

Figure 6.4.4 Well-differentiated papillary mesothelial tumor with tubules in stroma of papillae.

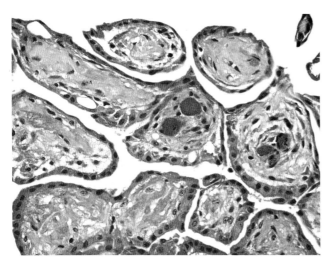

Figure 6.4.5   Well-differentiated papillary mesothelial tumor. Papillae are lined by a single layer of low-cuboidal cells.

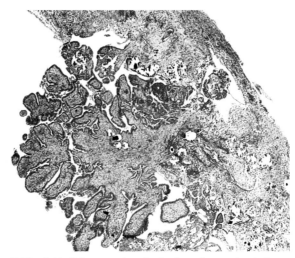

Figure 6.4.6   Epithelial-type noninvasive implant of serous borderline tumor simulating well-differentiated papillary mesothelial tumor.

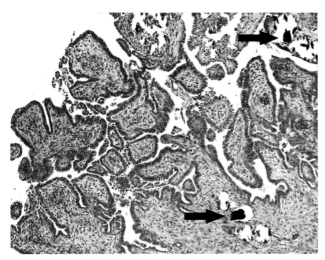

Figure 6.4.7   Epithelial-type noninvasive implant of serous borderline tumor simulating well-differentiated papillary mesothelial tumor (*same case as Fig. 6.4.6*). Psammoma bodies are also present (*arrows*).

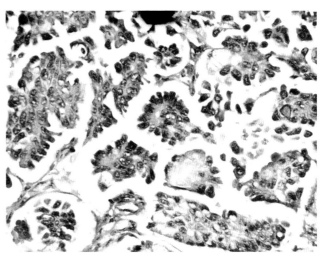

Figure 6.4.8   Low-grade serous carcinoma with micropapillae.

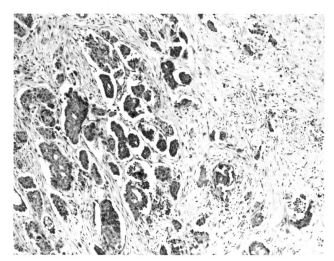

Figure 6.4.9 Low-grade serous carcinoma.

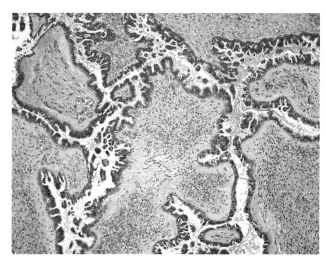

Figure 6.4.10 Serous borderline tumor with epithelial stratification and detached epithelial clusters.

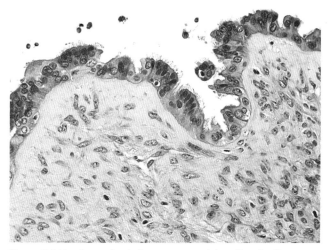

Figure 6.4.11 Serous borderline tumor containing ciliated cells.

	High-Grade Serous Carcinoma	Malignant Mesothelioma
Age	Postmenopausal (mean age, late 50s to early 60s)	Mean, 46 y
Location	Intra-abdominal/pelvic sites	Intra-abdominal/pelvic sites
Symptoms	Abdominal pain	Abdominal/pelvic pain and weight loss
Signs	Abdominal distension; pelvic mass; ascites, intra-abdominal/pelvic carcinomatosis; elevated serum CA-125	Ascites; diffuse peritoneal involvement by multiple nodules and plaques; pelvic mass
Etiology	Majority derive from serous tubal intraepithelial carcinoma (STIC), usually of fimbrial origin; nearly all have *TP53* mutations; a substantial proportion have either germline or somatic mutation in *BRCA1*, *BRCA2*, or other homologous recombination repair genes or epigenetic silencing of these genes; high levels of genomic instability	There is a reported association with asbestos exposure; however, the exact level of association with asbestos for female peritoneal cases unclear; somatic mutations or homozygous deletion of *BAP1* is common; *BAP1* germline mutations occur in a small subset; less common genetic alterations: *CDKN2A* homozygous deletion and mutations of *NF2*, *SETD2*, and *DDX3X*
Histology	1. Complex papillary, glandular, and solid architecture with marked epithelial stratification, irregular slit-like spaces, and stromal invasion *(Figs. 6.5.1-6.5.4)*	1. Can have admixture of tubular, papillary, and solid patterns; lesser degree of epithelial stratification than in serous carcinoma; irregular slit-like spaces can be seen but are not as characteristic as in serous carcinoma; may be surface-based growth, but invasion should be present; biphasic, sarcomatoid, and deciduoid patterns can occur; inflammatory infiltrates frequently present *(Figs. 6.5.6-6.5.9)*
	2. Papillae may be large and broad, fine and complex, or micropapillary	2. Variable appearance of papillae; they are less complex than in serous carcinoma *(Fig. 6.5.9)*; stromal cores of papillae more frequently hyalinized than in serous carcinoma
	3. Glands may have nonspecific appearance or pseudoendometrioid morphology	3. Glands may have tubular or adenomatoid tumor-like appearance
	4. Cells may be cuboidal or columnar with variable amount of cytoplasm	4. Epithelioid cells; usually more abundant eosinophillic cytoplasm than seen in serous carcinoma *(Fig. 6.5.8)*
	5. Nuclei are round, large, pleomorphic with prominent nucleoli; large hyperchromatic "monster"/bizarre cells may be seen; chromatin may be vesicular *(Fig. 6.5.5)*	5. Nuclei more uniform than in serous carcinoma with lower degree of atypia *(Fig. 6.5.10)*
	6. High mitotic rate	6. Mitotic rate usually low
	7. +/− Psammoma bodies	7. Psammoma bodies present in a minority of cases; when present, typically less abundant than can be seen in serous carcinoma

	High-Grade Serous Carcinoma	**Malignant Mesothelioma**
Special studies	• Calretinin: negative or nondiffuse expression • PAX8: positive • WT-1: positive • MOC-31/Ber-EP4/Claudin-4: positive • ER/PR: positive	• Calretinin: diffuse expression • PAX8: negative • WT-1: positive • MOC-31/Ber-EP4/Claudin-4: negative • ER/PR: negative
Treatment	Hysterectomy and bilateral salpingo-oophorectomy, including debulking of all grossly visible disease and chemotherapy	Surgery, including debulking of all grossly visible disease and chemotherapy
Prognosis	Stage III patients have 5-y survival of 45%-50% if optimally debulked; suboptimal debulking has 20%-30% 5-y survival	5-y survival: 34%-63%

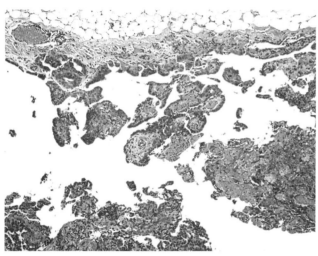

Figure 6.5.1   High-grade serous carcinoma with papillary architecture involving the surface of the omentum.

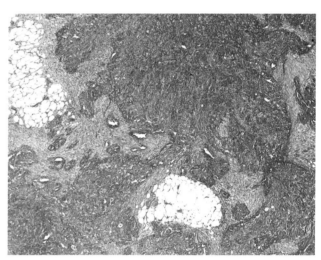

Figure 6.5.2   High-grade serous carcinoma. The tumor invades the omentum and displays solid and glandular architecture.

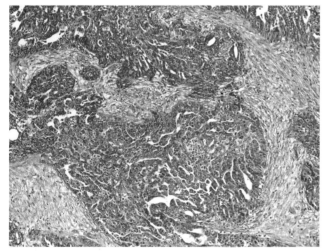

Figure 6.5.3   High-grade serous carcinoma showing epithelial complexity with irregular slit-like spaces.

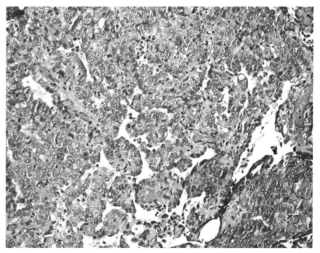

Figure 6.5.4   High-grade serous carcinoma with epithelial stratification and tufting.

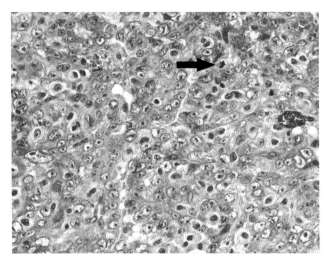

Figure 6.5.5 High-grade serous carcinoma exhibiting pleomorphic nuclei and mitotic activity (*arrow*).

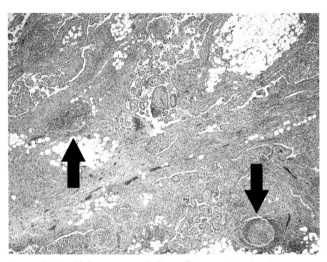

Figure 6.5.6 Malignant mesothelioma. The tumor invades the omentum and displays a papillary pattern and lymphoid aggregates (*arrows*).

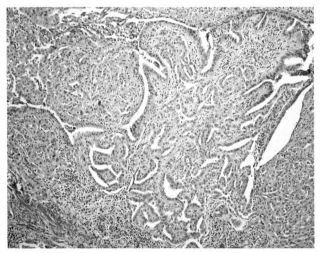

Figure 6.5.7 Malignant mesothelioma with tubulopapillary architecture.

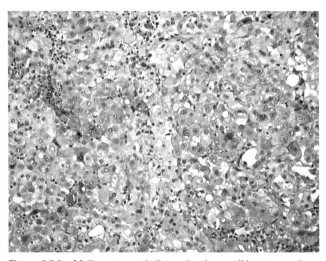

Figure 6.5.8 Malignant mesothelioma showing a solid pattern and deciduoid appearance.

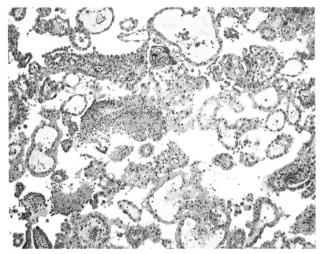

Figure 6.5.9 Malignant mesothelioma with simple papillae. They are mostly lined by a single layer of cells without the degree of epithelial complexity and stratification seen in high-grade serous carcinoma.

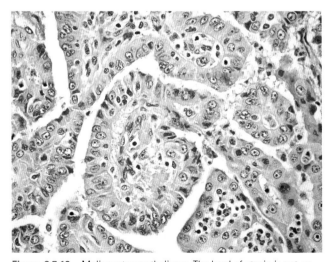

Figure 6.5.10 Malignant mesothelioma. The level of atypia is not as severe as in high-grade serous carcinoma.

	Keratin Granulomas	Metastatic Endometrioid Carcinoma With Squamous Differentiation
Age	Variable, ranging from pre- to postmenopausal	Most are postmenopausal
Location	Serosal/peritoneal surfaces	Serosal/peritoneal surfaces; involvement of lymph nodes and intra-abdominal/pelvic organs may also be present
Symptoms	Nonspecific; patients will have concurrent uterine or ovarian endometrioid carcinoma; symptoms attributable to uterine or ovarian tumor	Symptoms attributable to uterine or ovarian tumor
Signs	Usually microscopic finding, but in a minority of cases may appear as granules or small nodules	Intra-abdominal/pelvic nodules or may be microscopic finding
Etiology	Exfoliated keratin from ovarian or endometrial endometrioid carcinomas with squamous differentiation, which implants onto serosal/peritoneal surfaces, forms granulomas, and simulates metastatic carcinoma	Metastatic carcinoma from uterine or ovarian carcinoma involving serosal/peritoneal surfaces
Histology	1. Granulomas composed of laminated keratin or ghost outlines of squamous cells without nuclei *(Figs. 6.6.1-6.6.4)* 2. No tumor cells (particularly glands, papillae, or solid components with tumor cells containing nuclei) 3. Granulomas surrounded by macrophages (including multinucleated giant cells) and other inflammatory cells *(Figs. 6.6.3-6.6.5)* 4. Granulomas separated by fibrous tissue	1. Squamous differentiation may be present *(Figs. 6.6.6-6.6.9)* 2. Tumor cells with nuclei will be present, including glandular, papillary, or solid differentiation *(Figs. 6.6.7 and 6.6.9)* 3. +/− Associated inflammatory response; however, typically not characterized by multinucleated giant cells 4. Desmoplastic reaction can be seen *(Fig. 6.6.6)*
Special studies	• CD68/CD163: (+) in histiocytes/giant cells • PAX8/ER/PR (−)	• CD68/CD163: variable depending on the presence of histiocytic reaction • PAX8/ER/PR (+)
Treatment	No specific treatment necessary	Depends on stage and anatomic site of primary tumor, but options include surgery, chemotherapy, and/or radiation therapy
Prognosis	Should not be considered metastatic carcinoma; does not qualify for upstaging the uterine or ovarian tumor; of no prognostic significance	Stage designation/prognosis for involvement of serosal/peritoneal surfaces depends on anatomic sites of metastasis and primary tumor (can range from FIGO II to IV)

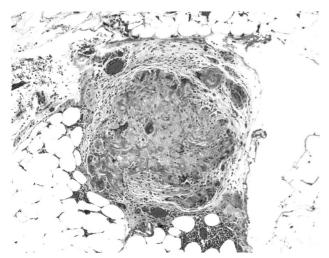

Figure 6.6.1   Keratin granuloma appearing as a small round nodule in the omentum.

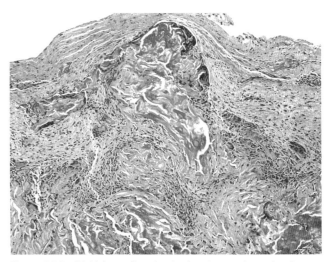

Figure 6.6.2   Multiple small coalescing keratin granulomas forming a nodule larger than the one seen in *Figure 6.6.1*.

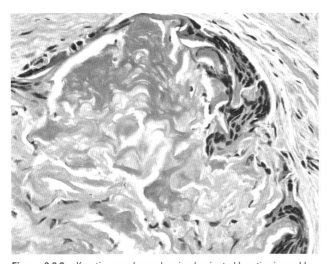

Figure 6.6.3   Keratin granuloma showing laminated keratin rimmed by compressed multinucleated giant cells.

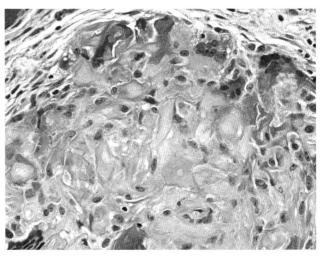

Figure 6.6.4   Keratin granuloma with ghost outlines of anucleated squamous cells. Macrophages are interspersed between squamous cells.

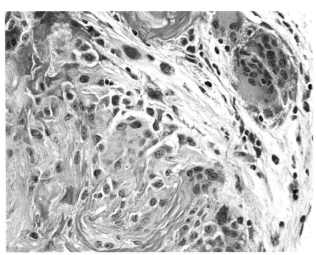

Figure 6.6.5   Keratin granuloma. A multinucleated giant cell is present in the upper right portion of the photograph, while mononucleated macrophages are present at the periphery of the keratin granuloma (**lower left**).

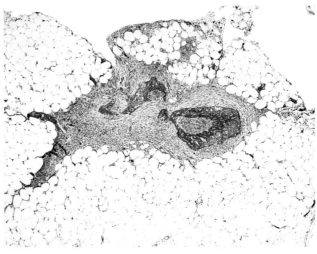

Figure 6.6.6   Metastatic endometrioid carcinoma with squamous differentiation, which can potentially simulate keratin granulomas at low-power magnification. Associated desmoplasia is present.

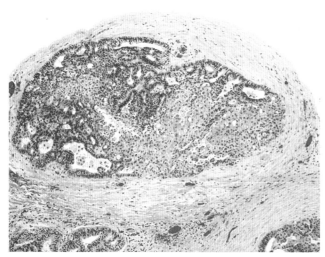

Figure 6.6.7   Metastatic endometrioid carcinoma with squamous differentiation. The nodular configuration is similar to that of a keratin granuloma, but admixed glandular elements, in addition to squamous differentiation, are seen.

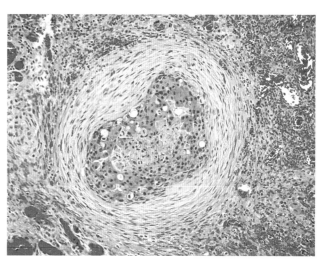

Figure 6.6.8   Metastatic endometrioid carcinoma with squamous differentiation. This focus is entirely composed of squamous differentiation without obvious glandular elements.

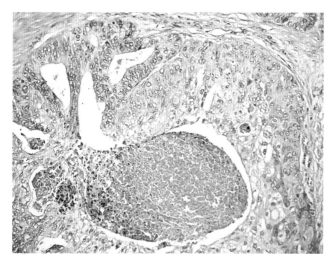

Figure 6.6.9   Metastatic endometrioid carcinoma with neoplastic glands containing intact nuclei (**left**) and squamous differentiation (**right**).

	Disseminated Peritoneal Leiomyomatosis	Metastatic Leiomyosarcoma
Age	Most are premenopausal; often associated with pregnancy	Usually, >50 y
Location	Serosal/peritoneal surfaces, including omentum	Intra-abdominal/pelvic sites with involvement of serosal/peritoneal surfaces, including omentum; parenchymal involvement of other organs, such as liver, lungs, and bowel, may be present
Symptoms	Often asymptomatic	May have prior history of uterine leiomyosarcoma, or may initially present with advanced stage (extrauterine) disease
Signs	Multiple nodules (typically <1 cm in size) within peritoneal cavity *(Fig. 6.7.1)*	May have uterine enlargement; intra-abdominal/pelvic masses; nodules often fewer and larger than disseminated peritoneal leiomyomatosis *(Fig. 6.7.7)*
Etiology	Unknown although thought to be hormonally related and that these multicentric lesions are clonal; also referred to as leiomyomatosis peritonealis disseminata; *MED12* mutations have been demonstrated	Metastasis from uterine leiomyosarcoma with involvement of intra-abdominal/pelvic sites
Histology	1. Circumscribed nodules, usually associated with serosal lining without invasion *(Figs. 6.7.2-6.7.4)* 2. Proliferation of smooth muscle, often with fascicular architecture *(Fig. 6.7.5)* 3. No nuclear atypia *(Fig. 6.7.6)* 4. No mitotic activity 5. No necrosis	1. Nodules may invade adjacent tissue 2. Diffuse architecture with sheets of tumor cells; often with fascicular architecture and spindle cell differentiation; can have epithelioid or myxoid features *(Fig. 6.7.8)* 3. Usually exhibits significant atypia (level of atypia in occasional cases may be deceptively bland) *(Fig. 6.7.9)* 4. Often mitotically active 5. May or may not have necrosis
Special studies	Of no use for this differential diagnosis	Of no use for this differential diagnosis
Treatment	Conservative management; surgical excision; success has been shown with GnRH agonists and aromatase inhibitors	Hysterectomy, +/− bilateral salpingo-oophorectomy, with excision of extrauterine masses; further treatment options include consideration of chemotherapy and/or radiation therapy
Prognosis	Benign	Stage dependent; 5-y survival: 15%-25%

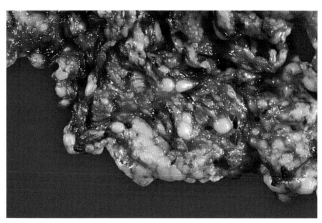

Figure 6.7.1   Disseminated peritoneal leiomyomatosis. Gross omental specimen involved by numerous small round nodules.

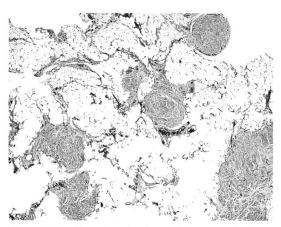

Figure 6.7.2   Disseminated peritoneal leiomyomatosis. The omentum is involved by multiple small round nodules of smooth muscle proliferation.

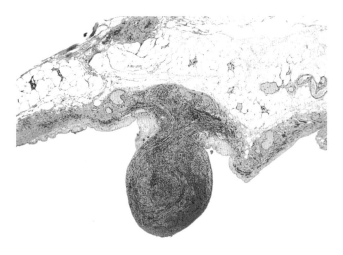

Figure 6.7.3   Disseminated peritoneal leiomyomatosis. The surface of the omentum is involved by a small round nodule of smooth muscle proliferation. The other lesional nodules are not shown in this photograph.

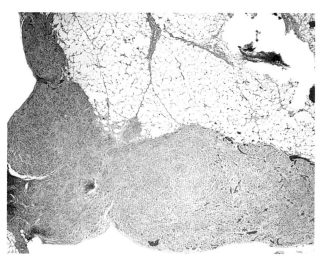

Figure 6.7.4   Disseminated peritoneal leiomyomatosis. Small nodules of smooth muscle proliferation coalesce to form a plaque covering the surface of the omentum.

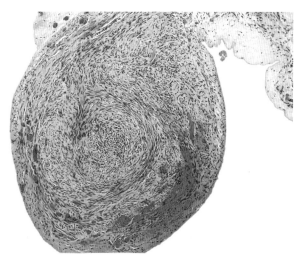

Figure 6.7.5   Disseminated peritoneal leiomyomatosis with fascicular architecture (*same case as Fig. 6.7.3*).

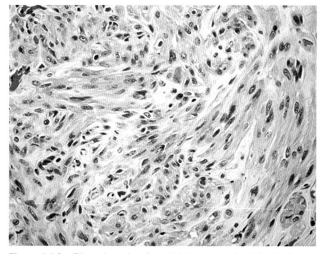

Figure 6.7.6   Disseminated peritoneal leiomyomatosis with spindle cells showing bland nuclei.

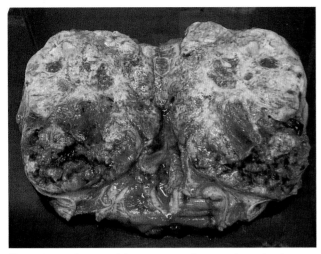

Figure 6.7.7 Recurrent leiomyosarcoma. Gross specimen showing a large mass with a heterogeneous cut surface (*contrast with Fig. 6.7.1*).

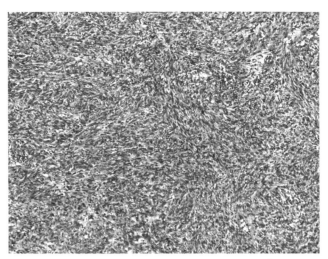

Figure 6.7.8 Metastatic leiomyosarcoma demonstrating diffuse cellular sheets with poorly formed fascicles.

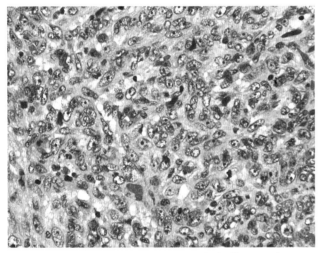

Figure 6.7.9 Metastatic leiomyosarcoma with significant atypia.

6.8

FLORID MESOTHELIAL HYPERPLASIA VS SECONDARY INVOLVEMENT BY OVARIAN LOW-GRADE SEROUS NEOPLASMS (IMPLANTS OF SEROUS BORDERLINE TUMOR/METASTATIC LOW-GRADE SEROUS CARCINOMA)

	Florid Mesothelial Hyperplasia	**Secondary Involvement by Ovarian Low-Grade Serous Neoplasms (Implants of Serous Borderline Tumor/ Metastatic Low-Grade Serous Carcinoma)**
Age	Variable	Usually peri- or postmenopausal
Location	Intra-abdominal/pelvic serosal/ peritoneal sites (often omentum); rarely, may involve subcapsular sinuses of lymph nodes	Serosal/peritoneal sites, ovaries, fallopian tubes, and/or lymph nodes
Symptoms	Dependent on underlying condition for which surgery was performed	Abdominal pain, but may be incidental finding
Signs	Mesothelial hyperplasia usually a microscopic finding, but small nodules can be seen; however, a concurrent ovarian epithelial tumor may be present	Dominant mass, intra-abdominal/pelvic carcinomatosis, and/or implants/tumor nodules
Etiology	Reactive proliferation of mesothelial cells; may be a response to ascites, inflammation, endometriosis, or tumors	Low-grade serous neoplasms (serous borderline tumor/ low-grade serous carcinoma) often harbor *BRAF/KRAS* mutations
Histology	1. Nodules or sheets of mesothelial cells predominantly coating serosal surfaces without invasion *(Fig. 6.8.1)* 2. Papillae may be seen but do not show the degree of architectural complexity or epithelial stratification as seen in serous tumors 3. Nests, tubules, and cords can be present within fibrous stroma, but their distribution is often linear and parallel to the surface without the haphazard arrangement seen in carcinoma *(Figs. 6.8.2 and 6.8.3)* 4. Lacks ciliated cells 5. No significant atypia *(Fig. 6.8.4)* 6. Associated inflammation may be present 7. Psammoma bodies typically not present 8. Nodular aggregates/sheets of mac-rophages with very few mesothelial cells may occur (in such cases, im-munohistochemical stains for CD68/ CD163 and pan-cytokeratin may be useful to demonstrate that the lesion of concern is not epithelial)	1. Carcinoma can exhibit nodular, sheet-like, or solid patterns; may involve serosal surfaces in plaque-like distribution or invade underlying tissue *(Fig. 6.8.6)* 2. Simple to complex papillary architecture with hierarchical branching of variably sized papillae, variable amount of fibrous stroma, and fine fibrovascular cores without invasion (typical serous borderline tumor); micropapillae with stromal invasion may be present (low-grade serous carcinoma) *(Fig. 6.8.6)* 3. Glands and nests with haphazard orientation and stromal invasion may be present (low-grade serous carcinoma); papillae, glands, and/or nests without stromal invasion can be seen (noninvasive implants of serous borderline tumor with or without desmoplastic stroma; desmoplastic noninvasive implants often show plaque-like distribution on serosal surfaces) *(Figs. 6.8.7-6.8.10)* 4. +/– Ciliated cells 5. Bland nuclei (atypia in carcinoma may be present but is low-grade) 6. Inflammation as part of stromal invasion in carcinoma may be present 7. +/– Psammoma bodies 8. Lesion of concern lacks aggregates/sheets of mac-rophages

	Florid Mesothelial Hyperplasia	**Secondary Involvement by Ovarian Low-Grade Serous Neoplasms (Implants of Serous Borderline Tumor/ Metastatic Low-Grade Serous Carcinoma)**
Special studies	• Calretinin: diffuse expression *(Fig. 6.8.5)* • PAX8: +/− • WT-1: positive • MOC-31/Ber-EP4/Claudin-4: negative • ER/PR: negative	• Calretinin: negative or nondiffuse expression • PAX8: positive • WT-1: positive • MOC-31/Ber-EP4/Claudin-4: positive • ER/PR: positive
Treatment	No therapy necessary	Surgical excision, including debulking of all grossly visible disease; further management options for low-grade serous carcinoma include observation, chemotherapy, or hormonal therapy
Prognosis	Benign	Serous borderline tumor with noninvasive implants: overall favorable outcome, but a subset will develop subsequent low-grade serous carcinoma; low-grade serous carcinoma: indolent with 5-/10-y survival ~75%/45%, respectively, for stage III

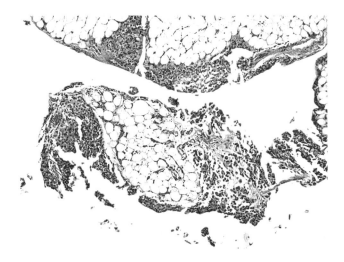

Figure 6.8.1   Mesothelial hyperplasia coating the surface of the omentum, including detached and irregular cellular fragments (**right of center**). This appearance at low-power magnification can be mistaken for secondary involvement by an ovarian serous tumor.

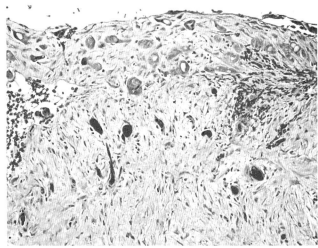

Figure 6.8.2   Mesothelial hyperplasia with linear distribution of tubules parallel to and immediately underneath the serosal surface.

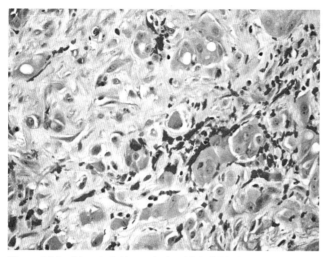

Figure 6.8.3 Mesothelial hyperplasia with individual cells and small clusters of cells, which can mimic serous carcinoma.

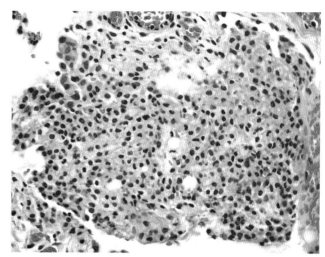

Figure 6.8.4 Sheets of mesothelial hyperplasia with focal artifactual round spaces simulating glandular differentiation of adenocarcinoma. The cellular population likely consists of an admixture of histiocytes and mesothelial cells.

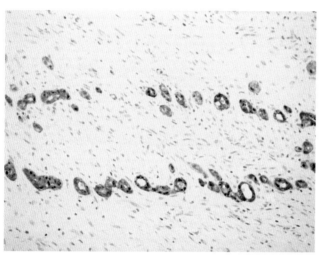

Figure 6.8.5 Mesothelial hyperplasia showing linear distribution of tubules with diffuse calretinin expression. Same case as *Figure 6.8.2*.

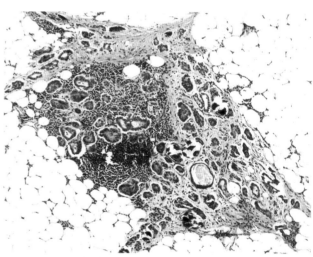

Figure 6.8.6 Low-grade serous carcinoma involving the omentum.

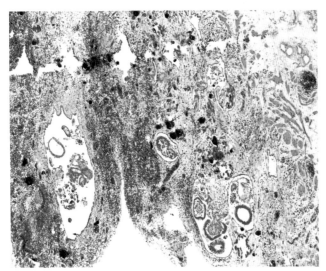

Figure 6.8.7 Noninvasive implants of serous borderline tumor. Medium-sized papillae within epithelial-lined spaces are present in a subserosal location.

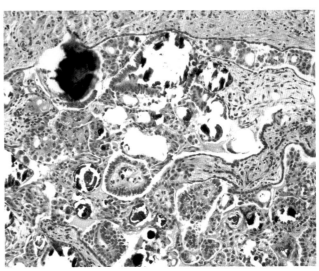

Figure 6.8.8 Noninvasive implants of serous borderline tumor. Detached papillae (with and without fibrovascular cores) and psammoma bodies are present.

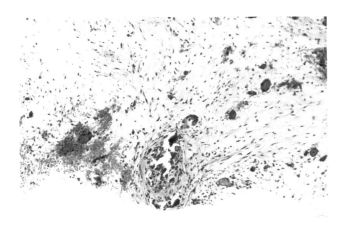

Figure 6.8.9 Desmoplastic noninvasive implants of serous borderline tumor simulating mesothelial hyperplasia at low-power magnification.

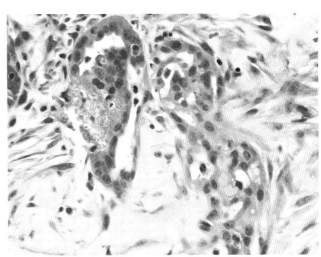

Figure 6.8.10 Desmoplastic noninvasive implants of serous borderline tumor. The cytologic features overlap with those of mesothelial hyperplasia.

	Metastatic Endometrioid Carcinoma	Endometriosis
Age	Most are postmenopausal	Usually pre- or perimenopausal
Location	Serosal/peritoneal surfaces; involvement of lymph nodes and intra-abdominal/pelvic organs may also be present	Extrauterine sites, including ovaries, uterine ligaments, rectovaginal septum, cul-de-sac, and pelvic or abdominal peritoneum
Symptoms	Symptoms attributable to uterine or ovarian tumor; the diagnosis of uterine/ovarian carcinoma may have been prior to a current serosal/peritoneal lesion	Dysmenorrhea, abdominal/pelvic pain, dyspareunia, and/or infertility; may be asymptomatic
Signs	Intra-abdominal/pelvic nodules, evidence of peritoneal carcinomatosis, or may be microscopic-only finding	Tender nodules in the cul-de-sac and uterosacral ligaments, and nonpigmented or pigmented lesions involving the peritoneum; can be a completely microscopic-only finding
Etiology	Metastatic carcinoma from uterine or ovarian carcinoma involving serosal/peritoneal surfaces	Ectopic extrauterine endometrial tissue with glands and stroma; most cases believed to be a result of retrograde menstruation
Histology	1. May be multifocal or a single focus *(Fig. 6.9.1)*	1. May be multifocal or a single focus; however, extensive distribution of lesional foci would be concerning for metastatic carcinoma
	2. May have nodular configuration or individual glands *(Fig. 6.9.1)*	2. Typically, foci are small and of microscopic size, but occasionally, endometriosis may produce a mass (polypoid endometriosis); individual glands will be present
	3. Crowded glands with haphazard arrangement or confluent architecture and cribriform growth can be seen *(Fig. 6.9.2)*	3. Glandular crowding or confluence should be absent except for the uncommon situation in which hyperplasia or carcinoma arises within endometriosis
	4. Squamous differentiation *(Fig. 6.9.3)* or papillary architecture may be present	4. No squamous differentiation/morular metaplasia or papillary architecture except for the uncommon situation in which hyperplasia or carcinoma arises within endometriosis
	5. Notable nuclear atypia or solid architecture may be evident in higher-grade tumors	5. Endometriotic glands show endometrioid features as seen in eutopic endometria *(Fig. 6.9.6)*; no atypia or solid architecture except for the uncommon situation in which carcinoma arises within endometriosis
	6. Associated desmoplastic stroma can be seen *(Figs. 6.9.3 and 6.9.4)*	6. No desmoplastic stroma; however, associated fibrosis and reactive stromal changes can be seen
	7. Absence of endometrial-type stroma *(Figs. 6.9.1-6.9.5)*	7. Intimately associated endometrial-type stroma is present between and/or around glands *(Fig. 6.9.7)*; the amount of stroma occasionally can be limited/attenuated making identification difficult *(Fig. 6.9.6)*; some cases may show distinct stromal capillaries, stromal hemorrhage *(Fig. 6.9.8)*, hemosiderin-laden macrophages, and/or necrotic pseudoxanthomatous nodules

	Metastatic Endometrioid Carcinoma	**Endometriosis**
Special studies	• Immunohistochemistry of no help for this differential diagnosis • Staining for CD10 to identify endometrial stroma (for endometriosis) may be nonspecific in this setting • Similarly, staining for ER/PR to identify endometrial stroma (for endometriosis) may be misleading as other tissues could have focal positivity	• Immunohistochemistry of no help for this differential diagnosis • Staining for CD10 to identify endometrial stroma (for endometriosis) may be nonspecific in this setting • Similarly, staining for ER/PR to identify endometrial stroma (for endometriosis) may be misleading as other tissues could have focal positivity
Treatment	Depends on stage and anatomic site of primary tumor, but options include surgery, chemotherapy, and/or radiation therapy	Surgical or hormonal/medical therapy
Prognosis	Stage designation/prognosis for involvement of serosal/peritoneal surfaces depends on anatomic sites of metastasis and primary tumor (can range from FIGO III to IV for uterine and II-IV for ovarian)	Benign

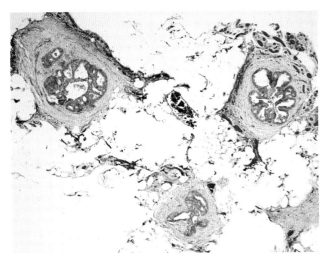

Figure 6.9.1   Multiple foci of metastatic endometrioid carcinoma with suggestion of nodular architecture.

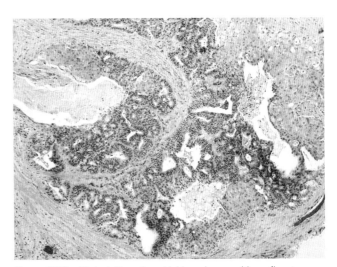

Figure 6.9.2   Metastatic endometrioid carcinoma with confluent glandular architecture.

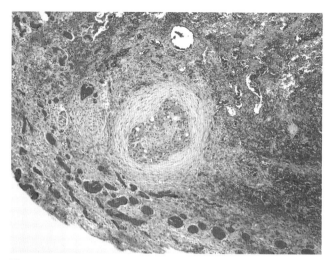

Figure 6.9.3 Metastatic endometrioid carcinoma. The gland in the center contains squamous differentiation, is surrounded by a rim of desmoplastic stroma, and the prominent hemorrhage could falsely suggest endometriosis at low-power magnification.

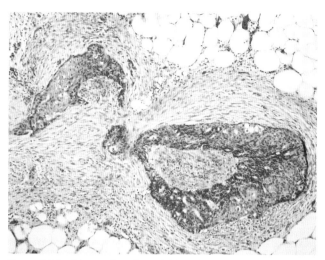

Figure 6.9.4 Metastatic endometrioid carcinoma with desmoplastic stroma.

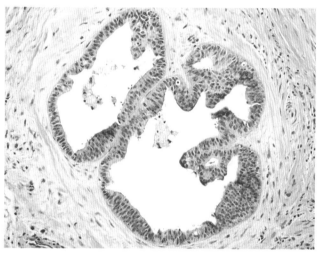

Figure 6.9.5 Metastatic endometrioid carcinoma. The glandular architecture could initially resemble endometriosis, but the lack of associated endometrial-type stroma with the presence of atypical endometrioid glands in this case is consistent with carcinoma.

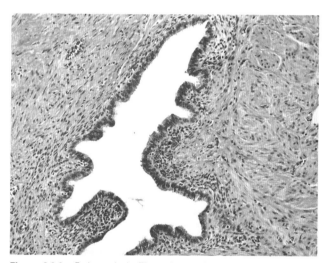

Figure 6.9.6 Endometriosis. The endometrioid gland in this case, which lacks atypia, is surrounded by a thin rim of endometrial-type stroma.

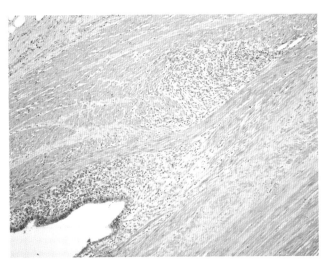

Figure 6.9.7   Endometriosis. The endometrial-type stroma in this case is more conspicuous than in *Figure 6.9.6.*

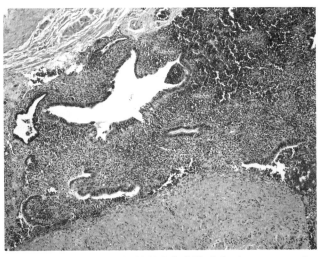

Figure 6.9.8   Endometriosis. Multiple individual glands are separated by abundant endometrial-type stroma. Stromal hemorrhage is also present.

SUGGESTED READINGS

6.1 and 6.2

Bell DA, Weinstock MA, Scully RE. Peritoneal implants of ovarian serous borderline tumors. Histologic features and prognosis. *Cancer.* 1988;62:2212-2222.

Bell KA, Smith Sehdev AE, Kurman RJ. Refined diagnostic criteria for implants associated with ovarian atypical proliferative serous tumors (borderline) and micropapillary serous carcinomas. *Am J Surg Pathol.* 2001;25:419-432.

Hannibal CG, Vang R, Junge J, et al. A nationwide study of serous "borderline" ovarian tumors in Denmark 1978–2002: centralized pathology review and overall survival compared with the general population. *Gynecol Oncol.* 2014;134:267-273.

Longacre TA, McKenney JK, Tazelaar HD, et al. Ovarian serous tumors of low malignant potential (borderline tumors): outcome-based study of 276 patients with long-term (> or =5-year) follow-up. *Am J Surg Pathol.* 2005;29:707-723.

Seidman JD, Bell DA, Crum CP, et al. Tumours of the ovary: epithelial tumours-serous tumours. In: Kurman RJ, Carcangiu ML, Herrington CS, Young RH, eds. *WHO Classification of Tumours of Female Reproductive Organs.* 4th ed. IARC Press; 2014:17-24.

Seidman JD, Kurman RJ. Ovarian serous borderline tumors: a critical review of the literature with emphasis on prognostic indicators. *Hum Pathol.* 2000;31:539-557.

Seidman JD, Soslow RA, Vang R, et al. Borderline ovarian tumors: diverse contemporary viewpoints on terminology and diagnostic criteria with illustrative images. *Hum Pathol.* 2004;35:918-933.

Vang R, Davidson B, Kong CS, et al. Tumours of the ovary: serous borderline tumour. In: WHO Classification of Tumours Editorial Board. *Female Genital Tumours. WHO Classification of Tumours.* 5th ed. International Agency for Research on Cancer; 2020:38-42.

Vang R, Gilks CB. Tumours of the peritoneum: serous borderline tumour. In: WHO Classification of Tumours Editorial Board. *Female Genital Tumours. WHO Classification of Tumours.* 5th ed. International Agency for Research on Cancer; 2020:184-185.

Vang R, Hannibal CG, Junge J, et al. Long-term behavior of serous borderline tumors subdivided into atypical proliferative tumors and non-invasive low-grade carcinomas: a population-based clinicopathologic study of 942 cases. *Am J Surg Pathol.* 2017;41:725-727.

Zinsser KR, Wheeler JE. Endosalpingiosis in the omentum: a study of autopsy and surgical material. *Am J Surg Pathol.* 1982;6:109-117.

6.3

Bell DA, Scully RE. Serous borderline tumors of the peritoneum. *Am J Surg Pathol.* 1990;14:230-239.

Biscotti CV, Hart WR. Peritoneal serous micropapillomatosis of low malignant potential (serous borderline tumors of the peritoneum). A clinicopathologic study of 17 cases. *Am J Surg Pathol.* 1992;16:467-475.

Gilks CB, Bell DA, Scully RE. Serous psammocarcinoma of the ovary and peritoneum. *Int J Gynecol Pathol.* 1990;9:110-121.

Talia KL, Fiorentino L, Scurry J, et al. A clinicopathologic study and descriptive analysis of "atypical endosalpingiosis". *Int J Gynecol Pathol.* 2020;39:254-260.

Weir MM, Bell DA, Young RH. Grade 1 peritoneal serous carcinomas: a report of 14 cases and comparison with 7 peritoneal serous psammocarcinomas and 19 peritoneal serous borderline tumors. *Am J Surg Pathol.* 1998;22:849-862.

6.4

Churg A, Allen T, Borczuk AC, et al. Well-differentiated papillary mesothelioma with invasive foci. *Am J Surg Pathol.* 2014;38:990-998.

Malpica A, Sant'Ambrogio S, Deavers MT, et al. Well-differentiated papillary mesothelioma of the female peritoneum: a clinicopathologic study of 26 cases. *Am J Surg Pathol.* 2012;36:117-127.

Quick CM, Solomon, DA, Wang J. Tumours of the peritoneum: well-differentiated papillary mesothelial tumour. In: WHO Classification of Tumours Editorial Board. *Female Genital Tumours. WHO Classification of Tumours.* 5th ed. International Agency for Research on Cancer; 2020:179-180.

6.5

Baker PM, Clement PB, Young RH. Malignant peritoneal mesothelioma in women: a study of 75 cases with emphasis on their morphologic spectrum and differential diagnosis. *Am J Clin Pathol.* 2005;123:724-737.

Gilks CB, Oliva E, Solomon DA. Tumours of the peritoneum: Mesothelioma. In: WHO Classification of Tumours Editorial Board. *Female Genital Tumours. WHO Classification of Tumours.* 5th ed. International Agency for Research on Cancer; 2020:181-183.

Husain AN, Colby TV, Ordóñez NG, et al. Guidelines for pathologic diagnosis of malignant mesothelioma 2017 update of the consensus statement from the International Mesothelioma Interest Group. *Arch Pathol Lab Med.* 2018;142:89-108.

Krasinskas AM, Borczuk AC, Hartman DJ, et al. Prognostic significance of morphological growth patterns and mitotic index of epithelioid malignant peritoneal mesothelioma. *Histopathology.* 2016;68:729-737.

Malpica A, Euscher ED, Marques-Piubelli ML, et al. Malignant mesothelioma of the peritoneum in women: a clinicopathologic study of 164 cases. *Am J Surg Pathol.* 2021;45:45-58.

Pavlisko EN, Liu B, Green C, et al. Malignant diffuse mesothelioma in women: a study of 354 cases. *Am J Surg Pathol.* 2020;44:293-304.

Seidman JD, Bell DA, Crum CP, et al. Tumours of the ovary: epithelial tumours-serous tumours. In: Kurman RJ, Carcangiu ML, Herrington CS, Young RH, eds. *WHO Classification of Tumours of Female Reproductive Organs.* 4th ed. IARC Press; 2014:17-24.

Soslow RA, Brenton JD, Davidson B, et al. Tumours of the ovary: high-grade serous carcinoma. In: WHO Classification of Tumours Editorial Board. *Female Genital Tumours. WHO Classification of Tumours.* 5th ed. International Agency for Research on Cancer; 2020:45-47.

Vang R, Ronnett BM. Metastatic and miscellaneous primary tumors of the ovary. In: Nucci MR, Oliva E, eds. *Gynecologic Pathology.* Elsevier; 2009:539-613.

6.6

Kim KR, Scully RE. Peritoneal keratin granulomas with carcinomas of endometrium and ovary and atypical polypoid adenomyoma of endometrium. A clinicopathological analysis of 22 cases. *Am J Surg Pathol.* 1990;14:925-932.

6.7

Ip PPC. Tumours of the peritoneum: Leiomyomatosis peritonealis disseminata. In: WHO Classification of Tumours Editorial Board. *Female Genital Tumours. WHO Classification of Tumours.* 5th ed. International Agency for Research on Cancer; 2020:188-189.

Quade BJ, McLachlin CM, Soto-Wright V, et al. Disseminated peritoneal leiomyomatosis. Clonality analysis by X chromosome inactivation and cytogenetics of a clinically benign smooth muscle proliferation. *Am J Pathol.* 1997;150:2153-2166.

Tavassoli FA, Norris HJ. Peritoneal leiomyomatosis (leiomyomatosis peritonealis disseminata): a clinicopathologic study of 20 cases with ultrastructural observations. *Int J Gynecol Pathol.* 1982;1:59-74.

6.8

Chikkamuniyappa S, Herrick J, Jagirdar JS. Nodular histiocytic/mesothelial hyperplasia: a potential pitfall. *Ann Diagn Pathol.* 2004;8:115-120.

Clement PB, Young RH. Florid mesothelial hyperplasia associated with ovarian tumors: a potential source of error in tumor diagnosis and staging. *Int J Gynecol Pathol.* 1993;12:51-58.

Oparka R, McCluggage WG, Herrington CS. Peritoneal mesothelial hyperplasia associated with gynaecological disease: a potential diagnostic pitfall that is commonly associated with endometriosis. *J Clin Pathol.* 2011;64:313-318.

Ordóñez NG, Ro JY, Ayala AG. Lesions described as nodular mesothelial hyperplasia are primarily composed of histiocytes. *Am J Surg Pathol.* 1998;22:285-292.

Vang R, Davidson B, Kong CS, et al. Tumours of the ovary: serous borderline tumour. In: WHO Classification of Tumours Editorial Board. *Female Genital Tumours. WHO Classification of Tumours.* 5th ed. International Agency for Research on Cancer; 2020:38-42.

6.9

Clement PB. The pathology of endometriosis: a survey of the many faces of a common disease emphasizing diagnostic pitfalls and unusual and newly appreciated aspects. *Adv Anat Pathol.* 2007;14:241-260.

Parker RL, Dadmanesh F, Young RH, et al. Polypoid endometriosis: a clinicopathologic analysis of 24 cases and a review of the literature. *Am J Surg Pathol.* 2004;28:285-297.

Stewart CJR, Ayhan A, Fukunaga M, et al. Endometriosis and derived tumours. In: WHO Classification of Tumours Editorial Board. *Female Genital Tumours. WHO Classification of Tumours.* 5th ed. International Agency for Research on Cancer; 2020: 170-173.

7

Fallopian Tube and Paratubal Region

	Papillary Tubal Hyperplasia	**Normal Tubal Mucosa**
Age	42 y (mean)	Any age
Location	Fallopian tube lumen and mucosa (does not uniformly involve all tubal mucosa)	Fallopian tube
Symptoms	None; may have coexisting ovarian serous borderline tumor	N/A
Signs	None; usually incidental finding; may have coexisting ovarian serous borderline tumor	N/A
Etiology	Not entirely known; possibly due to inflammatory injury of tubal mucosa; a putative precursor of serous borderline tumor, implants, and endosalpingiosis	N/A
Histology	1. More papillary complexity than normal mucosa, varying from slight to marked *(Figs. 7.1.1-7.1.3)* 2. Epithelial stratification, small papillae (with fibrovascular cores) budding from tubal mucosa, and detached epithelial clusters in tubal lumen *(Figs. 7.1.1-7.1.5)* 3. Psammoma bodies (salpingoliths) (either free floating in tubal lumen or present within stroma or epithelium of mucosa) *(Figs. 7.1.4-7.1.6)* 4. Background tubal mucosa may have salpingitis or distortion of the plical architecture	1. No papillary complexity *(Figs. 7.1.7-7.1.9)* 2. No epithelial stratification, small papillae (with fibrovascular cores) budding from tubal mucosa, or detached epithelial clusters in tubal lumen *(Figs. 7.1.7-7.1.10)* 3. No psammoma bodies (salpingoliths) 4. Background tubal mucosa may have salpingitis or distortion of the plical architecture
Special studies	Immunohistochemistry of no help for this differential diagnosis	Immunohistochemistry of no help for this differential diagnosis
Treatment	None needed	N/A
Prognosis	Benign; risk (if any) of subsequent serous borderline tumor unknown	N/A

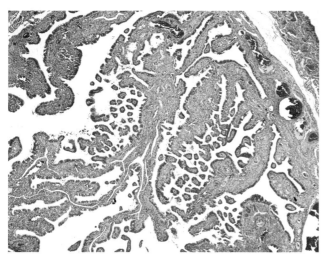

Figure 7.1.1   Papillary tubal hyperplasia with marked papillary complexity.

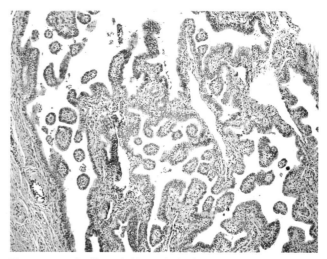

Figure 7.1.2   Papillary tubal hyperplasia showing papillae branching into numerous small ones.

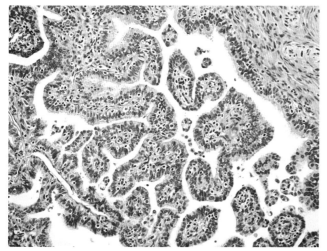

Figure 7.1.3   Papillary tubal hyperplasia (*same case as Fig. 7.1.2*). The small papillae have cytologic features identical to the background mucosa.

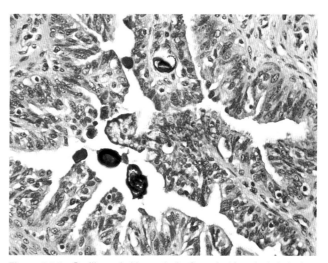

Figure 7.1.4   Papillary tubal hyperplasia. Some foci (*particularly in the* **upper right corner**) show epithelial stratification. Psammoma bodies (salpingoliths) are present within the lumen and stroma.

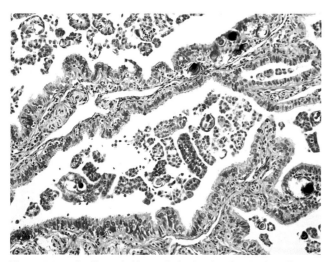

Figure 7.1.5   Papillary tubal hyperplasia showing detached small epithelial clusters within the lumen. Psammoma bodies (salpingoliths) are associated with some of these clusters but are also present within stroma of the background mucosa.

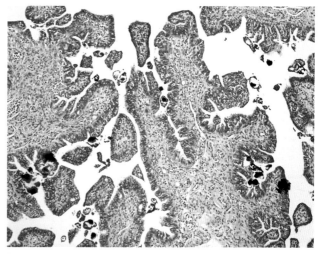

Figure 7.1.6   Papillary tubal hyperplasia. Psammoma bodies (salpingoliths) are associated with papillae in the lumen and within background stroma. The degree of papillary and mucosal complexity is beyond that encountered in normal mucosa.

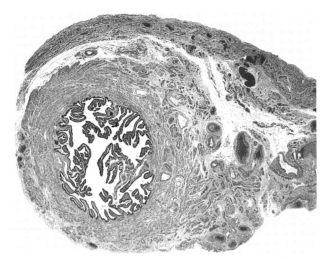

Figure 7.1.7   Normal fallopian tube. The papillary architecture is orderly and within normal limits.

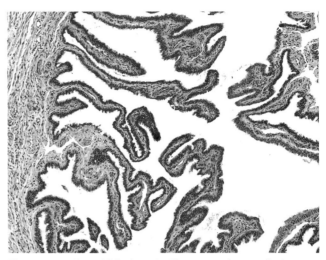

Figure 7.1.8   Normal fallopian tube. The mucosa does not display abnormal papillary branching.

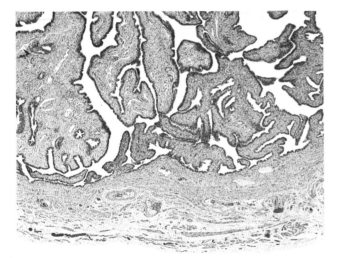

Figure 7.1.9   Normal fallopian tube. The plicae are wider and slightly more irregular than in *Figure 7.1.8*, but the mucosal architecture is otherwise unremarkable.

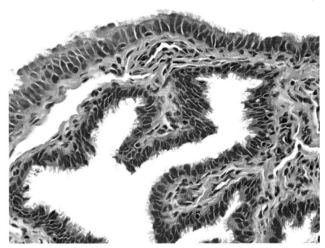

Figure 7.1.10   Normal fallopian tube. The mucosa is not stratified.

7.2

FALLOPIAN TUBE PAPILLOMA VS WELL-DIFFERENTIATED TUBAL NEOPLASM (FIGO GRADE 1 ENDOMETRIOID CARCINOMA/LOW-GRADE SEROUS CARCINOMA/SEROUS BORDERLINE TUMOR)

	Fallopian Tube Papilloma	Well-Differentiated Tubal Neoplasm (FIGO Grade 1 Endometrioid Carcinoma/Low-Grade Serous Carcinoma/Serous Borderline Tumor)
Age	Premenopausal	Peri- or postmenopausal
Location	Fallopian tube lumen	Fallopian tube (may also have extratubal involvement)
Symptoms	None expected but data limited; may be incidental finding	Symptoms attributable to adnexal mass
Signs	Small intraluminal mass; hydrosalpinx also may be present	Adnexal mass; extratubal involvement may be present
Etiology	Unknown	Low-grade serous neoplasms (serous borderline tumor/low-grade serous carcinoma) often harbor *BRAF/KRAS* mutations; evolution from endometriosis to endometrioid carcinoma with *CTNNB1, PTEN, PIK3CA*, and/or *ARID1A* mutations and/or microsatellite instability; data for serous and endometrioid tumors are based on ovarian cases
Histology	1. "Adenomatous" appearance with complex, but orderly, papillary pattern (+/− epithelial stratification); no invasion of underlying tissue; overall architecture vaguely resembles normal mucosa but with much more papillary architecture *(Figs. 7.2.1-7.2.3)*; no psammoma bodies (salpingoliths) 2. Papillae (with branching) have villous appearance and fine fibrovascular cores *(Fig. 7.2.3)* 3. No glandular confluence, solid architecture, squamous differentiation, or endometriosis 4. Contains ciliated and secretory cells similar to normal tubal mucosa *(Fig. 7.2.4)* 5. No atypia 6. No mitotic activity	1. Hierarchical papillary branching and stratification with detached epithelial tufts in typical serous borderline tumor *(Fig. 7.2.5)*; stromal invasion with micropapillary architecture in low-grade serous carcinoma *(Fig. 7.2.6)*; +/− psammoma bodies in either type of serous tumor 2. FIGO grade 1 endometrioid carcinoma can have villoglandular architecture *(Fig. 7.2.7)* 3. Endometrioid carcinoma may have glandular confluence, solid areas (<5% of tumor), squamous differentiation, or endometriosis *(Figs. 7.2.8 and 7.2.9)* 4. Tubal-type epithelium will be present in serous tumors; endometrioid carcinoma can have tubal differentiation with ciliated cells, although other areas should have classic endometrioid cell types *(Fig. 7.2.10)* 5. Some degree of atypia (but not significant) in low-grade serous or endometrioid tumors 6. Low mitotic index
Special studies	Immunohistochemistry of no help for this differential diagnosis, although WT-1 expression is expected	Immunohistochemistry of no help for this differential diagnosis, although endometrioid carcinomas usually lack WT-1 expression
Treatment	None needed	Histologic type and stage dependent
Prognosis	Presumably benign (outcome data limited)	Histologic type and stage dependent

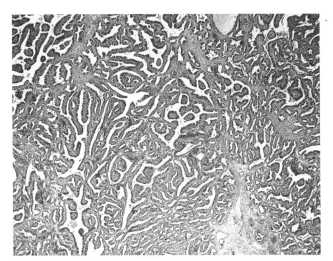

Figure 7.2.1   Fallopian tube papilloma with complex papillary architecture.

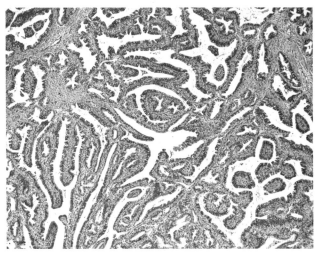

Figure 7.2.2   Fallopian tube papilloma demonstrating orderly papillary pattern.

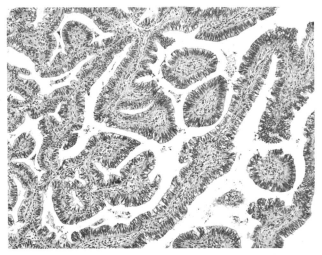

Figure 7.2.3   Fallopian tube papilloma with slender and branching papillae, which resemble normal tubal mucosa.

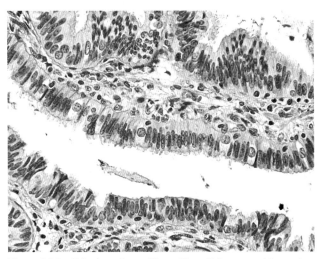

Figure 7.2.4   Fallopian tube papilloma. The cellular composition and appearance are similar to normal tubal mucosa.

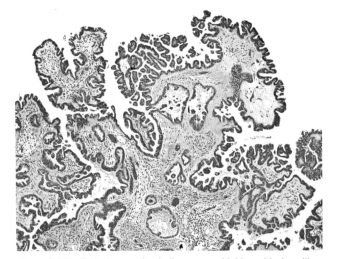

Figure 7.2.5   Typical serous borderline tumor with hierarchical papillary branching, stratification, and detached epithelial tufts.

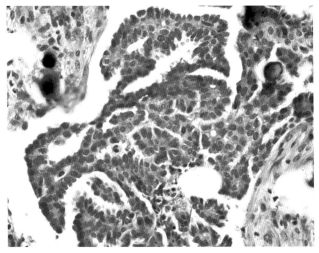

Figure 7.2.6   Low-grade serous carcinoma with complex micropapillary architecture, irregular slit-like spaces, and psammoma bodies.

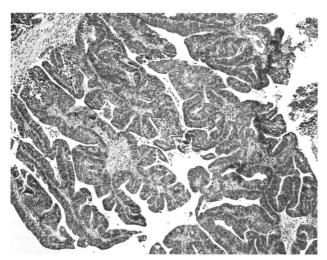

Figure 7.2.7 FIGO grade 1 endometrioid carcinoma with complex villoglandular architecture.

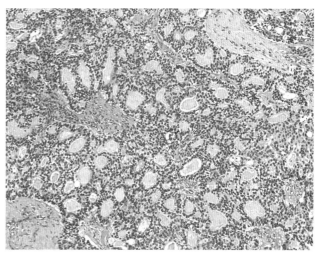

Figure 7.2.8 FIGO grade 1 endometrioid carcinoma with cribriform pattern.

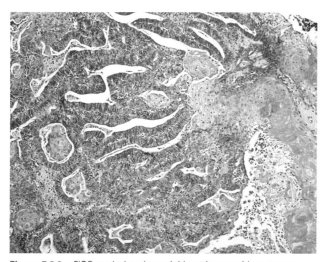

Figure 7.2.9 FIGO grade 1 endometrioid carcinoma with squamous differentiation.

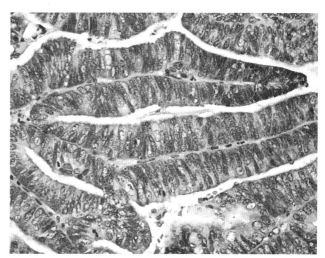

Figure 7.2.10 FIGO grade 1 endometrioid carcinoma with pseudostratified epithelium, columnar cells, flat luminal border, and absence of ciliated cells.

	Serous Tubal Intraepithelial Carcinoma (STIC)	Nondiagnostic Mucosal Atypia
Age	Usually peri- or postmenopausal	Variable
Location	Tubal mucosa, typically in fimbriated end	Tubal mucosa, +/− fimbriated end
Symptoms	None if an isolated finding; symptoms related to tubal/ovarian/peritoneal high-grade serous carcinoma if concurrently present	None if an isolated finding; symptoms related to an underlying condition leading to salpingectomy
Signs	None if an isolated finding (STIC is microscopic in size and does not create a grossly visible lesion); may be associated with a tubal/ovarian/peritoneal high-grade serous carcinoma	None if an isolated finding (mucosal atypia is microscopic in size and does not create a grossly visible lesion); may be associated with a tubal/ovarian/peritoneal high-grade serous carcinoma
Etiology	Arises from tubal mucosa (presumably as a progression pathway through "p53 signatures" and atypical lesions intermediate between p53 signature and STIC) via *TP53* mutations as an early event; +/− *BRCA* mutations	May be nonneoplastic alteration of reactive/reparative nature or preneoplastic step intermediate between "p53 signature" and STIC; also referred to as tubal intraepithelial lesion in transition and serous tubal intraepithelial lesion
Histology	1. Epithelial stratification; +/− detached clusters *(Figs. 7.3.1 and 7.3.2)* 2. Irregular luminal surface *(Figs. 7.3.2 and 7.3.3)* 3. Nuclear enlargement, nuclear rounding, increased nuclear-to-cytoplasmic ratios, nuclear molding, abnormal chromatin (hyperchromasia, irregularly distributed chromatin, or vesicular chromatin), irregular nuclear membranes, loss of polarity, and/or prominent nucleoli *(Figs. 7.3.2 and 7.3.3)* 4. Mitotic activity and/or apoptotic bodies 5. Loss of ciliated cells 6. Variable combinations of the above features	1. Can have some degree of epithelial stratification with detached clusters *(Figs. 7.3.8-7.3.13)* 2. May have some degree of irregular luminal surface 3. Can have some degree of nuclear enlargement, nuclear rounding, increased nuclear-to-cytoplasmic ratios, nuclear molding, abnormal chromatin (hyperchromasia, irregularly distributed chromatin, or vesicular chromatin), irregular nuclear membranes, loss of polarity, and/or prominent nucleoli *(Figs. 7.3.9, 7.3.10, 7.3.12, 7.3.13)* 4. Usually no mitotic activity or apoptotic bodies 5. Ciliated cells usually present but may be absent 6. Above features usually not as sufficiently abnormal as in STIC, but morphologic features of mucosal atypia can significantly overlap with the spectrum seen in STIC

	Serous Tubal Intraepithelial Carcinoma (STIC)	**Nondiagnostic Mucosal Atypia**
Special studies	• p53: aberrant pattern (diffuse moderate-to-strong staining [>75% cells] or complete absence of expression ["null pattern"]) *(Figs. 7.3.4 and 7.3.5)* • Ki-67 proliferation index: high (≥10% positive cells) *(Figs. 7.3.6 and 7.3.7)* • To qualify for a diagnosis of STIC, must have significant atypia, aberrant p53 pattern, and high Ki-67 index	• p53: may have aberrant pattern as in STIC or wild-type pattern (focal or patchy staining) • Ki-67 proliferation index: may have high Ki-67 as in STIC or low index (<10% positive cells) • Atypical lesions not qualifying as STIC do not fulfill all three criteria (significant atypia, aberrant p53 pattern, and high Ki-67 index)
Treatment	Limited data, but chemotherapy usually not administered	None
Prognosis	Probably best considered as uncertain malignant potential for isolated STIC; data in literature are limited (short follow-up for many cases, relatively limited number of cases, and existing data heavily weighted toward *BRCA* germline-mutated rather than sporadic cases); however, a subset of women are at risk for subsequent development of high-grade serous carcinoma (a recent meta-analysis of *BRCA* germline-mutated cases shows 5- and 10-y estimated risks of progression of 11% and 28%, respectively)	Unknown but expected favorable outcome

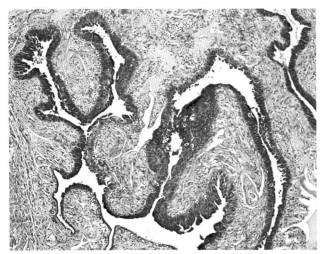

Figure 7.3.1 Serous tubal intraepithelial carcinoma with stratified epithelium (*contrast with normal mucosa*, **bottom center**).

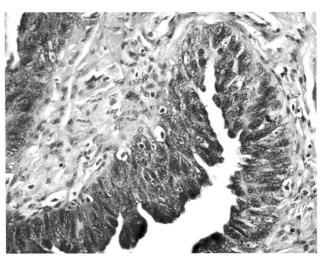

Figure 7.3.2 Serous tubal intraepithelial carcinoma with stratified epithelium and marked nuclear atypia (*same case as Fig. 7.3.1*).

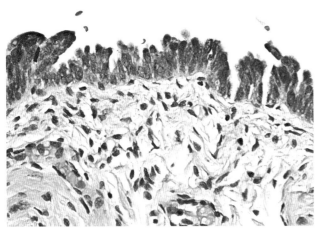

Figure 7.3.3 Serous tubal intraepithelial carcinoma with irregular luminal surface and hyperchromasia.

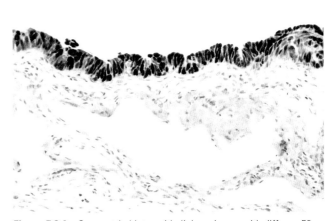

Figure 7.3.4 Serous tubal intraepithelial carcinoma with diffuse p53 expression (*same case as Fig. 7.3.3*).

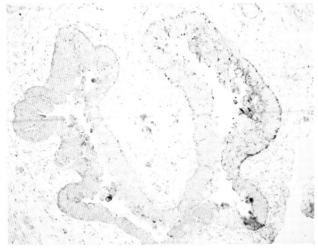

Figure 7.3.5 Serous tubal intraepithelial carcinoma with complete loss of p53 nuclear expression ("null pattern") (*same case as Fig. 7.3.2*).

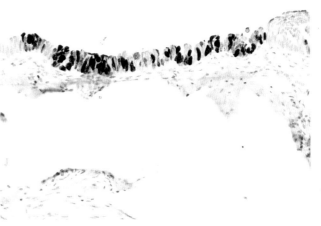

Figure 7.3.6 Serous tubal intraepithelial carcinoma with high Ki-67 proliferation index (*same case as Fig. 7.3.3*).

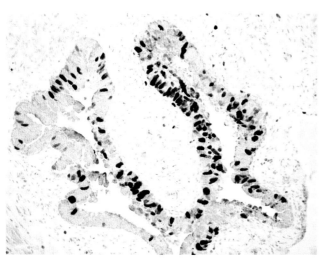

Figure 7.3.7   Serous tubal intraepithelial carcinoma with high Ki-67 proliferation index (*same case as Fig. 7.3.2*).

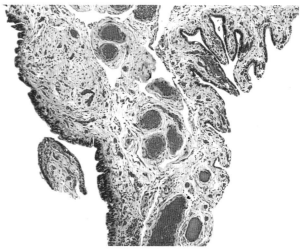

Figure 7.3.8   Nondiagnostic mucosal atypia with stratified epithelium (**lower left**) (*contrast with normal mucosa*, **upper right**).

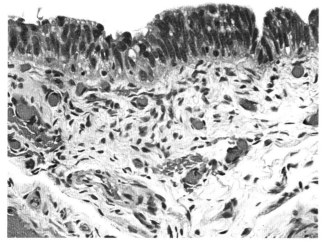

Figure 7.3.9   Nondiagnostic mucosal atypia. The epithelium is stratified and displays slightly coarse chromatin, a suggestion of nuclear molding, and loss of cilia; however, the morphologic features are insufficiently developed for a diagnosis of serous tubal intraepithelial carcinoma (*same case as Fig. 7.3.8*).

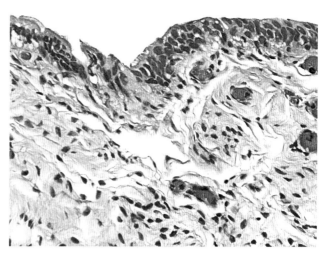

Figure 7.3.10   Nondiagnostic mucosal atypia (**upper right**). The epithelium shows stratification, nuclear rounding, loss of cilia, and slight nuclear enlargement (*contrast with normal mucosa*, **upper left**).

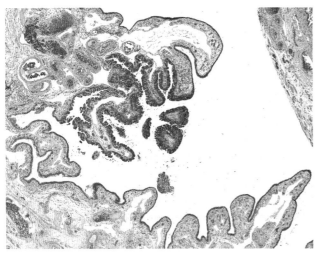

Figure 7.3.11 Nondiagnostic mucosal atypia. The low-power magnification appearance can suggest the possibility of serous tubal intraepithelial carcinoma. Some detached epithelial clusters are present.

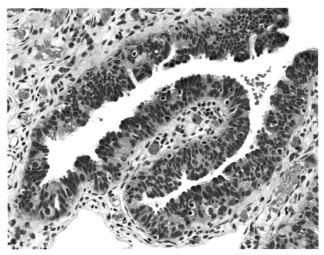

Figure 7.3.12 Nondiagnostic mucosal atypia (*same case as Fig. 7.3.11*). Epithelial stratification and slight nuclear enlargement are present. Note the presence of ciliated cells.

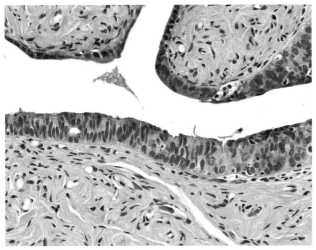

Figure 7.3.13 Nondiagnostic mucosal atypia. Some stratification and nuclear molding are seen. Occasional nuclei are mildly enlarged. Ciliated cells are difficult to identify. Cases such as this would require immunohistochemistry for p53 and Ki-67 to evaluate for the possibility of serous tubal intraepithelial carcinoma.

	Serous Tubal Intraepithelial Carcinoma (STIC)	Mucosal Transitional Cell Metaplasia
Age	Usually peri- or postmenopausal	Variable
Location	Tubal mucosa, typically in fimbriated end	Tubal mucosa, typically in fimbriated end
Symptoms	None if an isolated finding; symptoms related to tubal/ovarian/peritoneal high-grade serous carcinoma if concurrently present	Incidental finding
Signs	None if an isolated finding (STIC is microscopic in size and does not create a grossly visible lesion); may be associated with a tubal/ovarian/peritoneal high-grade serous carcinoma	Incidental finding (microscopic in size; does not create a grossly visible lesion)
Etiology	Arises from tubal mucosa (presumably as a progression pathway through "p53 signatures" and atypical lesions intermediate between p53 signature and STIC) via *TP53* mutations as an early event; +/− *BRCA* mutations	Not applicable; transitional cell metaplasia is commonly found at the fallopian tube-peritoneal junction and may be a normal finding
Histology	1. Epithelial stratification; +/− detached clusters *(Figs. 7.4.1-7.4.6)* 2. Irregular luminal surface *(Figs. 7.4.3, 7.4.5, and 7.4.6)* 3. Nuclear enlargement, nuclear rounding, increased nuclear-to-cytoplasmic ratios, nuclear molding, abnormal chromatin (hyperchromasia, irregularly distributed chromatin, or vesicular chromatin), irregular nuclear membranes, loss of polarity, and/or prominent nucleoli *(Figs. 7.4.4-7.4.6)* 4. Mitotic activity and/or apoptotic bodies 5. Loss of ciliated cells 6. Variable combinations of the above features	1. Epithelial stratification *(Figs. 7.4.7-7.4.10)* 2. Smooth luminal surface *(Figs. 7.4.7 and 7.4.8)* 3. Round to oval and uniform nuclei with pale chromatin, longitudinal nuclear grooves, and abundant cytoplasm; no atypia *(Figs. 7.4.8 and 7.4.9)* 4. No mitotic activity or apoptotic bodies 5. Usually lack ciliated cells 6. Does not show combination of morphologic findings seen in STIC
Special studies	• p53: aberrant pattern (diffuse moderate-to-strong staining [>75% cells] or complete absence of expression ["null pattern"]) • Ki-67 proliferation index: high (≥10% positive cells) • To qualify for a diagnosis of STIC, must have significant atypia, aberrant p53 pattern, and high Ki-67 index • WT-1 (+) • GATA3 expected to be (−)	• No aberrant p53 pattern • No increased Ki-67 index • Does not fulfill all three criteria for STIC (significant atypia, aberrant p53 pattern, and high Ki-67 index) • WT-1 expected to be (−) • GATA3 expected to be (+)
Treatment	Limited data, but chemotherapy usually not administered	None

	Serous Tubal Intraepithelial Carcinoma (STIC)	Mucosal Transitional Cell Metaplasia
Prognosis	Probably best considered as uncertain malignant potential for isolated STIC; data in literature are limited (short follow-up for many cases, relatively limited number of cases, and existing data heavily weighted toward *BRCA* germline-mutated rather than sporadic cases); however, a subset of women are at risk for subsequent development of high-grade serous carcinoma (a recent meta-analysis of *BRCA* germline-mutated cases shows 5- and 10-y estimated risks of progression of 11% and 28%, respectively)	Benign

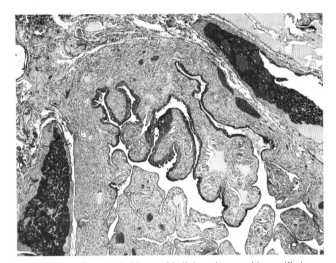

Figure 7.4.1   Serous tubal intraepithelial carcinoma with stratified epithelium (**center**) (*contrast with normal mucosa*, **bottom**).

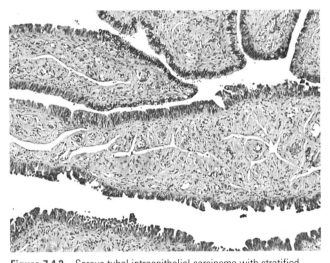

Figure 7.4.2   Serous tubal intraepithelial carcinoma with stratified epithelium (**center and bottom**) (*contrast with normal mucosa*, **top center**).

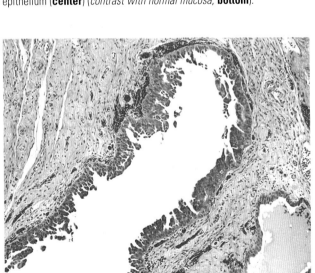

Figure 7.4.3   Serous tubal intraepithelial carcinoma with stratified epithelium and irregular luminal surface.

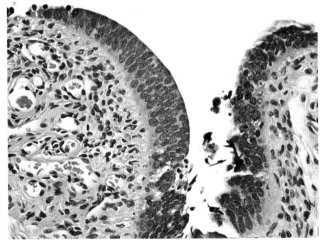

Figure 7.4.4   Serous tubal intraepithelial carcinoma with stratified epithelium, round nuclei showing coarse chromatin, and lack of ciliated cells. The **center and upper left** portions have a flat luminal surface.

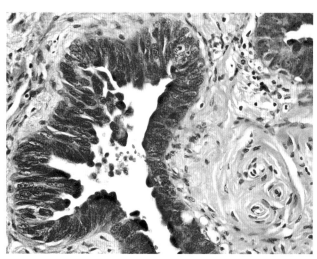

Figure 7.4.5   Serous tubal intraepithelial carcinoma with stratified epithelium, irregular luminal surface, and notable nuclear atypia.

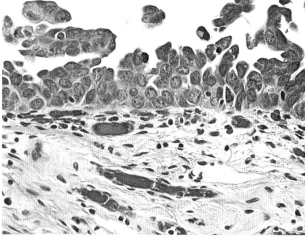

Figure 7.4.6   Serous tubal intraepithelial carcinoma with stratified epithelium, irregular luminal surface, cellular detachment, and marked nuclear atypia.

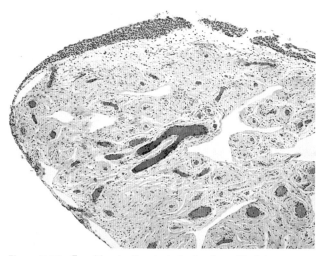

Figure 7.4.7   Transitional cell metaplasia showing epithelial stratification and flat luminal surface.

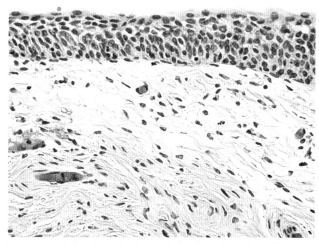

Figure 7.4.8   Transitional cell metaplasia with epithelial stratification, flat luminal surface, and absence of nuclear atypia. Longitudinal nuclear grooves are present.

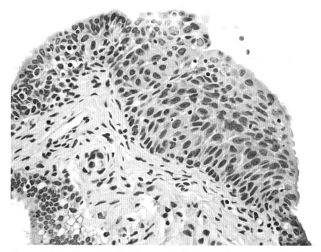

Figure 7.4.9   Transitional cell metaplasia. The nuclear-to-cytoplasmic ratio is not as high as in *Figure 7.4.8*. Some longitudinal nuclear grooves are barely evident.

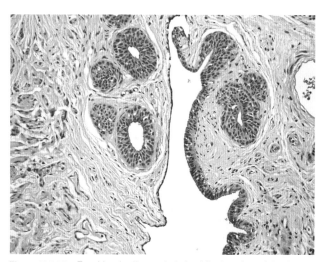

Figure 7.4.10   Transitional cell metaplasia involving invaginated glands. Slight epithelial stratification is present. The foci of transitional cell metaplasia are adjacent to the tuboperitoneal junction (the peritoneum/mesothelium is represented by the single layer with a flat lining in the **center**).

	Secretory Cell Outgrowth (SCOUT)	Serous Tubal Intraepithelial Carcinoma (STIC)
Age	Usually peri- or postmenopausal	Usually peri- or postmenopausal
Location	Tubal mucosa, involving distal or proximal fallopian tube; a subset of SCOUTs (p53 signatures [see below]) typically occur in fimbriated end	Tubal mucosa, typically in fimbriated end
Symptoms	More common in cases with tubal/ovarian/peritoneal high-grade serous carcinoma compared with controls but can be an incidental finding	None if an isolated finding; may be associated with a tubal/ovarian/peritoneal high-grade serous carcinoma
Signs	Incidental finding (microscopic in size; does not create a grossly visible lesion); can be found in cases with tubal/ovarian/peritoneal high-grade serous carcinoma	None if an isolated finding (STIC is microscopic in size and does not create a grossly visible lesion); may be associated with a tubal/ovarian/peritoneal high-grade serous carcinoma
Etiology	Related to *PAX2* dysregulation; SCOUTs may be involved in the pathway leading to the development of serous tubal intraepithelial carcinoma (STIC), but the exact relationship between SCOUTs without p53 overexpression and p53 signature is unclear (p53 signatures can be considered a subset of SCOUTs that demonstrates diffuse p53 expression [ie, p53(+) SCOUTs]; however, the usage of the term "SCOUTs" often implies SCOUTs without aberrant p53 expression [ie, p53-wild-type SCOUTs]); for p53 signatures (see below), genotoxic injury of tubal mucosa may be etiologic; it has been proposed that p53 signatures are the earliest step in pathogenesis of STIC, but p53 signatures are common in both women with *BRCA* germline mutations and controls; p53 signatures show evidence of DNA damage, and a subset have *TP53* mutations (SCOUTs without p53 overexpression do not show evidence of DNA damage or *TP53* mutations)	Arises from tubal mucosa (presumably as a progression pathway through "p53 signatures" and atypical lesions intermediate between p53 signature and STIC) via *TP53* mutations as an early event; +/− *BRCA* mutations

	Secretory Cell Outgrowth (SCOUT)	Serous Tubal Intraepithelial Carcinoma (STIC)
Histology	1. Discrete linear segments of mucosa composed mostly of secretory cells; often without ciliated cells *(Figs. 7.5.1 and 7.5.2)* 2. May have pseudostratification; often thicker than normal mucosa 3. Flat luminal surface 4. Cuboidal to columnar cells without atypia *(Fig. 7.5.2)* 5. No mitotic activity or apoptotic bodies 6. Does not show combination of morphologic findings seen in STIC	1. Loss of ciliated cells *(Figs. 7.5.5-7.5.10)* 2. Epithelial stratification; +/− detached clusters *(Figs. 7.5.9 and 7.5.10)* 3. Irregular luminal surface *(Figs. 7.5.6 and 7.5.10)* 4. Nuclear enlargement, nuclear rounding, increased nuclear-to-cytoplasmic ratios, nuclear molding, abnormal chromatin (hyperchromasia, irregularly distributed chromatin, or vesicular chromatin), irregular nuclear membranes, loss of polarity, and/or prominent nucleoli *(Figs. 7.5.9 and 7.5.10)* 5. Mitotic activity and/or apoptotic bodies *(Fig. 7.5.8)* 6. Variable combinations of the above features
Special studies	• p53: a subset of SCOUTs will have diffuse staining involving a linear stretch of ≥12 consecutive secretory cells ("p53 signature" [*see above*]) *(Figs. 7.5.3 and 7.5.4)* • Ki-67 proliferation index: low (<10% positive cells) • Does not fulfill all three criteria for STIC (significant atypia, aberrant p53 pattern, and high Ki-67 index)	• p53: aberrant pattern (diffuse moderate-to-strong staining [>75% cells] or complete absence of expression ["null pattern"]) • Ki-67 proliferation index: high (≥10% positive cells) • To qualify for a diagnosis of STIC, must have significant atypia, aberrant p53 pattern, and high Ki-67 index
Treatment	None	Limited data, but chemotherapy usually not administered
Prognosis	Benign; the terms SCOUT and p53 signature should be reserved only for research and not be used in the pathology report	Probably best considered as uncertain malignant potential for isolated STIC; data in literature are limited (short follow-up for many cases, relatively limited number of cases, and existing data heavily weighted toward *BRCA* germline-mutated rather than sporadic cases); however, a subset of women are at risk for subsequent development of high-grade serous carcinoma (a recent meta-analysis of *BRCA* germline-mutated cases shows 5- and 10-y estimated risks of progression of 11% and 28%, respectively)

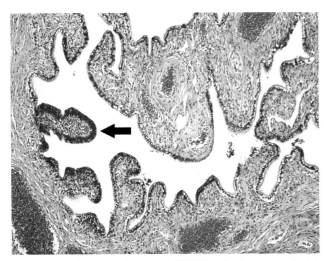

Figure 7.5.1 Secretory cell outgrowth (SCOUT). A focal secretory cell–rich segment (*arrow*) appears darker than the adjacent mucosa, which can simulate serous tubal intraepithelial carcinoma at low-power magnification.

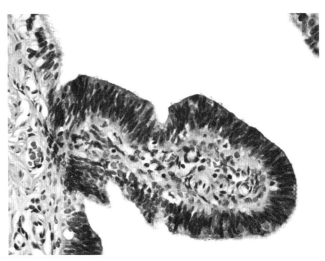

Figure 7.5.2 Secretory cell outgrowth (SCOUT). Same case as *Figure 7.5.1*. Despite the significant reduction in ciliated cells, atypia is not present.

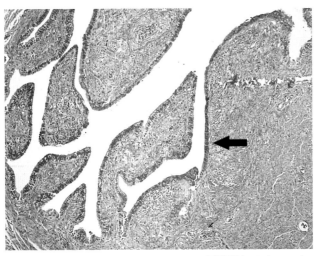

Figure 7.5.3 p53(+)-Secretory cell outgrowth (SCOUT) (p53 signature). A segment of mucosa (*arrow*) lacks ciliated cells and appears more darkly staining compared with other regions of mucosa in this photograph. Atypia is absent (high-power magnification not shown). See text for details regarding terminology.

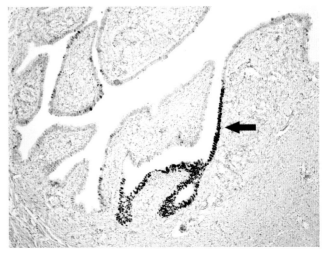

Figure 7.5.4 p53(+)-Secretory cell outgrowth (SCOUT) (p53 signature). The same focus in *Figure 7.5.3* (*arrow*) shows a contiguous segment of p53-positive cells without intervening p53-negative cells. See text for details regarding terminology.

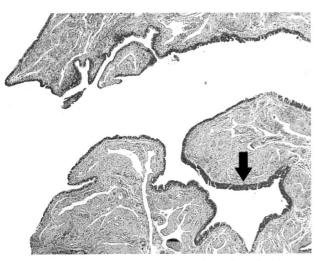

Figure 7.5.5 Serous tubal intraepithelial carcinoma (*arrow*) with stratified epithelium. This segment stains more darkly than adjacent mucosa below and to the left of the *arrow*.

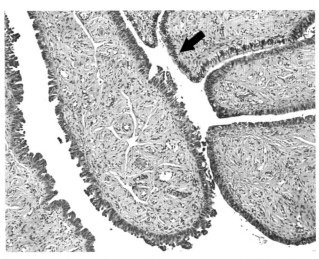

Figure 7.5.6 Serous tubal intraepithelial carcinoma with stratified epithelium and irregular luminal surface. Contrast with normal mucosa (*arrow*).

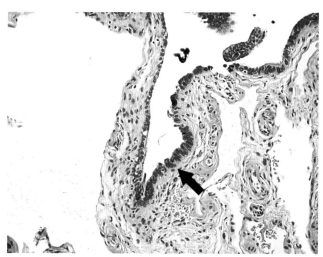

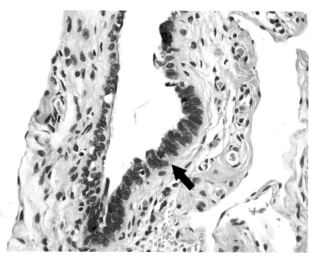

Figure 7.5.7   Attenuated focus of serous tubal intraepithelial carcinoma (*arrow*). Serous tubal intraepithelial carcinomas with nonstratified epithelium may not be obvious at low-power magnification due to their attenuated nature. Contrast with segment of normal mucosa to the **left** of the attenuated serous tubal intraepithelial carcinoma.

Figure 7.5.8   Attenuated serous tubal intraepithelial carcinoma (*same case as Fig. 7.5.7*). A mitotic figure is present (*arrow*).

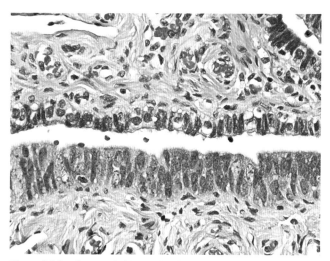

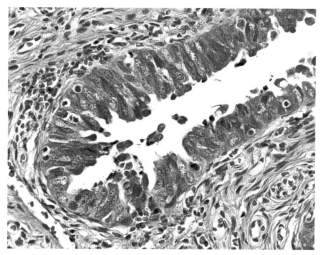

Figure 7.5.9   Serous tubal intraepithelial carcinoma **(bottom)** with stratification, nuclear rounding, marked atypia, and loss of cilia. Normal mucosa is present **(top)**.

Figure 7.5.10   Serous tubal intraepithelial carcinoma with stratification, marked atypia, irregular luminal surface, and cellular detachment.

7 FALLOPIAN TUBE AND PARATUBAL REGION

	Salpingitis Isthmica Nodosa	Invasive Carcinoma
Age	Usually premenopausal	Usually peri- or postmenopausal
Location	Isthmus region of fallopian tube	Fallopian tube; early high-grade serous carcinoma preferentially arises within the fimbriated end
Symptoms	Incidental finding	Symptoms related to adnexal mass
Signs	Incidental microscopic finding or small nodules (ranging up to 1-2 cm) within the isthmus region; often bilateral	Adnexal mass; may have extratubal disease
Etiology	A pseudoinfiltrative diverticular lesion; etiology unknown, but postinflammatory architectural distortion and an adenomyosis-like process are possibilities	Precursors: serous tubal intraepithelial carcinoma (high-grade serous carcinoma); serous borderline tumor (low-grade serous carcinoma); and endometriosis (endometrioid carcinoma)
Histology	1. Round to elongated glands penetrate into the muscular wall of the fallopian tube; glands circumferentially swirl around dilated central lumen of fallopian tube *(Figs. 7.6.1-7.6.5)* 2. Glands lined by single layer of tubal-type epithelium *(Fig. 7.6.6)* 3. Ciliated cells present *(Fig. 7.6.6)* 4. No atypia 5. No mitotic activity 6. No desmoplasia, but chronic inflammation may be present	1. Complex papillary architecture, confluent glandular growth, and/or infiltrating glands or solid nests *(Figs. 7.6.7-7.6.9)* 2. Neoplastic epithelium consists of serous- or endometrioid-type cells, often with stratification 3. Ciliated cells usually absent; some endometrioid carcinomas can have tubal differentiation with ciliated cells 4. Atypia present (marked in high-grade serous carcinoma; low-grade atypia in low-grade serous or endometrioid carcinoma) *(Fig. 7.6.10)* 5. Mitotic index high in high-grade serous carcinoma; low index in low-grade serous or endometrioid carcinoma 6. Desmoplastic response often present
Special studies	• p53: no aberrant expression pattern • Ki-67 proliferation index: low	• p53: aberrant expression pattern (diffuse or complete absence of expression or rare cytoplasmic pattern) in high-grade serous carcinoma; no aberrant pattern in low-grade serous or endometrioid carcinoma • Ki-67 proliferation index: high in high-grade serous carcinoma; low in low-grade serous or endometrioid carcinoma
Treatment	None	Histologic type and stage dependent
Prognosis	Benign, but infertility and ectopic pregnancy are complications	Histologic type and stage dependent

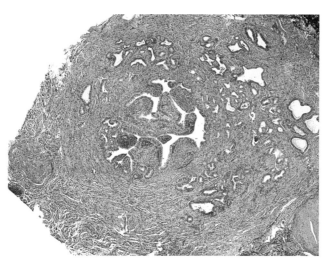

Figure 7.6.1   Salpingitis isthmica nodosa. Glands penetrate into the muscular wall of the fallopian tube and circumferentially swirl around the lumen **(center)**.

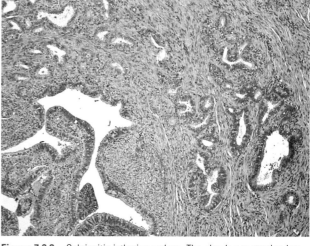

Figure 7.6.2   Salpingitis isthmica nodosa. The glands penetrating into the muscular wall of the fallopian tube (**upper left** *and* **right half** *of photograph*) do not show a direct connection with the mucosa of the lumen (**lower left**), but the overall appearance is consistent with a diverticular process.

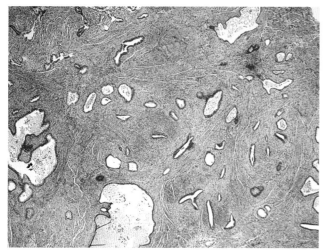

Figure 7.6.3   Salpingitis isthmica nodosa. The glands penetrate through the muscular wall of the fallopian tube (*the distorted lumen is present at the* **left***, and the serosa is present at the* **upper right**).

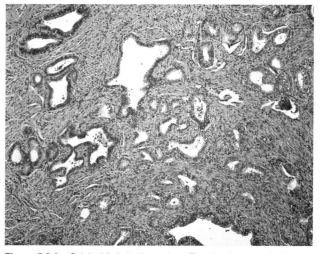

Figure 7.6.4   Salpingitis isthmica nodosa. The glands are markedly crowded and suggestive of haphazard arrangement. Some glands are small and tubular, while others are large and cystically dilated.

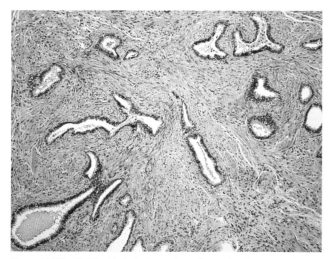

Figure 7.6.5   Salpingitis isthmica nodosa. Some glands are round, while others are elongated.

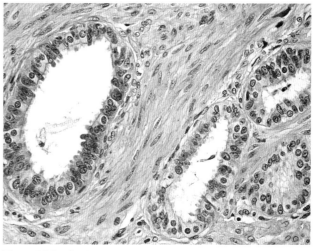

Figure 7.6.6   Salpingitis isthmica nodosa showing tubal-type epithelium, ciliated cells, and absence of atypia.

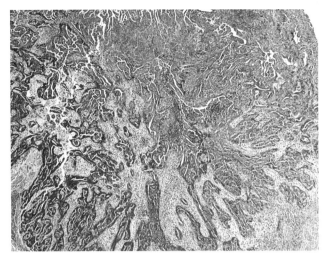

Figure 7.6.7   Invasive high-grade serous carcinoma with infiltrative complex glands.

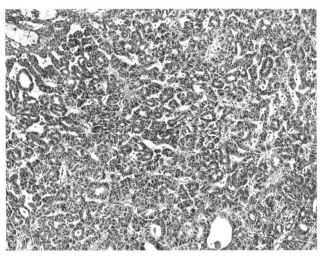

Figure 7.6.8   Invasive endometrioid carcinoma with confluence of tubular glands.

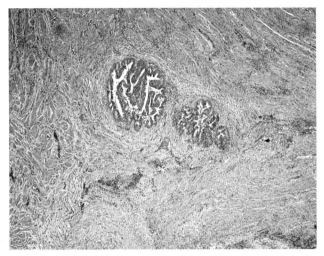

Figure 7.6.9   Endometrioid carcinoma with glands invading wall of fallopian tube. The main body of the tumor is not shown in this photograph.

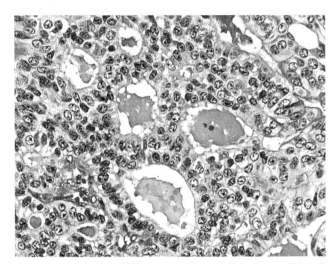

Figure 7.6.10   Invasive FIGO grade 1 endometrioid carcinoma. Although this is a low-grade tumor, the degree of atypia is greater than that encountered in salpingitis isthmica nodosa.

	Detached Fragments of Endometrial Carcinoma Within Tubal Lumen	FIGO Stage III Endometrial Carcinoma Involving Fallopian Tube
Age	Usually postmenopausal	Usually postmenopausal
Location	Fallopian tube lumen	Fallopian tube mucosa, wall, and/or serosa
Symptoms	No specific symptoms related to detached fragments of endometrial carcinoma within tubal lumen; usually present with vaginal bleeding (endometrial carcinoma)	May or may not have pelvic pain specifically related to tubal involvement
Signs	Microscopic finding	May have gross mass involving the fallopian tube or be microscopic finding
Etiology	Detached fragments of endometrial carcinoma (particularly for low-grade endometrial tumors [eg, FIGO grades 1-2 endometrioid carcinoma] in the setting of a robotic hysterectomy or hysteroscopy) within fallopian tube lumen (without adherence to or involvement of mucosa); most likely represent artifactual displacement (contaminant) due to intraoperative uterine manipulation	True secondary involvement (direct extension or metastasis) of fallopian tube by endometrial carcinoma
Histology	1. Fragments of endometrial carcinoma within lumen of fallopian tube *(Figs. 7.7.1-7.7.3)* 2. No adherence to or involvement of fallopian tube mucosa, wall, or serosa *(Figs. 7.7.2 and 7.7.3)* 3. Endometrial primary may be of any histologic type/grade	1. +/− Fragments of endometrial carcinoma within lumen of fallopian tube 2. Adherence to or involvement of fallopian tube mucosa, wall, and/or serosa *(Figs. 7.7.3-7.7.7)* 3. Endometrial primary may be of any histologic type/grade
Special studies	Immunohistochemistry of no help for this differential diagnosis	Immunohistochemistry of no help for this differential diagnosis
Treatment	This finding alone does not warrant upstaging	Postsurgical therapy: chemotherapy and/or radiation therapy
Prognosis	Clinical significance unknown; for high-grade endometrial tumors (eg, serous carcinoma, FIGO grade 3 endometrioid carcinoma, etc.), the presence of intraluminal fragments of endometrial carcinoma is statistically associated with peritoneal metastases; 5-y survival for stage I endometrial carcinoma: 75%-88%	5-y survival for stage IIIA endometrial carcinoma: ~58%

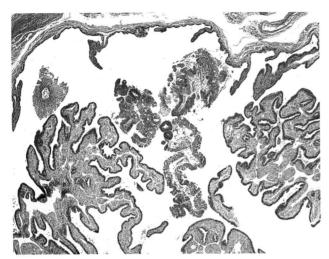

Figure 7.7.1   Detached fragments of endometrial carcinoma within lumen of fallopian tube.

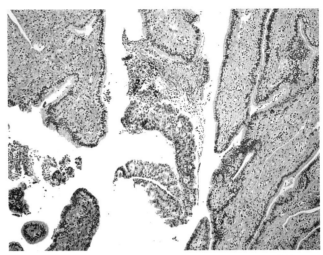

Figure 7.7.2   Detached fragments of endometrial carcinoma within lumen of fallopian tube. The fragments do not directly involve the mucosa.

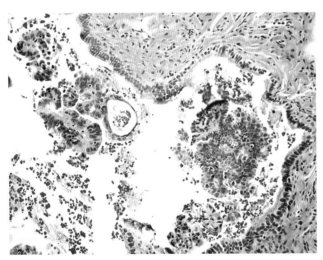

Figure 7.7.3   Detached fragments of endometrial carcinoma with metaplastic-like features within lumen of fallopian tube. The fragments do not directly involve the mucosa.

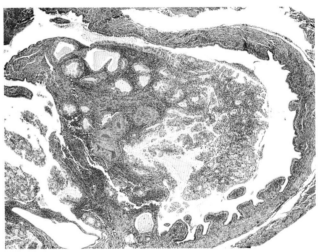

Figure 7.7.4   Endometrial carcinoma with secondary involvement of the fallopian tube. Although some fragments are detached within the tubal lumen, others directly involve the mucosa.

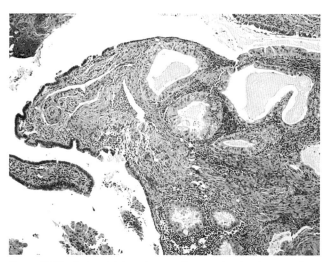

Figure 7.7.5   Endometrial carcinoma with secondary involvement of the fallopian tube. Tumor involves both the epithelium and stroma of the plicae.

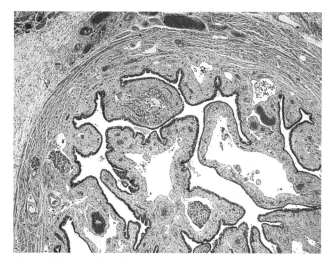

Figure 7.7.6   Multifocal lymphovascular space and stromal invasion of the fallopian tube by undifferentiated endometrial carcinoma.

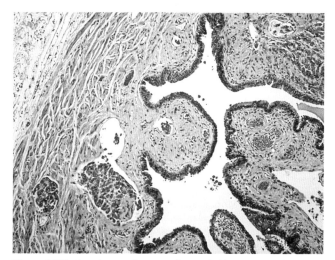

Figure 7.7.7   Lymphovascular space (**lower left**) and stromal (**upper right**) invasion of the fallopian tube by undifferentiated endometrial carcinoma (*same case as Fig. 7.7.6*).

	Adenomatoid Tumor	Metastatic Nongynecologic Carcinoma
Age	Pre-, peri-, or postmenopausal	Usually peri- or postmenopausal
Location	Fallopian tube, subserosal; can be seen within adnexal soft tissue; occasionally, uterine serosa and myometrium	Variety of primary sites, including lower gastrointestinal tract, stomach/upper gastrointestinal tract/pancreaticobiliary region, and breast
Symptoms	Usually an incidental finding	May have a history of prior or concurrent adenocarcinoma
Signs	Usually 1- to 2-cm nodule within wall of fallopian tube; typically unilateral	Fallopian tube may be involved by a mass or tumor may be only microscopic; may have extrafallopian tube tumor within pelvis or abdomen; may be uni- or bilateral
Etiology	Benign mesothelial tumor originating from serosal mesothelium; *TRAF7* mutations are common	Secondary involvement of fallopian tube from a variety of primary sites
Histology	1. Relatively circumscribed 2. Proliferation of tubules, some of which are slightly dilated, through muscular wall of fallopian tube *(Figs. 7.8.1-7.8.4)* 3. Tubules are lined by single layer of low-cuboidal to flat eosinophilic cells *(Fig. 7.8.2)* 4. Nuclei are bland; no mitotic activity 5. Tubules may be empty *(Fig. 7.8.3)* or contain pale fluid (mucin dissipates upon formalin fixation, but mucin may be present in tubules at the time of frozen section) *(Fig. 7.8.4)* 6. Cytoplasm may contain small vacuoles 7. Thin cytoplasmic strands bridge the lumen of tubules *(Fig. 7.8.3)* 8. Stroma may be fibrous or hyalinized or contain lymphoid aggregates *(Figs. 7.8.5 and 7.8.6)* 9. No lymphovascular space invasion	1. Can have circumscribed or infiltrative border 2. Tumor frequently involves serosa but can also involve the mucosa and wall of the fallopian tube; may also have signet ring cells, glands, papillae, and solid sheets and expansion of the stromal compartment of the plicae by tumor *(Figs. 7.8.7-7.8.10)* 3. Glands and papillae lined by columnar to cuboidal cells with simple or complex epithelium; signet ring cells can simulate tubules of adenomatoid tumor 4. Atypia and mitotic activity may be evident; however, nuclei may be deceptively bland, and mitotic figures might be difficult to find 5. Mucin present within signet ring cells *(Fig. 7.8.8)* 6. +/– Cytoplasmic vacuoles 7. No cytoplasmic strands bridging lumen of the tubules/glands 8. Stroma may be desmoplastic or unaltered 9. Lymphovascular space invasion may be present, particularly in the stroma of the plicae
Special studies	• Calretinin: diffuse expression • WT-1: positive • MOC-31: negative • Ber-EP4: negative • Claudin-4: negative	• Calretinin: nondiffuse pattern of expression (negative, focal, or patchy) • WT-1: negative • MOC-31: positive • Ber-EP4: positive • Claudin-4: positive
Treatment	None	Dependent on primary site
Prognosis	Benign	Poor

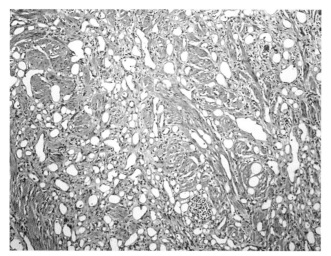

Figure 7.8.1 Adenomatoid tumor with tubules permeating through muscular wall of fallopian tube.

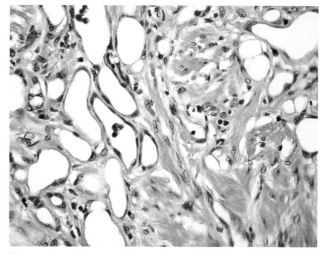

Figure 7.8.2 Adenomatoid tumor. Tubules are lined by single layer of flat cells with bland nuclei.

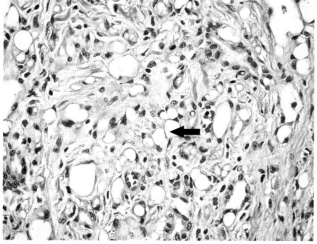

Figure 7.8.3 Adenomatoid tumor. Some tubules are small and may simulate metastatic signet ring cell carcinoma, but the lumens are empty. A thin cytoplasmic bridge is present (*arrow*).

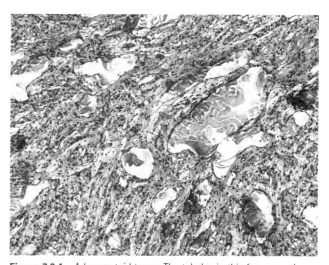

Figure 7.8.4 Adenomatoid tumor. The tubules in this frozen section are filled with mucin, which dissipates upon formalin fixation (*see Fig. 7.8.5*). This appearance at the time of frozen section can mimic metastatic mucinous carcinoma.

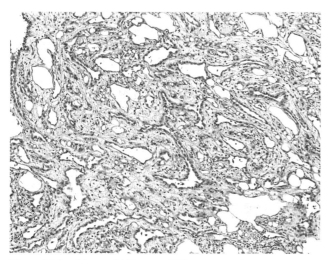

Figure 7.8.5 Adenomatoid tumor with loose stroma (*permanent section from same case as Fig. 7.8.4*).

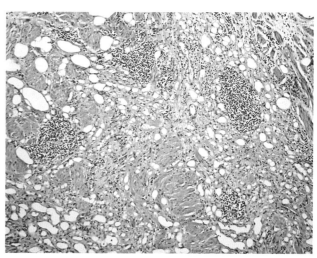

Figure 7.8.6 Adenomatoid tumor with lymphoid aggregates.

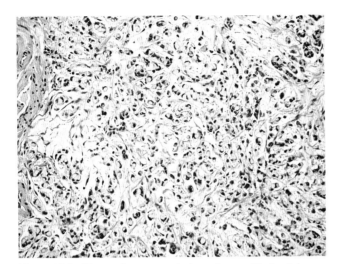

Figure 7.8.7 Metastatic nongynecologic carcinoma with signet ring cells infiltrating through the fallopian tube wall.

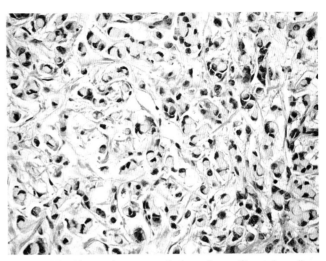

Figure 7.8.8 Metastatic nongynecologic carcinoma. Signet ring cells are filled with mucin.

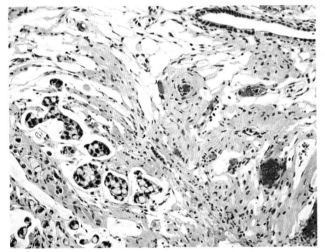

Figure 7.8.9 Metastatic nongynecologic carcinoma with solid nests of cells and signet ring cell differentiation and extracellular mucin within the stroma. Normal fallopian tube mucosa is present in the **upper right corner**.

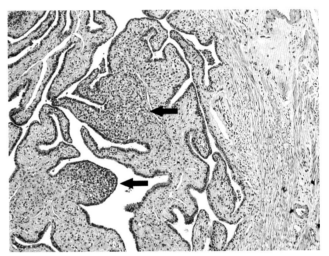

Figure 7.8.10 Metastatic nongynecologic (breast lobular) carcinoma (*arrows*) with stromal expansion of the plicae.

	Metastatic Nongynecologic Carcinoma	**Primary Tubal Carcinoma**
Age	Usually peri- or postmenopausal	Usually peri- or postmenopausal
Location	Variety of primary sites, including lower gastrointestinal tract, stomach/upper gastrointestinal tract/pancreaticobiliary region, and breast	Fallopian tube; early high-grade serous carcinoma preferentially arises within the fimbriated end
Symptoms	May have history of prior or concurrent adenocarcinoma	Symptoms related to adnexal mass
Signs	Fallopian tube may be involved by a mass, or tumor may be only microscopic; may have extrafallopian tube tumor within pelvis or abdomen; may be uni- or bilateral	Adnexal mass; may have extratubal disease; may be uni- or bilateral
Etiology	Secondary involvement of fallopian tube from a variety of primary sites	Precursors: serous tubal intraepithelial carcinoma (STIC) (*TP53* mutation, high-grade serous carcinoma); serous borderline tumor (low-grade serous carcinoma); and endometriosis (endometrioid carcinoma)
Histology	1. Tumor frequently involves serosa but can also involve the mucosa and wall of the fallopian tube *(Fig. 7.9.1)*; expansion of the stromal compartment of the plicae by tumor may be present *(Fig. 7.9.2)*; tumor can involve mucosa of fimbriated end mimicking STIC *(Fig. 7.9.3)* 2. Tumor composed of signet ring cells, glands, papillae, and/or solid sheets *(Figs. 7.9.4 and 7.9.5)* 3. Glands and papillae lined by columnar to cuboidal cells with simple or complex epithelium; mucinous differentiation may be present 4. Atypia and mitotic activity may be evident; however, nuclei may be deceptively bland, and mitotic figures might be difficult to find 5. Dissecting extracellular mucin may be present in stroma 6. No psammoma bodies 7. Lymphovascular space invasion may be present, particularly in the stroma of the plicae *(Fig. 7.9.5)*	1. Tumor preferentially involves mucosa and wall of fallopian tube rather than serosal-predominant distribution, but bulky tumor may obliterate the underlying fallopian tube; high-grade serous carcinoma may have associated STIC in fimbriated end mucosa *(Fig. 7.9.6)* 2. Complex papillary architecture, confluent glandular growth, and/or infiltrating solid nests *(Figs. 7.9.7 and 7.9.8)* 3. Neoplastic epithelium consists of serous- or endometrioid-type cells, often with stratification; squamous metaplasia may be present in endometrioid carcinoma *(Figs. 7.9.9 and 7.9.10)* 4. Atypia present (marked in high-grade serous carcinoma; low-grade atypia in low-grade serous or endometrioid carcinoma); mitotic index high in high-grade serous carcinoma; low index in low-grade serous or endometrioid carcinoma 5. No dissecting mucin 6. Psammoma bodies may be present with serous carcinoma 7. +/− Lymphovascular space invasion

	Metastatic Nongynecologic Carcinoma	**Primary Tubal Carcinoma**
Special studies	• WT-1: negative • PAX8: negative • ER/PR: negative (positive in breast carcinoma, which is also positive for GATA-3) • CK7/CK20 coordinate expression (nonlower gastrointestinal tract): CK7 > CK20 • CK7/CK20 coordinate expression (lower gastrointestinal tract): CK7 < CK20 • SATB2: positive in lower gastrointestinal tract tumors	• WT-1: positive (serous carcinoma) • PAX8: positive • ER/PR: usually positive • CK7/CK20 coordinate expression: CK7 > CK20 • SATB2: negative
Treatment	Dependent on primary site	Histologic type and stage dependent
Prognosis	Poor	Histologic type and stage dependent

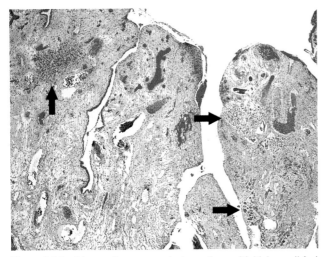

Figure 7.9.1   Metastatic nongynecologic carcinoma. Multiple small foci of carcinoma (*arrows*) involve the stroma of the plicae.

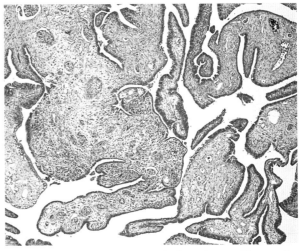

Figure 7.9.2   Metastatic nongynecologic carcinoma with expansion of the stroma of the plicae.

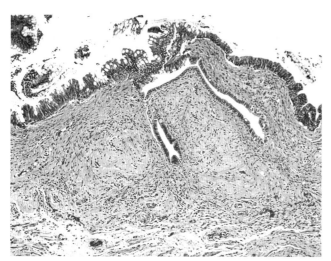

Figure 7.9.3   Secondary involvement by low-grade appendiceal mucinous neoplasm. The lesion exhibits intraepithelial spread in the mucosa of the fallopian tube (**top**), which contrasts with normal mucosa (**center**). If goblet cells are not appreciated in this lesion, it may simulate serous tubal intraepithelial carcinoma.

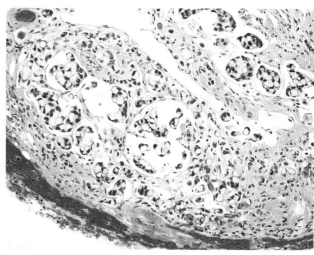

Figure 7.9.4   Metastatic nongynecologic carcinoma with signet ring cell differentiation.

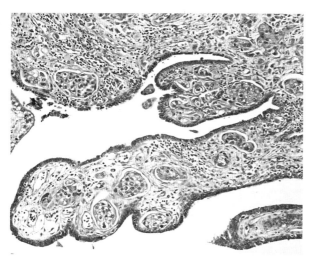

Figure 7.9.5   Metastatic nongynecologic carcinoma with solid nests and lymphovascular space invasion (*same case as Fig. 7.9.2*).

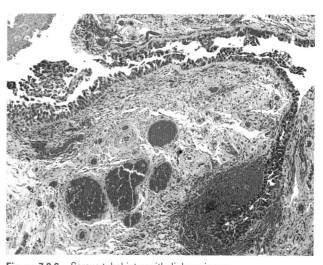

Figure 7.9.6   Serous tubal intraepithelial carcinoma.

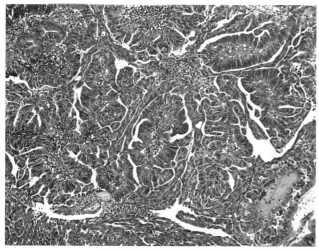

Figure 7.9.7   Primary fallopian tube high-grade serous carcinoma with complex papillary architecture and irregular slit-like spaces.

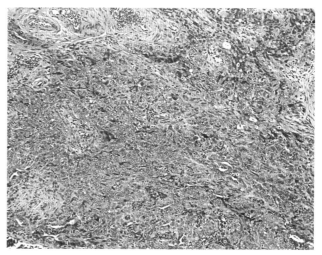

Figure 7.9.8   Primary fallopian tube high-grade serous carcinoma with solid architecture.

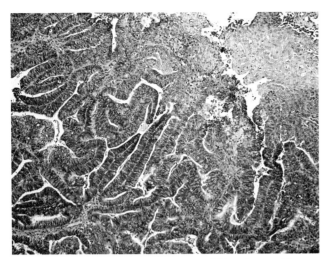

Figure 7.9.9 Primary fallopian tube endometrioid carcinoma with complex villoglandular architecture and squamous differentiation (**upper right**).

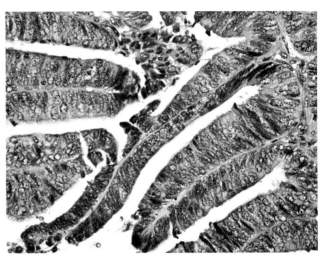

Figure 7.9.10 Primary fallopian tube endometrioid carcinoma with classic cytologic features.

	Female Adnexal Tumor of Wolffian Origin (FATWO)	Endometrioid Carcinoma
Age	Variable age range with mean age in 40s	Variable age range, but most patients are peri- or postmenopausal
Location	Usually broad ligament; can also arise within the ovary	Fallopian tube, paratubal, or ovarian locations
Symptoms	Abdominal pain or discovered as incidental finding	Symptoms attributable to pelvic mass
Signs	Palpable mass or discovered as incidental finding; usually unilateral and confined to primary site; mean size 6 cm but may be microscopic finding	Mass in fallopian tube or paratubal region; variable size; may have locally advanced or metastatic disease
Etiology	Thought to arise from wolffian duct remnants; various molecular alterations have been observed, but no highly consistent genetic changes have been demonstrated; tumors with certain histologic features overlapping with what has been traditionally classified as FATWO (specifically, epithelioid cords/trabeculae, myxoid stroma, and tubular/cystic/cribriform/microacinar architecture) have been shown to harbor *STK11* alterations and a frequent association with Peutz-Jeghers syndrome; the designation "*STK11* adnexal tumor" has been proposed for such cases; however, it is unclear whether this is a unique subset of FATWO vs a distinct entity	Evolution from endometriosis to endometrioid carcinoma with *CTNNB1*, *PTEN*, *PIK3CA*, and/or *ARID1A* mutations and/or microsatellite instability
Histology	1. Combination of growth patterns: tubular (open or solid tubules), cystic, diffuse/solid, lobulated, sieve-like/retiform, and/or adenomatoid-like *(Figs. 7.10.1-7.10.4)*; also referred to as "wolffian tumor" 2. Tubular lumens and sieve-like spaces may have colloid-like material; lacks other confirmatory features typical of endometrioid carcinoma 3. Cuboidal, flat, and/or spindle cells; cells usually have scant cytoplasm *(Fig. 7.10.5)* 4. No associated endometriosis or coexisting endometrioid carcinoma of uterus 5. Bland nuclei; mitotic index usually low 6. Fibrous or hyalinized stroma *(Fig. 7.10.6)*	1. Lacks the combination of features typically seen in FATWO; however, some cases may have a FATWO-like appearance 2. Histologic appearance similar to its uterine counterpart, including classic endometrioid glandular differentiation, villoglandular architecture, squamous and other types of metaplastic-like differentiation, and/or sertoliform architecture *(Figs. 7.10.7-7.10.9)* 3. Mostly columnar and cuboidal cells, but a proportion of oxyphilic and spindle cells may be seen *(Fig. 7.10.10)* 4. Background of endometriosis within the tumor or elsewhere in the pelvis may be seen; synchronous endometrioid carcinoma in the uterus may be present 5. Grade can vary from FIGO 1 to 3 depending on degree of solid growth and nuclear atypia 6. Stroma may be nonspecific or desmoplastic

	Female Adnexal Tumor of Wolffian Origin (FATWO)	**Endometrioid Carcinoma**
Special studies	• Pancytokeratin and CD10 usually positive • Calretinin and low molecular weight cytokeratin often positive but may be negative • CK7 and inhibin: can be positive or negative • ER, PR, and EMA: frequently negative • PAX8: available data suggest PAX8 is negative, but experience is limited	• Pancytokeratin positive; CD10 variable • Calretinin variable; low molecular weight cytokeratin positive • CK7 usually positive; inhibin negative • ER and PR frequently positive; EMA positive • PAX8: usually positive
Treatment	Surgery	Surgery; additional therapy is stage and grade dependent
Prognosis	Usually benign; malignant types have been reported; criteria for predicting behavior are ill defined, but malignant FATWOs frequently have atypia and mitotic activity, although reliable histologic distinction between benign and malignant types is not possible in all cases	Stage and grade dependent

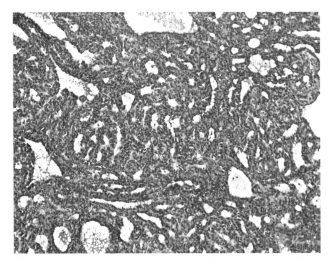

Figure 7.10.1   Female adnexal tumor of wolffian origin (FATWO) with open tubules.

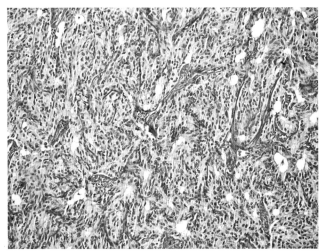

Figure 7.10.2   Female adnexal tumor of wolffian origin (FATWO) with open and closed tubules.

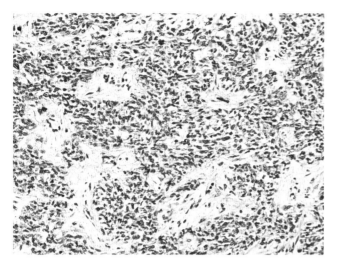

Figure 7.10.3   Female adnexal tumor of wolffian origin (FATWO) with solid pattern and slight spindle cell differentiation.

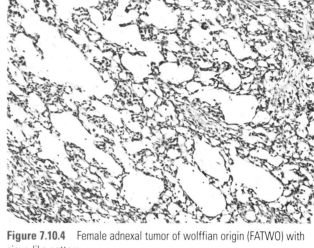

Figure 7.10.4   Female adnexal tumor of wolffian origin (FATWO) with sieve-like pattern.

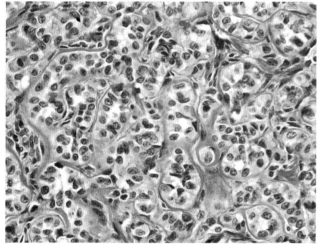

Figure 7.10.5   Female adnexal tumor of wolffian origin (FATWO) with mostly solid tubules and bland nuclei.

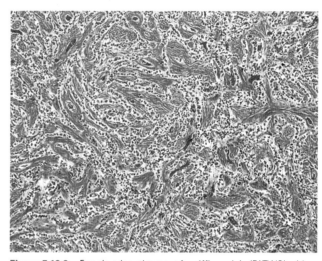

Figure 7.10.6   Female adnexal tumor of wolffian origin (FATWO) with solid tubules/cords and hyalinized bands.

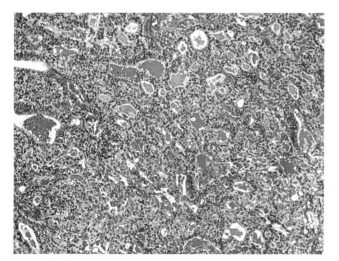

Figure 7.10.7   Endometrioid carcinoma demonstrating glandular confluence.

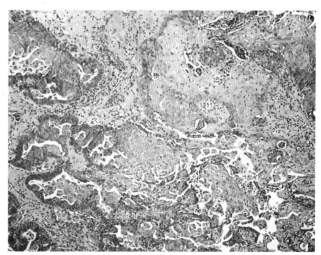

Figure 7.10.8   Endometrioid carcinoma with squamous differentiation.

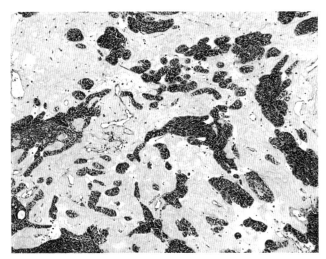

Figure 7.10.9   Endometrioid carcinoma with sertoliform pattern resembling female adnexal tumor of wolffian origin (FATWO).

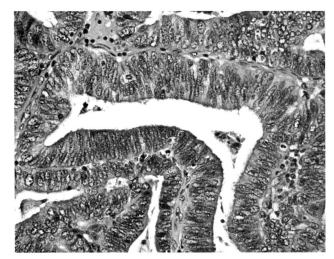

Figure 7.10.10   Endometrioid carcinoma with glands showing columnar cells and pseudostratification.

SUGGESTED READINGS

7.1

Kurman RJ, Vang R, Junge J, et al. Papillary tubal hyperplasia: the putative precursor of ovarian atypical proliferative (borderline) serous tumors, noninvasive implants, and endosalpingiosis. *Am J Surg Pathol.* 2011;35:1605-1614.

Seidman JD, Yemelyanova A, Zaino RJ, et al. The fallopian tube-peritoneal junction: a potential site of carcinogenesis. *Int J Gynecol Pathol.* 2011;30:4-11.

Vang R, Shih IM, Kurman RJ. Fallopian tube precursors of ovarian low- and high-grade serous neoplasms. *Histopathology.* 2013;62:44-58.

7.2

Alvarado-Cabrero I, Wilkinson N. Tumours of the fallopian tube: serous adenofibroma and papilloma of the fallopian tube. In: WHO Classification of Tumours Editorial Board, ed. *Female Genital Tumours. WHO Classification of Tumours.* 5th ed. International Agency for Research on Cancer; 2020:217.

Gisser SD. Obstructing fallopian tube papilloma. *Int J Gynecol Pathol.* 1986;5:179-102.

Vang R. Diseases of the fallopian tube and paratubal region. In: Kurman RJ, Ellenson LH, Ronnett BM, eds. *Blaustein's Pathology of the Female Genital Tract.* 7th ed. Springer; 2019:649-714.

7.3-7.5

Chen EY, Mehra K, Mehrad M, et al. Secretory cell outgrowth, PAX2 and serous carcinogenesis in the Fallopian tube. *J Pathol.* 2010;222:110-116.

Conner JR, Meserve E, Pizer E, et al. Outcome of unexpected adnexal neoplasia discovered during risk reduction salpingo-oophorectomy in women with germ-line BRCA1 or BRCA2 mutations. *Gynecol Oncol.* 2014;132:280-286.

Crum CP, Davidson B, Konishi I, et al. Tumours of the fallopian tube: high-grade serous carcinoma. In: WHO Classification of Tumours Editorial Board, ed. *Female Genital Tumours. WHO Classification of Tumours.* 5th ed. International Agency for Research on Cancer; 2020:219-220.

Lee Y, Miron A, Drapkin R, et al. A candidate precursor to serous carcinoma that originates in the distal fallopian tube. *J Pathol.* 2007;211:26-35.

Morrison JC, Blanco LZ Jr, Vang R, et al. Incidental serous tubal intraepithelial carcinoma and early invasive serous carcinoma in the non-prophylactic setting: analysis of a case series. *Am J Surg Pathol.* 2015;39:442-453.

Patrono MG, Iniesta MD, Malpica A, et al. Clinical outcomes in patients with isolated serous tubal intraepithelial carcinoma (STIC): a comprehensive review. *Gynecol Oncol.* 2015;139:568-572.

Powell CB, Swisher EM, Cass I, et al. Long term follow up of BRCA1 and BRCA2 mutation carriers with unsuspected neoplasia identified at risk reducing salpingo-oophorectomy. *Gynecol Oncol.* 2013;129:364-371.

Przybycin CG, Kurman RJ, Ronnett BM, et al. Are all pelvic (non-uterine) serous carcinomas of tubal origin? *Am J Surg Pathol.* 2010;34:1407-1416.

Quick CM, Ning G, Bijron J, et al. PAX2-null secretory cell outgrowths in the oviduct and their relationship to pelvic serous cancer. *Mod Pathol.* 2012;25:449-455.

Rabban JT, Crawford B, Chen LM, et al. Transitional cell metaplasia of fallopian tube fimbriae: a potential mimic of early tubal carcinoma in risk reduction salpingo-oophorectomies from women with BRCA mutations. *Am J Surg Pathol.* 2009;33:111-119.

Seidman JD, Krishnan J, Yemelyanova A, et al. Incidental serous tubal intraepithelial carcinoma and non-neoplastic conditions of the fallopian tubes in grossly normal adnexa: a clinicopathologic study of 388 completely embedded cases. *Int J Gynecol Pathol.* 2016;35:423-429.

Seidman JD, Sherman ME, Bell KA, et al. Salpingitis, salpingoliths and serous tumors of the ovaries: is there a connection? *Int J Gynecol Pathol.* 2002;21:101-107.

Steenbeek MP, van Bommel MHD, Bulten J, et al. Risk of peritoneal carcinomatosis after risk-reducing salpingo-oophorectomy: a systematic review and individual patient data meta-analysis. *J Clin Oncol.* 2022;40:1879-1891.

Van der Hoeven NMA, Van Wijk K, Bonfrer SE, et al. Outcome and prognostic impact of surgical staging in serous tubal intraepithelial carcinoma: a cohort study and systematic review. *Clin Oncol (R Coll Radiol).* 2018;30:463-471.

Vang R. Diseases of the fallopian tube and paratubal region. In: Kurman RJ, Ellenson LH, Ronnett BM, eds. *Blaustein's Pathology of the Female Genital Tract.* 7th ed. Springer; 2019:649-714.

Vang R, Shih IM, Kurman RJ. Fallopian tube precursors of ovarian low- and high-grade serous neoplasms. *Histopathology.* 2013;62:44-58.

Vang R, Visvanathan K, Gross A, et al. Validation of an algorithm for the diagnosis of serous tubal intraepithelial carcinoma. *Int J Gynecol Pathol.* 2012;31:243-253.

Visvanathan K, Vang R, Shaw P, et al. Diagnosis of serous tubal intraepithelial carcinoma based on morphologic and immunohistochemical features: a reproducibility study. *Am J Surg Pathol.* 2011;35:1766-1775.

7.6

Bolaji II, Oktaba M, Mohee K, et al. An odyssey through salpingitis isthmica nodosa. *Eur J Obstet Gynecol Reprod Biol.* 2015;184:73-79.

Vang R. Diseases of the fallopian tube and paratubal region. In: Kurman RJ, Ellenson LH, Ronnett BM, eds. *Blaustein's Pathology of the Female Genital Tract.* 7th ed. Springer; 2019:649-714.

7.7

Albright BB, Black JD, Passarelli R, et al. Associated characteristics and impact on recurrence and survival of free-floating tumor fragments in the lumen of fallopian tubes in Type I and Type II endometrial cancer. *Gynecol Oncol Rep.* 2018;23:28-33.

Delair D, Soslow RA, Gardner GJ, et al. Tumoral displacement into fallopian tubes in patients undergoing robotically assisted hysterectomy for newly diagnosed endometrial cancer. *Int J Gynecol Pathol.* 2013;32:188-192.

Felix AS, Sinnott JA, Vetter MH, et al. Detection of endometrial cancer cells in the fallopian tube lumen is associated with adverse prognostic factors and reduced survival. *Gynecol Oncol.* 2018;150:38-43.

Rodriquez M, Felix AS, Brett MA, et al. Associations between intraluminal tumor cell involvement in serially examined fallopian tubes and endometrial carcinoma characteristics and outcomes. *Int J Gynecol Pathol.* 2022;41(5):520-529.

Stewart CJ, Doherty DA, Havlat M, et al. Transtubal spread of endometrial carcinoma: correlation of intra-luminal tumour cells with tumour grade, peritoneal fluid cytology, and extra-uterine metastasis. *Pathology.* 2013;45:382-387.

7.8 and 7.9

Goode B, Joseph NM, Stevers M, et al. Adenomatoid tumors of the male and female genital tract are defined by TRAF7 mutations that drive aberrant NF-kB pathway activation. *Mod Pathol.* 2018;31:660-673.

Hes O, Perez-Montiel DM, Alvarado Cabrero I, et al. Thread-like bridging strands: a morphologic feature present in all adenomatoid tumors. *Ann Diagn Pathol.* 2003;7:273-277.

Rabban JT, Vohra P, Zaloudek CJ. Nongynecologic metastases to fallopian tube mucosa: a potential mimic of tubal high-grade serous carcinoma and benign tubal mucinous metaplasia or nonmucinous hyperplasia. *Am J Surg Pathol.* 2015;39:35-51.

Roma AA. Metastatic gastric adenocarcinoma primarily presenting in the fallopian tube. *Ann Diagn Pathol.* 2012;16:63-66.

Sangoi AR, McKenney JK, Schwartz EJ, et al. Adenomatoid tumors of the female and male genital tracts: a clinicopathological and immunohistochemical study of 44 cases. *Mod Pathol.* 2009;22:1228-1235.

Stewart CJ, Leung YC, Whitehouse A. Fallopian tube metastases of non-gynaecological origin: a series of 20 cases emphasizing patterns of involvement including intra-epithelial spread. *Histopathology.* 2012;60:E106-E114.

Vang R. Diseases of the fallopian tube and paratubal region. In: Kurman RJ, Ellenson LH, Ronnett BM, eds. *Blaustein's Pathology of the Female Genital Tract.* 7th ed. Springer; 2019:649-714.

Wachter DL, Wünsch PH, Hartmann A, et al. Adenomatoid tumors of the female and male genital tract. A comparative clinicopathologic and immunohistochemical analysis of 47 cases emphasizing their site-specific morphologic diversity. *Virchows Arch.* 2011;458:593-602.

7.10

Bennett JA, Ritterhouse LL, Furtado LV, et al. Female adnexal tumors of probable Wolffian origin: morphological, immunohistochemical, and molecular analysis of 15 cases. *Mod Pathol.* 2020;33:734-47.

Bennett JA, Young RH, Howitt BR, et al. A distinctive adnexal (usually paratubal) neoplasm often associated with Peutz-Jeghers syndrome and characterized by STK11 alterations (STK11 Adnexal Tumor): a report of 22 cases. *Am J Surg Pathol.* 2021;45:1061-1074.

Cossu A, Casula M, Paliogiannis P, et al. Female adnexal tumors of probable wolffian origin (FATWO): a case series with next-generation sequencing mutation analysis. *Int J Gynecol Pathol.* 2017;36:575-581.

Daya D, Young RH, Scully RE. Endometrioid carcinoma of the fallopian tube resembling an adnexal tumor of probable wolffian origin: a report of six cases. *Int J Gynecol Pathol.* 1992;11:122-130.

Devouassoux-Shisheboran M, Silver SA, Tavassoli FA. Wolffian adnexal tumor, so-called female adnexal tumor of probable Wolffian origin (FATWO): immunohistochemical evidence in support of a Wolffian origin. *Hum Pathol.* 1999;30:856-863.

Goyal A, Masand RP, Roma AA. Value of PAX-8 and SF-1 immunohistochemistry in the distinction between female adnexal tumor of probable wolffian origin and its mimics. *Int J Gynecol Pathol.* 2016;35:167-175.

Hou Y, Yang B, Zhang G. Female adnexal tumor of probable wolffian origin. *Arch Pathol Lab Med.* 2022;146:166-171.

Kariminejad MH, Scully RE. Female adnexal tumor of probable Wolffian origin. A distinctive pathologic entity. *Cancer.* 1973;31:671-677.

Mirkovic J, Dong F, Sholl LM, et al. Targeted genomic profiling of female adnexal tumors of probable wolffian origin (FATWO). *Int J Gynecol Pathol.* 2019;38:543-551.

Navani SS, Alvarado-Cabrero I, Young RH, et al. Endometrioid carcinoma of the fallopian tube: a clinicopathologic analysis of 26 cases. *Gynecol Oncol.* 1996;63:371-378.

8

Gestational Trophoblastic Disease

	Nonmolar Hydropic Abortus	Partial Hydatidiform Mole
Age	Reproductive years (15-46 y)	Reproductive years (13-45 y)
Location	Uterus; occasionally ectopic in fallopian tubes	Uterus; rarely ovaries and fallopian tubes
Symptoms	Usual presentation as missed or incomplete abortion	Usual presentation as missed or incomplete abortion in late first or early second trimester
Signs	Usual presentation as missed or incomplete abortion	Usual presentation as missed or incomplete abortion; may have focal cystic changes on ultrasound; serum β-hCG may be elevated
Etiology	Early pregnancy loss; multifactorial, including chromosomal aberrations other than diandric triploidy	Diandric triploid conception with nearly all being dispermic
Histology	1. Enlarged, hydropic chorionic villi; usually not as large as in partial moles 2. Villi tend to be more symmetrically rounded than in partial moles but can be occasionally slightly irregular *(Figs. 8.1.1-8.1.3)* 3. Usually no villous trophoblastic hyperplasia, but occasional focal mild hyperplasia can be seen *(Fig. 8.1.4)*; villi have polarization of trophoblast *(Fig. 8.1.5)* 4. Trophoblastic inclusions in villi typically absent 5. Nucleated red blood cells may be present in villi 6. Fetal parts may be present	1. Enlarged, hydropic chorionic villi; may be larger than in nonmolar cases *(Fig. 8.1.6)* 2. Variably irregular villous contours ("scalloping") *(Fig. 8.1.7)* 3. Variable villous trophoblastic hyperplasia *(Fig. 8.1.8)*; often greater than in nonmolar cases but may be limited and mild *(Figs. 8.1.9 and 8.1.10)*; villi lack polarization of trophoblast 4. Focal trophoblastic inclusions in villi may be present *(Fig. 8.1.11)* 5. Nucleated red blood cells may be present in villi 6. Fetal parts may be present
Special studies	• p57 immunohistochemistry not helpful for this differential diagnosis ([+] in villous cytotrophoblast and stroma); occasionally, false-negative staining may occur due to poor fixation/degenerative changes • Genotyping: biparental diploid (or tetraploid); uncommonly, genotyping may reveal mosaic/chimeric or digynic triploid conception • Usual karyotype, XX or XY; trisomies can occur	• p57 immunohistochemistry not helpful for this differential diagnosis ([+] in villous cytotrophoblast and stroma); occasionally, false-negative staining may occur due to poor fixation/degenerative changes • Genotyping: almost always diandric triploid, rarely triandric tetraploid • XXY most common karyotype followed by XXX and XYY
Treatment	Dilation and evacuation/curettage	Dilation and evacuation/curettage; follow-up with serum β-hCG measurement; contraception during follow-up period
Prognosis	Unremarkable	Risk of persistent gestational trophoblastic disease and subsequent choriocarcinoma, 0.5%-5% and <0.5%, respectively

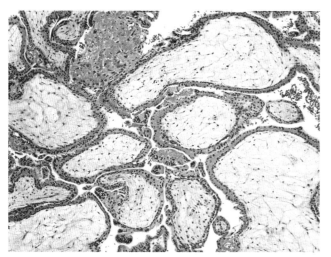

Figure 8.1.1 Nonmolar hydropic abortus with mostly round chorionic villi. Only minimal and limited trophoblastic hyperplasia is noted.

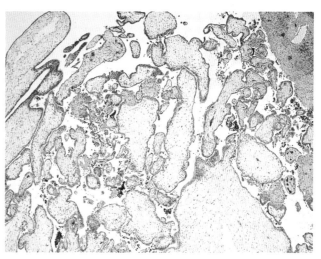

Figure 8.1.2 Nonmolar hydropic abortus with slightly irregular villi. This case was digynic triploid by genotyping, which is incompatible with a diagnosis of a partial mole (the latter is diandric triploid by definition). Digynic triploid conceptions can have some abnormal villous morphology that can histologically overlap with a partial mole.

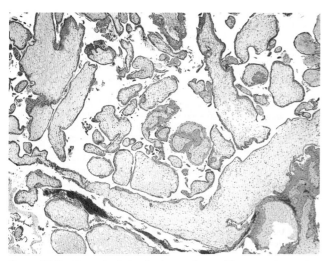

Figure 8.1.3 Nonmolar hydropic abortus. Some villi are mostly round, while others are slightly irregular. This morphology can create concern for a partial mole. However, no appreciable trophoblastic hyperplasia is present.

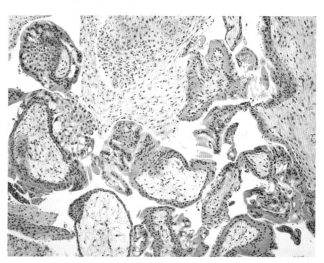

Figure 8.1.4 Nonmolar hydropic abortus with some degree of trophoblastic hyperplasia. This case was biparental diploid by genotyping but also had trisomy of chromosome 13. Trisomies can be associated with abnormal villous morphology, which histologically mimics a partial mole.

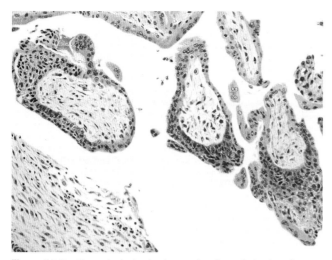

Figure 8.1.5 Nonmolar hydropic abortus showing polarization of trophoblast.

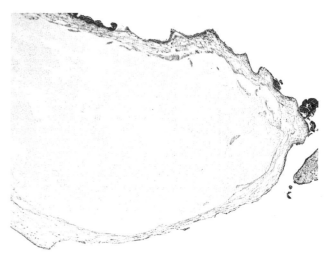

Figure 8.1.6 Partial hydatidiform mole with enlarged molar villus containing a cistern.

8 GESTATIONAL TROPHOBLASTIC DISEASE

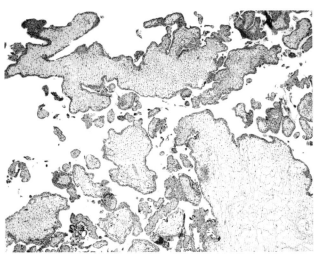

Figure 8.1.7 Partial hydatidiform mole with villous scalloping.

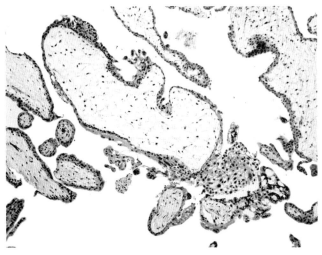

Figure 8.1.8 Partial hydatidiform mole with trophoblastic hyperplasia.

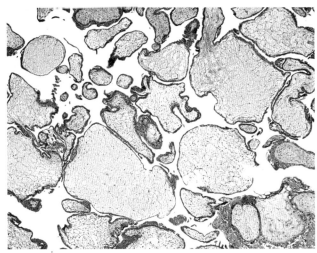

Figure 8.1.9 Partial hydatidiform mole. Some villi are round as in nonmolar hydropic abortuses. However, some villi demonstrate mild scalloping. Mild trophoblastic hyperplasia is noted in the **lower right**.

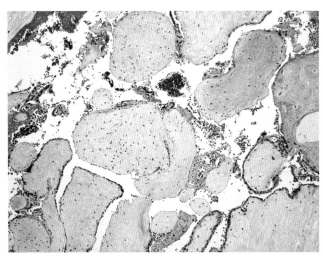

Figure 8.1.10 Partial hydatidiform mole, status post methotrexate therapy, with fibrotic villi and no appreciable trophoblastic hyperplasia. This case was diandric triploid by genotyping and shows features that can be seen in partial moles treated with methotrexate.

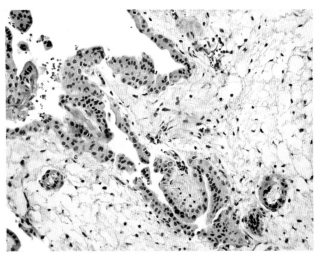

Figure 8.1.11 Partial hydatidiform mole with trophoblastic inclusions.

	Partial Mole	Complete Mole (Including the Early Variant)
Age	Reproductive years (13-45 y)	14-55 y
Location	Uterus; rarely ovaries and fallopian tubes	Uterus; rarely ovaries and fallopian tubes
Symptoms	Usual presentation as missed or incomplete abortion in late first or early second trimester	Usual presentation as missed or incomplete abortion in late first or early second trimester; can have hyperemesis
Signs	Usual presentation as missed or incomplete abortion; may have focal cystic changes on ultrasound; serum β-hCG may be elevated	Usual presentation as missed or incomplete abortion; uterus can be enlarged; may have preeclampsia or hyperthyroidism; may have snow storm pattern without the presence of fetus on ultrasound; serum β-hCG can be markedly elevated
Etiology	Diandric triploid conception with nearly all being dispermic	Androgenetic diploid conception with most being monospermic; rare recurrent, familial, and biparental complete moles due to *NALP7/NLRP7* or *KHDC3L* mutations have been described
Histology	1. Enlarged, hydropic chorionic villi 2. Variably irregular villous contours ("scalloping") *(Fig. 8.2.1)* 3. Villous cisterns may be present 4. Villous stroma usually not myxoid and typically lacks "canalicular" vascular pattern 5. Villous stroma may contain mild amount of apoptotic debris but not as abundant as in some complete moles 6. Variable villous trophoblastic hyperplasia *(Figs. 8.2.2 and 8.2.3)*; not as marked or circumferential as in complete moles 7. Atypical exaggerated implantation site usually absent 8. Focal trophoblastic inclusions in villi may be present 9. Nucleated red blood cells may be present in villi *(Fig. 8.2.4)* 10. Fetal parts may be present	1. Enlarged, hydropic chorionic villi; may be larger than in partial moles 2. Typically do not have irregular villous contours ("scalloping") as seen in partial moles; early complete moles may have bulbous "cauliflower-like" shapes 3. Villous cisterns may be present 4. Villous stroma may be myxoid with "canalicular" vascular pattern 5. Villous stroma may contain abundant apoptotic debris 6. Marked villous trophoblastic hyperplasia (typically circumferential) *(Figs. 8.2.6-8.2.9)*; often greater than in partial moles; hyperplasia in early complete moles may be limited 7. Atypical exaggerated implantation site may be seen 8. Focal trophoblastic inclusions in villi may be present 9. Nucleated red blood cells absent in villi 10. Fetal parts absent except in rare cases of complete moles arising in multiple gestation pregnancies *(Fig. 8.2.10)*

	Partial Mole	**Complete Mole (Including the Early Variant)**
Special studies	• p57 immunohistochemistry (+) in villous cytotrophoblast and stroma *(Fig. 8.2.5)*; occasionally, false-negative staining may occur due to poor fixation/degenerative changes • Genotyping: almost always diandric triploid, rarely triandric tetraploid • XXY most common karyotype followed by XXX and XYY	• p57 immunohistochemistry (−) in villous cytotrophoblast and stroma *(Figs. 8.2.9-8.2.11)*; ≤10% cells may show retained staining • Genotyping: almost always androgenetic diploid, rarely androgenetic tetraploid; rare cases may show a biparental genotype (recurrent, familial, and biparental complete moles) • Karyotype in majority of cases, XX; minority are XY
Treatment	Dilation and evacuation/curettage; follow-up with serum β-hCG measurement; contraception during follow-up period	Dilation and evacuation/curettage; follow-up with serum β-hCG measurement; contraception during follow-up period; chemotherapy for cases in which serum β-hCG does not return to normal
Prognosis	Risk of persistent gestational trophoblastic disease and subsequent choriocarcinoma, 0.5%-5% and <0.5%, respectively	Risk of persistent gestational trophoblastic disease and subsequent choriocarcinoma, 15%-29% and 2%-3%, respectively; heterozygous/dispermic complete moles are clinically more aggressive than homozygous/monospermic cases

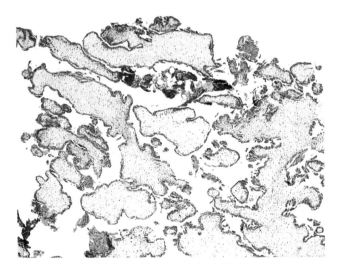

Figure 8.2.1 Partial hydatidiform mole with scalloping.

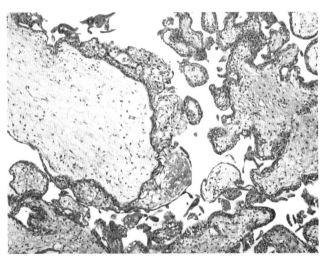

Figure 8.2.2 Partial hydatidiform mole with notable trophoblastic hyperplasia.

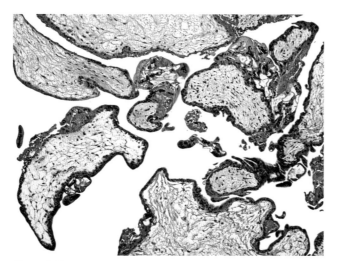

Figure 8.2.3 Partial hydatidiform mole with mild trophoblastic hyperplasia.

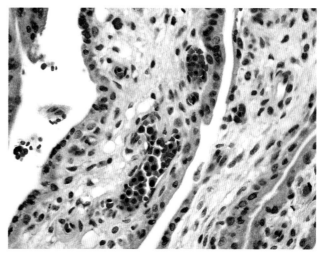

Figure 8.2.4 Partial hydatidiform mole with nucleated red blood cells within molar villi.

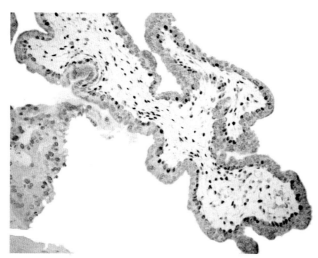

Figure 8.2.5 Partial hydatidiform mole. p57 immunostain shows positivity in the cytotrophoblast layer and stroma of a molar villus.

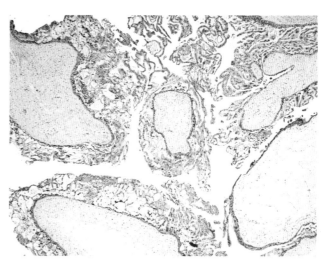

Figure 8.2.6 Complete hydatidiform mole with circumferential villous trophoblastic hyperplasia.

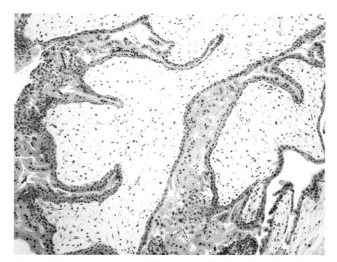

Figure 8.2.7 Complete hydatidiform mole with circumferential villous trophoblastic hyperplasia.

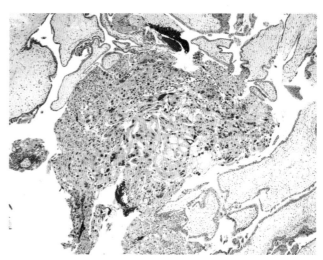

Figure 8.2.8 Complete hydatidiform mole with marked villous trophoblastic hyperplasia.

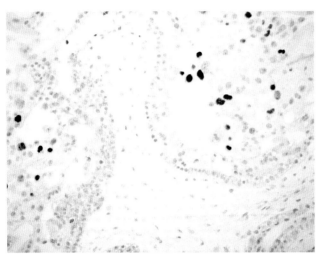

Figure 8.2.9   Complete hydatidiform mole. p57 immunostain shows loss of expression in the cytotrophoblast layer and stroma of a molar villus. Note that intervillous intermediate trophoblast (seen on either side of the villus) is positive in complete moles serving as a positive internal control.

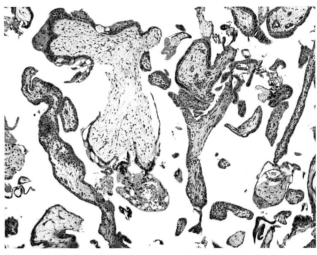

Figure 8.2.10   Complete hydatidiform mole arising in the setting of a twin pregnancy. The combination of two types of villi (complete mole [**left**] and normal [**right**]) can be mistaken for a partial mole.

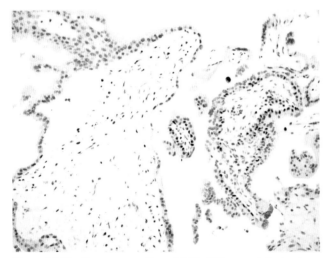

Figure 8.2.11   Same case as *Figure 8.2.10*. p57 immunostain showing loss of expression in the cytotrophoblast layer and stroma of a molar villus (**left**) and positivity in the nonmolar villus (**center and right**). Failure to recognize two morphologically different populations can result in incorrect interpretation of the immunostain and misclassification as a partial mole because of some positivity in the specimen.

	Early Complete Hydatidiform Mole	Nonmolar Hydropic Abortus
Age	14-55 y	Reproductive years (15-46 y)
Location	Uterus; rarely ovaries and fallopian tubes	Uterus; occasionally ectopic in fallopian tubes
Symptoms	Usual presentation as missed or incomplete abortion in first trimester	Usual presentation as missed or incomplete abortion
Signs	Usual presentation as missed or incomplete abortion; serum β-hCG can be normal or elevated	Usual presentation as missed or incomplete abortion
Etiology	Androgenetic diploid conception with most being monospermic; rare recurrent, familial, and biparental complete moles due to *NALP7/NLRP7* or *KHDC3L* mutations have been described	Early pregnancy loss
Histology	1. Enlarged, hydropic chorionic villi 2. Villi may have bulbous "cauliflower-like" shapes *(Fig. 8.3.1)* 3. Villous cisterns may be present *(Fig. 8.3.2)* 4. Villous stroma often myxoid with "canalicular" vascular pattern *(Fig. 8.3.3)* 5. Villous stroma often contains abundant apoptotic debris *(Fig. 8.3.3)* 6. Villous trophoblastic hyperplasia can be marked and may be circumferential; however, hyperplasia in early complete moles can be limited *(Figs. 8.3.4 and 8.3.5)*; villi lack polarization of trophoblast 7. Atypical exaggerated implantation site may be seen *(Fig. 8.3.6)* (exaggerated implantation sites associated with complete moles have greater cytologic atypia than in nonmolar cases) 8. Focal trophoblastic inclusions in villi may be present 9. Nucleated red blood cells absent in villi 10. Fetal parts absent except in rare cases of complete moles arising in multiple gestation pregnancies	1. Enlarged, hydropic chorionic villi 2. Villi tend to be symmetrically rounded but can be occasionally slightly irregular *(Fig. 8.3.8)* 3. No villous cisterns 4. Villous stroma often lacks both myxoid appearance and "canalicular" vascular pattern 5. Villous stroma often lacks abundant apoptotic debris 6. Usually no villous trophoblastic hyperplasia *(Fig. 8.3.8)*, but occasional focal mild proliferation can be seen; however, early nonmolar abortuses can show exuberant trophoblastic proliferation *(Fig. 8.3.9)*; villi have polarization of trophoblast *(Fig. 8.3.10)* 7. Atypical exaggerated implantation site absent 8. Trophoblastic inclusions in villi typically absent 9. Nucleated red blood cells may be present in villi 10. Fetal parts may be present

	Early Complete Hydatidiform Mole	**Nonmolar Hydropic Abortus**
Special studies	• p57 immunohistochemistry (−) in villous cytotrophoblast and stroma *(Fig. 8.3.7)*; ≤10% cells may show retained staining • Genotyping: almost always androgenetic diploid, rarely androgenetic tetraploid; rare cases may show a biparental genotype (recurrent, familial, and biparental complete moles) • Karyotype in majority of cases, XX; minority are XY	• p57 immunohistochemistry (+) in villous cytotrophoblast and stroma *(Fig. 8.3.11)*; occasionally, false-negative staining may occur due to poor fixation/degenerative changes • Genotyping: biparental diploid (or tetraploid); uncommonly, genotyping may reveal mosaic/chimeric or digynic triploid conception • Usual karyotype, XX or XY; trisomies can occur
Treatment	Dilation and evacuation/curettage; follow-up with serum β-hCG measurement; contraception during follow-up period; chemotherapy for cases in which serum β-hCG does not return to normal	Dilation and evacuation/curettage
Prognosis	Risk of persistent gestational trophoblastic disease and subsequent choriocarcinoma, 15%-29% and 2%-3%, respectively; heterozygous/dispermic complete moles are clinically more aggressive than homozygous/monospermic cases	Unremarkable

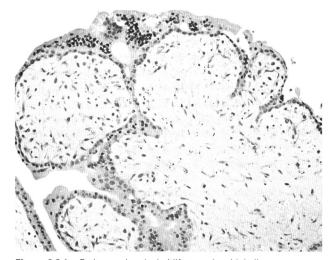

Figure 8.3.1   Early complete hydatidiform mole with bulbous "cauliflower-like" villous shapes.

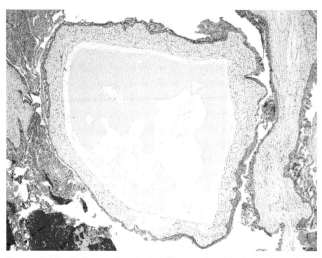

Figure 8.3.2   Early complete hydatidiform mole with cistern formation.

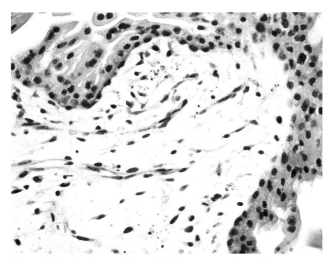

Figure 8.3.3   Early complete hydatidiform mole with myxoid stroma, canalicular vessels, and apoptotic debris within a villus.

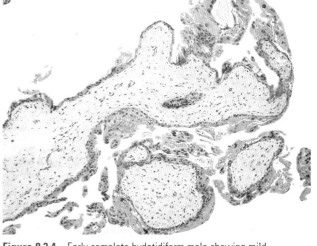

Figure 8.3.4   Early complete hydatidiform mole showing mild trophoblastic hyperplasia. Note that the hyperplasia is nonpolarized.

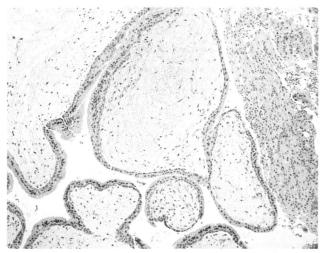

Figure 8.3.5   Early complete hydatidiform mole. In this field, the villi are round without evident trophoblastic hyperplasia, mimicking a nonmolar hydropic abortus.

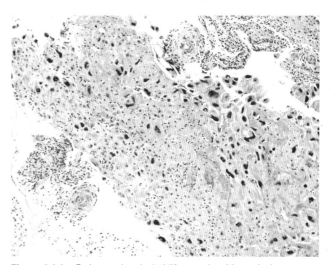

Figure 8.3.6   Early complete hydatidiform mole with atypical implantation site.

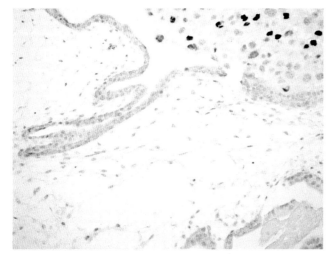

Figure 8.3.7   Early complete hydatidiform mole. p57 immunostain shows loss of expression in the villous cytotrophoblast layer and villous stromal cells. Adjacent to the villus is an intervillous trophoblastic island with p57 expression serving as a positive internal control.

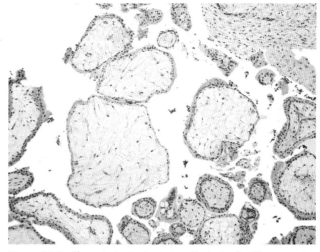

Figure 8.3.8   Nonmolar hydropic abortus. The hydropic villi are round without trophoblastic hyperplasia.

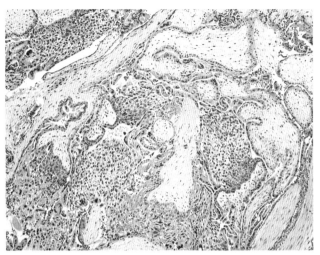

Figure 8.3.9 Nonmolar hydropic abortus. This early/immature conception exhibits much greater trophoblastic proliferation than is usually seen in a later-date nonmolar hydropic abortus. However, early/immature conceptions can simulate an early complete mole.

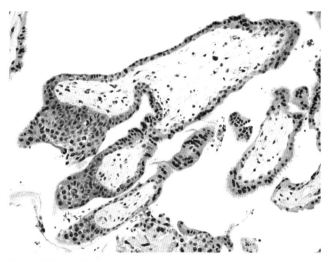

Figure 8.3.10 Nonmolar hydropic abortus with polarized trophoblast.

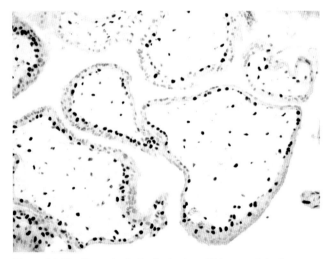

Figure 8.3.11 Nonmolar hydropic abortus. p57 immunostain shows positivity in the villous cytotrophoblast layer and villous stromal cells.

	Complete Hydatidiform Mole With Atypical Trophoblastic Hyperplasia	Choriocarcinoma
Age	14-55 y	Reproductive years
Location	Uterus; rarely ovaries and fallopian tubes	Often in uterus; occasionally in the fallopian tube or ovary
Symptoms	Usual presentation as missed or incomplete abortion in late first or early second trimester; can have hyperemesis	Vaginal bleeding
Signs	Usual presentation as missed or incomplete abortion; uterus can be enlarged; may have preeclampsia or hyperthyroidism; may have snow storm pattern without the presence of fetus on ultrasound; serum β-hCG can be markedly elevated	Serum β-hCG is markedly elevated; may have persistent gestational trophoblastic disease
Etiology	Androgenetic diploid conception with most being monospermic; rare recurrent, familial, and biparental complete moles due to *NALP7/NLRP7* or *KHDC3L* mutations have been described	A subset of cases have an antecedent complete mole, but many choriocarcinomas develop after a normal pregnancy
Histology	1. Molar villi are present with marked circumferential trophoblastic hyperplasia, which may be extensive *(Fig. 8.4.1)*	1. Molar villi may or may not be present; some investigators do not accept a diagnosis of choriocarcinoma in the presence of molar villi (however, choriocarcinoma in the presence of normal villi, such as an intraplacental choriocarcinoma, is accepted *[Figs. 8.4.5 and 8.4.6]*), while others do accept a diagnosis of choriocarcinoma in a background of a complete mole
	2. Detached fragments of atypical trophoblast may qualitatively resemble choriocarcinoma *(Figs. 8.4.2-8.4.4)*	2. The atypical trophoblast proliferation contains sheets of trimorphic malignant cells, which include cytotrophoblast, intermediate trophoblast, and syncytiotrophoblast; the architecture of these intimately admixed populations resembles the arrangement seen in their normal counterparts, in which cytotrophoblast are rimmed by syncytiotrophoblast *(Figs. 8.4.7 and 8.4.8)*; tissue invasion *(Fig. 8.4.9)*, hemorrhage, and necrosis are present; lymphovascular space invasion is frequent
	3. Atypical trophoblast lack tissue invasion	3. Criteria for diagnosing choriocarcinoma in the setting of a complete mole: cytologically malignant trophoblastic proliferation, separate from molar villi and morphologically indistinguishable from choriocarcinoma, must display evidence of tissue invasion; this diagnosis is extremely challenging, particularly in curettage specimens

	Complete Hydatidiform Mole With Atypical Trophoblastic Hyperplasia	Choriocarcinoma
Special studies	• p57 immunohistochemistry (−) in villous cytotrophoblast and stroma; ≤10% cells may show retained staining • Genotyping: almost always androgenetic diploid, rarely androgenetic tetraploid; rare cases may show a biparental genotype (recurrent, familial, and biparental complete moles) • Karyotype in majority of cases, XX; minority are XY	• p57 immunohistochemistry (−) in villous cytotrophoblast and stroma (if villi are present), as the type of mole that a choriocarcinoma typically arises within is the complete type • Genotyping: can be androgenetic or biparental; androgenetic ones are often associated with a genetically related concurrent or prior complete mole, and, thus, of molar-type; biparental choriocarcinomas typically are of intraplacental origin • Complex karyotypes can occur; majority of cases will have XX sex chromosome component; most cases lack a Y chromosome
Treatment	Dilation and evacuation/curettage; follow-up with serum β-hCG measurement; contraception during follow-up period; chemotherapy for cases in which serum β-hCG does not return to normal	Chemotherapy
Prognosis	Risk of persistent gestational trophoblastic disease and subsequent choriocarcinoma, 15%-29% and 2%-3%, respectively; heterozygous/dispermic complete moles are clinically more aggressive than homozygous/monospermic cases	Favorable outcome with chemotherapy

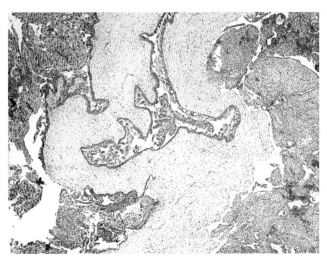

Figure 8.4.1   Complete hydatidiform mole with atypical trophoblastic hyperplasia (**left**). Molar villi are present in the **center** of this field, while gestational endometrium is located on the **right**.

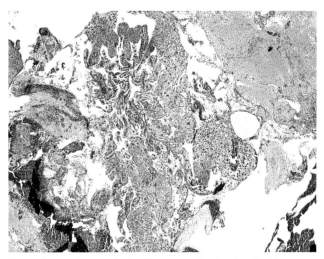

Figure 8.4.2   Complete hydatidiform mole showing detached fragments of atypical trophoblast.

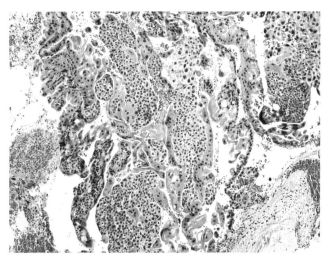

Figure 8.4.3   Same case as *Figure 8.4.2*. Intimate arrangement of two populations of trophoblast qualitatively identical to choriocarcinoma.

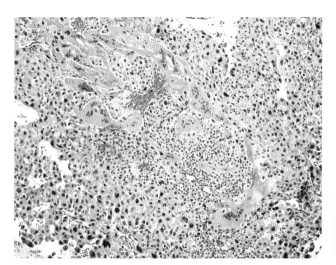

Figure 8.4.4   Complete hydatidiform mole with sheets of atypical trophoblast, which can simulate choriocarcinoma.

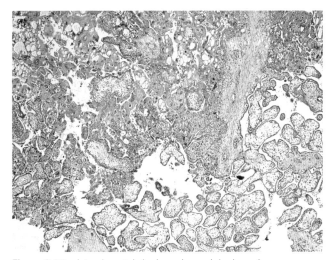

Figure 8.4.5   Intraplacental choriocarcinoma (*choriocarcinoma*, **upper left**; *term placenta*, **lower right**).

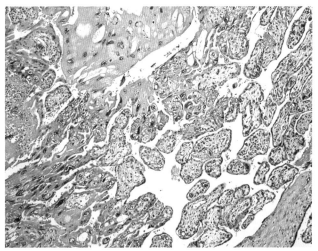

Figure 8.4.6   Same case as *Figure 8.4.5* (*choriocarcinoma*, **upper left**; *term placenta*, **lower right**).

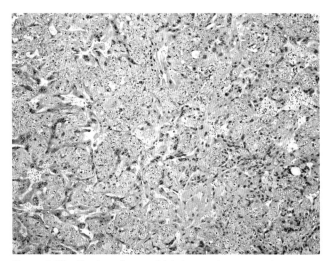

Figure 8.4.7 Choriocarcinoma with intimate arrangement of two populations of trophoblast.

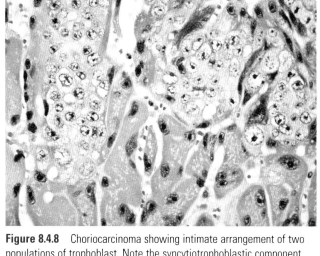

Figure 8.4.8 Choriocarcinoma showing intimate arrangement of two populations of trophoblast. Note the syncytiotrophoblastic component with abundant amphophilic cytoplasm rims the mononuclear component.

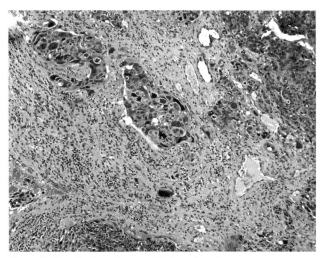

Figure 8.4.9 Choriocarcinoma with tissue invasion.

	Mosaic/Chimeric Conception	Partial Hydatidiform Mole
Age	Reproductive years (18-45 y)	Reproductive years (13-45 y)
Location	Uterus	Uterus; rarely ovaries and fallopian tubes
Symptoms	Usual presentation as missed or incomplete abortion in late first or early second trimester	Usual presentation as missed or incomplete abortion in late first or early second trimester
Signs	Usual presentation as missed or incomplete abortion; may have ultrasound findings suggesting a molar pregnancy; serum β-hCG may be elevated if coexisting complete hydatidiform mole is present	Usual presentation as missed or incomplete abortion; may have focal cystic changes on ultrasound; serum β-hCG may be elevated
Etiology	Conception resulting in mixture of two cell lines (one androgenetic, the other biparental) arising by either mosaicism (mitotic error in a single zygote) or chimerism (fusion of two different zygotes)	Diandric triploid conception with nearly all being dispermic
Histology	1. Enlarged, hydropic chorionic villi *(Fig. 8.5.1)* 2. Variably sized and irregularly shaped villi 3. Some villi will have hypercellular stroma *(Fig. 8.5.2)* 4. Villous cisterns may be present 5. Focal trophoblastic inclusions in villi may be present 6. Nonmolar mosaic/chimeric villi lack trophoblastic hyperplasia; villi have polarization of trophoblast 7. Coexisting component of complete hydatidiform mole will be present in some cases *(Figs. 8.5.3 and 8.5.4)* 8. Nucleated red blood cells may be present in nonmolar villi 9. Fetal parts may be present	1. Enlarged, hydropic chorionic villi 2. Variably irregular villous contours ("scalloping") *(Fig. 8.5.7)* 3. No villi with hypercellular stroma 4. Villous cisterns may be present 5. Focal trophoblastic inclusions in villi may be present 6. Variable villous trophoblastic hyperplasia *(Fig. 8.5.8)*; may be limited and mild; villi lack polarization of trophoblast 7. No component of complete mole 8. Nucleated red blood cells may be present in villi 9. Fetal parts may be present

	Mosaic/Chimeric Conception	**Partial Hydatidiform Mole**
Special studies	• p57 immunohistochemistry (in individual nonmolar villi): discordant pattern ([+] in villous cytotrophoblast [biparental population], [−] in villous stroma [androgenetic population]) *(Fig. 8.5.5)* • p57 immunohistochemistry (component of complete mole, if present): (−) in villous cytotrophoblast and stroma *(Fig. 8.5.6)* • Genotyping (nonmolar villi; >1 villous area should be analyzed): excess of paternal alleles with variable paternal:maternal allele ratios, >2:1 • Genotyping (component of complete mole, if present): androgenetic diploid • FISH analysis (nonmolar villous component): both cytotrophoblast and stroma are usually diploid (often XX in both cell types), but discordant ploidy between cytotrophoblast vs stroma can occur	• p57 immunohistochemistry (+) in villous cytotrophoblast and stroma *(Fig. 8.5.9)*; occasionally, false-negative staining may occur due to poor fixation/degenerative changes • Genotyping: almost always diandric triploid, rarely triandric tetraploid • XXY most common karyotype followed by XXX and XYY
Treatment	Dilation and evacuation/curettage; for cases without a molar component, follow-up with serum β-hCG measurement is recommended because of the presence of an androgenetic cell line; contraception during follow-up period; cases with a component of a complete mole should be managed accordingly	Dilation and evacuation/curettage; follow-up with serum β-hCG measurement; contraception during follow-up period
Prognosis	For cases without a molar component, outcome data are limited; cases with a component of complete mole would be expected to have prognosis similar to conventional complete moles	Risk of persistent gestational trophoblastic disease and subsequent choriocarcinoma, 0.5%-5% and <0.5%, respectively

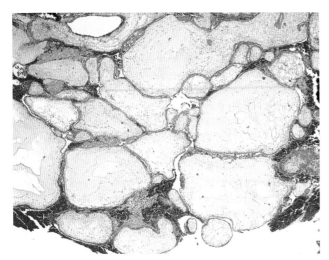

Figure 8.5.1   Mosaic/chimeric conception with large and hydropic chorionic villi. No trophoblastic hyperplasia is present.

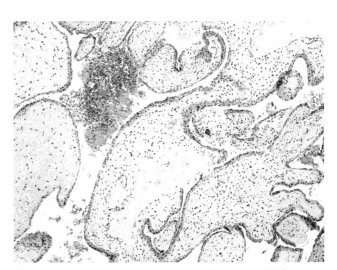

Figure 8.5.2   Mosaic/chimeric conception with hydropic villi. Some have hypocellular villous stroma, while others have increased stromal cellularity. Slight villous irregularity is present, which can create concern for a partial hydatidiform mole.

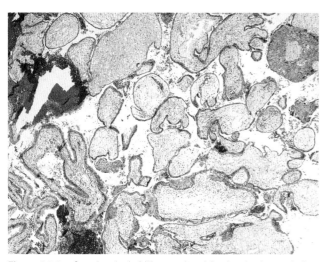

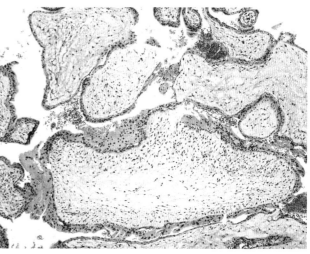

Figure 8.5.3   Complete hydatidiform mole arising in a background of a mosaic/chimeric conception. The villi in the **lower portion** of this field have trophoblastic hyperplasia (component of complete mole), while villi in the **upper portion** lack trophoblastic hyperplasia (component of nonmolar mosaic/chimeric conception).

Figure 8.5.4   Same case as *Figure 8.5.3*. The villus in the **lower portion** of this field has trophoblastic hyperplasia (component of complete mole), while villi in the **upper portion** lack trophoblastic hyperplasia (component of nonmolar mosaic/chimeric conception).

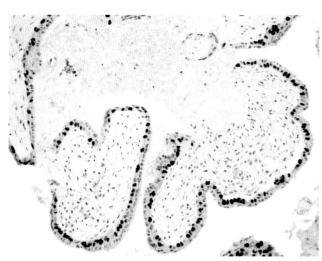

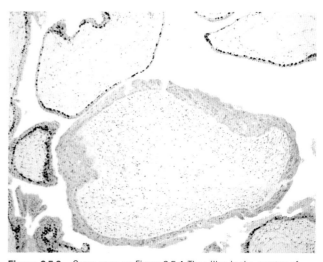

Figure 8.5.5   Mosaic/chimeric conception. p57 immunostain shows a characteristic pattern with expression in the cytotrophoblast layer but loss of expression in the villous stroma.

Figure 8.5.6   Same case as *Figure 8.5.4*. The villus in the **center** of this field with trophoblastic hyperplasia (component of complete mole) exhibits loss of p57 expression in the cytotrophoblast layer and villous stroma, while the other villi lacking trophoblastic hyperplasia (component of nonmolar mosaic/chimeric conception) show the characteristic pattern of p57 expression seen in nonmolar mosaic/chimeric conceptions, in which p57 is expressed in the cytotrophoblast layer with loss of expression in the villous stroma (compare with *Fig. 8.5.5*).

8   GESTATIONAL TROPHOBLASTIC DISEASE

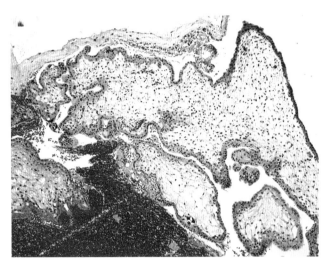

Figure 8.5.7   Partial hydatidiform mole with scalloping. No trophoblastic hyperplasia is present in this field.

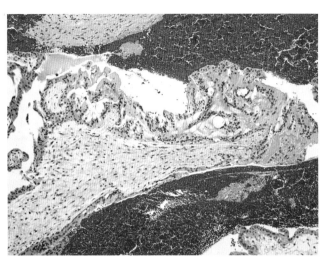

Figure 8.5.8   Partial hydatidiform mole with trophoblastic hyperplasia.

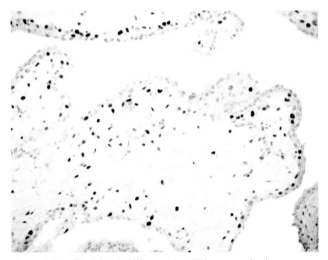

Figure 8.5.9   Partial hydatidiform mole. p57 immunostain shows positivity in the cytotrophoblast layer and villous stroma.

	Exaggerated Implantation Site	Placental Site Trophoblastic Tumor
Age	Reproductive years	20-63 y; typically young
Location	Uterus	Uterus
Symptoms	No specific symptoms; incidental finding usually in products of conception specimen	Vaginal bleeding; missed abortion
Signs	No specific symptoms; incidental finding usually in products of conception specimen; does not produce a mass	Serum β-hCG may be mildly to moderately elevated; gross mass may be evident
Etiology	Implantation site changes within the spectrum of intermediate trophoblast during pregnancy	Trophoblast neoplasia with differentiation toward implantation-type intermediate trophoblast
Histology	1. No separation of myometrial bundles by sheets of lesional cells 2. Mononucleated implantation-type intermediate trophoblastic cells infiltrate decidua and myometrium *(Figs. 8.6.1 and 8.6.2)*; cells are often epithelioid with abundant eosinophilic cytoplasm but can be spindle shaped *(Fig. 8.6.3)* 3. May have abundant multinucleated intermediate trophoblastic cells *(Figs. 8.6.4 and 8.6.5)* 4. Lesional cells can infiltrate vascular walls 5. Can have some degree of nuclear atypia, which can overlap with placental site trophoblastic tumor (molar-associated implantation sites can have greater atypia than in nonmolar cases) *(Fig. 8.6.6)* 6. No mitotic activity 7. Chorionic villi may be present elsewhere in specimen	1. Aggregates to sheets of tumor cells, which separate myometrial bundles *(Figs. 8.6.8 and 8.6.9)* 2. Mononucleated implantation-type intermediate trophoblastic tumor cells; large polygonal to round cells, occasionally spindled; abundant amphophilic, eosinophilic, or clear cytoplasm 3. Multinucleated tumor cells can be present in a scattered fashion but not as numerous as in some exaggerated implantation sites 4. Tumor cells can replace vascular walls 5. Nuclei are atypical, large, and irregular with hyperchromasia *(Fig. 8.6.10)* 6. Mitotically active, but mitotic index is generally low (usually 2-4 mitotic figures per 10 high-power fields) 7. Specimens typically lack villi
Special studies	• HLA-G/Ki-67 double stain: no increased proliferation in HLA-G(+) cells (HLA-G [+] in intermediate trophoblastic cells, [−] in lymphocytes, decidua, and myometrium); hydroxyl-delta-5-steroid dehydrogenase (HSD3B1) or cytokeratin can be used instead of HLA-G *(Fig. 8.6.7)* • Molar-associated implantation sites can have higher proliferation index (5%-30%) than in nonmolar cases	• HLA-G/Ki-67 double stain: tumor cells have increased proliferation index (usually 5%-30%); hydroxyl-delta-5-steroid dehydrogenase (HSD3B1) or cytokeratin can be used instead of HLA-G *(Fig. 8.6.11)*

	Exaggerated Implantation Site	**Placental Site Trophoblastic Tumor**
Treatment	None	Hysterectomy, +/− chemotherapy
Prognosis	Unremarkable	70% survival at 10 y; a subset of cases exhibit recurrent disease and/or die of disease; advanced FIGO stage, antecedent pregnancy of ≥48 mo, and clear cytoplasm are independent risk factors

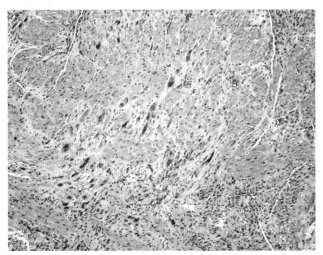

Figure 8.6.1   Implantation site showing usual architectural pattern with infiltration into myometrium.

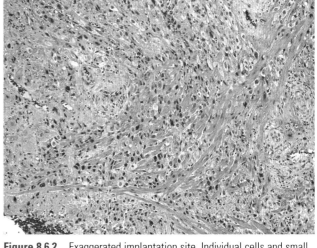

Figure 8.6.2   Exaggerated implantation site. Individual cells and small clusters of cells infiltrate between muscle fibers, which can create concern for placental site trophoblastic tumor.

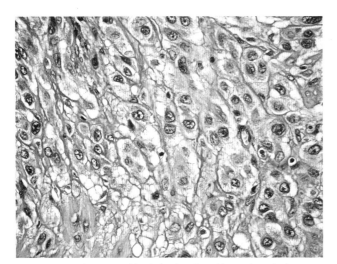

Figure 8.6.3   Exaggerated implantation site with usual cytologic features. Epithelioid cells show mild nuclear atypia. The degree of cellularity in this focus is slightly greater than in most cases but can simulate placental site trophoblastic tumor if taken out of context.

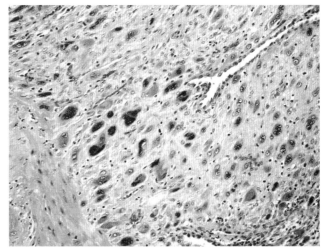

Figure 8.6.4   Implantation site with abundant multinucleated intermediate trophoblastic cells.

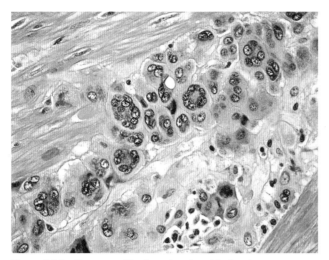

Figure 8.6.5 Exaggerated implantation site with abundant multinucleated intermediate trophoblastic cells.

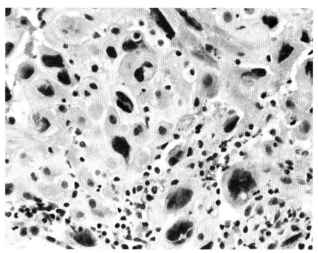

Figure 8.6.6 Atypical exaggerated implantation site associated with a complete hydatidiform mole. Exaggerated implantation sites associated with complete moles can show greater cytologic atypia compared with those unassociated with complete moles. Here, the degree of hyperchromasia can mimic the cytologic features of placental site trophoblastic tumor.

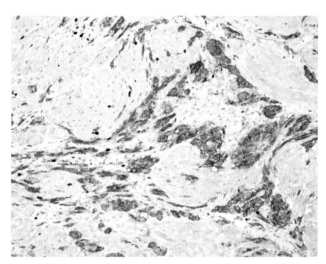

Figure 8.6.7 Exaggerated implantation site. An HLA-G/Ki-67 double stain shows no proliferation (brown chromogen) within the HLA-G(+) intermediate trophoblastic cells (red chromogen). Performing only the Ki-67 stain by itself can create confusion since associated lymphocytes will be positive.

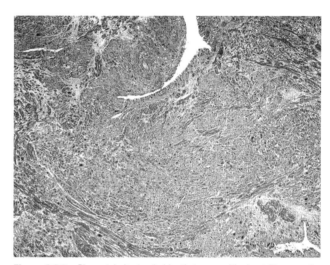

Figure 8.6.8 Placental site trophoblastic tumor with sheet-like growth.

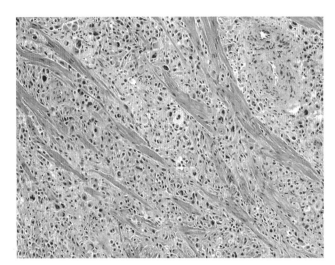

Figure 8.6.9 Placental site trophoblastic tumor. Classic pattern showing wide trabeculae separating nonneoplastic muscle fibers.

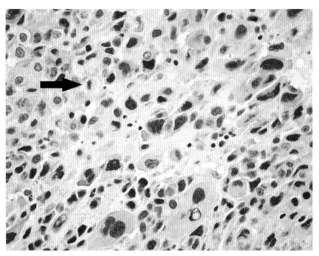

Figure 8.6.10 Placental site trophoblastic tumor with nuclear atypia greater than in most exaggerated implantation sites. A mitotic figure is present (*arrow*).

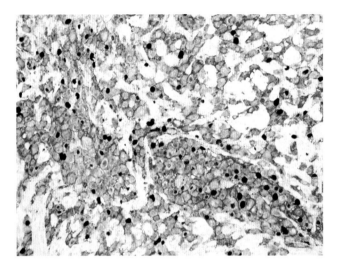

Figure 8.6.11 Placental site trophoblastic tumor. An HLA-G/Ki-67 double stain shows increased proliferation (brown chromogen) within the HLA-G(+) intermediate trophoblastic cells (red chromogen). Performing only the Ki-67 stain by itself can create confusion since associated lymphocytes will be positive.

	Placental Site Nodule/Plaque	Epithelioid Trophoblastic Tumor
Age	Reproductive years; occasionally may be seen in older women many years after pregnancy	15-48 y; typically young
Location	Uterus (endometrium or endocervical mucosa)	Uterus, often in cervix or lower uterine segment
Symptoms	No specific symptoms; incidental finding usually in endometrial or endocervical curettages	Vaginal bleeding
Signs	No specific symptoms; incidental finding usually in endometrial or endocervical curettages; does not produce a mass, but placental site plaques are >1 cm in size	Serum β-hCG may be mildly to moderately elevated; gross mass may be evident
Etiology	Chorionic-type intermediate trophoblast resulting from prior pregnancy	Trophoblast neoplasia with differentiation toward chorionic-type intermediate trophoblast; atypical placental site nodule/plaque has been proposed as a precursor
Histology	1. Well-circumscribed nodules or plaques *(Fig. 8.7.1)* 2. Single cells and cords/clusters of lesional cells separated by abundant hyalinized stroma *(Fig. 8.7.2)* 3. Central necrosis may be present *(Fig. 8.7.3)* 4. Low degree of cellularity 5. Epithelioid cells with enlarged and hyperchromatic but smudgy nuclei *(Fig. 8.7.4)* (The term "atypical placental site nodule/plaque" has been proposed for lesions characterized by larger size/more abundant lesional tissue, more extensive plaque-like growth, increased cellularity with more cohesive nests and cords of cells, a greater extent/distribution of necrosis, increased atypia, mitotic activity, and/or a Ki-67 proliferation index greater than usually encountered in typical placental site nodule/plaque; however, criteria for the exact distinction between atypical placental site nodule/plaque and an emerging intermediate trophoblastic tumor are ill defined) *(Fig. 8.7.5)* 6. Abundant eosinophilic to scant clear cytoplasm 7. Mitotic figures are rare 8. No calcifications	1. Nodular growth pattern 2. Nests, cords, and sheets of tumor cells within hyalinized stroma *(Fig. 8.7.7)* 3. Geographic necrosis is frequent; isolated nodules of cellular tumor with a central vessel are frequent within necrosis *(Fig. 8.7.8)* 4. Frequently highly cellular 5. Epithelioid cells with moderate nuclear atypia; fine chromatin with small nucleoli *(Fig. 8.7.9)* 6. Abundant eosinophilic to clear cytoplasm 7. Variable mitotic index (0-9 mitotic figures per 10 high-power fields) 8. Calcifications typically present *(Fig. 8.7.10)*

	Placental Site Nodule/Plaque	Epithelioid Trophoblastic Tumor
Special studies	HLA-G/Ki-67 double stain: proliferation in HLA-G(+) cells is low (<8%) (HLA-G [+] in intermediate trophoblastic cells, [−] in lymphocytes, decidua, and myometrium); hydroxyl-delta-5-steroid dehydrogenase (HSD3B1) or cytokeratin can be used instead of HLA-G *(Fig. 8.7.6)*	HLA-G/Ki-67 double stain: tumor cells have increased proliferation index (usually >10%); hydroxyl-delta-5-steroid dehydrogenase (HSD3B1) or cytokeratin can be used instead of HLA-G
Treatment	None for typical placental site nodule/plaque; further clinical evaluation and follow-up (if diagnosed on curettage) are warranted for atypical placental site nodule/plaque	Hysterectomy, +/− chemotherapy
Prognosis	Unremarkable for typical placental site nodule/plaque; 14% of atypical placental site nodules/plaques are associated with concurrent or subsequent malignant gestational trophoblastic disease	Survival approaches 100% and is 50%-60% for cases without and with metastases, respectively; high mitotic index (>6 mitotic figures per 10 high-power fields) is a poor prognostic factor

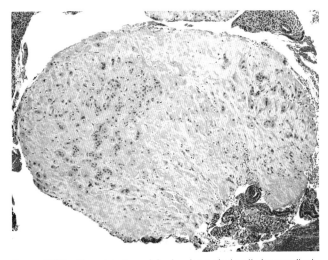

Figure 8.7.1 Placental site nodule showing typical well-circumscribed appearance.

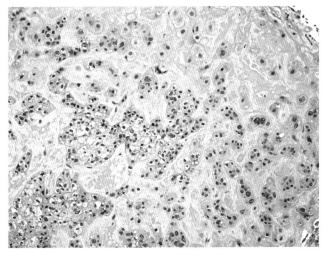

Figure 8.7.2 Placental site nodule with individual cells, small clusters, and cords.

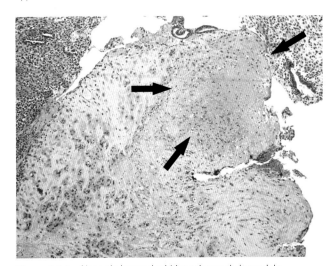

Figure 8.7.3 Necrosis (*arrows*) within a placental site nodule.

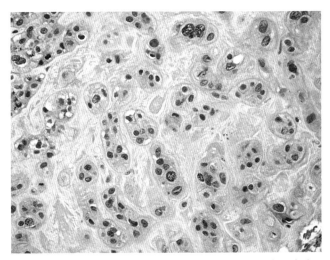

Figure 8.7.4 Placental site nodule containing small nests of atypical epithelioid cells within hyalinized stroma.

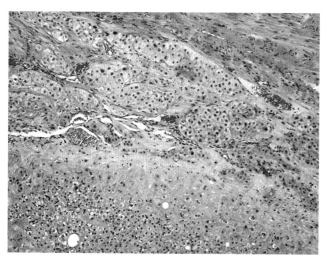

Figure 8.7.5 Atypical placental site plaque showing a greater degree of cellularity than in typical cases.

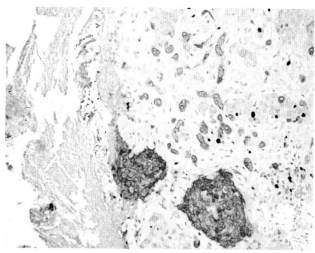

Figure 8.7.6 Placental site nodule. An HLA-G/Ki-67 double stain shows no proliferation (brown chromogen) within the HLA-G(+) intermediate trophoblastic cells (red chromogen). Performing only the Ki-67 stain by itself can create confusion since associated lymphocytes will be positive. Note that chorionic-type intermediate trophoblast (such as placental site nodule/plaque or epithelioid trophoblastic tumor) does not have as much robust staining for HLA-G as do implantation-type intermediate trophoblast (such as exaggerated implantation site or placental site trophoblastic tumor).

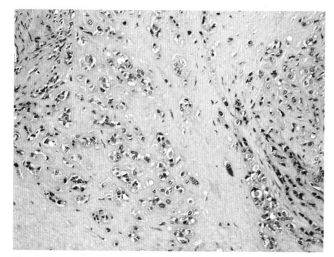

Figure 8.7.7 Epithelioid trophoblastic tumor with clusters of tumor cells within hyalinized stroma mimicking placental site nodule/plaque.

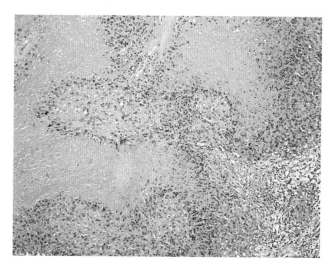

Figure 8.7.8 Epithelioid trophoblastic tumor showing geographic necrosis with preserved small tumor nodules within necrotic zones.

8 GESTATIONAL
TROPHOBLASTIC DISEASE

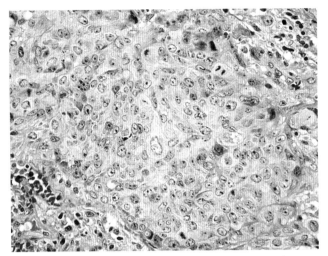

Figure 8.7.9   Epithelioid trophoblastic tumor. Epithelioid cells show a greater degree of atypia than in placental site nodule/plaque.

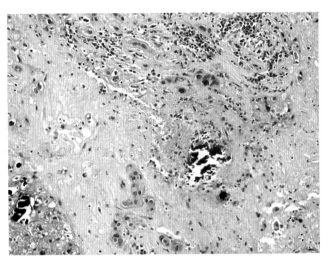

Figure 8.7.10   Epithelioid trophoblastic tumor with calcifications.

	Placental Site Trophoblastic Tumor	Epithelioid Trophoblastic Tumor
Age	20-63 y; typically young	15-48 y; typically young
Location	Uterus, usually corpus	Uterus, often in cervix or lower uterine segment
Symptoms	Vaginal bleeding; missed abortion	Vaginal bleeding
Signs	Serum β-hCG may be mildly to moderately elevated; gross mass may be evident	Serum β-hCG may be mildly to moderately elevated; gross mass may be evident
Etiology	Trophoblast neoplasia with differentiation toward implantation-type intermediate trophoblast	Trophoblast neoplasia with differentiation toward chorionic-type intermediate trophoblast; atypical placental site nodule/plaque has been proposed as a precursor
Histology	1. Infiltrative growth pattern; aggregates to sheets of tumor cells, which separate myometrial bundles (Figs. 8.8.1 and 8.8.2); hyaline material can be present but is usually found in vascular walls 2. Necrosis usually absent 3. Large, pleomorphic, and polygonal to round epithelioid cells, occasionally spindled 4. Abundant amphophilic, eosinophilic, or clear cytoplasm 5. Nuclei are moderately to markedly atypical, large, and irregular with hyperchromasia (Fig. 8.8.3) 6. Tumor cells can replace vascular walls (Fig. 8.8.4) 7. Mitotically active, but mitotic index is generally low (usually 2-4 mitotic figures per 10 high-power fields) 8. Calcifications absent 9. Rarely, mixed placental site trophoblastic tumor-epithelioid trophoblastic tumor can occur	1. Expansile/pushing growth pattern with nodular architecture; nests, cords, and sheets of tumor cells within hyalinized stroma (Fig. 8.8.5) 2. Geographic necrosis is frequent (Fig. 8.8.6); isolated small nodules of cellular tumor with a central vessel are frequent within necrosis (Fig. 8.8.7) 3. Smaller, round, and uniform epithelioid cells 4. Abundant eosinophilic to clear cytoplasm 5. Mild to moderate nuclear atypia; fine chromatin with small nucleoli (Fig. 8.8.8) 6. No vascular invasion 7. Variable mitotic index (0-9 mitotic figures per 10 high-power fields) 8. Calcifications typically present (Fig. 8.8.9) 9. Rarely, mixed epithelioid trophoblastic tumor-placental site trophoblastic tumor can occur
Special studies	• HLA-G/Ki-67 double stain: tumor cells have increased proliferation index (usually 5%-30%) (HLA-G [+] in intermediate trophoblastic cells, [−] in lymphocytes and myometrium); hydroxyl-delta-5-steroid dehydrogenase (HSD3B1) or cytokeratin can be used instead of HLA-G • Diffusely (+) for hPL and CD146 • p63(−)	• HLA-G/Ki-67 double stain: tumor cells have increased proliferation index (usually >10%); hydroxyl-delta-5-steroid dehydrogenase (HSD3B1) or cytokeratin can be used instead of HLA-G • Limited expression of hPL and CD146 • Diffusely (+) for p63

	Placental Site Trophoblastic Tumor	**Epithelioid Trophoblastic Tumor**
Treatment	Hysterectomy, +/− chemotherapy	Hysterectomy, +/− chemotherapy
Prognosis	70% survival at 10 y; a subset of cases exhibit recurrent disease and/or die of disease; advanced FIGO stage, antecedent pregnancy of ≥48 mo, and clear cytoplasm are independent risk factors	Survival approaches 100% and is 50%-60% for cases without and with metastases, respectively; high mitotic index (>6 mitotic figures per 10 high-power fields) is a poor prognostic factor

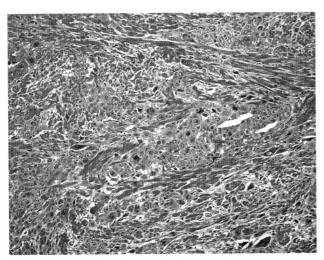

Figure 8.8.1 Placental site trophoblastic tumor with tumor nests separating nonneoplastic smooth muscle bundles.

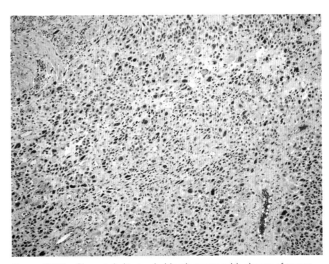

Figure 8.8.2 Placental site trophoblastic tumor with sheets of tumor cells architecturally similar to epithelioid trophoblastic tumor.

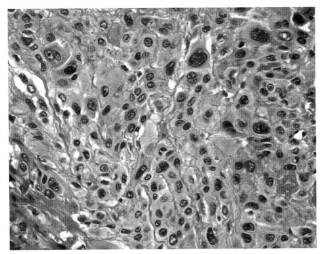

Figure 8.8.3 Placental site trophoblastic tumor with atypical epithelioid cells cytologically similar to epithelioid trophoblastic tumor; however, the nuclei of placental site trophoblastic tumor tend to be more hyperchromatic.

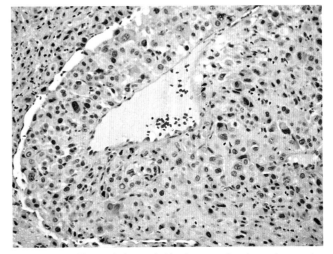

Figure 8.8.4 Placental site trophoblastic tumor showing replacement of vessel wall with tumor cells.

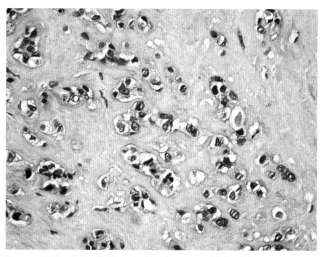

Figure 8.8.5 Epithelioid trophoblastic tumor with hyalinized stroma.

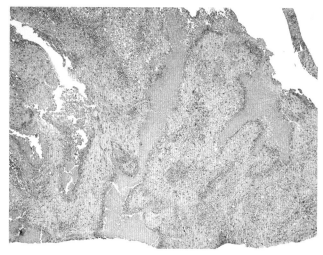

Figure 8.8.6 Epithelioid trophoblastic tumor with geographic necrosis.

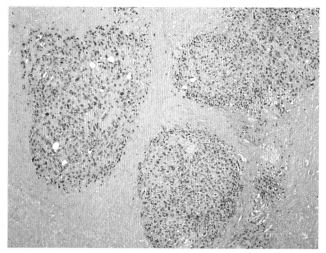

Figure 8.8.7 Epithelioid trophoblastic tumor with preserved small tumor nodules within necrotic zones.

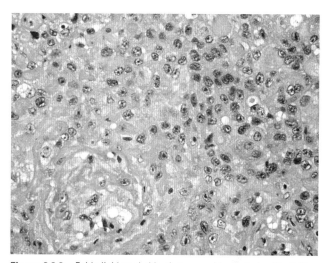

Figure 8.8.8 Epithelioid trophoblastic tumor with atypical epithelioid cells cytologically similar to placental site trophoblastic tumor; however, the nuclei of epithelioid trophoblastic tumor tend to have paler chromatin with evident nucleoli. Also, a minimal amount of hyalinized stroma is noted between tumor cells.

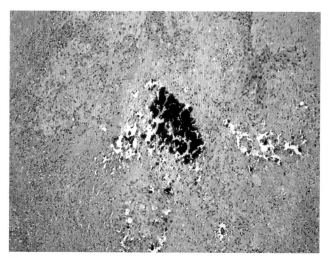

Figure 8.8.9 Epithelioid trophoblastic tumor with calcifications.

	Placental Site Trophoblastic Tumor	Leiomyosarcoma/Atypical Leiomyoma
Age	20-63 y; typically young	Usually >50 for leiomyosarcoma; most women in 30s or 40s for atypical leiomyoma
Location	Uterus, usually corpus	Usually uterus; extrauterine pelvic primaries are uncommon
Symptoms	Vaginal bleeding; missed abortion	Vaginal bleeding; pelvic pain
Signs	Serum β-hCG may be mildly to moderately elevated; gross mass may be evident	Serum β-hCG not elevated; gross mass may be evident
Etiology	Trophoblast neoplasia with differentiation toward implantation-type intermediate trophoblast	Leiomyosarcoma: pathogenesis unclear but probably arises *de novo* rather than from malignant transformation of leiomyoma, although cases of the latter have been described; various chromosomal aberrations; subsets contain mutations of *TP53*, *ATRX*, and *MED12* (the frequency of *MED12* mutations is much lower than in leiomyomas)
Histology	1. Infiltrative growth pattern; aggregates to sheets of tumor cells, which separate myometrial bundles *(Fig. 8.9.1)* 2. Necrosis usually absent 3. Large, pleomorphic, and polygonal to round epithelioid cells, occasionally spindled *(Figs. 8.9.2 and 8.9.3)* 4. Multinucleated tumor cells can be present 5. Abundant amphophilic, eosinophilic, or clear cytoplasm 6. Nuclei are moderately to markedly atypical, large, and irregular with hyperchromasia 7. Tumor cells can replace vascular walls *(Fig. 8.9.4)*; hyaline material can be present in vascular walls 8. Mitotically active, but mitotic index is generally low (usually 2-4 mitotic figures per 10 high-power fields) 9. No myxoid features	1. Usually pushing border, but infiltrative patterns may be seen at periphery of tumor *(Figs. 8.9.5 and 8.9.6)*; tumor cells arranged in fascicles *(Fig. 8.9.7)* 2. Necrosis frequently but not always present in leiomyosarcoma; hyaline/infarct type necrosis can be present in atypical leiomyoma 3. Usually spindle cells, but epithelioid-predominant tumors occur uncommonly *(Figs. 8.9.8 and 8.9.9)* 4. Multinucleated tumor cells can be present 5. Eosinophilic cytoplasm 6. Moderate to severe nuclear atypia; some cases may have uniform pattern of moderate atypia 7. Tumor cells do not replace vascular walls *(Fig. 8.9.10)*; hyaline material not present in vascular walls 8. Variable mitotic index (high in leiomyosarcoma, low in atypical leiomyoma) 9. Some cases may have a myxoid component
Special studies	• HLA-G, CD146, HSD3B1, hPL, GATA-3 (+) • Smooth muscle actin, desmin (−) • Cytokeratin usually diffusely (+)	• HLA-G, CD146, HSD3B1, hPL, GATA-3 (−) • Smooth muscle actin, desmin (+) • Cytokeratin usually (−), but some cases may have expression (typically not diffuse)
Treatment	Hysterectomy, +/− chemotherapy	Hysterectomy (+/− chemotherapy, +/− radiation therapy) for leiomyosarcoma; hysterectomy or myomectomy for atypical leiomyoma

	Placental Site Trophoblastic Tumor	**Leiomyosarcoma/Atypical Leiomyoma**
Prognosis	70% survival at 10 y; a subset of cases exhibit recurrent disease and/or die of disease; advanced FIGO stage, antecedent pregnancy of ≥48 mo, and clear cytoplasm are independent risk factors	15%-25% (all stages) and 40%-70% (stages I-II) 5-y survivals for leiomyosarcoma; prognosis dependent on stage and other risk factors; 2% of atypical leiomyomas recur

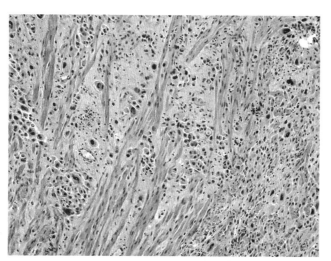

Figure 8.9.1   Placental site trophoblastic tumor with tumor nests characteristically separating nonneoplastic smooth muscle bundles. However, incorrect interpretation of nonneoplastic smooth muscle bundles as spindle cell differentiation within the tumor can cause misclassification as a smooth muscle tumor.

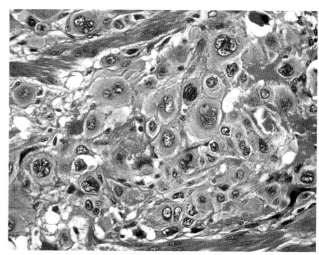

Figure 8.9.2   Placental site trophoblastic tumor with usual epithelioid morphology.

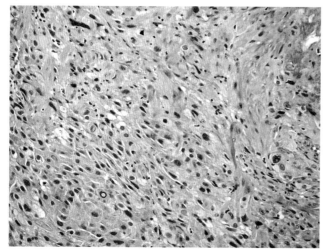

Figure 8.9.3   Placental site trophoblastic tumor with slight suggestion of spindle cell morphology, which can potentially simulate a smooth muscle tumor.

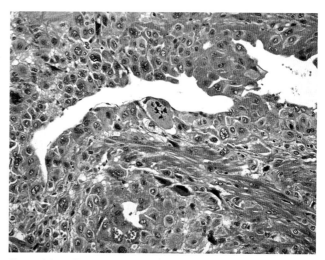

Figure 8.9.4   Placental site trophoblastic tumor showing replacement of vessel wall with tumor cells.

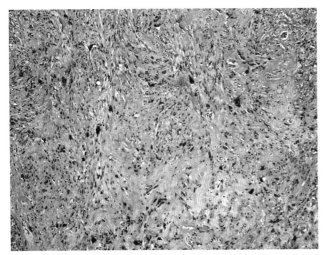

Figure 8.9.5 Atypical leiomyoma. The growth pattern in this case can mimic a placental site trophoblastic tumor.

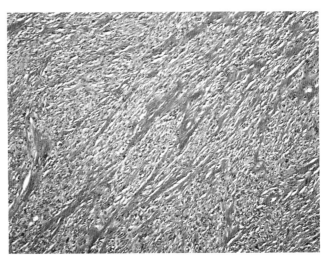

Figure 8.9.6 Leiomyosarcoma. The pattern of hyalinization between tumor cells in this case can create architectural overlap with the pattern of separation of nonneoplastic smooth muscle bundles in placental site trophoblastic tumor.

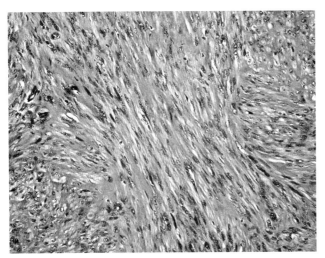

Figure 8.9.7 Atypical leiomyoma with fascicle formation.

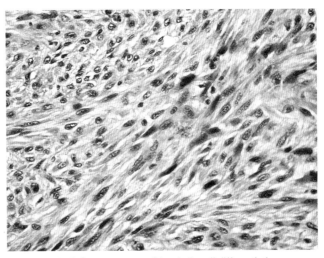

Figure 8.9.8 Leiomyosarcoma with spindle cell differentiation.

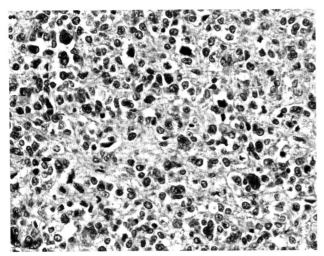

Figure 8.9.9 Epithelioid leiomyosarcoma with cytologic features resembling the epithelioid morphology of a placental site trophoblastic tumor.

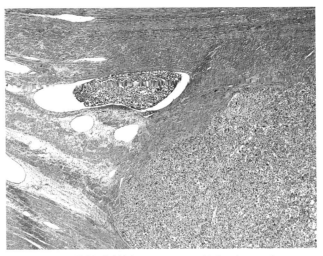

Figure 8.9.10 Epithelioid leiomyosarcoma with lymphovascular space invasion. The tumor is present within the lymphovascular space lumen as opposed to the pattern seen in placental site trophoblastic tumor, in which tumor cells replace the wall of the vessel.

	Epithelioid Trophoblastic Tumor	Squamous Cell Carcinoma
Age	15-48 y; typically young	55 y (median age)
Location	Uterus, often in cervix or lower uterine segment	Cervix
Symptoms	Vaginal bleeding	Can be asymptomatic for small tumors; abnormal vaginal bleeding
Signs	Serum β-hCG may be mildly to moderately elevated; gross mass may be evident	Serum β-hCG not elevated; gross mass may be evident; may have prior abnormal Pap smear or cervical biopsy; HPV(+) testing on liquid-based Pap smear
Etiology	Trophoblast neoplasia with differentiation toward chorionic-type intermediate trophoblast; atypical placental site nodule/plaque has been proposed as a precursor	HPV results in development of HSIL in cervix, which then undergoes further malignant transformation with invasion of stroma
Histology	1. Expansile/pushing growth pattern with nodular architecture; nests, cords, and sheets of tumor cells within hyalinized stroma *(Fig. 8.10.1)*; no papillary architecture 2. No keratinization, but hyalinized stroma can mimic keratinization 3. No associated HSIL, but tumor colonization of mucosa can simulate HSIL 4. Geographic necrosis is frequent; isolated small nodules of cellular tumor with a central vessel are frequent within necrosis *(Fig. 8.10.2)* 5. Relatively small, round, and uniform epithelioid cells 6. Abundant eosinophilic to clear cytoplasm; no intercellular bridges 7. Mild to moderate nuclear atypia; fine chromatin with small nucleoli *(Figs. 8.10.3 and 8.10.4)* 8. Variable mitotic index (0-9 mitotic figures per 10 high-power fields) 9. Calcifications typically present *(Fig. 8.10.5)*	1. Infiltrative pattern with haphazard arrangement of irregular nests within desmoplastic stroma *(Fig. 8.10.6)*; sheet-like and papillary architecture can be seen in some cases *(Figs. 8.10.7 and 8.10.8)* 2. Definitive keratinization may be present in some cases *(Fig. 8.10.9)* 3. Associated HSIL may be present 4. Necrosis can be present but is infrequent 5. Medium to large epithelioid cells, which may be pleomorphic 6. Variable amount of cytoplasm, from scant (basaloid appearance) to abundant; usually eosinophilic cytoplasm but occasionally may be clear (glycogenated); intercellular bridges may be seen *(Figs. 8.10.10 and 8.10.11)* 7. Variable nuclear atypia 8. Variable mitotic activity 9. Calcifications absent

	Epithelioid Trophoblastic Tumor	Squamous Cell Carcinoma
Special studies	• HLA-G, HSD3B1, GATA-3 (+)	• HLA-G, CD146, HSD3B1, hPL (−); GATA-3 may be positive but with less extensive expression than epithelioid trophoblastic tumor
	• Limited expression of hPL and CD146 • Inhibin may be occasionally (+) • p63/p40 (+) (These markers are not helpful for this differential diagnosis) • CK18(+) in 100% of cases • CK5/6 usually (−) • p16(−) or focal/patchy staining • No detectable HPV by *in situ* hybridization	• Inhibin often negative • p63/p40(+) (These markers are not helpful for this differential diagnosis) • CK18(+) in 60% of cases • CK5/6 often (+) • Diffusely (+) for p16 • (+) HPV by *in situ* hybridization (HPV may be undetectable by this method in some cases)
Treatment	Hysterectomy, +/− chemotherapy	Stage dependent: may include hysterectomy, chemotherapy, and/or radiation therapy
Prognosis	Survival approaches 100% and is 50%-60% for cases without and with metastases, respectively; high mitotic index (>6 mitotic figures per 10 high-power fields) is a poor prognostic factor	5-y survival: 90%-95% (stage I) and <50% (stage II+), respectively

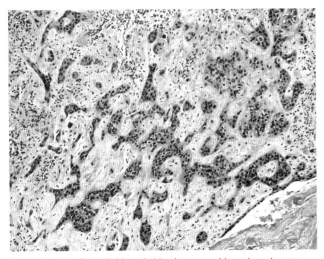

Figuro 8.10.1   Cpithelioid trophoblastic tumor with cords and nests, which can simulate squamous cell carcinoma.

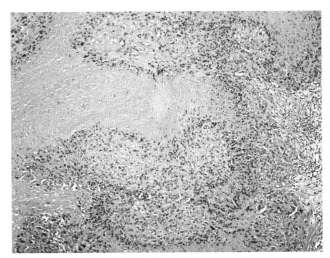

Figure 8.10.2   Epithelioid trophoblastic tumor with geographic necrosis and preserved small tumor nodules within necrotic zones.

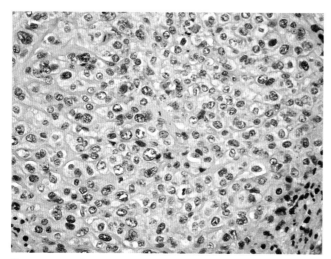

Figure 8.10.3 Epithelioid trophoblastic tumor with usual cytologic features. Minimal hyalinized stroma can be detected between tumor cells.

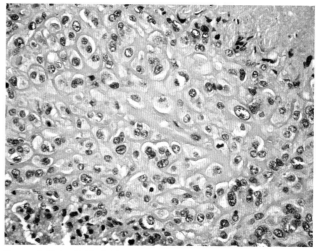

Figure 8.10.4 Epithelioid trophoblastic tumor with usual cytologic features. More hyalinized stroma is evident between tumor cells compared with *Figure 8.10.3.*

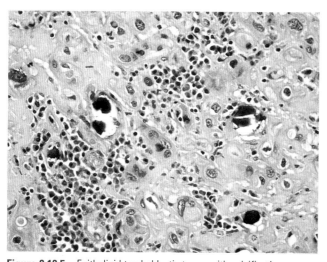

Figure 8.10.5 Epithelioid trophoblastic tumor with calcifications.

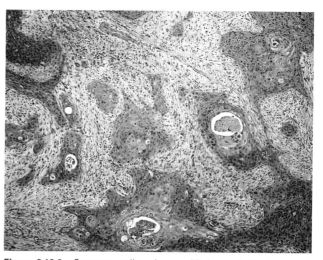

Figure 8.10.6 Squamous cell carcinoma with desmoplastic stroma and haphazard arrangement of nests.

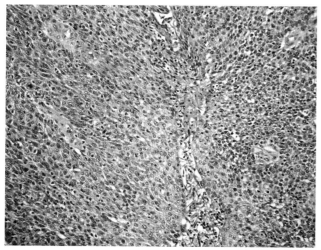

Figure 8.10.7 Squamous cell carcinoma with sheets of tumor cells.

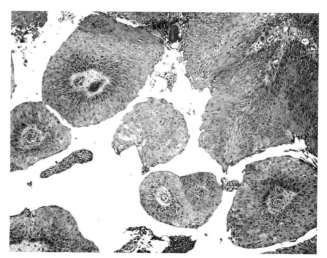

Figure 8.10.8 Squamous cell carcinoma with papillary architecture.

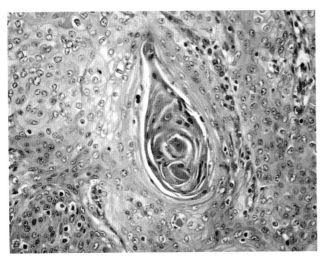

Figure 8.10.9   Squamous cell carcinoma with keratinization in the form of a keratin pearl.

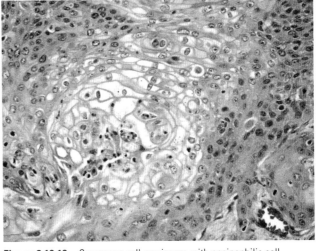

Figure 8.10.10   Squamous cell carcinoma with eosinophilic cell membranes and glycogenation.

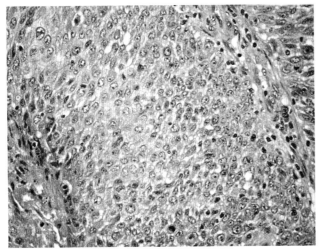

Figure 8.10.11   Squamous cell carcinoma showing cytologic features mimicking epithelioid trophoblastic tumor.

	Choriocarcinoma	Intermediate Trophoblastic Tumor
Age	Reproductive years (rare postmenopausal cases); typically young	15-63 y; typically young
Location	Often in uterus; occasionally in the fallopian tube or ovary	Uterus (corpus, cervix, or lower uterine segment)
Symptoms	Vaginal bleeding	Vaginal bleeding; missed abortion
Signs	Serum β-hCG is markedly elevated; may have persistent gestational trophoblastic disease	Serum β-hCG may be mildly to moderately elevated
Etiology	A subset of cases have an antecedent complete mole, but many choriocarcinomas develop after a normal pregnancy	Trophoblast neoplasia with differentiation toward intermediate trophoblast (placental site trophoblastic tumor or epithelioid trophoblastic tumor)
Histology	1. Infiltrative growth pattern; sheets of tumor cells; no fibrinoid change in vascular walls	1. Infiltrative or expansile/pushing growth pattern; may have nodular architecture; may have aggregates to sheets of tumor cells (which separate myometrial bundles) *(Fig. 8.11.6)*, nests, or cords; hyaline material can be found in vascular walls; cells may be within hyalinized stroma
	2. Extensive hemorrhage and necrosis	2. Necrosis can be present or absent; when present, may have geographic pattern; isolated small nodules of cellular tumor with a central vessel may be present within necrosis *(Fig. 8.11.7)*; no extensive hemorrhage
	3. The tumor consists of sheets of trimorphic cells, which include cytotrophoblast, intermediate trophoblast, and syncytiotrophoblast; the architecture of these intimately admixed populations resembles the arrangement seen in their normal counterparts, in which cytotrophoblast are rimmed by syncytiotrophoblast; variable cell size and shape *(Figs. 8.11.1-8.11.5)*	3. Monomorphic cell population; tumor cells may be large, pleomorphic, and polygonal to round with epithelioid shapes (occasionally spindled) or may be relatively small, round, and uniform with epithelioid morphology; scattered multinucleated intermediate trophoblastic cells can be present
	4. Scant to abundant pale to amphophilic cytoplasm	4. Abundant amphophilic, eosinophilic, or clear cytoplasm
	5. Marked nuclear atypia	5. Nuclei may be moderately to markedly atypical, large, and irregular with hyperchromasia or mildly to moderately atypical with fine chromatin and small nucleoli *(Figs. 8.11.8 and 8.11.9)*
	6. Intravascular invasion may be seen	6. Tumor cells can replace vascular walls, or vascular invasion may be absent
	7. High mitotic activity, including atypical mitotic figures	7. Variable mitotic index (0-9 mitotic figures per 10 high-power fields)
	8. No calcifications	8. Calcifications may be present or absent *(Fig. 8.11.10)*
	9. Mixed choriocarcinoma-intermediate trophoblastic tumor can occur	9. Mixed choriocarcinoma-intermediate trophoblastic tumor can occur

	Choriocarcinoma	**Intermediate Trophoblastic Tumor**
Special studies	Immunohistochemistry mostly of no help for this differential diagnosis, although staining for β-hCG is usually more extensive than in intermediate trophoblastic tumors, and the Ki-67 index is usually >90%	Immunohistochemistry mostly of no help for this differential diagnosis, although staining for β-hCG is usually less extensive, and the Ki-67 index is typically not as high compared with choriocarcinoma
Treatment	Chemotherapy	Hysterectomy, +/− chemotherapy
Prognosis	Highly favorable outcome with chemotherapy; aggressive if untreated	Intermediate trophoblastic tumors are not as responsive to chemotherapy as choriocarcinoma; a subset of cases exhibit recurrent disease and/or die of disease (prognosis dependent on stage and other risk factors)

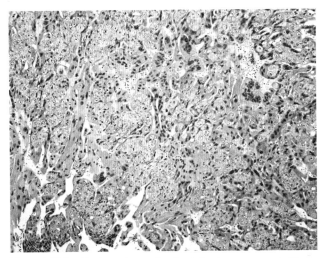

Figure 8.11.1   Choriocarcinoma showing intimate arrangement of two populations of trophoblast.

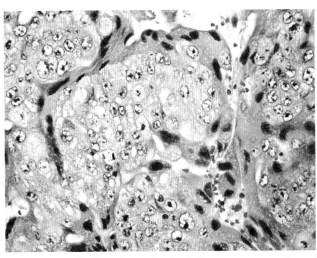

Figure 8.11.2   Choriocarcinoma showing intimate arrangement of two populations of trophoblast. Note the syncytiotrophoblastic component with abundant amphophilic cytoplasm rims the mononuclear component.

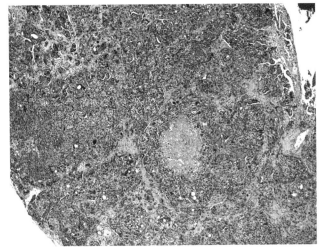

Figure 8.11.3   Choriocarcinoma. The limited number of syncytiotrophoblast and presence of nested growth pattern can mimic some intermediate trophoblastic tumors.

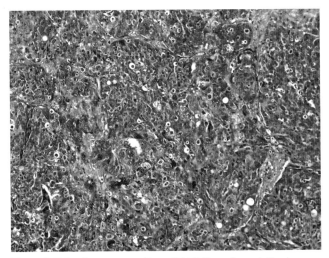

Figure 8.11.4   Same case as *Figure 8.11.3*. The cell population is predominantly mononuclear with very few syncytiotrophoblast.

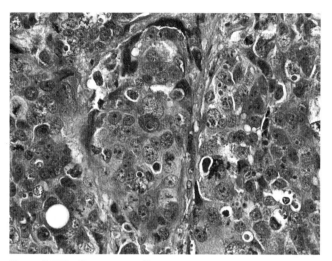

Figure 8.11.5   Same case as *Figures 8.11.3* and *8.11.4*. The limited syncytiotrophoblast can result in misclassification as an intermediate trophoblastic tumor.

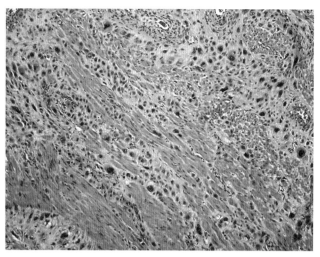

Figure 8.11.6   Placental site trophoblastic tumor with tumor nests separating nonneoplastic smooth muscle bundles.

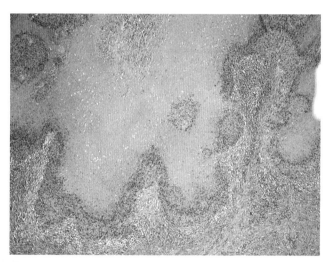

Figure 8.11.7   Epithelioid trophoblastic tumor with geographic necrosis.

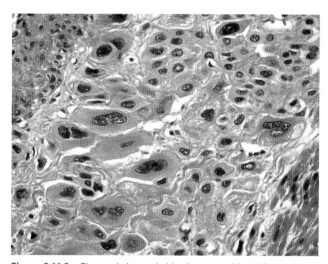

Figure 8.11.8   Placental site trophoblastic tumor with atypical epithelioid cells and hyperchromatic nuclei, overlapping with the cytologic features of some choriocarcinomas.

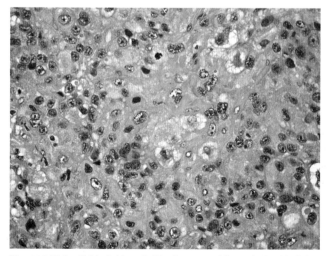

Figure 8.11.9   Epithelioid trophoblastic tumor with atypical epithelioid cells. Note the pale chromatin and small nucleoli typical of epithelioid trophoblastic tumor. Also, hyalinized stroma can be seen between tumor cells.

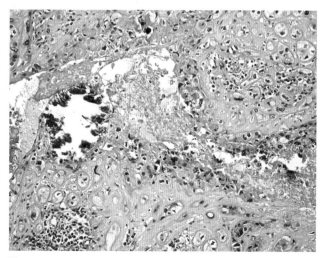

Figure 8.11.10   Epithelioid trophoblastic tumor with calcifications.

8 GESTATIONAL TROPHOBLASTIC DISEASE

	Choriocarcinoma	Poorly Differentiated Endometrial Carcinoma
Age	Reproductive years (rare postmenopausal cases); typically young	Usually postmenopausal
Location	Often in uterus; occasionally in the fallopian tube or ovary	Uterus
Symptoms	Vaginal bleeding; may have prior molar pregnancy	Vaginal bleeding; pelvic pain; usually no prior molar pregnancy
Signs	Serum β-hCG is markedly elevated; may have persistent gestational trophoblastic disease	Serum β-hCG not elevated; +/− pelvic mass
Etiology	A subset of cases have an antecedent complete mole, but many choriocarcinomas develop after a normal pregnancy	Endometrioid carcinoma: unopposed estrogen stimulation drives the development of hyperplasia, which then progresses to carcinoma
Histology	1. Sheets of tumor cells *(Fig. 8.12.1)*; no glandular, papillary, or squamous differentiation 2. No background of endometrial hyperplasia 3. Extensive hemorrhage and necrosis 4. Tumor consists of sheets of trimorphic cells, which include cytotrophoblast, intermediate trophoblast, and syncytiotrophoblast; the architecture of these intimately admixed populations resembles the arrangement seen in their normal counterparts, in which cytotrophoblast are rimmed by syncytiotrophoblast *(Figs. 8.12.2-8.12.4)* 5. Scant to abundant pale to amphophilic cytoplasm 6. Marked nuclear atypia	1. Areas of solid architecture will be present *(Figs. 8.12.6-8.12.8)*, but focal glandular, papillary, or squamous differentiation may be seen *(Figs. 8.12.9 and 8.12.10)* 2. Background of endometrial hyperplasia may be seen 3. May have necrosis 4. No trimorphic populations or syncytiotrophoblast *(Fig. 8.12.11)* (rare carcinomas can have choriocarcinomatous differentiation); cohesive sheets of epithelioid cells in endometrioid carcinoma; discohesive sheets of epithelioid cells in undifferentiated carcinoma 5. Usually scant cytoplasm with increased nuclear:cytoplasm ratio 6. Variable nuclear atypia, but usually high grade
Special studies	• Cytokeratin (+) • (+) for trophoblast markers (β-hCG, HLA-G, CD146, HSD3B1, inhibin, hPL, GATA-3) *(Fig. 8.12.5)* • Genotyping of gestational choriocarcinoma: presence of nonmaternal (presumed paternal) chromosome complements	• Cytokeratin (+) • (−) for trophoblast markers (β-hCG, HLA-G, CD146, HSD3B1, inhibin, hPL, GATA-3) ([+] β-hCG can be seen in the rare carcinomas with choriocarcinomatous differentiation) • Genotyping of somatic-type carcinoma with choriocarcinomatous differentiation: absence of nonmaternal (presumed paternal) chromosome complements
Treatment	Chemotherapy	Stage and risk factor dependent: hysterectomy, +/− chemotherapy, +/− radiation therapy
Prognosis	Highly favorable outcome with chemotherapy; aggressive if untreated	Stage and risk factor dependent: 75%-88% and 15%-69% 5-y survivals for stages I and II+, respectively (all histologic types)

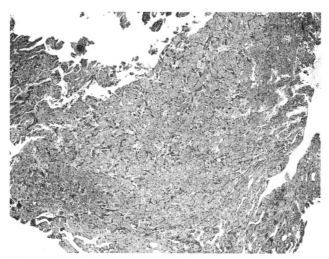

Figure 8.12.1   Choriocarcinoma with predominantly sheet-like architecture that can resemble a poorly differentiated carcinoma at low-power magnification.

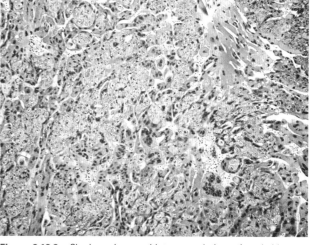

Figure 8.12.2   Choriocarcinoma with two populations of trophoblast. The gland-like spaces in this case can simulate an adenocarcinoma if the two characteristic trophoblast populations are not recognized.

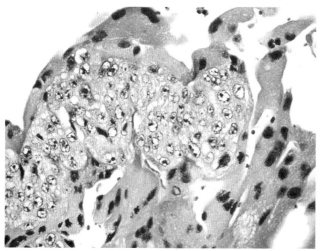

Figure 8.12.3   Choriocarcinoma showing intimate arrangement of two populations of trophoblast. Note the syncytiotrophoblastic component with abundant amphophilic cytoplasm rims the mononuclear component.

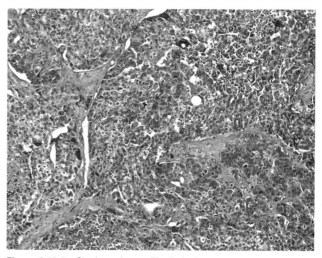

Figure 8.12.4   Choriocarcinoma. The limited number of syncytiotrophoblast and presence of nested growth pattern can mimic a poorly differentiated carcinoma.

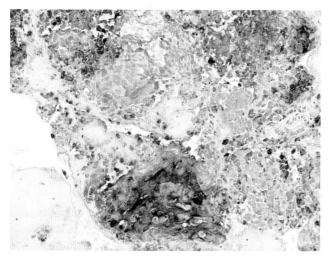

Figure 8.12.5   Choriocarcinoma with positive β-hCG immunostain.

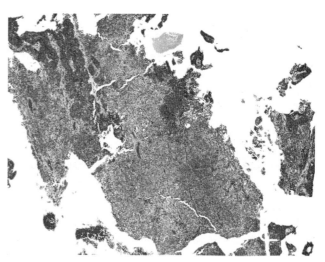

Figure 8.12.6   FIGO grade 3 endometrioid carcinoma with solid architecture.

8   GESTATIONAL TROPHOBLASTIC DISEASE

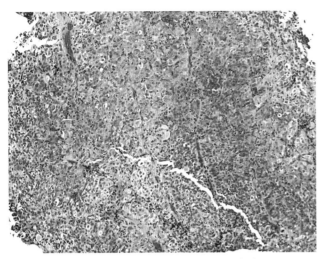

Figure 8.12.7   Same case as *Figure 8.12.6*. This histologic appearance can overlap with some choriocarcinomas that have a predominantly monomorphic cell composition.

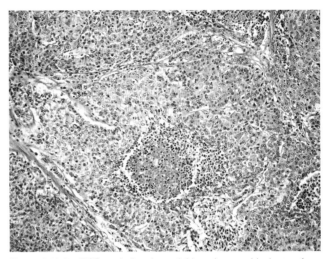

Figure 8.12.8   FIGO grade 3 endometrioid carcinoma with sheets of tumor and focal necrosis.

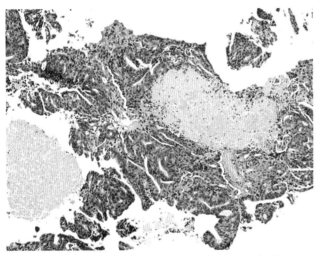

Figure 8.12.9   FIGO grade 3 endometrioid carcinoma with focal glandular differentiation.

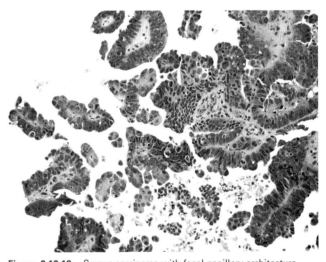

Figure 8.12.10   Serous carcinoma with focal papillary architecture.

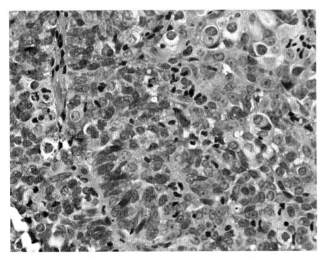

Figure 8.12.11   FIGO grade 3 endometrioid carcinoma. Note the monomorphic population without syncytiotrophoblast.

SUGGESTED READINGS

8.1-8.5

Banet N, DeScipio C, Murphy KM, et al. Characteristics of hydatidiform moles: analysis of a prospective series with p57 immunohistochemistry and molecular genotyping. *Mod Pathol.* 2014;27:238-254.

Buza N, Hui P. Partial hydatidiform mole: histologic parameters in correlation with DNA genotyping. *Int J Gynecol Pathol.* 2013;32:307-315.

Buza N, McGregor SM, Barroilhet L, et al. Paternal uniparental isodisomy of tyrosine hydroxylase locus at chromosome 11p15.4: spectrum of phenotypical presentations simulating hydatidiform moles. *Mod Pathol.* 2019;32:1180-1188.

Bynum J, Murphy KM, DeScipio C, et al. Invasive complete hydatidiform moles: analysis of a case series with genotyping. *Int J Gynecol Pathol.* 2016;35:134-141.

Castrillon DH, Sun D, Weremowicz S, et al. Discrimination of complete hydatidiform mole from its mimics by immunohistochemistry of the paternally imprinted gene product p57KIP2. *Am J Surg Pathol.* 2001;25:1225-1230.

Gaillot-Durand L, Patrier S, Aziza J, et al. p57-discordant villi in hydropic products of conception: a clinicopathological study of 70 cases. *Hum Pathol.* 2020;101:18-30.

Gupta M, Vang R, Yemelyanova AV, et al. Diagnostic reproducibility of hydatidiform moles: ancillary techniques (p57 immunohistochemistry and molecular genotyping) improve morphologic diagnosis for both recently trained and experienced gynecologic pathologists. *Am J Surg Pathol.* 2012;36:1747-1760.

Joseph NM, Pineda C, Rabban JT. DNA genotyping of nonmolar donor egg pregnancies with abnormal villous morphology: allele zygosity patterns prevent misinterpretation as complete hydatidiform mole. *Int J Gynecol Pathol.* 2018;37:191-197.

Keep D, Zaragoza MV, Hassold T, et al. Very early complete hydatidiform mole. *Hum Pathol.* 1996;27:708-713.

Khawajkie Y, Mechtouf N, Nguyen NMP, et al. Comprehensive analysis of 204 sporadic hydatidiform moles: revisiting risk factors and their correlations with the molar genotypes. *Mod Pathol.* 2020;33:880-892.

Kim KR, Park BH, Hong YO, et al. The villous stromal constituents of complete hydatidiform mole differ histologically in very early pregnancy from the normally developing placenta. *Am J Surg Pathol.* 2009;33:176-185.

Lewis GH, DeScipio C, Murphy KM, et al. Characterization of androgenetic/biparental mosaic/chimeric conceptions, including some with a molar component: morphology, p57 immunohistochemistry, molecular genotyping, and risk of persistent gestational trophoblastic disease. *Int J Gynecol Pathol.* 2013;32:199-214.

McConnell TG, Murphy K, Hafez M, et al. Diagnosis and subclassification of hydatidiform moles using p57 immunohistochemistry and molecular genotyping: validation and prospective analysis in routine and consultation practice settings with development of an algorithmic approach. *Am J Surg Pathol.* 2009;33:805-817.

Murphy KM, McConnell TG, Hafez MJ, et al. Molecular genotyping of hydatidiform moles: analytic validation of a multiplex short tandem repeat assay. *J Mol Diagn.* 2009;11:598-605.

Nguyen NMP, Khawajkie Y, Mechtouf N, et al. The genetics of recurrent hydatidiform moles: new insights and lessons from a comprehensive analysis of 113 patients. *Mod Pathol.* 2018;31:1116-1130.

Redline RW, Hassold T, Zaragoza M. Determinants of villous trophoblastic hyperplasia in spontaneous abortions. *Mod Pathol.* 1998;11:762-768.

Ronnett BM. Hydatidiform moles: ancillary techniques to refine diagnosis. *Arch Pathol Lab Med.* 2018;142:1485-1502.

Ronnett BM, DeScipio C, Murphy KM. Hydatidiform moles: ancillary techniques to refine diagnosis. *Int J Gynecol Pathol.* 2011;30:101-116.

Savage J, Adams E, Veras E, et al. Choriocarcinoma in women: analysis of a case series with genotyping. *Am J Surg Pathol.* 2017;41:1593-1606.

Vang R, Gupta M, Wu LSF, et al. Diagnostic reproducibility of hydatidiform moles: ancillary techniques (p57 immunohistochemistry and molecular genotyping) improve morphologic diagnosis. *Am J Surg Pathol.* 2012;36:443-453.

Xing D, Adams E, Huang J, et al. Refined diagnosis of hydatidiform moles with p57 immunohistochemistry and molecular genotyping: updated analysis of a prospective series of 2217 cases. *Mod Pathol.* 2021;34:961-982.

Xing D, Miller K, Beierl K, et al. Loss of p57 expression in conceptions other than complete hydatidiform mole: a case series with emphasis on the etiology, genetics, and clinical significance. *Am J Surg Pathol.* 2022;46:18-32.

Zheng XZ, Qin XY, Chen SW, et al. Heterozygous/dispermic complete mole confers a significantly higher risk for post-molar gestational trophoblastic disease. *Mod Pathol.* 2020;33(10):1979-1988.

8.6-8.12

Baergen RN, Rutgers JL, Young RH, et al. Placental site trophoblastic tumor: a study of 55 cases and review of the literature emphasizing factors of prognostic significance. *Gynecol Oncol.* 2006;100:511-520.

Banet N, Gown AM, Shih IeM, et al. GATA-3 expression in trophoblastic tissues: an immunohistochemical study of 445 cases, including diagnostic utility. *Am J Surg Pathol.* 2015;39:101-108.

Bower M, Brock C, Fisher RA, et al. Gestational choriocarcinoma. *Ann Oncol.* 1995;6:503-508.

Buza N, Hui P. Genotyping diagnosis of gestational trophoblastic disease: frontiers in precision medicine. *Mod Pathol.* 2021;34:1658-1672.

Chou YY, Jeng YM, Mao TL. HSD3B1 is a specific trophoblast-associated marker not expressed in a wide spectrum of tumors. *Int J Gynecol Cancer.* 2013;23:343-347.

Davis MR, Howitt BE, Quade BJ, et al. Epithelioid trophoblastic tumor: a single institution case series at the New England Trophoblastic Disease Center. *Gynecol Oncol.* 2015;137:456-461.

Huettner PC, Gersell DJ. Placental site nodule: a clinicopathologic study of 38 cases. *Int J Gynecol Pathol.* 1994;13:191-198.

Kalhor N, Ramirez PT, Deavers MT, et al. Immunohistochemical studies of trophoblastic tumors. *Am J Surg Pathol.* 2009;33:633-638.

Kaur B, Short D, Fisher RA, et al. Atypical placental site nodule (APSN) and association with malignant gestational trophoblastic disease; a clinicopathologic study of 21 cases. *Int J Gynecol Pathol.* 2015;34:152-158.

Kurman RJ, Shih IeM. Discovery of a cell: reflections on the checkered history of intermediate trophoblast and update on its nature and pathologic manifestations. *Int J Gynecol Pathol.* 2014;33:339-347.

Mao TL, Kurman RJ, Huang CC, et al. Immunohistochemistry of choriocarcinoma: an aid in differential diagnosis and in elucidating pathogenesis. *Am J Surg Pathol.* 2007;31:1726-1732.

Mao TL, Kurman RJ, Jeng YM, et al. HSD3B1 as a novel trophoblast-associated marker that assists in the differential diagnosis of trophoblastic tumors and tumorlike lesions. *Am J Surg Pathol.* 2008;32:236-242.

Mao TL, Seidman JD, Kurman RJ, et al. Cyclin E and p16 immunoreactivity in epithelioid trophoblastic tumor—an aid in differential diagnosis. *Am J Surg Pathol.* 2006;30:1105-1110.

Ober WB, Edgcomb JH, Price EB Jr. The pathology of choriocarcinoma. *Ann N Y Acad Sci.* 1971;172:299-426.

Rawish KR, Buza N, Zheng W, et al. Endometrial carcinoma with trophoblastic components: clinicopathologic analysis of a rare entity. *Int J Gynecol Pathol.* 2018;37:174-190.

Shih IM, Kurman RJ. Epithelioid trophoblastic tumor: a neoplasm distinct from choriocarcinoma and placental site trophoblastic tumor simulating carcinoma. *Am J Surg Pathol.* 1998;22:1393-1403.

Shih IM, Kurman RJ. Expression of melanoma cell adhesion molecule in intermediate trophoblast. *Lab Invest.* 1996;75:377-388.

Shih IM, Kurman RJ. p63 expression is useful in the distinction of epithelioid trophoblastic and placental site trophoblastic tumors by profiling trophoblastic subpopulations. *Am J Surg Pathol.* 2004;28:1177-1183.

Shih IM, Kurman RJ. The pathology of intermediate trophoblastic tumors and tumor-like lesions. *Int J Gynecol Pathol.* 2001;20:31-47.

Shih IM, Seidman JD, Kurman RJ. Placental site nodule and characterization of distinctive types of intermediate trophoblast. *Hum Pathol.* 1999;30:687-694.

Shih IeM. Trophogram, an immunohistochemistry-based algorithmic approach, in the differential diagnosis of trophoblastic tumors and tumorlike lesions. *Ann Diagn Pathol.* 2007;11:228-234.

Singer G, Kurman RJ, McMaster MT, et al. HLA-G immunoreactivity is specific for intermediate trophoblast in gestational trophoblastic disease and can serve as a useful marker in differential diagnosis. *Am J Surg Pathol.* 2002;26:914-920.

Smith HO, Kohorn E, Cole LA. Choriocarcinoma and gestational trophoblastic disease. *Obstet Gynecol Clin North Am.* 2005;32:661-684.

Young RH, Kurman RJ, Scully RE. Placental site nodules and plaques. A clinicopathologic analysis of 20 cases. *Am J Surg Pathol.* 1990;14:1001-1009.

INDEX